Pediatric Dermatology

A Quick Reference Guide

5th Edition

Section on Dermatology
American Academy of Pediatrics

Editors
Daniel P. Krowchuk, MD, FAAP
Anthony J. Mancini, MD, FAAP, FAAD

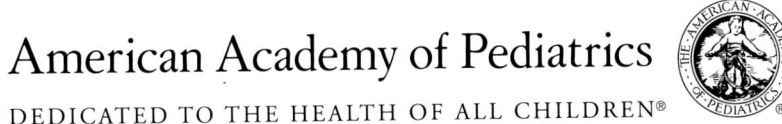

American Academy of Pediatrics Publishing Staff
Mary Lou White, *Chief Product and Services Officer/SVP, Membership, Marketing, and Publishing*
Mark Grimes, *Vice President, Publishing*
Mary Kelly, *Senior Editor, Professional/Clinical Publishing*
Heather Babiar, MS, *Senior Editor, Professional/Clinical Publishing*
Laura Underhile, *Senior Editor, Professional/Clinical Publishing*
Grace Klooster, *Editorial Assistant*
Jason Crase, *Senior Manager, Production and Editorial Services*
Theresa Wiener, *Production Manager, Clinical and Professional Publications*
Leesa Levin-Doroba, *Production Manager, Practice Management*
Mary Louise Carr, MBA, *Marketing Manager, Clinical Publications*

Published by the American Academy of Pediatrics
345 Park Blvd
Itasca, IL 60143
Telephone: 630/626-6000
Facsimile: 847/434-8000
www.aap.org

The American Academy of Pediatrics is an organization of 67,000 primary care pediatricians, pediatric medical subspecialists, and pediatric surgical specialists dedicated to the health, safety, and well-being of all infants, children, adolescents, and young adults.

While every effort has been made to ensure the accuracy of this publication, the American Academy of Pediatrics does not guarantee that it is accurate, complete, or without error.

The recommendations in this publication do not indicate an exclusive course of treatment or serve as a standard of medical care. Variations, taking into account individual circumstances, may be appropriate.

Statements and opinions expressed are those of the authors and not necessarily those of the American Academy of Pediatrics.

Any websites, brand names, products, or manufacturers are mentioned for informational and identification purposes only and do not imply an endorsement by the American Academy of Pediatrics (AAP). The AAP is not responsible for the content of external resources. Information was current at the time of publication.

The publishers have made every effort to trace the copyright holders for borrowed materials. If they have inadvertently overlooked any, they will be pleased to make the necessary arrangements at the first opportunity.

This publication has been developed by the American Academy of Pediatrics. The contributors are expert authorities in the field of pediatrics. No commercial involvement of any kind has been solicited or accepted in the development of the content of this publication. Disclosures: Dr Ingrid Polcari has disclosed a financial relationship as an advisory board member with Verrica. Dr Anthony Mancini has disclosed a financial relationship as a consultant with ParaPRO, a financial relationship as a speaker with Sanofi/Genzyme, a financial relationship as a consultant with Verrica, a financial relationship as an advisory board member with Dermavant, and a financial relationship as an advisory board member with Arcutis. Dr Deepti Gupta has disclosed a financial relationship as a consultant with Noblepharma and a financial relationship as an author with UpToDate. Dr Fred Ghali has disclosed a financial relationship with Sanofi Regeneron as a speaker; a financial relationship with Verrica Pharmaceuticals as an advisory board member; a financial relationship with Fred Ghali as a stockholder; a financial relationship with Arcutis Pharmaceuticals as an advisory board member; a financial relationship with Dermavant as an advisory board member; a financial relationship with Galderma Labs as a speaker; a financial relationship with ACRC Clinical Trials as a principal investigator and should be recused from the topics of Acne, Atopic Dermatitis, and molluscum contaigiousum. Any other disclosures were reviewed and determined not relevant to the work related to The Pediatric Dermatology Reference Guide. Disclosures are reviewed and mitigated through a Conflict-of-Interest process that consists of reviewing pertinent information which is then used to decide what action is required to maintain content integrity. There may be instances where no action is necessary. This process has been approved by the AAP Board of Directors.

Every effort has been made to ensure that the drug selection and dosages set forth in this publication are in accordance with the current recommendations and practice at the time of publication. It is the responsibility of the health care professional to check the package insert of each drug for any change in indications or dosage and for added warnings and precautions.

Every effort is made to keep *Pediatric Dermatology: A Quick Reference Guide* consistent with the most recent advice and information available from the American Academy of Pediatrics.

Please visit www.aap.org/errata for an up-to-date list of any applicable errata for this publication.

Special discounts are available for bulk purchases of this publication. Email Special Sales at nationalaccounts@aap.org for more information.

© 2025 American Academy of Pediatrics

All rights reserved. No part of this publication may be reproduced, stored in a retrieval system, or transmitted in any form or by any means—electronic, mechanical, photocopying, recording, or otherwise—without prior permission from the publisher (locate title at https://ebooks.aappublications.org and click on © Get Permissions; you may also fax the permissions editor at 847/434-8780 or email permissions@aap.org). No permission is necessary to make single copies of quick references sheets for noncommercial, educational purposes. First edition published 2009; second, 2011; third, 2016; fourth, 2021.

Printed in the United States of America

3-368/0125   1 2 3 4 5 6 7 8 9 10

MA1172

ISBN: 978-1-61002-777-9

eISBN: 978-1-61002-779-3

EPUB: 978-1-61002-778-6

Cover and publication design by LSD DESIGN, LLC

Library of Congress Control Number: 2024941842

Equity, Diversity, and Inclusion Statement

The American Academy of Pediatrics is committed to principles of equity, diversity, and inclusion in its publishing program. Editorial boards, author selections, and author transitions (publication succession plans) are designed to include diverse voices that reflect society as a whole. Editor and author teams are encouraged to actively seek out diverse authors and reviewers at all stages of the editorial process. Publishing staff are committed to promoting equity, diversity, and inclusion in all aspects of publication writing, review, and production.

Reviewers/Contributors

Editors

Daniel P. Krowchuk, MD, FAAP
Professor Emeritus of Pediatrics and Dermatology
Wake Forest University School of Medicine
Winston-Salem, NC

Anthony J. Mancini, MD, FAAP, FAAD
Professor of Pediatrics and Dermatology
Northwestern University Feinberg School of Medicine
Head and Associate Program Director, Division of Pediatric Dermatology
Ann & Robert H. Lurie Children's Hospital of Chicago
Chicago, IL

Associate Editors

Latanya T. Benjamin, MD, FAAD
Associate Professor of Pediatric Dermatology
Department of Women's & Children's Health
Director, Communication, Compassion, & Collaborative Care Thread
Florida Atlantic University
Boca Raton, FL

Fred Ghali, MD
Private Practice
Pediatric Dermatology of North Texas
Grapevine, TX

Deepti Gupta, MD, FAAP
Associate Professor of Pediatrics
Division of Dermatology
Seattle Children's Hospital
University of Washington School of Medicine
Seattle, WA

Brandon D. Newell, MD, FAAP
Children's Mercy Kansas City, Division of Dermatology
Associate Professor of Pediatrics
University of Missouri–Kansas City
Kansas City, MO

Ingrid C. Polcari, MD, FAAP
Associate Professor of Pediatrics and Dermatology
University of Minnesota
Minneapolis, MN

Duri Yun, MD, MPH
Assistant Professor of Pediatrics and Dermatology
Northwestern University Feinberg School of Medicine
Ann & Robert H. Lurie Children's Hospital of Chicago
Chicago, IL

The editors wish to thank Steven D. Resnick, MD, FAAP, FAAD, for his contributions to the first edition of this book; J. Thomas Badgett, MD, PhD, FAAP, for his contributions to the first 2 editions of this book; Amy Jo Nopper, MD, FAAP, FAAD, and Michael L. Smith, MD, FAAP, FAAD, for their contributions to the first 3 editions of this book; Patricia A. Treadwell, MD, FAAP, FAAD, for her contributions to the first 4 editions of this book; Anna L. Bruckner, MD, FAAP, FAAD, for her contributions to the second through fourth editions of this book; and Lucia Z. Diaz, MD, and Emily Gurnee, MD, for their contributions to the fourth edition of this book.

American Academy of Pediatrics Board of Directors Reviewer
Patricia M. Purcell, MD, MBA, FAAP

Reviewers
Committee on Infectious Diseases
Council on Adolescent Health
Council on Environmental Health and Climate Change
Council on Genetics
Section on Allergy and Immunology
Section on Clinical Pharmacology and Therapeutics
Section on Dermatology
Section on Neurology
Section on Rheumatology

American Academy of Pediatrics
Melissa Marx
Manager, Section on Dermatology

To our families—Heidi and Will; Nicki, Mallory, Christopher, Mackenzie, and Alexander—whose ongoing understanding and support again made this project possible.

Contents

Foreword xv
Editors' Note xvi
Figure Credits xvii

CHAPTER 1 — **Approach to the Patient With a Rash** 1
CHAPTER 2 — **Diagnostic Techniques** 15
CHAPTER 3 — **Therapeutics** 21

Dermatitis

CHAPTER 4 — **Atopic Dermatitis** 33
CHAPTER 5 — **Contact Dermatitis (Irritant and Allergic)** 47
CHAPTER 6 — **Juvenile Plantar Dermatosis** 61

Acne

CHAPTER 7 — **Acne Vulgaris** 67
CHAPTER 8 — **Neonatal and Infantile Acne** 79
CHAPTER 9 — **Periorificial Dermatitis** 83

Skin Infections

Localized Viral Infections

CHAPTER 10 — **Herpes Simplex** 89
CHAPTER 11 — **Herpes Zoster** 99
CHAPTER 12 — **Molluscum Contagiosum** 105
CHAPTER 13 — **Warts** 111

Systemic Viral Infections

CHAPTER 14 — **Erythema Infectiosum/Human Parvovirus B19 Infection (Fifth Disease)** 121
CHAPTER 15 — **Gianotti-Crosti Syndrome** 127
CHAPTER 16 — **Hand, Foot, and Mouth Disease (HFMD) and Other Enteroviral Exanthems** 131
CHAPTER 17 — **Measles** 141
CHAPTER 18 — **Papular-Purpuric Gloves-and-Socks Syndrome (PPGSS)** 147
CHAPTER 19 — **Roseola Infantum (Exanthem Subitum)** 151
CHAPTER 20 — **Rubella** 155
CHAPTER 21 — **Unilateral Laterothoracic Exanthem (ULE)** 161
CHAPTER 22 — **Varicella** 165

Localized Bacterial Infections

CHAPTER 23 — **Acute Paronychia** **173**
CHAPTER 24 — **Blistering Distal Dactylitis** **177**
CHAPTER 25 — **Ecthyma** **181**
CHAPTER 26 — **Folliculitis/Furunculosis/Carbunculosis** **185**
CHAPTER 27 — **Impetigo** **191**
CHAPTER 28 — **Perianal Bacterial Dermatitis** **197**

Systemic Bacterial, Rickettsial, or Spirochetal Infections With Skin Manifestations

CHAPTER 29 — **Lyme Disease** **205**
CHAPTER 30 — **Meningococcemia** **211**
CHAPTER 31 — **Rocky Mountain Spotted Fever (RMSF)** **217**
CHAPTER 32 — **Scarlet Fever** **223**
CHAPTER 33 — **Staphylococcal Scalded Skin Syndrome (SSSS)** **231**
CHAPTER 34 — **Toxic Shock Syndrome (TSS)** **237**

Fungal and Yeast Infections

CHAPTER 35 — *Candida* **245**
CHAPTER 35A — **Angular Cheilitis/Perlèche** **247**
CHAPTER 35B — **Candidal Diaper Dermatitis** **251**
CHAPTER 35C — **Chronic Paronychia** **255**
CHAPTER 35D — **Neonatal/Congenital Candidiasis** **259**
CHAPTER 35E — **Thrush** **263**
CHAPTER 36 — **Onychomycosis** **267**
CHAPTER 37 — **Tinea Capitis** **271**
CHAPTER 38 — **Tinea Corporis** **281**
CHAPTER 39 — **Tinea Cruris** **287**
CHAPTER 40 — **Tinea Pedis** **291**
CHAPTER 41 — **Tinea Versicolor** **297**

Infestations and Bites

CHAPTER 42 — **Cutaneous Larva Migrans** **305**
CHAPTER 43 — **Head Lice** **309**
CHAPTER 44 — **Insect Bites and Papular Urticaria** **315**
CHAPTER 45 — **Scabies** **325**
CHAPTER 46 — **Cercarial Dermatitis (Swimmer's Itch)** **333**

Papulosquamous Diseases

- CHAPTER 47 — **Lichen Nitidus** 341
- CHAPTER 48 — **Lichen Planus (LP)** 345
- CHAPTER 49 — **Lichen Striatus**..349
- CHAPTER 50 — **Pityriasis Lichenoides**..353
- CHAPTER 51 — **Pityriasis Rosea** 359
- CHAPTER 52 — **Psoriasis** 363
- CHAPTER 53 — **Pityriasis Rubra Pilaris (PRP)**................................373
- CHAPTER 54 — **Seborrheic Dermatitis** 377

Vascular Lesions

- CHAPTER 55 — **Cutis Marmorata**...385
- CHAPTER 56 — **Cutis Marmorata Telangiectatica Congenita (CMTC)**.........387
- CHAPTER 57 — **Infantile Hemangioma**...393
- CHAPTER 58 — **Kasabach-Merritt Phenomenon** 407
- CHAPTER 59 — **Pernio/Chilblains** 411
- CHAPTER 60 — **Pyogenic Granuloma** 417
- CHAPTER 61 — **Telangiectasias** 421
- CHAPTER 62 — **Vascular Malformations** 427

Disorders of Pigmentation

Hypopigmentation
- CHAPTER 63 — **Albinism** 441
- CHAPTER 64 — **Pigmentary Mosaicism, Hypopigmented**.....................445
- CHAPTER 65 — **Pityriasis Alba** 451
- CHAPTER 66 — **Postinflammatory Hypopigmentation**........................455
- CHAPTER 67 — **Vitiligo**...459

Hyperpigmentation
- CHAPTER 68 — **Acanthosis Nigricans** 467
- CHAPTER 69 — **Acquired Melanocytic Nevi** 471
- CHAPTER 70 — **Café au Lait Macules**...477
- CHAPTER 71 — **Congenital Melanocytic Nevi (CMN)** 481
- CHAPTER 72 — **Ephelides** 487
- CHAPTER 73 — **Lentigines** 489
- CHAPTER 74 — **Congenital Dermal Melanocytosis**.............................493
- CHAPTER 75 — **Melanonychia Striata** 497
- CHAPTER 76 — **Pigmentary Mosaicism, Hyperpigmented** 501

Lumps and Bumps

- CHAPTER 77 — **Cutaneous Mastocytosis** ... 509
- CHAPTER 78 — **Dermoid Cysts** ... 517
- CHAPTER 79 — **Epidermal Nevi** ... 521
- CHAPTER 80 — **Granuloma Annulare** ... 525
- CHAPTER 81 — **Juvenile Xanthogranuloma** ... 529
- CHAPTER 82 — **Pilomatricoma** ... 533
- CHAPTER 83 — **Spitz Nevus** ... 539

Bullous Diseases

- CHAPTER 84 — **Childhood Dermatitis Herpetiformis** ... 545
- CHAPTER 85 — **Epidermolysis Bullosa (EB)** ... 551
- CHAPTER 86 — **Linear IgA Dermatosis** ... 561

Genodermatoses

- CHAPTER 87 — **Ichthyosis** ... 569
- CHAPTER 88 — **Incontinentia Pigmenti** ... 577
- CHAPTER 89 — **Neurofibromatosis (NF)** ... 583
- CHAPTER 90 — **Tuberous Sclerosis Complex (TSC)** ... 591
- CHAPTER 91 — **Ectodermal Dysplasia** ... 599

Hair Disorders

- CHAPTER 92 — **Alopecia Areata** ... 605
- CHAPTER 93 — **Androgenetic Alopecia** ... 615
- CHAPTER 94 — **Hypertrichosis and Hirsutism** ... 619
- CHAPTER 95 — **Loose Anagen Syndrome** ... 623
- CHAPTER 96 — **Telogen Effluvium** ... 629
- CHAPTER 97 — **Traction Alopecia** ... 635
- CHAPTER 98 — **Trichotillomania** ... 639

Skin Disorders in Neonates/Infants

- CHAPTER 99 — **Aplasia Cutis Congenita** ... 649
- CHAPTER 100 — **Collodion Baby** ... 655
- CHAPTER 101 — **Diaper Dermatitis** ... 659
- CHAPTER 102 — **Eosinophilic Pustular Folliculitis** ... 669
- CHAPTER 103 — **Erythema Toxicum** ... 671
- CHAPTER 104 — **Infantile Acropustulosis** ... 675
- CHAPTER 105 — **Intertrigo** ... 677
- CHAPTER 106 — **Miliaria** ... 681

CHAPTER 107 — **Nevus Sebaceus (of Jadassohn)** **685**
CHAPTER 108 — **Transient Neonatal Pustular Melanosis**. **689**
CHAPTER 109 — **Subcutaneous Fat Necrosis (SFN)**. **693**

Acute Drug/Toxic Reactions

CHAPTER 110 — **Drug Hypersensitivity Syndrome**. **701**
CHAPTER 111 — **Erythema Multiforme (EM)** **707**
CHAPTER 112 — **Exanthematous and Urticarial Drug Reactions** **713**
CHAPTER 113 — **Fixed Drug Eruption** **719**
CHAPTER 114 — **Serum Sickness–Like Reaction** **723**
CHAPTER 115 — **Stevens-Johnson Syndrome (SJS),** *Mycoplasma pneumoniae*–**Induced Rash and Mucositis (MIRM), and Reactive Infectious Mucocutaneous Eruption (RIME)**. **729**
CHAPTER 116 — **Toxic Epidermal Necrolysis (TEN)** **737**
CHAPTER 117 — **Urticaria** **743**

Cutaneous Manifestations of Rheumatologic Diseases

CHAPTER 118 — **Juvenile Dermatomyositis (JDM)** **751**
CHAPTER 119 — **Morphea (Localized Scleroderma)**. **761**
CHAPTER 120 — **Systemic Lupus Erythematosus (SLE)**. **777**

Nutritional Dermatoses

CHAPTER 121 — **Acrodermatitis Enteropathica (AE)** **795**
CHAPTER 122 — **Kwashiorkor** **801**

Other Disorders

CHAPTER 123 — **Erythema Nodosum** **809**
CHAPTER 124 — **Henoch-Schönlein Purpura**. **813**
CHAPTER 125 — **Kawasaki Disease**. **821**
CHAPTER 126 — **Langerhans Cell Histiocytosis** **829**
CHAPTER 127 — **Lichen Sclerosus et Atrophicus (LSA)** **837**
CHAPTER 128 — **Polymorphous Light Eruption**. **843**
CHAPTER 129 — **Confluent and Reticulated Papillomatosis (CARP)**. **849**
CHAPTER 130 — **Hyperhidrosis** **853**

Index **857**

Foreword

Concerns relating to the skin are common reasons for parents to seek medical care for their children. Data from several sources indicate that up to 20% of child visits to pediatricians or family physicians involve a dermatologic problem as the primary reason for the visit, a secondary concern, or an incidental finding on physical examination. The volume of skin-related concerns and the supply-demand crunch for dermatologic referrals mandate that primary care physicians who care for children are prepared to recognize, diagnose, and treat common cutaneous disorders.

This guide was originally designed to be a practical, easy-to-use tool for the busy practitioner, and we hope that this fifth edition continues to meet these goals. As with past editions, it is not an exhaustive reference; rather, it provides a concise summary of many common dermatologic disorders, with a standardized format that includes a brief background, physical findings, diagnostic modalities, and treatment approaches. Each chapter includes a useful Look-alikes table to assist in differential diagnosis and, when applicable, a Resources for Families section that provides links to patient information or support groups. Chapters to help enhance skills in recognizing and describing skin disorders, performing and interpreting diagnostic tests, and managing skin disease also are included. The accompanying color photographs have been selected to illustrate some cardinal features of each disorder. In this edition, in addition to updating material from the fourth edition, we have added new chapters on androgenetic alopecia, collodion baby, hypertrichosis and hirsutism, melanonychia striata, and pernio/chilblains. We have also supplied new links to useful patient resources and added or replaced numerous clinical images. We have striven to incorporate as many clinical photographs of disease presentations in skin of color as possible.

We hope this guide continues to fulfill an important need for the pediatric practitioner who wants a quick dermatology reference.

D.P.K. and A.J.M.

Editors' Note

The information contained in this text has been gleaned from reviews of multiple scientific papers and textbooks. The materials have been synthesized into what we hope is a coherent, easy-to-read style. Individual references have not been included in an effort to keep the size of this work practical for a quick reference guide. Some key textbook references are listed here, and we invite the reader to refer to updated medical publications for further information or contemporary scientific updates.

Daniel P. Krowchuk, MD, FAAP
Anthony J. Mancini, MD, FAAP, FAAD

Textbook References

Bolognia JL, Schaffer JV, Cerroni L, eds. *Dermatology.* 5th ed. Elsevier; 2024

Eichenfield LF, Frieden IJ, Mathes E, Zaenglein A, eds. *Neonatal and Infant Dermatology.* 3rd ed. Elsevier Saunders; 2014

Paller AS, Mancini AJ. *Hurwitz Clinical Pediatric Dermatology: A Textbook of Skin Disorders of Childhood and Adolescence.* 6th ed. Elsevier; 2022

Figure Credits

All figures not included in the following list are courtesy of the American Academy of Pediatrics. Special thanks to Daniel P. Krowchuk, MD, FAAP; Anthony J. Mancini, MD, FAAP, FAAD; J. Thomas Badgett, MD, PhD, FAAP; Anna L. Bruckner, MD, FAAP, FAAD; Fred Ghali, MD, FAAP; Amy Jo Nopper, MD, FAAP, FAAD; Ingrid C. Polcari, MD, FAAP; Steven D. Resnick, MD, FAAP, FAAD; Michael L. Smith, MD, FAAP, FAAD; and Patricia A. Treadwell, MD, FAAP, FAAD.

AAFP
Figure 40.3

AAP
Figure 35D.2 from Jani S, Ariss R, Chawla S. A preterm infant with a characteristic erythematous and scaly rash after birth. *Neoreviews*. 2020;21(7):e495–e498.

Figure 121.3 reprinted with permission from Leonard D, Koca R, Acun C, et al. Visual diagnosis: three infants who have perioral and acral skin lesions. *Pediatr Rev*. 2007;28(8):312–318.

Figure 14.1 from *Red Book Online Visual Library*. Courtesy of H. Cody Meissner, MD, FAAP.

The American Journal of Medicine blog
Figure 25.2

Latanya T. Benjamin, MD, FAAD, FAAP
Figures 67.4, 75.1

Black & Brown Skin
Figure 22.2

Canadian Medical Association Journal
Figure 121.4 from Leung AKC, Leong KF, Lam JM. Acrodermatitis enteropathica in a 3-month-old boy. *CMAJ*. 2021;193(7):E243.

Case Reports in Pediatrics
Figure 56.4 from Leung AKC, Lam JM, Leong KF. Cutis marmorata telangiectatica congenita associated with hemiatrophy. *Case Rep Pediatr*. 2020;2020:88138909.

Centers for Disease Control and Prevention
Figures 20.1

DermNet
Figures 81.3, 107.2

Elsevier
Figures 2.7, 35A.2, 37.2, 37.3, 57.10, 60.2, 101.9, 125.4, 125.6. Reprinted with permission from Elsevier. From Paller AS, Mancini AJ. *Hurwitz Clinical Pediatric Dermatology: A Textbook of Skin Disorders of Childhood and Adolescence*. 3rd ed. Elsevier Saunders; 2006.
Figure 125.5. Reprinted with permission from Elsevier. From Mancini AJ. Childhood exanthems: a primer and update for the dermatologist. *Adv Dermatol*. 2000;16:3–38.
Figure 73.1 from Cohen BA. *Pediatric Dermatology*. 3rd ed. Elsevier Mosby; 2005.

Alexander W. Fender, MD
Figure 23.2

Alan B. Fleischer Jr, MD
Figure 84.1

Frontiers in Immunology
Figure 84.3. Antiga E, Maglie R, Quintarelli L, et al. Dermatitis herpetiformis: novel perspectives. *Front Immunol.* 2019;(10):1290.

Laurence Givner, MD
Figure 101.11

Chad Haldeman-Englert, MD
Figures 122.1, 122.2, 122.3

Kristen Hook, MD
Figures 91.1, 91.2

Kimberly Horii, MD
Figures 92.3, 97.1

Sheilagh Maguiness, MD
Figures 115.4, 115.5

McGraw-Hill
Figure 98.4 from Usatine RP, Sabella C, Smith MA, Mayeaux Jr EJ, Chumley HS, Appachi E. *The Color Atlas of Pediatrics.* McGraw-Hill Education.

National Health Service, United Kingdom
Figure 59.4

Brandon D. Newell, MD
Figures 52.2, 52.6, 52.7, 52.9, 52.10, 59.1–59.3, 76.3, 76.4, 83.2, 84.2, 92.5, 95.3, 96.3, 98.7, 98.8, 118.4, 118.5, 118.7, 119.2, 119.3, 119.8, 119.10, 120.1, 120.3, 120.4, 130.1, 130.2

Pediatric Dermatology
Figure 109.3 from Siegel LH, Alonso CF, Tuazon CFR, et al. Subcutaneous fat necrosis of the newborn: a retrospective study of 32 infants and care algorithm. *Pediatr Dermatol.* 2023;40(3):413–421

Ingrid C. Polcari, MD, FAAP
Figures 51.3, 54.4, 85.5, 93.1, 93.2, 94.1, 94.2, 111.1, 111.4, 124.4, 124.5

Howard Pride, MD
Figures 13.1, 13.5, 15.1, 17.2, 22.2

Mary Rimsza, MD
Figures 20.2, 103.1

Paul J. Sagerman, MD
Figures 98.2, 108.3

Walt W. Tunnesen Jr, MD
Figure 1.10

Anthony J. Vivian, FRCS, FRCOphth
Figure 89.5

Albert Yan, MD
Figures 7.8, 101.5

Duri Yun, MD
Figures 9.3, 10.2, 12.2, 13.2, 13.3, 13.4, 16.6, 53.1

CHAPTER 1

Approach to the Patient With a Rash

Introduction

- ▶ Recognizing and describing skin lesions accurately is essential to the diagnosis and differential diagnosis of skin disorders.
- ▶ The first step is to identify the primary lesion, defined as the earliest lesion and the lesion most characteristic of the disease.
- ▶ Next note the distribution, arrangement, and color of primary lesions, along with any secondary change (eg, crusting or scaling).
- ▶ If feasible, uploading some photographs of the rash to the electronic medical record can be very helpful, especially in cases in which the diagnosis is uncertain or the condition requires longitudinal follow-up.

Types of Primary Lesions

- ▶ Flat lesions
  - Macule: a small (<1 cm), circumscribed area of color change without elevation or depression of the skin (Figure 1.1).
  - Patch: a larger (≥1 cm) area of color change without skin elevation or depression (Figure 1.2).
- ▶ Elevated lesions
  - Solid lesions
    - Papule: lesion less than 1 cm in diameter (Figure 1.3).
    - Nodule: lesion 0.5 to 2.0 cm in diameter, most of which is below the skin surface (Figure 1.4).
    - Tumor: deeper than a nodule and larger than 2 cm in diameter.
    - Wheals: pink, rounded, or flat-topped elevations due to edema in the skin (Figure 1.5).
    - Plaques: plateau-shaped structures often formed by the coalescence of papules; larger than 1 cm in diameter (Figure 1.6).

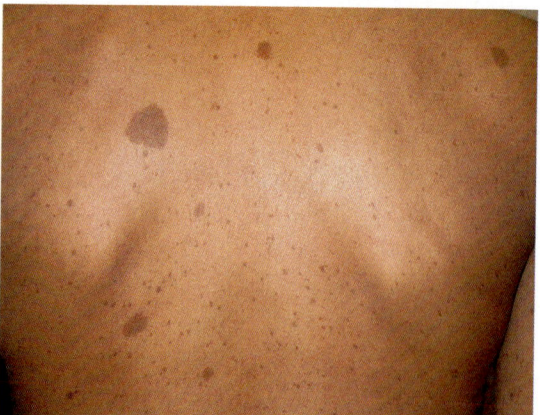

Figure 1.1. Café au lait macules (spots) in a patient who has neurofibromatosis type 1.

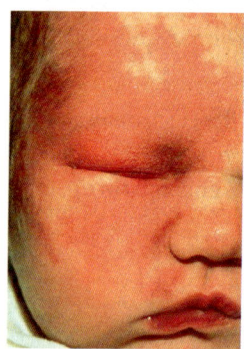

Figure 1.2. A port-wine stain—a vascular patch.

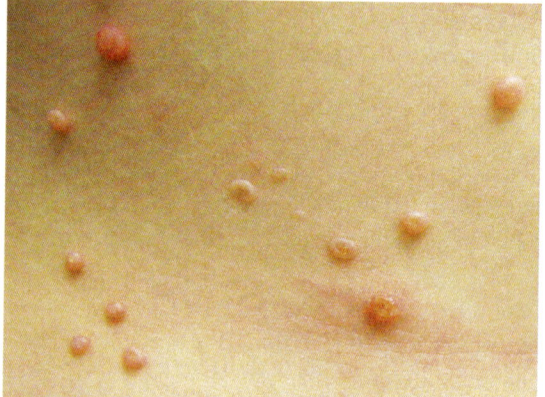

Figure 1.3. Molluscum contagiosum. There are erythematous and skin-colored papules.

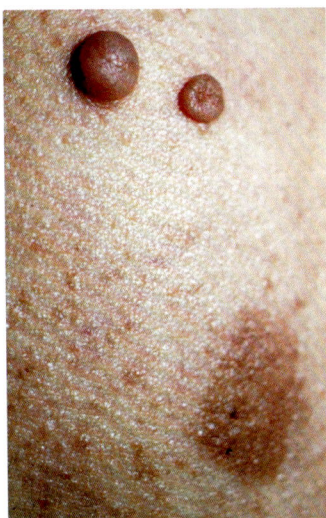

Figure 1.4. Nodules that are neurofibromas in a patient who has neurofibromatosis type 1.

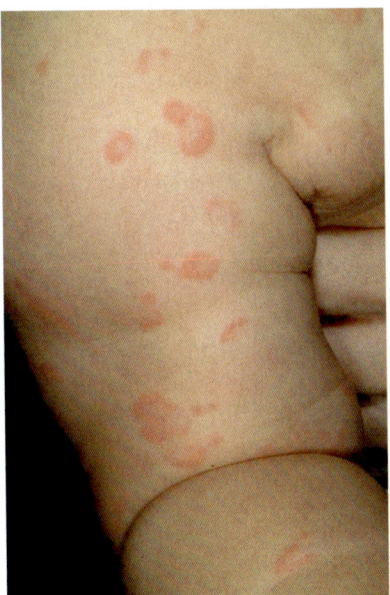

Figure 1.5. Pink wheals in a patient who has urticaria.

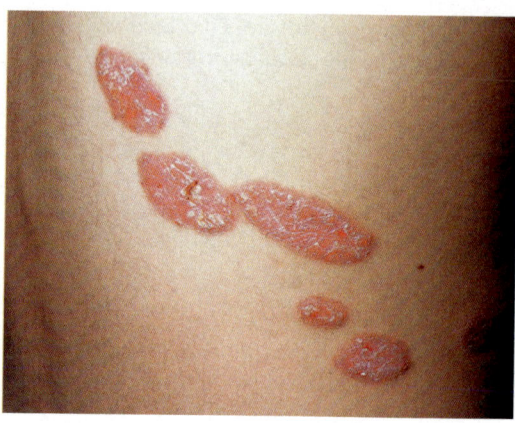

Figure 1.6. Scaling plaques, plateau-like lesions, are observed in psoriasis.

- Fluid-filled lesions
  - Vesicles: smaller than 1 cm in diameter and filled with serous or clear fluid (Figure 1.7).
  - Bullae: 1 cm or larger in diameter and typically filled with serous or clear fluid (Figure 1.8).
  - Pustules: smaller than 1 cm in diameter and filled with purulent material (Figure 1.9).
  - Abscesses: 1 cm or larger and filled with purulent material.
  - Cysts: 0.5 cm or larger in diameter; sacs containing fluid or semisolid material (unlike in bullae, the material within a cyst is not visible from the surface).
- Depressed lesions
  - Erosions: superficial loss of epidermis with a moist base (Figure 1.10).
  - Ulcers: deeper lesions extending into the dermis or below (Figure 1.11).

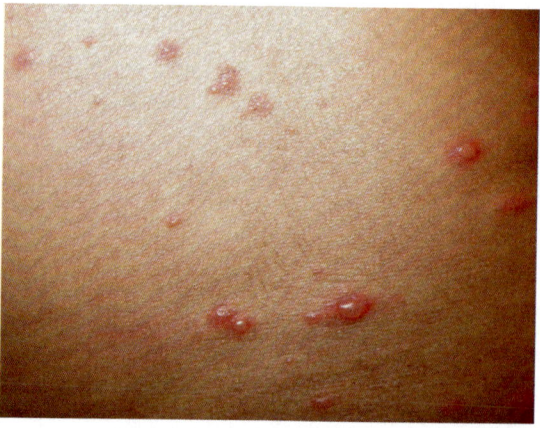

Figure 1.7. Vesicles, as seen here in varicella, are filled with serous or clear fluid.

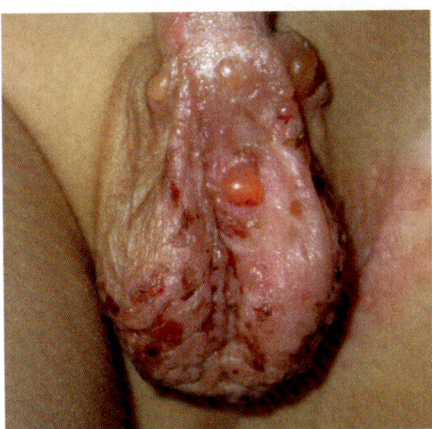

Figure 1.8. Bullae, filled with clear fluid, are observed in chronic bullous disease of childhood.

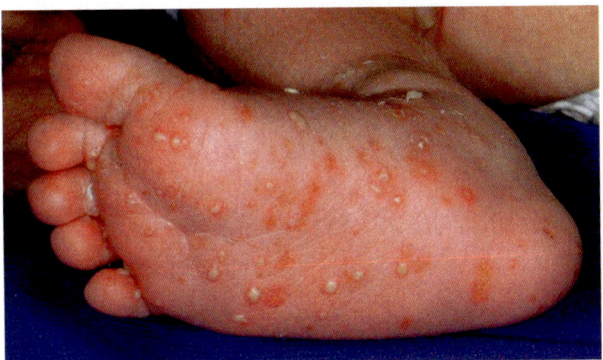

Figure 1.9. Pustules are filled with purulent material. This infant has congenital cutaneous candidiasis.

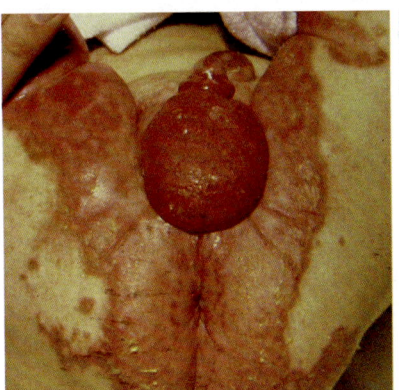

Figure 1.10. Erosions, as seen in this infant who has acrodermatitis enteropathica, indicate a superficial loss of epidermis.

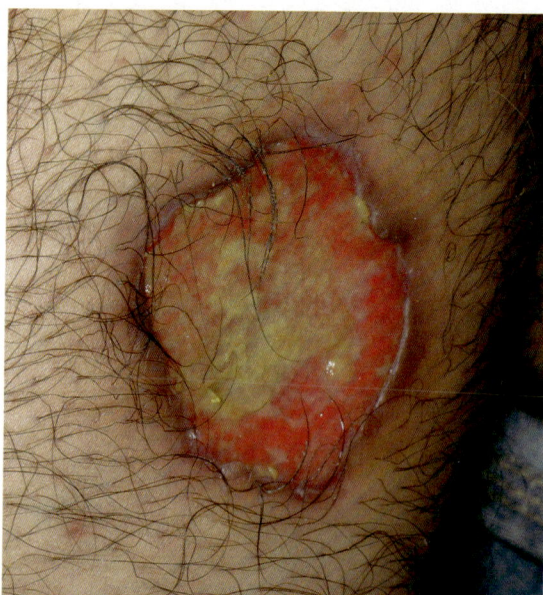

Figure 1.11. An ulcer occurs when there has been loss of epidermal and dermal tissues. In the patient shown here, the ulcer is the result of pyoderma gangrenosum.

Distribution of Lesions

Certain disorders are characterized by unique patterns of lesion distribution. For example

- Atopic dermatitis in children and adolescents typically involves the antecubital or popliteal fossae.
- Seborrheic dermatitis in adolescents commonly involves not only the scalp but also the eyebrows and nasolabial folds.
- Lesions of psoriasis are often seen in areas that are traumatized, such as the extensor surfaces of the elbows and knees.
- Acne is limited to the face, back, shoulders, and chest, sites of the highest concentrations of pilosebaceous follicles.

Arrangement of Lesions

The arrangement of lesions also may provide a clue to diagnosis. Some examples include

- ▶ Linear: allergic contact dermatitis due to plants (eg, poison ivy) (Figure 1.12), lichen striatus, and incontinentia pigmenti; may also occur in epidermal nevi, psoriasis, and warts.
- ▶ Grouped: herpes simplex virus infection (Figure 1.13), warts, molluscum contagiosum, and microcystic lymphatic malformation.
- ▶ Dermatomal: herpes zoster (Figure 1.14).
- ▶ Annular (ie, ring-shaped with central clearing): tinea corporis (Figure 1.15), granuloma annulare, erythema migrans, and lupus erythematosus.

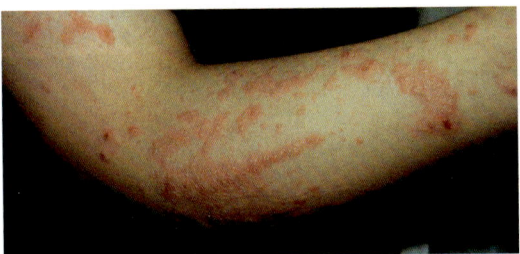

Figure 1.12. A linear arrangement of papules or vesicles often occurs in allergic contact dermatitis due to poison ivy.

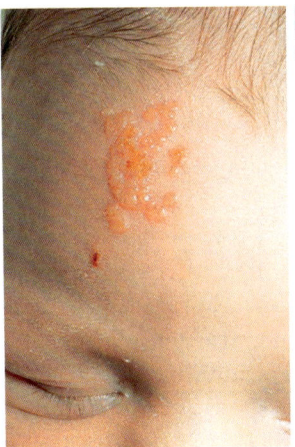

Figure 1.13. Grouped vesicles are characteristic of herpes simplex virus infection on the skin.

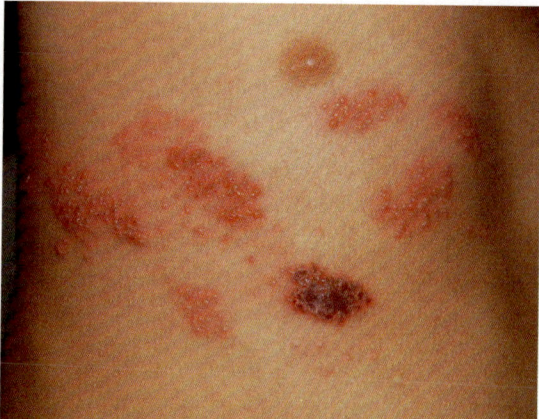

Figure 1.14. The lesions of herpes zoster appear in a dermatomal distribution.

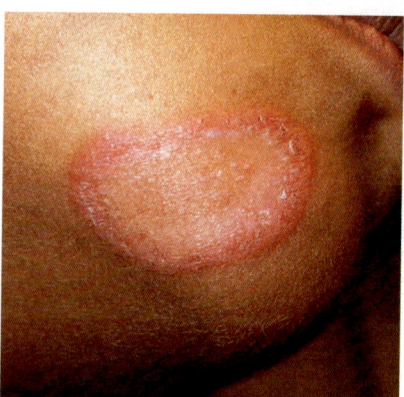

Figure 1.15. An annular (ring-shaped with central clearing) plaque is typical of tinea corporis.

Color

- Erythematous: pink or red. When erythematous lesions are observed, it is important to note whether they blanch. If the red cells are within vessels, as occurs in urticaria, compression of the skin forces the cells into deeper vessels, and blanching occurs. However, if the cells are outside vessels, as occurs in forms of vasculitis, blanching will not occur. Non-blanching lesions are termed *petechiae*, *purpura*, or *ecchymoses*. Also note that in individuals with skin of color, erythema may be more difficult to appreciate.
- Hyperpigmented: tan, brown, or black.
- Hypopigmented: amount of pigment decreased but not entirely absent (as seen with postinflammatory pigmentary alteration).
- Depigmented: all pigment absent (as occurs in vitiligo).

Secondary Changes

Alterations in the skin that may accompany primary lesions include

- Excoriation: a superficial loss of skin (ie, an erosion) caused by scratching, picking, or rubbing.
- Crusting: dried fluid; commonly seen after rupture of vesicles or bullae (as occurs with the honey-colored crust of impetigo).
- Scaling: epidermal fragments that are characteristic of several disorders, including fungal infections (eg, tinea corporis) and psoriasis.
- Atrophy: an area of surface depression due to absence of the epidermis, dermis, or subcutaneous fat; atrophic skin often is thin and wrinkled. Examples include steroid atrophy, morphea, and atrophoderma.
- Lichenification: thickening of the skin from chronic rubbing or scratching (as occurs in atopic dermatitis); as a result, typical skin markings and creases appear more prominent (Figure 1.16).

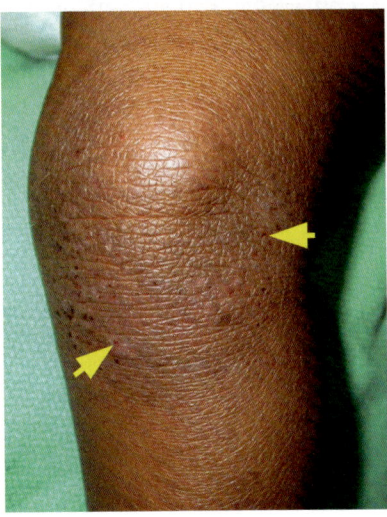

Figure 1.16. Lichenification. The typical skin markings are very prominent due to chronic scratching. Also note the tiny erosions (arrows), some of which have formed crusts.

Appearance Differences in Skin of Color

- The degree of skin pigmentation often influences the appearance of certain dermatologic disorders. In patients with darker skin tones, erythema may be difficult to appreciate or virtually absent (Figure 1.17) or may appear violaceous, brown, gray, blue, or black.

- Postinflammatory hypo- or hyperpigmentation occurs commonly in patients with darker skin tones (Figures 1.17 and 1.18). These pigmentary disturbances may be troubling for patients and may take months to resolve.

- In patients with darker skin tones, lesion morphology also may differ from that seen in patients with less pigmentation. In atopic dermatitis and pityriasis rosea, for example, lesions may be papular (often follicular in nature, resembling goose bumps) rather than patches or plaques (Figures 1.19 and 1.20). In patients with atopic dermatitis, somewhat larger, flat-topped (lichenoid) papules may be observed (Figure 1.21). These papules may occasionally appear more violaceous.

- Some additional disorders that may appear different in patients with darker skin tones compared with patients with lighter skin tones include
  - Capillary malformations: port-wine stains may appear more brown or reddish-brown and may be mistaken for café au lait macules.
  - Infantile hemangiomas: superficial infantile hemangiomas may appear violaceous rather than bright red, and deep infantile hemangiomas may lack the characteristic blue color seen in patients with lighter skin tones.
  - Morbilliform drug eruptions: in patients with darker skin tones the erythematous macules and papules may be difficult to appreciate.
  - Psoriasis: plaques may appear violaceous or hyperpigmented.
  - Urticaria: wheals may appear more skin-colored or pale rather than erythematous.
  - Viral exanthems: in patients with darker skin tones the erythematous macules may be difficult to appreciate.

Chapter 1: Approach to the Patient With a Rash

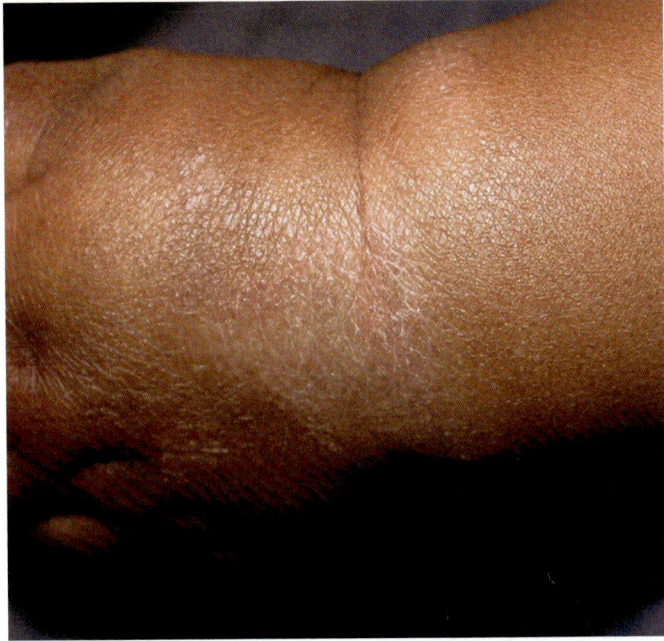

Figure 1.17. Subtle erythema and postinflammatory hypopigmentation in an infant with skin of color who has atopic dermatitis.

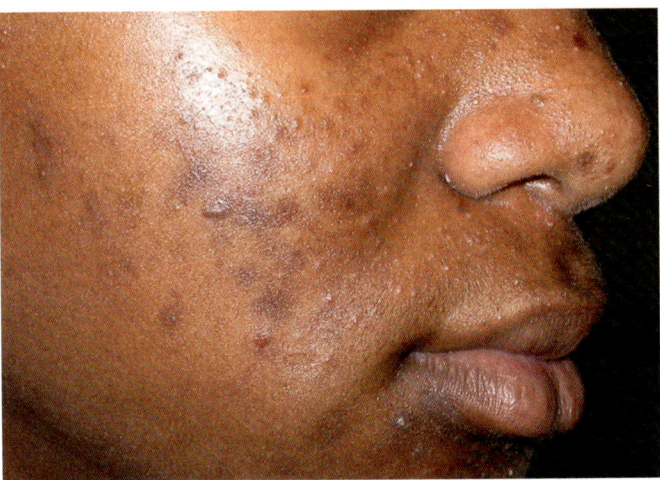

Figure 1.18. Postinflammatory hyperpigmentation in an adolescent with skin of color who has acne.

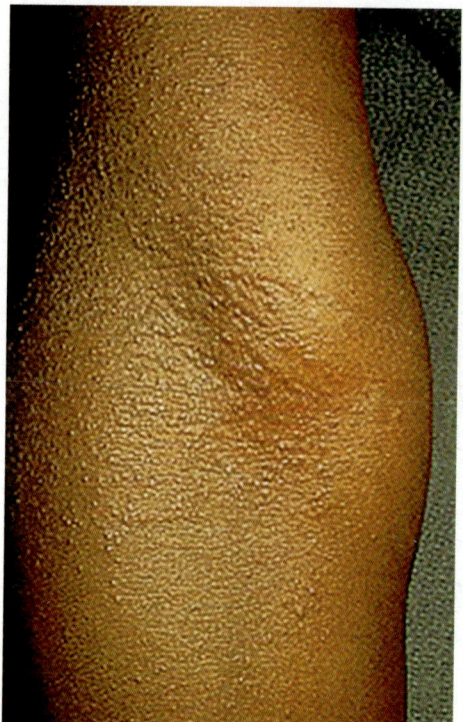

Figure 1.19. Tiny follicular papules in an adolescent with skin of color who has atopic dermatitis. Reproduced with permission from Krowchuk DP. Practical aspects of the diagnosis and management of atopic dermatitis. *Pediatr Ann.* 1987;16(1):57–66.

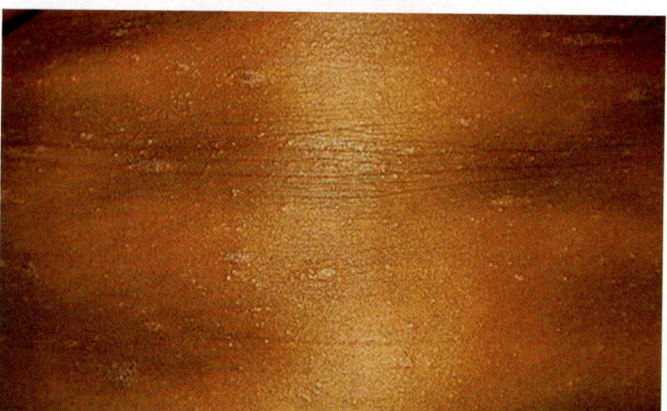

Figure 1.20. Abdomen of a patient with skin of color who has pityriasis rosea. There are tiny follicular papules and oval thin plaques with erythema that is more subtle and associated central hyperpigmentation in several lesions.

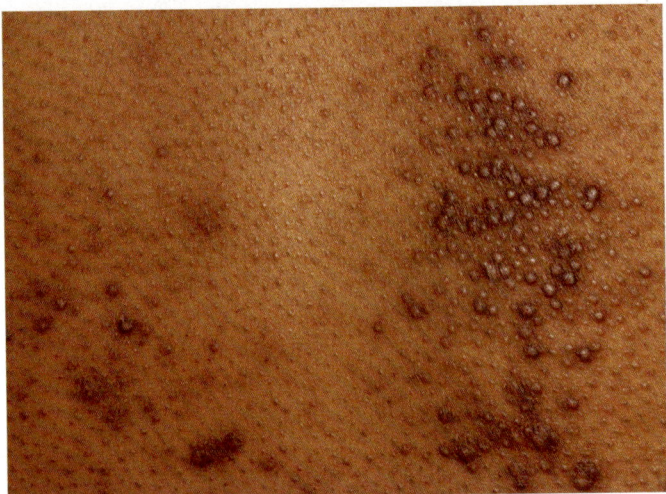

Figure 1.21. In some patients with skin of color who have atopic dermatitis, areas of disease activity may appear as slightly larger, flat-topped (lichenoid), violaceous papules.

CHAPTER 2

Diagnostic Techniques

Introduction

Several procedures can assist the clinician in diagnosing skin problems. Discussed here are the potassium hydroxide (KOH) preparation, fungal culture, mineral oil preparation for scabies, and Wood lamp examination.

KOH Preparation

Used to identify fungal elements (eg, spores, hyphae, pseudohyphae) in skin, hair, or nail samples. The procedure is as follows:

- Using the edge of a glass microscope slide or #15 scalpel blade, scrape the skin and collect fragments or hair remnants on a second glass microscope slide. Preparing the area first with alcohol may be useful in helping debris stick to the blade or slide.
- If sampling a nail, use a scalpel blade to scrape the underside of the nail (or its surface if superficial infection is suspected) and collect the debris obtained.
- Cover the specimen on the glass slide with a coverslip.
- Apply 1 to 2 drops of 10% to 20% KOH to the edge of the coverslip. Capillary action will draw the liquid under the entire coverslip.
- Gently heat the slide with an alcohol lamp or match, taking care to avoid boiling, which causes the KOH to crystallize and makes interpretation of the preparation difficult.
- Gently compress the coverslip to separate skin fragments further.
- Scan the preparation initially under low power (using the 10× objective lens).
- Examine any suspicious areas under higher power (using a 40× objective lens) for
   - Branching hyphae or spores: characteristic of dermatophyte infections of the skin or nails (eg, tinea corporis, tinea pedis, tinea cruris, onychomycosis) (Figure 2.1).

- Spores within hair fragments (ie, an endothrix infection): characteristic of the most common form of tinea capitis in the United States caused by *Trichophyton tonsurans* (Figure 2.2). If tinea capitis is caused by *Microsporum canis* (approximately 5% of all cases), hyphae or spores will be seen on the outside of hair shafts (ie, an ectothrix infection).
- Pseudohyphae and spores: seen in infections with *Candida* species (Figure 2.3).
- Spores and short hyphae (ie, "spaghetti and meatballs"): seen in tinea versicolor (Figure 2.4).

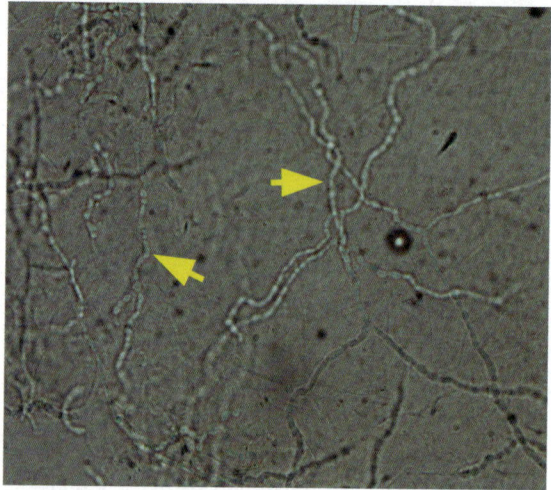

Figure 2.1. Potassium hydroxide preparation showing branching hyphae (arrows).

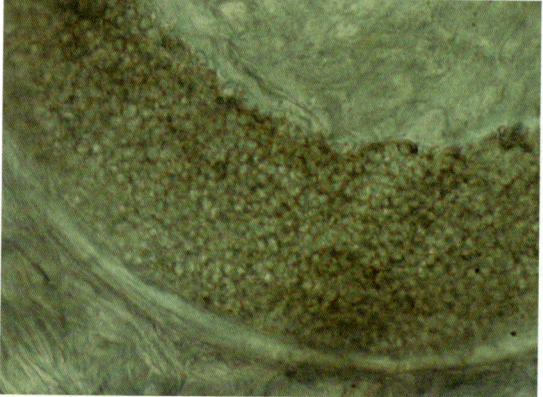

Figure 2.2. Potassium hydroxide preparation in tinea capitis caused by *Trichophyton tonsurans*. The hair fragment is filled with small spheres (ie, arthrospores).

Chapter 2: Diagnostic Techniques

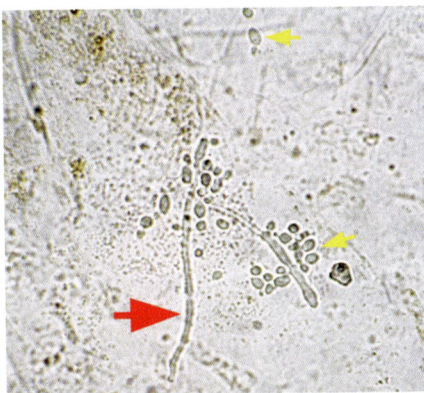

Figure 2.3. Pseudohyphae (red arrow) and spores (yellow arrows) are characteristic of infection caused by *Candida* species.

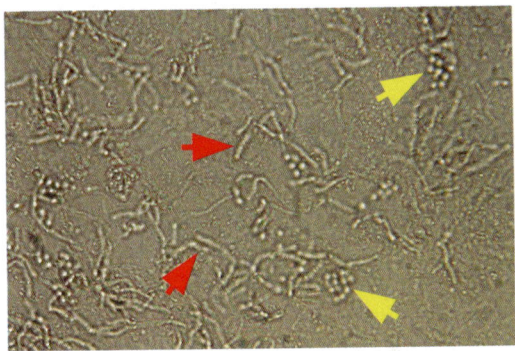

Figure 2.4. In tinea versicolor, the potassium hydroxide preparation reveals short hyphae (red arrows) and spores (yellow arrows) (ie, "spaghetti and meatballs").

Fungal Culture

- Sampling techniques
  - If sampling the skin, use the edge of a glass microscope slide or #15 scalpel, scrape the lesion, and collect scale on a glass microscope slide.
  - If sampling a nail, use a scalpel blade to scrape the underside of the nail (or its surface if superficial infection is suspected), and collect the debris on a glass microscope slide or folded sheet of paper; alternatively, use a nail clipper to obtain nail clippings.
  - If sampling the scalp, moisten a cotton-tipped applicator with tap water, rub the affected area of the scalp, and inoculate the fungal culture medium with the swab. If fungal culture medium is not available, a Culturette swab system (or other system) may be used to collect and transport the specimen to the laboratory.

- Transfer the material collected to the fungal medium (typically dermatophyte test medium or Mycosel agar) and process appropriately.
  - Leave the cap slightly loose to permit air entry.
  - If fungal culture medium is not available, transfer the specimen in a sterile glass tube or other container to the laboratory.
- In the presence of a pathogenic fungus, dermatophyte test medium will change from yellow to red in 1 to 2 weeks (Figure 2.5).

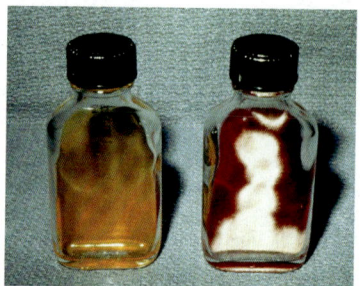

Figure 2.5. Uninoculated dermatophyte test medium is yellow (left). In the presence of a pathogenic fungus, the medium becomes red (right).

Mineral Oil Preparation for Scabies

- Place a small drop of mineral oil on a suspicious burrow, papule, or vesicle that has not been traumatized by the patient. Recent data suggest that debris from under fingernails (if present and accessible) may also be high yield for mineral oil examination.
- Using a #15 scalpel blade oriented parallel to the skin surface, scrape the lesion. Because scabies mites live in the epidermis, it is not necessary to scrape deeply; however, some bleeding is common with the procedure. For fingernail debris, a Hyfrecator tip, curet, or small cerumen extractor can be used to collect the specimen.
- Transfer the material to a drop of mineral oil on a glass microscope slide.
- Repeat the process for several other suspicious lesions.
- Cover the sample on the glass slide with a coverslip (add a few more drops of mineral oil if necessary for uniform distribution).
- Examine at low power for the presence of mites, eggs, or fecal material (Figures 2.6 and 2.7).

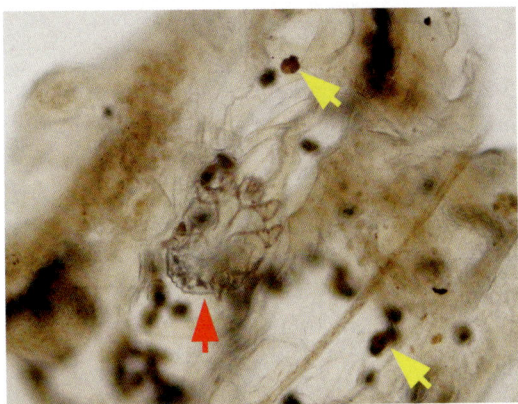

Figure 2.6. Newly hatched mite (red arrow) and fecal material (yellow arrows) on a mineral oil preparation.

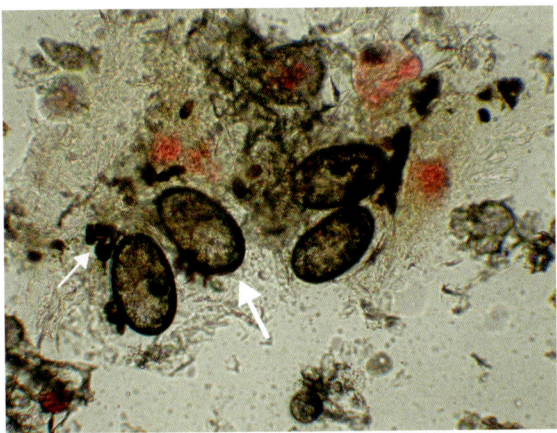

Figure 2.7. A mineral oil preparation in a patient who has scabies reveals eggs (large arrow) and mite fecal material (ie, scybala) (small arrow).

Wood Lamp Examination

Examination of the skin with a Wood lamp in a darkened room may assist in the diagnosis of several conditions.

- Erythrasma (a superficial *Corynebacterium* infection): affected areas fluoresce coral red.
- Tinea capitis: Wood lamp examination is useful in the recognition of only a minority of cases (perhaps 5%) of tinea capitis caused by *Microsporum* species (Figure 2.8). Green fluorescence does not occur when infections are caused by *T tonsurans*.
- Tinea versicolor (caused by yeasts of the genus *Malassezia* [formerly *Pityrosporum*]): affected areas may fluoresce yellow gold.
- Diseases characterized by hypopigmentation or depigmentation: in individuals who are lightly pigmented, examining the skin with a Wood lamp may assist in identifying lesions of vitiligo or ash-leaf macules of tuberous sclerosis.

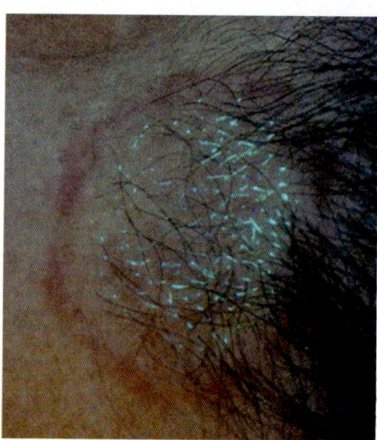

Figure 2.8. Wood lamp examination in tinea capitis caused by *Microsporum canis*. There is green fluorescence of affected hairs.

CHAPTER 3

Therapeutics
I. Selection and Use of Topical Corticosteroids

Introduction

▶ Topical corticosteroids exert their effect through many mechanisms, including anti-inflammatory, immunosuppressive, antiproliferative, and vasoconstrictive effects.

▶ Preparations may be grouped according to relative potency (Table 3.1). Differences in potency between groups are not linear. For example, hydrocortisone (group 7) has a relative potency of less than 1; triamcinolone (group 4), 75; and clobetasol propionate (group 1), 1,869.

Table 3.1. Selected Topical Corticosteroids by Potency

Group	Generic Name (Vehicles; Concentration)
Group 1 (most potent)	• Augmented betamethasone dipropionate (ointment; 0.05%). • Clobetasol propionate (cream, ointment, foam; 0.05%). • Diflorasone diacetate (ointment; 0.05%). • Fluocinonide (cream; 0.1%). • Halobetasol propionate (cream, ointment, lotion; 0.05%).
Group 2	• Amcinonide (ointment; 0.1%). • Augmented betamethasone dipropionate (cream, lotion; 0.05%). • Fluocinonide (cream, ointment, gel, solution; 0.05%). • Mometasone furoate (ointment; 0.1%).
Group 3	• Amcinonide (cream, lotion; 0.1%). • Betamethasone valerate (foam; 0.12%). • Diflorasone diacetate (cream; 0.05%). • Fluticasone propionate (ointment; 0.005%). • Triamcinolone acetonide (ointment; 0.1%).
Group 4	• Fluocinolone acetonide (ointment; 0.025%). • Hydrocortisone valerate (ointment; 0.2%). • Mometasone furoate (cream, lotion; 0.1%). • Triamcinolone acetonide (cream; 0.1%).

(continued)

Table 3.1. (continued)	
Group	**Generic Name (Vehicles; Concentration)**
Group 5	• Betamethasone valerate (cream; 0.1%). • Fluocinolone acetonide (cream; 0.025%). • Fluticasone propionate (cream; 0.05%). • Hydrocortisone valerate (cream; 0.2%). • Prednicarbate (cream; 0.1%).
Group 6	• Alclometasone dipropionate (cream, ointment; 0.05%). • Desonide (cream, ointment, gel, foam; 0.05%). • Fluocinolone acetonide (solution, oil; 0.01%).
Group 7 (least potent)	• Hydrocortisone (cream, ointment; 1%, 2.5%).

Adapted with permission from Eichenfield LF, Friedlander SF. Coping with chronic dermatitis. *Contemp Pediatr.* 1998;15(10):53–80 and Eichenfield LF, Boguniewicz M, Simpson EL, et al. Translating atopic dermatitis management guidelines into practice for primary care providers. *Pediatrics.* 2015;136(3):554–565.

Selecting and Prescribing a Topical Corticosteroid

Consider the following factors when selecting a topical corticosteroid (Table 3.2):

▶ How old is the patient?
- In general, a less potent preparation is required in infants than in older children or adolescents. For example, for the management of flares of atopic dermatitis, a low-potency preparation (eg, hydrocortisone ointment 1% or 2.5%) usually is sufficient in an infant, whereas in an adolescent, a mid-potency (eg, triamcinolone 0.1%) or high-potency (eg, mometasone 0.1%) product is needed.

▶ What area will be treated?
- Absorption of steroids varies with the thickness of the skin in various regions of the body.
- Absorption is greatest in areas where the skin is thin (eg, face, perineum) and lowest where the skin is thick (eg, palms, soles). Thus, only a low-potency preparation should be used on the face, whereas a mid-potency (or high-potency) product will be needed to manage dermatitis on the feet.
- Absorption is also increased in occluded or warm and opposed areas of skin. Hence, in areas such as the axillae, groin, or diapered area of an infant, low-potency preparations are typically recommended.

▶ What vehicle should be selected?

- Creams: tolerated by most patients but can be drying, and, occasionally, their ingredients may cause burning or contact dermatitis.
- Ointments: the most effective vehicle, especially for thickened or lichenified skin; increase the absorption and potency ranking of the steroid; generally are preservative free and less likely to cause contact or irritant dermatitis; have a greasy feel that may not be tolerated by some patients. Ointments are the preferred vehicle for most dermatologists in most situations.
- Lotions: cosmetically pleasing because they do not leave a greasy feel; tend to sting on open or damaged skin.
- Gels: usually for hair-bearing areas; may cause stinging or burning.

▶ How much should you dispense?
- For treatment of a self-limited condition involving a small area, prescribing a small tube (eg, 15 g) will be sufficient; however, if the process is more extensive or chronic, larger amounts will be needed. Some rules that will help include the following:
  – One gram of product will cover a 10-cm by 10-cm area (perhaps 30% more coverage if an ointment is used rather than a cream). Note that 0.5 g is the amount of cream dispensed from a standard tube that extends from the tip of the adult finger to the flexural crease overlying the volar distal interphalangeal joint.
  – In an older child (6–10 years of age), it is estimated that it takes
    - 1 g to cover the face and neck.
    - 1.25 g to cover the hand and arm.
    - 1.75 g to cover the chest and abdomen.
    - 2.25 g to cover the foot and leg.
  – Thus, when managing a chronic condition like atopic dermatitis that involves a significant portion of the body, prescribing amounts of 227 or 454 g (0.5 or 1 lb), rather than small tubes, may be necessary.

▶ Cost
- As with other medications, the cost of topical corticosteroids varies widely and often is influenced by the patient's insurance formulary. Although proprietary corticosteroids typically are more expensive than generics, generics are not always inexpensive. There are insufficient data, however, to enable direct comparison of efficacy and bioavailability of branded versus generic preparations.

Table 3.2. Guidelines for Selecting Corticosteroid Potency

Potency	Guideline
Low	• Infant (any body site) or young child. • Face, perineum, axillae in patient of any age.
Moderate	• Child (exclusive of face) with moderate to severe disease. • Adolescent (exclusive of face or anatomically occluded areas [eg, axillae, genitalia]).
High	• Used primarily by dermatologists. • Most often used in the management of severe or lichenified (thickened) dermatoses and/or those involving the feet or hands.

Adverse Effects

When used appropriately, topical corticosteroids are very safe; however, using too potent a preparation, particularly in an inappropriate location or for too long, may result in adverse effects.

▶ Local adverse effects: atrophy, striae, pigmentary changes, easy bruising, hypertrichosis, and acne-like eruptions. To prevent these effects, use only low-potency preparations on the face, axillae, and groin (including the diaper area); limit the duration of use of all corticosteroids; and use high-potency preparations very discriminatingly.

▶ Systemic adverse effects: hypothalamic-pituitary-adrenal axis suppression, Cushing syndrome, growth retardation, glaucoma, and cataracts. Systemic adverse effects are most likely to occur when very potent agents are used (even for short periods) or when moderately potent preparations are used over large areas of the body for long periods, especially in young infants, where the ratio of skin to body surface area is larger.

Frequency of Application

▶ Typically twice daily as needed.

II. Selection and Use of Moisturizers

Introduction

- Moisturizers (also known as emollients or lubricants) are designed to hydrate the skin by creating a barrier and preventing evaporation.
- In patients who have atopic dermatitis, moisturizers can reduce the need for corticosteroids.

Selecting a Moisturizer

Traditional moisturizers are available as ointments, creams, or lotions. Barrier repair agents also are available.

- Ointments
  - Water-in-oil emulsions are most occlusive and are the best moisturizers.
  - Have a greasy feel that some patients find unpleasant.
  - Because they generally are preservative free, they are less likely to cause allergic contact or irritant contact dermatitis.
  - Some examples include Aquaphor ointment, CeraVe healing ointment, and petrolatum (eg, Vaseline pure petroleum jelly).
- Creams
  - Oil-in-water emulsions that often are more cosmetically pleasing than ointments.
  - Some examples include CeraVe cream, Cetaphil cream, Eucerin cream, and Vanicream.
- Lotions
  - Oil-in-water emulsions containing more water than creams have.
  - Cosmetically pleasing but least effective as moisturizers.
  - Some examples include CeraVe lotion, Cetaphil lotion, Curel lotion, DML lotion, Eucerin lotion, Keri lotion, Lubriderm lotion, and Moisturel lotion.
- Barrier repair agents
  - A variety of over-the-counter (eg, CeraVe, Cetaphil Restoraderm) and prescription (eg, Atopiclair, EpiCeram, Hylatopic) barrier repair agents exist that may help reduce the severity of atopic dermatitis and play an adjunctive therapeutic role. These agents include products with ceramides, filaggrin degradation products, natural moisturizing factors, avenanthramides, glycyrrhetinic acid, shea nut derivatives, and palmitamide monoethanolamine.

- Although the exact role of these agents is unclear, they may play a role in active disease (usually in conjunction with anti-inflammatory agents such as corticosteroids and calcineurin inhibitors) and as maintenance agents.
- Prescription barrier repair agents may be expensive.

Adverse Effects

Preservatives, antimicrobial agents, or fragrances contained in moisturizers, or products that are lanolin based, may cause allergic or irritant contact dermatitis.

Frequency of Application

▶ Apply 2 to 3 times daily as needed (at least 1 application should immediately follow a bath or shower while the skin is still damp, when possible).

▶ Lotions and creams may need to be applied more often than ointments.

▶ If the patient is using a topical corticosteroid, topical calcineurin inhibitor, topical phosphodiesterase 4 inhibitor, or topical Janus kinase inhibitor, apply these agents first, followed by the moisturizer.

III. Cryotherapy

Introduction

Cryotherapy uses liquid nitrogen (or another cryogen) to destroy skin lesions through tissue necrosis. In pediatrics, it is commonly used to treat warts.

Selecting a Cryogen

- Liquid nitrogen is the most effective cryogen, with an achieved temperature of approximately −195 °C (−319 °F).
- If cryotherapy will be performed infrequently, products that use other cryogens (eg, dimethyl ether and propane [eg, Histofreezer]) may be more economical for a practice because they have a long shelf life, although their effectiveness and freeze effect (temperature approximately −57 °C [−70.6 °F]) are significantly lower than those of liquid nitrogen.
- Some cryotherapy devices can be purchased by patients without a prescription. They also contain dimethyl ether and propane.

Procedure

- Liquid nitrogen usually is applied with a spray device or a cotton swab that is dipped into the liquid nitrogen and then applied to the skin.
    - Standard cotton-tipped applicators do not work well because the tight wrap of the cotton does not allow liquid nitrogen to be absorbed.
    - To make an applicator, wrap additional cotton onto the tip of an applicator, shaping it to a point.
- Liquid nitrogen should be applied to the lesion until a white ring (the ice ball) extends 1 to 3 mm beyond the margin of the wart. Once the ring appears, stop cryotherapy. The lesion will then thaw and return to typical color within 30 seconds. Some experts advise a second or third treatment after initial thawing (freeze-thaw cycles).
- Patients should be advised that within 1 to 2 days a blister may form. Once the blister ruptures, the area should be cleansed twice daily and a topical antibiotic and a bandage applied.
- Any remaining wart can be treated with a keratolytic that contains salicylic acid. Repeat cryotherapy may be performed in 2 to 4 weeks if necessary.

IV. Sun Protection

Elements of Sun Protection

- Minimize prolonged outdoor activities between 10:00 am and 4:00 pm when possible.
- Wear protective clothing, such as a wide-brimmed hat, long-sleeved shirt, and long pants. Many manufacturers produce sun-protective clothing with a UV protection factor (approximately equivalent to the sun protection factor [SPF]) of 30 or more.
- Use a sunscreen regularly.
  - Choose a product with an SPF of 30 or more that has UV-A and UV-B protection (ie, is labeled broad-spectrum). SPF is a measure of protection from UV-B. At present, there is no rating system for UV-A protection. With respect to the safety of sunscreen active ingredients, consider the following:
    - Zinc oxide and titanium dioxide (physical [inorganic] sunscreen ingredients) are generally recognized as safe and effective by the US Food and Drug Administration (FDA); trolamine salicylate and para-aminobenzoic acid are not. For the remaining 12 chemical (organic) sunscreens used in products commercially available in the United States, the FDA has requested more data to determine whether they merit classification as generally recognized as safe and effective.
    - Studies conducted by the FDA demonstrate that chemical (organic) sunscreen active ingredients may be absorbed systemically. The clinical significance of these findings is unknown, but additional study is needed to understand the implications, if any. Pending these investigations, the FDA encourages individuals to continue using these sunscreens.
    - Concern exists that chemical sunscreens, like oxybenzone, may have estrogenic and antiandrogenic effects. Oxybenzone also may inhibit the migration of neural crest cells during embryogenesis. Women with high levels of urine oxybenzone had a greater than expected risk of giving birth to neonates with Hirschsprung disease. For the present, physical (inorganic) sunscreens should be recommended during pregnancy, and breastfeeding mothers may wish to avoid using oxybenzone-containing sunscreens.

- Oxybenzone and octinoxate have been implicated in damage to coral reefs and some fish populations, and their use has been banned in Hawaii.
- In 2021, an independent laboratory (Valisure) reported finding benzene, a known carcinogen, in 27% of 294 commercially available sunscreens, primarily sprays. The clinical significance of this finding is not known.

- Consider a product that is not alcohol based (ie, will not cause stinging) and that is labeled non-acnegenic or noncomedogenic (ie, to prevent worsening acne in adolescents).
- Apply liberally (using too little may reduce the SPF), ideally 30 minutes before beginning outdoor activities, even on cloudy days.
- Apply every 2 hours, as well as after swimming or activities resulting in significant sweating.
- Although there are limited data on the safety of sunscreen use in infants younger than 6 months, there is no evidence that applying small amounts is associated with adverse long-term effects. Therefore, in situations in which other sun protection strategies may be inadequate or unfeasible, it is reasonable to apply sunscreen to exposed areas of the skin in young infants.
- Products with a combination of sunscreen ingredients and the insect repellent N,N-diethyl-3-methylbenzamide should be avoided because of differences in recommended application frequencies, unnecessary repellent exposure, and potential toxicity.

▶ To prevent cataracts and ocular melanoma, wear sunglasses that are labeled as blocking 100% of UV-A and UV-B rays.

Dermatitis

CHAPTER 4 — **Atopic Dermatitis** 33

CHAPTER 5 — **Contact Dermatitis (Irritant and Allergic)** 47

CHAPTER 6 — **Juvenile Plantar Dermatosis** 61

CHAPTER 4

Atopic Dermatitis

Introduction/Etiology/Epidemiology

- Most common chronic pediatric skin disorder, affecting as many as 15% of children.
- Cause unknown but appears to be the result of a complex interplay among immune dysregulation, barrier dysfunction, and the environment.
- Strong genetic predisposition; many patients have personal or family history of atopy.
- Generally begins during infancy or childhood; 90% of those ultimately affected present before 5 years of age.
- Children who have atopic dermatitis are susceptible to certain cutaneous bacterial and viral infections.
  - Increased adherence of *Staphylococcus aureus* to the skin and reduced production of antimicrobial peptides may explain the high rates of colonization with and infection due to this bacterium.
  - Altered T-cell function may explain the predisposition of children to develop molluscum contagiosum, eczema herpeticum, and eczema vaccinatum.

Signs and Symptoms

- Characterized by pruritus with resultant scratching that leads to excoriations and lichenification.
- The distribution of lesions varies with the patient's age, and their appearance is related to the degree of skin pigmentation.
  - Infants and toddlers: involvement of the face, trunk, and extensor extremities (Figures 4.1 and 4.2).
  - Childhood: lesions are concentrated in flexural areas, such as the antecubital and popliteal fossae, wrists, and ankles (Figures 4.3 and 4.4). Some children exhibit round, crusted lesions (ie, nummular [coin-shaped] eczema) (Figure 4.5); in older children, the feet may be involved (Figure 4.6).

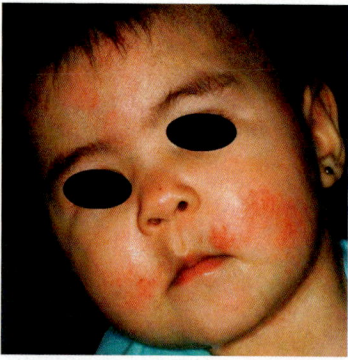

Figure 4.1. Erythematous patches on the face of an infant who has atopic dermatitis.

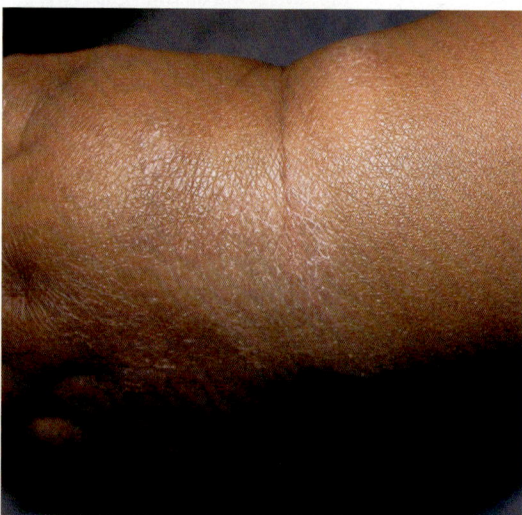

Figure 4.2. Hypopigmented patch on the dorsum of the wrist in an infant with skin of color who has atopic dermatitis.

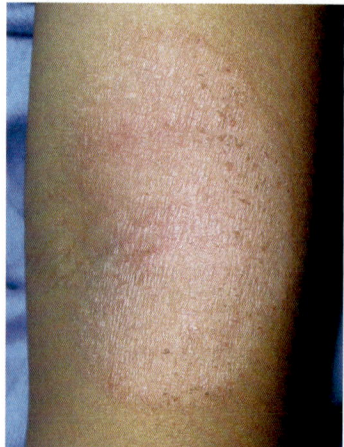

Figure 4.3. Erythematous lichenified patch in the antecubital fossa in childhood atopic dermatitis.

Chapter 4: Atopic Dermatitis 35

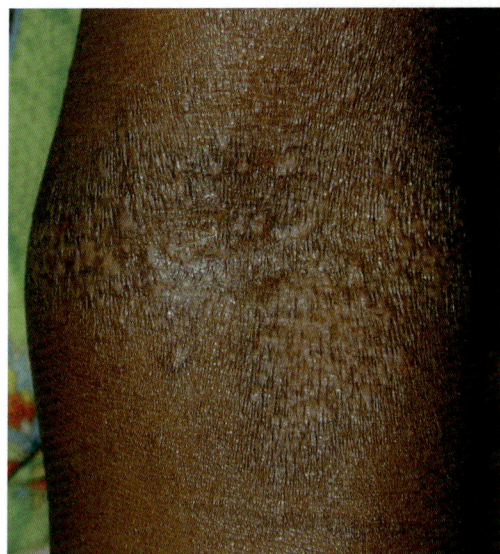

Figure 4.4. Chronic atopic dermatitis in the antecubital fossa in a patient with skin of color.

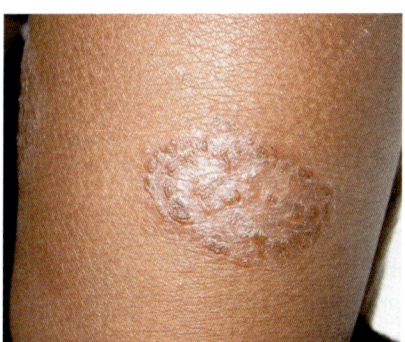

Figure 4.5. Oval crusted lesion of nummular eczema.

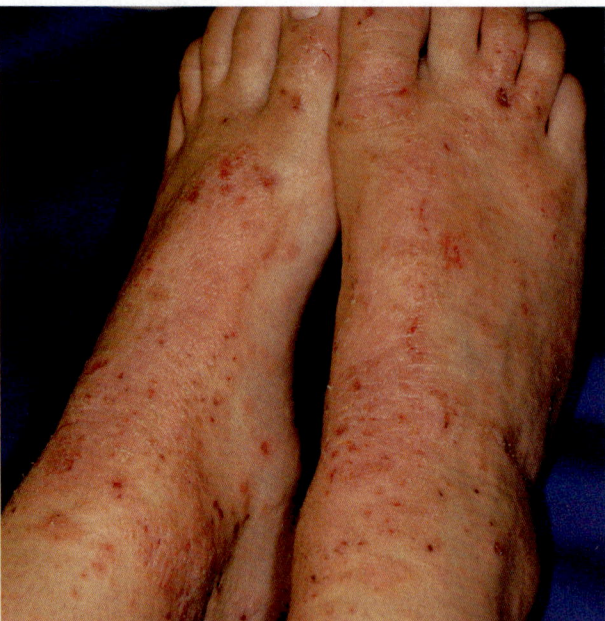

Figure 4.6. Involvement of the feet in atopic dermatitis: erythema, lichenification, scaling, and numerous erosions and crusts.

- Adolescents continue to exhibit a flexural distribution but often develop lesions on the hands, face, and neck (Figure 4.7).
- In individuals who have less pigment, lesions are erythematous, somewhat scaly or crusted papules, patches, or thin plaques. In people with skin of color, erythema is less obvious, the eruption often is more papular (Figure 4.8), and postinflammatory hypopigmentation or hyperpigmentation often is present (see Figure 4.2).

Chapter 4: Atopic Dermatitis

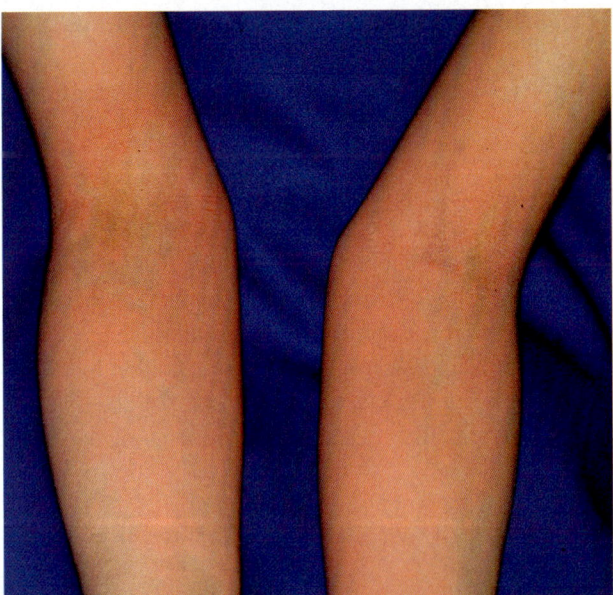

Figure 4.7. Erythematous patches in the antecubital fossae of an adolescent who has atopic dermatitis.

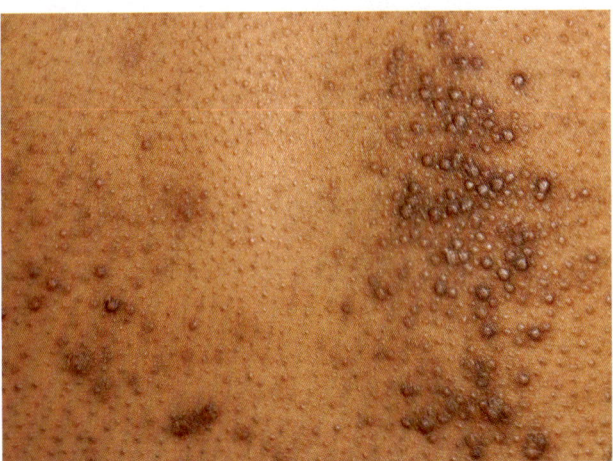

Figure 4.8. Papular atopic dermatitis. In persons with skin of color, lesions of atopic dermatitis often are composed of flat-topped (ie, lichenoid) papules.

- Other cutaneous variations that serve as clues to diagnosis include the following:
  - Morgan folds (atopic pleats): prominent skinfolds located beneath the lower eyelids.
  - Dry skin (xerosis).
  - Hyper-linearity of the palms and soles.
  - Lichenification: thickened skin with prominent creases (see Figure 4.3).
  - Keratosis pilaris: papules centered about follicles that have a central core of keratin debris and, at times, surrounding erythema (Figure 4.9); lesions usually located on the upper outer arms, face, and thighs.
  - Pityriasis alba: small, poorly defined areas of hypopigmentation located on the face or elsewhere (Figure 4.10).
  - Ichthyosis vulgaris: polygonal scales, most commonly involving the lower extremities (Figure 4.11).

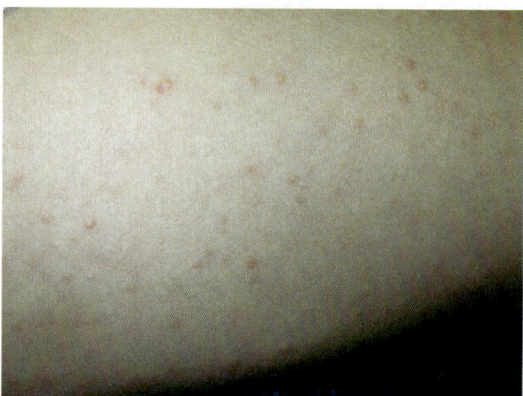

Figure 4.9. Keratosis pilaris: follicular papules that have a central core of keratin debris.

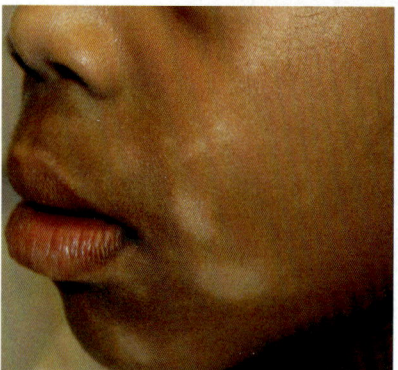

Figure 4.10. Ill-defined hypopigmented macules are characteristic of pityriasis alba.

Chapter 4: Atopic Dermatitis

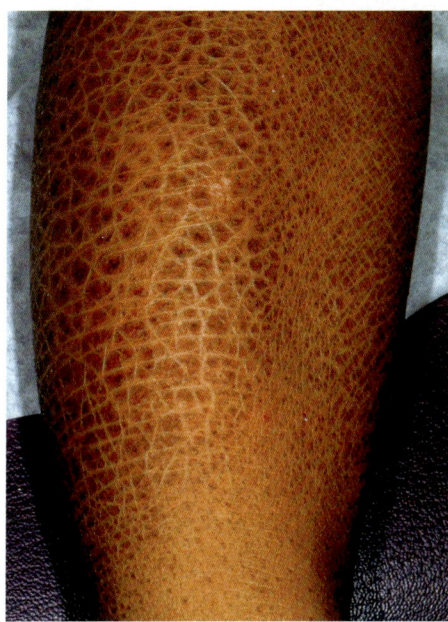

Figure 4.11. Polygonal scales with a pasted-on appearance located on the lower extremities are characteristic of ichthyosis vulgaris, a condition commonly associated with atopic dermatitis.

Look-alikes

Disorder	Differentiating Features
Contact dermatitis	• Location corresponds to exposure to contact allergen (eg, earlobes in those with sensitivity to nickel used in earrings). • Configuration may be unusual (eg, linear in plant dermatitis).
Psoriasis	• Erythematous papules and plaques with thick, silvery scale. • Scaling of scalp common; pitting of nails may be observed. • Pruritus much less common or less severe than in atopic dermatitis. • Extensor (rather than flexural) surfaces of knees and elbows common sites of involvement.
Scabies	• Papules often larger than those in atopic dermatitis. • Linear burrows present. • Beyond infancy, lesions concentrated in interdigital spaces, in wrist flexures, on penis and scrotum, or on areolae. • Other family members may be affected.
Seborrheic dermatitis	• Erythematous, greasy, scaling patches involving the eyebrows, nasolabial folds, and intertriginous areas (eg, postauricular areas; axillae; and, in infants, the diaper area). • Scaling of scalp common. • Most often seen in infants younger than 1 year or after adrenarche; less common in prepubertal children. • Pruritus often minimal.
Tinea corporis	• Often annular, with central clearing. • Pruritus often absent.

How to Make the Diagnosis

- The diagnosis is made clinically based on the presence of 3 or more of the following signs or symptoms: typical morphology and distribution of lesions, pruritus, chronic relapsing course, and a family or personal history of atopic disorders.
- The presence of associated features (discussed previously) provides support for the diagnosis.

Treatment

(See Also Stepwise Management for Atopic Dermatitis)

Daily Measures

Hydrate Skin and Prevent Pruritus

- Daily bathing is desirable, if less than 10 minutes and warm (not hot) water is used.
- Apply an emollient as needed to control dry skin; most effective timing is when applied immediately after bathing (while skin is still moist). Application often is recommended at least once daily, but this will vary with the individual and environmental factors (eg, during warm weather months in humid conditions an emollient may not be needed).
  - Lotions (eg, CeraVe, Cetaphil, Curel, Eucerin, Lubriderm, Moisturel, Aveeno) work well for most individuals, although preservatives (found in some) occasionally cause stinging or skin reactions.
  - Creams (eg, CeraVe, Cetaphil, Eucerin, Vanicream, Moisturel, Aveeno) moisturize better than lotions and do not leave as greasy a feel, which may be a benefit in older patients.
  - Ointments (eg, Aquaphor, Vaseline, CeraVe) are very good moisturizers but because of their greasy feel may not be well tolerated by some.
- During colder months when humidity is low, one may consider using a vaporizer in the patient's room at night (taking care to cleanse the device regularly and avoid moisture contact with walls [which could promote mold growth]).
- Use a fragrance-free, non-soap cleanser. Examples include synthetic detergent (ie, syndet) cleansers in bar (eg, Cetaphil Bar, Dove Bar) or liquid (eg, Dove Liquid) forms or lipid-free cleansers (eg, Aquanil, CeraVe, Cetaphil).

▶ Use an additive-free (fragrance- and dye-free) detergent for laundering clothes (eg, All Free Clear, Ivory Snow, Tide Free and Gentle). If a fabric softener is used, it too should be additive free.
▶ Wear cotton clothing next to the skin when possible.

Table 4.1. Stepwise Management for Atopic Dermatitis

	Non-Lesional[a]	Mild	Moderate	Severe
Daily Management and Maintenance	Basic management • Moisturizer • Warm baths or showers • Avoid triggers (allergens, irritants) • Consider comorbidities	Basic management • Moisturizer • Warm baths or showers • Dilute bleach bath or equivalent twice per week • Antibiotics, if needed • Avoid triggers (allergens, irritants) • Consider comorbidities	Basic management + topical anti-inflammatory medication to potential problem areas • Maintenance TCS or • Maintenance TCI or • Maintenance crisaborole	Basic management + referral to AD specialist for other treatment options • Phototherapy (approved for ≥12 years) • Dupilumab (approved for ≥6 months) • Upadacitinib (approved for ≥12 years) • Abrocitinib (approved for ≥12 years) • Systemic immunosuppressant agent
Management During Acute Flares		Apply TCS (low to medium potency) to inflamed skin (consider TCI, crisaborole, ruxolitinib)	Apply TCS (medium to high potency)/TCI/crisaborole/ruxolitinib to inflamed skin. If not improved in 7 days consider the following: • Nonadherence • Incorrect diagnosis • Infection (*Staphylococcus aureus* or herpes simplex virus) • Contact allergy • Referral	

Abbreviations: AD, atopic dermatitis; TCI, topical calcineurin inhibitor; TCS, topical corticosteroid.
[a] A number of severity rating scales exist. Some examples include Patient-Oriented Eczema Measure (POEM), SCORing Atopic Dermatitis (SCORAD), Three Item Severity (TIS) score, and Eczema Area and Severity Index (EASI).
Adapted from Boguniewicz M, Fonacier L, Guttman-Yassky E, Ong PY, Silverberg J, Farrar JR. Atopic dermatitis yardstick: practical recommendations for an evolving therapeutic landscape. *Ann Allergy Asthma Immunol*. 2018;120(1): 10.e2–22.e2.

When the Disease Flares
Reduce Inflammation
Apply a topical corticosteroid twice daily as needed. Ointments are preferred over creams because they tend to be more effective and better tolerated (although some patients prefer creams because they are less greasy). The selection and use of these agents is discussed in detail in Chapter 3. Systemic corticosteroids rarely are necessary for the management of atopic dermatitis.

- Infants (or treatment of the face in a patient of any age): use a low-potency preparation (eg, hydrocortisone 1% or 2.5%).
- Young children (exclusive of the face): use a low-potency preparation (eg, hydrocortisone 1% or 2.5%) or, if necessary, a mid-potency preparation (eg, triamcinolone 0.025% or 0.1%, fluocinolone 0.025%).
- Older children and adolescents (exclusive of the face): use a mid-potency preparation (eg, triamcinolone 0.1%); a high-potency agent (eg, mometasone 0.1%, fluocinonide 0.05%) may be needed for resistant, non-facial areas during a flare.
- Once symptoms have improved, the corticosteroid may be withdrawn and a moisturizer continued regularly. However, applying a corticosteroid once or twice weekly at locations prone to exacerbations can reduce relapses and increase the time to the next flare.

Control Pruritus/Optimize Nighttime Sleep
Administer a bedtime dose of a first-generation antihistamine (eg, hydroxyzine 0.5–1 mg/kg, diphenhydramine 1.25 mg/kg) to provide sedation, improve sleep, and reduce scratching; daytime doses may occasionally be needed but should be lower (to avoid sedation). Alternatively, some practitioners use a nonsedating agent (eg, cetirizine) for daytime coverage in school-aged children, although evidence of its benefit is controversial.

Control Infection
If there is evidence of secondary bacterial infection (eg, crusting, pustules, oozing [Figure 4.12]), consider administering an oral antistaphylococcal antibiotic (eg, cephalexin or other agent on the basis of local antibiotic resistance patterns) for 7 to 10 days. If no improvement is noted within 48 hours, consider skin swab for bacterial culture to assess for resistant organisms (eg, methicillin-resistant *S aureus*) and treat appropriately. At this time, most *S aureus* isolates from patients with atopic dermatitis in the United States remain methicillin sensitive.

If infection is limited to very focal areas, a prescription topical antimicrobial agent (eg, mupirocin, retapamulin, ozenoxacin) may be useful.

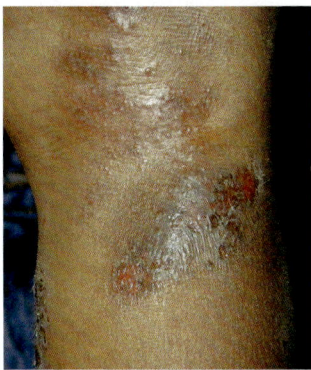

Figure 4.12. Erosions, weeping, and crusting are observed when lesions of atopic dermatitis become secondarily infected.

Other Measures

▶ Non-corticosteroid topical calcineurin inhibitors (eg, tacrolimus [Protopic], pimecrolimus [Elidel]).
  - Reduce inflammation and avoid potential local or systemic corticosteroid adverse effects.
  - Are used as second-line agents in patients older than 2 years for whom topical corticosteroids fail or when avoidance of more potent topical corticosteroid is desired (eg, treatment of the face). The US Food and Drug Administration advises using these agents only for active areas of dermatitis and discourages long-term application.
    – May be used as monotherapy twice daily or in conjunction with topical corticosteroids (eg, a topical corticosteroid is applied morning and afternoon and the topical calcineurin inhibitor at bedtime).
    – Once symptoms have improved, application of a topical calcineurin inhibitor 2 to 3 times weekly at locations prone to exacerbations can reduce relapses.

▶ Non-corticosteroid phosphodiesterase inhibitor (eg, crisaborole [Eucrisa]): nonsteroidal anti-inflammatory agent not associated with local or systemic corticosteroid adverse effects. It is approved for children 3 months of age or older and is applied twice daily to affected areas. Some burning may be reported with application.

▶ Non-corticosteroid Janus kinase inhibitor (eg, ruxolitinib, [Opzelura]): nonsteroidal anti-inflammatory agent not associated with local or systemic corticosteroid adverse effects. It is approved for use in those 12 years of age or older who have mild to moderate atopic dermatitis and is applied twice daily to affected areas.

- Control *S aureus* colonization: may be useful for those with severe or recalcitrant disease. Consider 1 or more of the following options: (1) twice weekly 5- to 10-minute baths to which standard (not concentrated) household bleach is added (½ cup in a full tub of water [40 gallons]), (2) use of a sodium hypochlorite bodywash (eg, CLn BodyWash) in the bath or shower, or (3) intranasal mupirocin (twice a day for 5 days).
- Wet-wrap therapy: method may be useful during severe flares of atopic dermatitis. A topical corticosteroid is applied to affected areas and covered with a moistened cotton suit (eg, pajamas); wet gauze strips; or a specially designed, commercially available garment, which is then covered with a dry outer layer (eg, dry pajamas). The wrap may be worn for several hours or up to 24 hours; on removal, emollient is applied. Once the disease flare improves, wet-wrap therapy is discontinued.
- Barrier repair agents
  - A variety of over-the-counter (eg, CeraVe, Cetaphil Restoraderm) and prescription (eg, Atopiclair, EpiCeram, Hylatopic) barrier repair agents exist that may help reduce the severity of atopic dermatitis and play an adjunctive therapeutic role. These agents include products with ceramides, filaggrin degradation products, natural moisturizing factors, avenanthramides, glycyrrhetinic acid, shea nut derivatives, and palmitamide monoethanolamine.
  - Although the exact role of these agents is unclear, they may play a role in active disease (usually in conjunction with anti-inflammatory agents such as corticosteroids and calcineurin inhibitors) and as maintenance agents.
  - Prescription barrier repair agents may be more expensive.
- Dietary manipulation
  - Breastfeeding for the first 3 to 4 months after birth reduces the incidence of atopic dermatitis in children during the first 2 years of life. Maternal antigen avoidance during pregnancy or lactation is not recommended as a strategy to prevent atopic dermatitis.
  - Although food allergies are common in children who have atopic dermatitis, rarely is food a trigger of the disease. Food allergy contributing to atopic dermatitis should be considered in children with moderate to severe disease that is recalcitrant to standard therapies and/or when there is a history of pruritus or rash occurring within 30 minutes of ingesting a food. The foods most often responsible are egg, peanut, and milk. Children in whom concern exists for food allergy triggering atopic dermatitis are best referred to an allergist for evaluation.

- House dust mite avoidance: Avoidance through frequent vacuuming and encasing pillows and mattresses with allergen-proof products may result in a modest reduction in the severity of atopic dermatitis. Such recommendations are reserved for patients with severe or recalcitrant disease.

Treating Associated Conditions

- Keratosis pilaris and ichthyosis vulgaris
  - Advise patients and families there is no cure and the course may be variable.
  - Use of an emollient or emollient with a keratolytic agent (eg, AmLactin, Lac-Hydrin, Carmol), applied twice daily as needed, may soften papules and make them less noticeable.
  - Good dry skin care is vital.
- Pityriasis alba
  - Apply an appropriate topical corticosteroid twice daily (eg, for the face, hydrocortisone 1%) for 2 to 3 weeks to treat any existing inflammation (topical calcineurin inhibitors or phosphodiesterase inhibitors may also be useful in this regard).
  - Sun protection should be recommended to reduce the contrast between typical skin (which will become darker with sun exposure) and affected skin (in which there is temporary melanocyte dysfunction).
  - The patient and family should be counseled that several months might be required for typical pigmentation to return.

Prognosis

- The prognosis for children with atopic dermatitis is good; 80% to 90% of infants experience a spontaneous resolution or improvement in symptoms by adolescence. However, until this time, the course is chronic and relapsing, an issue that should be discussed with patients and parents.

When to Worry or Refer

- Consider referral to a dermatologist for patients who have severe or extensive disease, do not respond to standard treatment, or have chronic or recurrent bacterial or viral (eg, molluscum contagiosum, herpes simplex virus) infections. Such patients may need light therapy, immunosuppressive agents, biologic therapy (eg, dupilumab), or small molecule therapy (eg, oral Janus kinase inhibitors like abrocitinib, upadacitinib). In addition, a dermatologist can discuss the potential role of newer and emerging therapies.

Resources for Families

- American Academy of Dermatology: Childhood eczema.
  https://www.aad.org/public/diseases/eczema/childhood
- American Academy of Dermatology: Eczema types: dyshidrotic eczema overview.
  https://www.aad.org/public/diseases/eczema/types/dyshidrotic-eczema
- American Academy of Pediatrics: HealthyChildren.org.
  www.HealthyChildren.org/eczema
- National Eczema Association: A national patient-oriented organization. The site contains information for patients and families, education for practitioners, and links to other resources.
  www.nationaleczema.org
- Society for Pediatric Dermatology: Patient handout on atopic dermatitis (eczema).
  https://pedsderm.net/for-patients-families/patient-handouts/#AtopicDerm
- WebMD: Information for families is contained in Skin Problems and Treatments.
  www.webmd.com/skin-problems-and-treatments/eczema/default.htm

CHAPTER 5

Contact Dermatitis (Irritant and Allergic)

I. Irritant Contact Dermatitis

Introduction/Etiology/Epidemiology

- Inflammatory reaction of the skin caused by physical contact with an irritating substance.
- Occurs in any individual exposed to a sufficient amount of the offending agent.
- Can be exacerbated by local physical factors (eg, diapering) and individual susceptibility (eg, diminished skin barrier function, as in atopic dermatitis).
- Common forms of irritant contact dermatitis include:
  - Irritant diaper dermatitis: most common presentation of irritant contact dermatitis in infancy (occurs in up to 20% of all infants); caused by friction, moisture, maceration, and occlusion. (See also Chapter 101, Diaper Dermatitis.)
  - Dry skin dermatitis (ie, asteatotic eczema or winter eczema): caused by low relative humidity and aggravated by soaps, excessive bathing or washing, and alcohol-containing lotions and solutions such as hand sanitizers.
  - Lip-licking dermatitis and thumb-sucking dermatitis: caused by wetting the skin frequently with saliva.
  - Berries, tomatoes, and citrus fruits are common causes of irritant contact dermatitis of the perioral skin in infants and toddlers.
- Irritant contact dermatitis is more common in children with underlying atopic dermatitis, presumably related to their diminished skin barrier function.

Signs and Symptoms

Irritant Diaper Dermatitis
- Affects convex surfaces of buttocks, upper inner thighs (Figure 5.1).
- Characteristically spares creases and folds.
- Sharply marginated erythema that becomes more deeply red with a "glazed" appearance.
- May have dermatitis along the diaper margins ("tidemark dermatitis").

Asteatotic Eczema
- Dry, rough skin with white, sometimes rectangular, scaling and variable erythema (Figure 5.2).
- Often associated with keratosis pilaris.

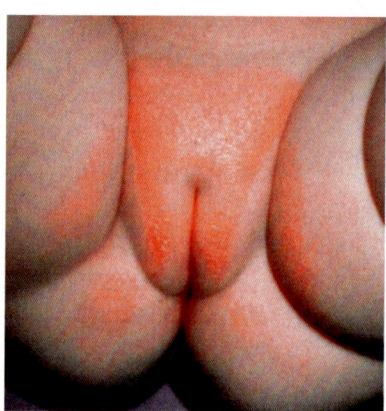

Figure 5.1. Irritant diaper dermatitis. Erythematous patches sparing the skinfolds.

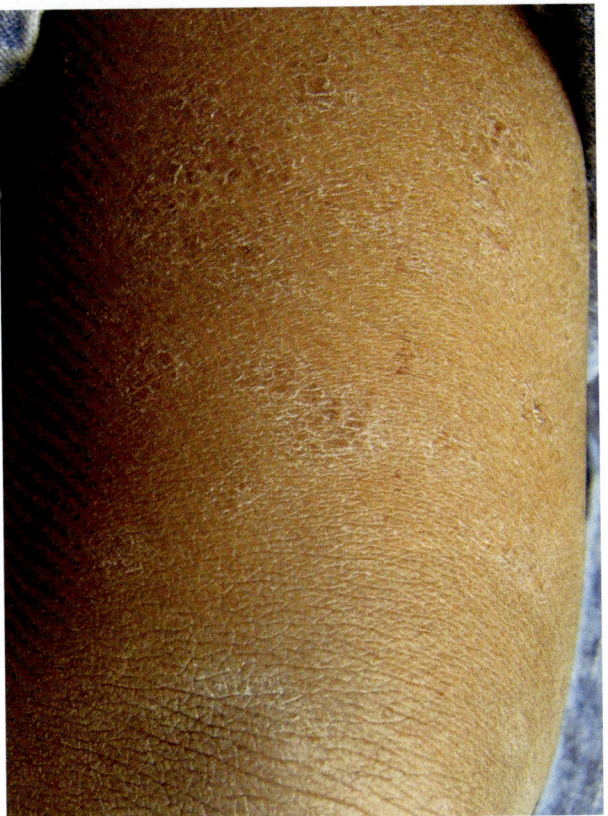

Figure 5.2. Asteatotic eczema is characterized by dry, rough skin with white rectangular scaling.

Look-alikes (See also Chapter 101, Diaper Dermatitis.)

Disorder	Differentiating Features
Irritant Diaper Dermatitis	
Candidiasis	• Erythematous patches that involve convexities and inguinal creases. • Satellite papules and pustules. • Scaling at margins of involved areas.
Seborrheic dermatitis	• Salmon-pink patches with greasy scale that involve the convexities and inguinal creases. • Involvement of scalp, face, postauricular creases, or chest may be present.
Bullous impetigo	• Flaccid blisters filled with clear or purulent fluid. • Blisters rupture rapidly, leaving round or oval crusted erosions with a rim of scale (collarettes).
Folliculitis	• Pustules with surrounding erythema centered on hair follicles.
Intertrigo	• Erythema and superficial erosions in inguinal creases.
Jacquet erosive dermatitis	• Well-defined shallow ulcers or ulcerated diaper dermatitis nodules.
Perianal bacterial dermatitis	• Well-defined, moist erythema surrounding the anus. • Pain and constipation may be present.
Langerhans cell histiocytosis	• Erythematous to brown papules and plaques, often with erosions; typically involving skin creases. • Erosions, petechiae, and hemorrhagic papules often present at examination, classically involving the scalp. • Seborrheic dermatitis-like eruption may be present and is poorly responsive to typical treatments. • Lymphadenopathy is often present; associated hepatosplenomegaly may be present.
Nutritional or metabolic disorders (eg, zinc deficiency, cystic fibrosis, biotin-dependent multiple carboxylase deficiency)	• Sharply marginated plaques with shiny, peeling scale. • Eruption often located in a periorificial (eg, perioral, perianal) and acral distribution. • Secondary bacterial and/or candidal infections are common. • Unresponsive to typical therapies. • May have associated diarrhea, alopecia, or failure to thrive.
Asteatotic Eczema	
Nummular eczema	• Well-defined, coin-shaped, scaly, pink plaques; may appear more pigmented in darker skin types. • History of atopic dermatitis often present.
Allergic contact dermatitis	• Rash located at site of antigen exposure. • Characteristic (eg, linear) or geographic patterns may be present. • History of exposure to antigen.
Atopic dermatitis	• Family history of atopic disorders (atopic dermatitis, allergic rhinitis, and/or asthma) usually present. • Eruption located in typical areas (eg, antecubital and popliteal fossae in a toddler or school-aged child).

How to Make the Diagnosis

- Irritant diaper dermatitis: the diagnosis is made clinically based on the typical appearance and distribution of the eruption.
- Asteatotic eczema: the diagnosis is made clinically based on the appearance of lesions; a history of using harsh, drying soaps; and its occurrence during times of low environmental humidity. Concomitant keratosis pilaris may be present.

Treatment of Irritant Contact Dermatitis

General Principles for All Types of Irritant Contact Dermatitis
- Decrease or eliminate contact with the irritant when feasible.
- Restore skin barrier function with emollients.
- Decrease inflammation with anti-inflammatory measures (typically topical corticosteroids).
- Treat secondary infection, if present.

Irritant Diaper Dermatitis
- Remove or minimize contactants (urine and feces) from skin surface by changing diapers frequently.
- Decrease skin maceration by considering superabsorbent disposable diapers.
- Specific measures include:
  - Gently cleanse with tap water or cotton balls or pads soaked in mineral oil; avoid scrubbing skin or using soaps; if diaper wipes are used, ensure that they are free of fragrance and allergens to decrease risk of secondary allergic contact dermatitis (ACD).
  - Use emollient ointments or barrier creams to protect skin surface (eg, zinc oxide ointment or paste, petrolatum).
  - Selectively use a low-potency topical corticosteroid (eg, 1% to 2.5% hydrocortisone ointment or cream) for active inflammation in a thin layer before application of emollient or barrier ointments.
  - Selectively use anti-candidal creams (eg, nystatin, an imidazole antifungal agent) if there is evidence of secondary candidiasis; apply a thin layer before application of emollient or barrier ointments.
  - Do not use combination topical therapies that contain potent topical steroids (eg, betamethasone-clotrimazole).

Asteatotic Eczema

- Restore skin barrier function and diminish trans-epidermal water loss.
- Apply emollients and moisturizers 1 to 2 times a day and after water exposure.
- Eliminate use of soaps and alcohol-based lotions and solutions as much as possible; when improved, reintroduce soaps that are superfatted or contain emollient ingredients.
- Selectively use low- or mid-potency topical corticosteroids for more severe cases.

Prognosis

- The prognosis for irritant dermatitis is excellent, provided appropriate treatment is instituted.
- Recurrences are common.

When to Worry or Refer

- Uncertainty about the diagnosis.
- Failure for therapy to work.

II. Allergic Contact Dermatitis (ACD)

Introduction/Etiology/Epidemiology

- ACD is an inflammatory immunologic reaction in the skin.
- Results from a biphasic, type IV hypersensitivity reaction (cell-mediated immunity), and the pathogenesis involves a sensitization phase and an elicitation phase.
- Skin changes may be noted within a few hours after exposure to a contact allergen or may take up to 1 week to become evident.
- A wide variety of natural and synthetic substances can produce ACD.
- Up to 20% of childhood dermatitis may be ACD and is likely underreported.
- Common sources of contact allergens in children include:
  - Plants, especially poison ivy, poison oak, and poison sumac (urushiol is the antigen in these plants).
  - Jewelry, belt buckles, clothing snaps, toys, or devices with metal (nickel).
  - Shoes (potassium dichromate).
  - Toilet seats (lacquered or painted wood, plastic, cleaning products; can result in irritant contact dermatitis or ACD).
  - Creams, lotions (quaternium-15, formaldehyde, lanolin) and topical antimicrobials (particularly neomycin and bacitracin found in triple antibiotic ointments).
  - Premoistened hygienic wipes containing preservatives such as methylisothiazolinone or methylchloroisothiazolinone.

Signs and Symptoms

- Acute ACD: presents as an abrupt, intensely pruritic, exudative dermatitis. Vesiculation and blister formation may be prominent in ACD to potent sensitizers like poison ivy (Figure 5.3).
- Chronic ACD: presents with scaling, lichenification, fissuring, and hyperpigmentation often due to less potent antigens (eg, nickel) (Figure 5.4).

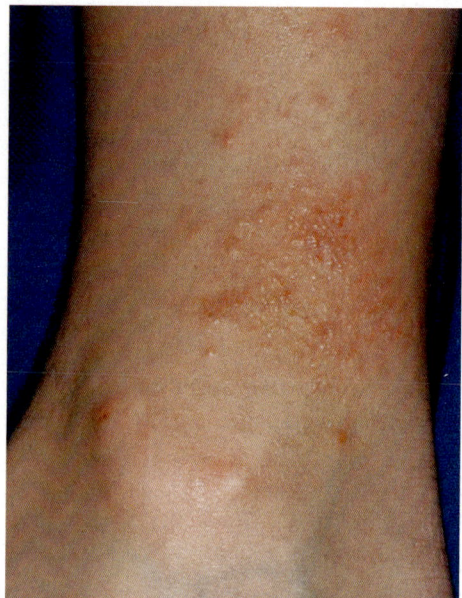

Figure 5.3. Multiple small vesicles overlying an erythematous plaque in a patient exposed to poison ivy.

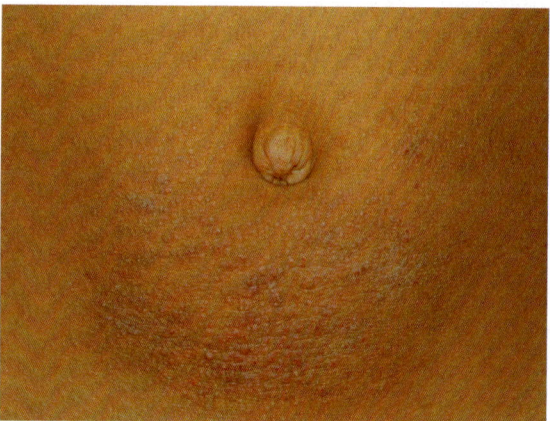

Figure 5.4. Contact dermatitis caused by nickel in a clothing snap or belt buckle affects the lower abdomen.

- ▶ Dermatitis typically is limited to the area(s) of skin in contact with the allergen.
  - Involvement at the site of contact with a wristwatch, clothing snap, belt buckle (see Figure 5.4), earring (Figure 5.5), or necklace suggests nickel allergy.
  - Involvement of the dorsum of the feet occurs in shoe dermatitis (often due to potassium dichromate in leather).
  - Sharply demarcated, symmetric involvement of the anterior lower legs occurs in children with shin guard ACD (occasionally is an ACD related to rubber components).
  - Symmetric involvement of the posterior thighs and buttocks in a circular pattern occurs in toilet seat dermatitis (Figure 5.6), which can arise due to allergic sensitization (essential oils in wood, varnish, paint), irritants (harsh cleaning products), or a combination of the 2.
  - Linearly arranged dermatitis or vesicles are characteristic of plant dermatitis, with distribution corresponding to the plant brushing in a streaky fashion against the skin (Figure 5.7).
  - Distribution can sometimes be misleading or confusing. Eyelid dermatitis may be caused by allergic contact sensitivity to components of nail polish (whereby the fingers may be spared, but the sensitive skin of the eyelids is affected) or nickel if metal eyelash curlers are used.
- ▶ A hypersensitivity or id reaction may occur in association with the primary ACD and presents with diffuse, symmetrically distributed pruritic papules on the extensor aspects of the arms (Figure 5.8), legs, and cheeks.

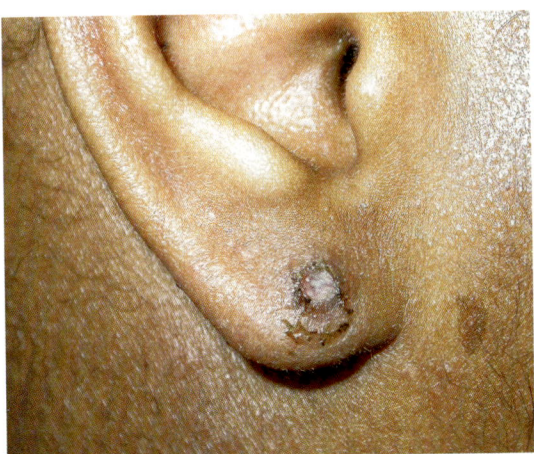

Figure 5.5. Nickel contact dermatitis at the site of an earring.

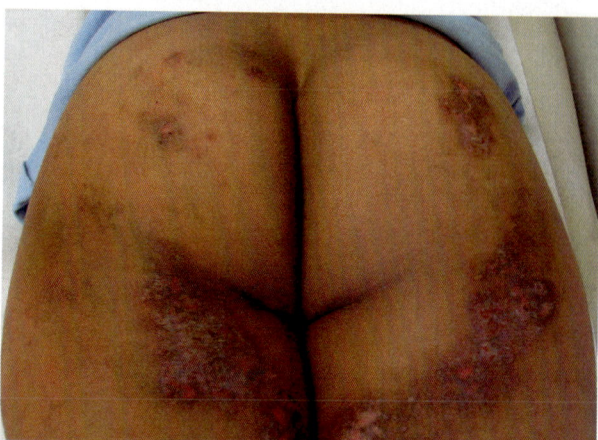

Figure 5.6. In toilet seat dermatitis, symmetric, eczematous lesions are seen on the posterior thighs and buttocks.

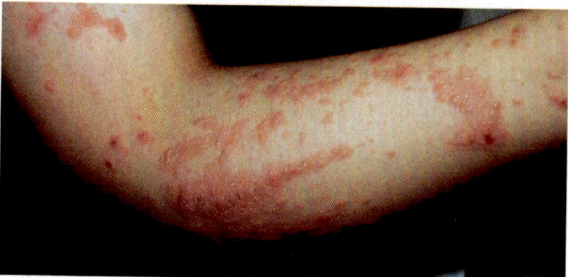

Figure 5.7. Vesicles and erythematous papules in a linear arrangement are often seen in allergic contact dermatitis caused by plants.

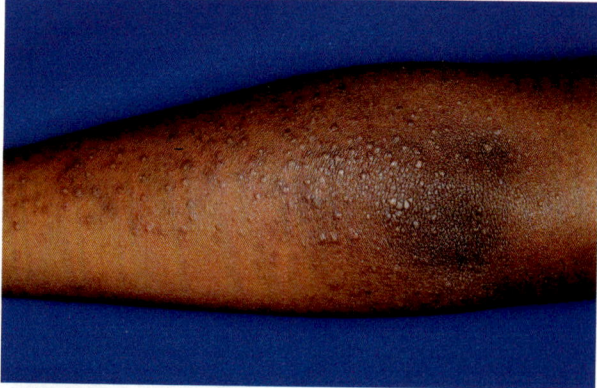

Figure 5.8. Id reaction. These itchy papules occurred on the extensor aspects of the arms and legs in a patient with allergic contact dermatitis to nickel.

- Once the ACD reaction occurs, the response to a strong allergen may last 2 to 3 weeks, even without further exposure.
- Continued appearance of new areas of dermatitis in episodes of poison ivy are more slowly evolving reactions in areas that received a lower dose of exposure to the allergen. The blister fluid of poison ivy lesions does not contain allergen and cannot spread the eruption.

Look-alikes

Disorder	Differentiating Features
Atopic dermatitis	• Typical distribution based on age of patient (eg, antecubital fossae in a child or adolescent). • Personal or family history of atopic dermatitis often present.
Irritant contact dermatitis	• Area of involvement often not as well defined as in allergic contact dermatitis. • Marked pruritus and blistering typically absent.
Seborrheic dermatitis	• Located in typical areas (eg, nasolabial folds, eyebrows, scalp). • Scale is greasy. • Sites of involvement may not be consistent with allergen exposure.
Herpes zoster	• May be confused with contact dermatitis due to plants. • Pain usually more prominent than pruritus. • Lesions typically distributed along a dermatome. • Viral culture, polymerase chain reaction technique, or direct fluorescent antibody testing may be valuable in differentiating the 2 conditions.

How to Make the Diagnosis

- Acute onset, extreme pruritus, and localized distribution of the dermatitis are often sufficient to make a clinical diagnosis of acute ACD.
- Chronic ACD can be more challenging to diagnose, but distribution of the eruption and history of potential exposures are key.
- Chronic, lichenified sub-umbilical dermatitis is nearly always related to nickel allergy from buckles or clothing snaps.
- Patch testing is the criterion standard for establishing the diagnosis. It is not needed for straightforward plant dermatitis or nickel allergy but may be essential to evaluate for other forms of ACD when the offending agent is less clear. Skin prick testing is not applicable to testing for ACD.

Treatment

- Contact allergen avoidance and topical corticosteroids are the mainstays of treatment for ACD.
  - Moderate- or high-potency agents are often necessary to produce a therapeutic response and may be needed 2 times daily for 1 to 2 weeks.
  - Wet dressings are a helpful adjunct for more severe cases.
- Facial, genital, and extensive ACD from potent allergens, such as poison ivy, require systemic corticosteroids. Prednisone at a dose of 1 mg/kg (up to 60 mg) as a single daily dose is prescribed and tapered over 2 to 3 weeks. This prolonged treatment course is necessary to avoid rebound exacerbation.
- Id reactions may be treated with low- to mid-potency topical corticosteroids and generally resolve concomitantly with successful treatment of the primary contact dermatitis.
- Identification and avoidance of the offending allergen is the goal of long-term management and, in some cases, requires patch testing to help identify the allergen involved.

Prognosis

- The prognosis is good, providing the responsible antigen is identified and avoided.

When to Worry or Refer

- Refer patients to a dermatologist when the diagnosis is uncertain.
- Refer patients who have recurrent or treatment-resistant contact dermatitis or those in whom an antigen has not been identified. Patch testing may be indicated in these patients.

Resources for Families

- American Academy of Dermatology: Eczema types: contact dermatitis tips for managing.
  https://www.aad.org/public/diseases/eczema/contact-dermatitis
- National Eczema Association: Contact dermatitis.
  https://nationaleczema.org/eczema/types-of-eczema/contact-dermatitis
- Society for Pediatric Dermatology: Patient handout on allergic contact dermatitis.
  https://pedsderm.net/for-patients-families/patient-handouts/#AllergicContactDermatitis

CHAPTER 6

Juvenile Plantar Dermatosis

Introduction/Etiology/Epidemiology

▶ Juvenile plantar dermatosis (also known as sweaty sock syndrome) is a dermatitis thought to be the result of friction (applied by footwear) and excessive sweating. Cycles of foot moisture (caused by excessive sweating and occlusion of the feet by socks and shoes) and evaporative drying (when footwear is removed) likely contribute.

▶ Usually affects young children and resolves by adolescence. The course is chronic and relapsing.

Signs and Symptoms

▶ Scaling and erythema of the plantar aspect of the forefeet and toes (especially the great toes) with sparing of the interdigital spaces (Figure 6.1).

▶ Fissures may occur (Figure 6.2) that, at times, may be deep and painful.

Look-alikes

Disorder	Differentiating Features
Tinea pedis	• Most commonly involves the interdigital spaces with scaling and fissuring. • Relapsing course uncommon. • Relatively uncommon before adolescence. • Concomitant onychomycosis may be present. • Potassium hydroxide examination of scrapings positive for fungal elements.
Contact dermatitis	• Usually affects the dorsum of the foot (although plantar foot may be involved as well).
Psoriasis	• Usually presents as erythematous plaques with thicker scale. • Lesions of psoriasis may be present elsewhere.
Pityriasis rubra pilaris	• Usually involves the soles diffusely (not just the distal feet) and the palms with thickening of the skin, scaling, and a yellow-orange color. • Lesions usually present elsewhere (especially elbows, knees).

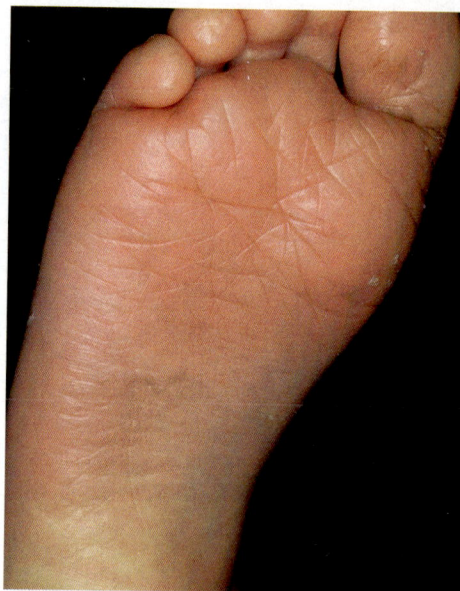

Figure 6.1. Erythema, scaling, and increased skin markings of the forefoot in juvenile plantar dermatosis.

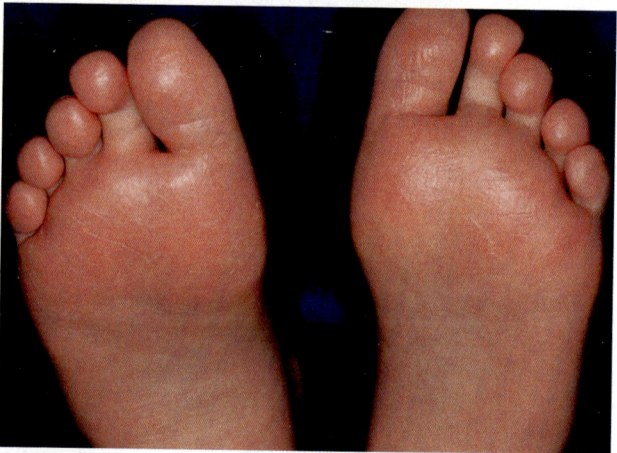

Figure 6.2. Scaling and fissuring of the forefeet in juvenile plantar dermatosis.

Treatment

- The goal of treatment is to reduce foot moisture and cycles of excessive moisture and drying.
  - Wear absorbent socks, preferably cotton.
  - Avoid occlusive shoes or boots.
  - Sprinkle absorbent powder in shoes.
  - Remove socks and shoes after arriving home and apply a moisturizing cream or ointment.
- A medium-potency (eg, triamcinolone) or high-potency (eg, fluocinonide) topical corticosteroid may be applied to control inflammation or pruritus.
- If painful fissures appear, a cyanoacrylate adhesive (eg, Super Glue, Krazy Glue) may be applied to seal the fissure (thereby reducing pain).
- If crusting or pustules appear, suggesting secondary staphylococcal infection, treat with an oral antibiotic according to local antibiotic resistance patterns.
- Topical antiperspirants or oral anticholinergic agents are occasionally used; the former may be limited by increased irritation.

Prognosis

- The prognosis is excellent, as the disorder typically resolves by adolescence.

When to Worry or Refer

- Consider referral for patients who do not respond to standard treatment measures.

Acne

CHAPTER 7 — **Acne Vulgaris** 67

CHAPTER 8 — **Neonatal and Infantile Acne** 79

CHAPTER 9 — **Periorificial Dermatitis** 83

CHAPTER 7

Acne Vulgaris

Introduction/Etiology/Epidemiology

- Most common skin disease that is treated by physicians.
- Affects approximately 45 million individuals in the United States, including at least 85% of all teenagers and young adults.
- Most often self-limited and tends to remit during early adulthood but can be a continuing problem for a significant subset of young and middle-aged adults.
- Has the potential for significant negative effect on quality of life, including poorer academic performance and higher unemployment rates.
- Successful treatment is generally associated with improved psychologic well-being.

Pathophysiology

- Result of a complex interaction between hormonal changes and their effects on the pilosebaceous unit (ie, specialized structures consisting of a hair follicle and sebaceous glands concentrated on the face, chest, and back).
- Onset at puberty as a result of increased androgen production.
- End-organ androgen hyperresponsiveness of the follicle probably also plays a role.

Multifactorial Pathogenesis

- Disordered function of the pilosebaceous unit with atypical follicular keratinization (tendency toward increased follicular plugging).
- Recent data suggest that inflammation of the skin is present even before comedone formation; therefore, acne is considered primarily an inflammatory disorder of the pilosebaceous unit.

- Increased circulating androgens play a role in promoting inflammation of the sebaceous gland in addition to sebaceous gland growth resulting in increased sebum production.
- This increased sebum milieu favors *Cutibacterium* (formerly *Propionibacterium*) *acnes* growth and likely contributes to the pathogenesis of acne via activation of the innate immune response via toll-like receptors, although this relationship continues to be explored.

Factors That May Exacerbate Acne

- Trauma: scrubbing the skin too vigorously or picking of lesions.
- Comedogenic cosmetics or other skin care products.
- Tight-fitting sports equipment.
- Medications: corticosteroids (topical, inhaled, and oral) and anabolic steroids, antiepileptic drugs, lithium, and progesterone-only contraceptives (eg, progesterone-only mini pill, progesterone intrauterine device, implantable progesterone).
- Syndromes associated with hormonal dysregulation such as polycystic ovary syndrome and Cushing syndrome may be associated with more severe acne.
- A high glycemic index diet and consumption of nonfat dairy may be associated with acne vulgaris.

Signs and Symptoms

Early on, acne lesions often appear on the forehead and middle third of the face (T-zone) and are obstructive (ie, comedones); inflammatory lesions tend to develop later and may occur on all areas of the face, neck, chest, and back.

- Comedonal lesions: often the first sign of acne, appearing before other signs of puberty.
  - Open comedones (blackheads): dilated follicles (Figure 7.1).
  - Closed comedones (whiteheads): white or skin-colored papules without surrounding erythema (Figure 7.2).
- Inflammatory lesions typically appear later in the course of acne vulgaris and vary from 1- to 2-mm micro-papules to nodules larger than 5 mm (Figure 7.3).

- Large (5–15 mm) inflammatory nodules and cysts occur in the most severe cases, and such nodulocystic presentations are most likely to lead to permanent scarring.
    - Mild, moderate, and severe inflammatory acne can be associated with disfiguring postinflammatory discoloration, which can appear red, violaceous, or grayish brown.
    - Pigmentary changes may persist for many months to years (Figure 7.4).

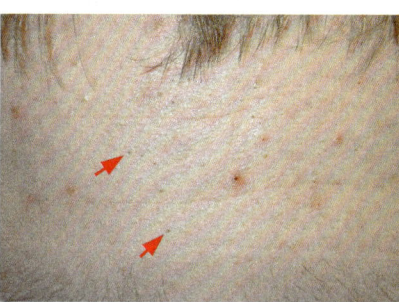

Figure 7.1. Open comedones (ie, blackheads; arrows) on the forehead.

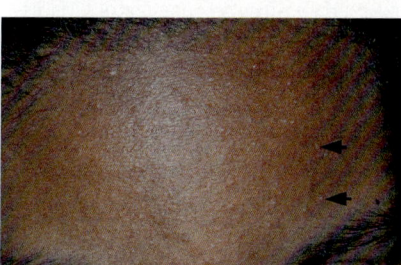

Figure 7.2. Closed comedones (arrows) are small white or skin-colored papules without surrounding erythema. This patient has mild acne.

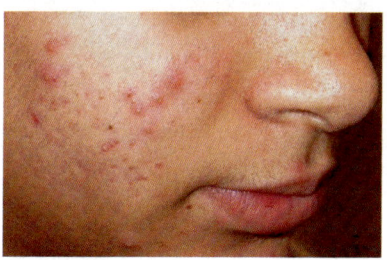

Figure 7.3. Inflammatory lesions are erythematous papules, pustules, or nodules. This patient has moderate acne. Note some mild early scarring.

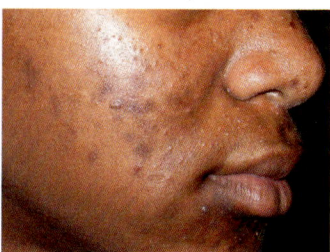

Figure 7.4. Patient with skin of color with moderate acne. As inflammatory lesions resolve, areas of hyperpigmentation persist. This may appear as violaceous to grayish brown color changes.

Look-alikes

In each of the conditions listed herein, comedones are absent.

Disorder	Differentiating Features
Acne rosacea	• Flushing and telangiectasias.
Angiofibromas (ie, adenoma sebaceum)	• Appears during childhood (earlier than acne). • Favors nose and medial aspect of cheeks. • Associated with tuberous sclerosis or multiple endocrine neoplasia type 1.
Flat warts	• Skin-colored to tan papules or small, thin plaques. • Koebnerization (lesions distributed in linear clusters) often present.
Gram-negative folliculitis	• Sudden worsening of acne in patient receiving long-term antibiotic treatment for acne vulgaris.
Keratosis pilaris	• Presents during infancy or early childhood. • Presence of a central keratin plug differentiates keratosis pilaris from acne. • Favors lateral aspects of cheeks (rather than T-zone) and may also be present on the extensor surfaces of upper arms, dorsal surfaces of thighs.
Miliaria rubra	• Erythematous, small papules often in occluded areas (eg, skinfolds). • Resolves rapidly.
Molluscum contagiosum	• Translucent papules, often with central umbilication. • Koebnerization (lesions distributed in linear clusters) often present.
Periorificial dermatitis	• Concentrated around mouth; nares; or, less commonly, eyes. • Often (but not always) history of preceding use of topical corticosteroids.
Malassezia (*Pityrosporum*) folliculitis	• Typically spares the face. • Potassium hydroxide preparation performed on pustule roof will demonstrate budding yeast.
Steroid acne	• Lesions have monomorphous appearance (ie, only papules without comedones). • Temporal relationship between onset or worsening of acne and corticosteroid therapy.

How to Make the Diagnosis

▶ The clinical diagnosis of acne vulgaris is usually straightforward.

Treatment

Options for acne treatment based on lesion type and disease severity are summarized in Figures 7.5, 7.6, and 7.7.

▶ Adolescents are anxious for improvement in their acne; however, patient education is key. Patients should be counseled that acne improvement is gradual and that 4 to 6 weeks or longer may be required to observe a benefit from treatment.

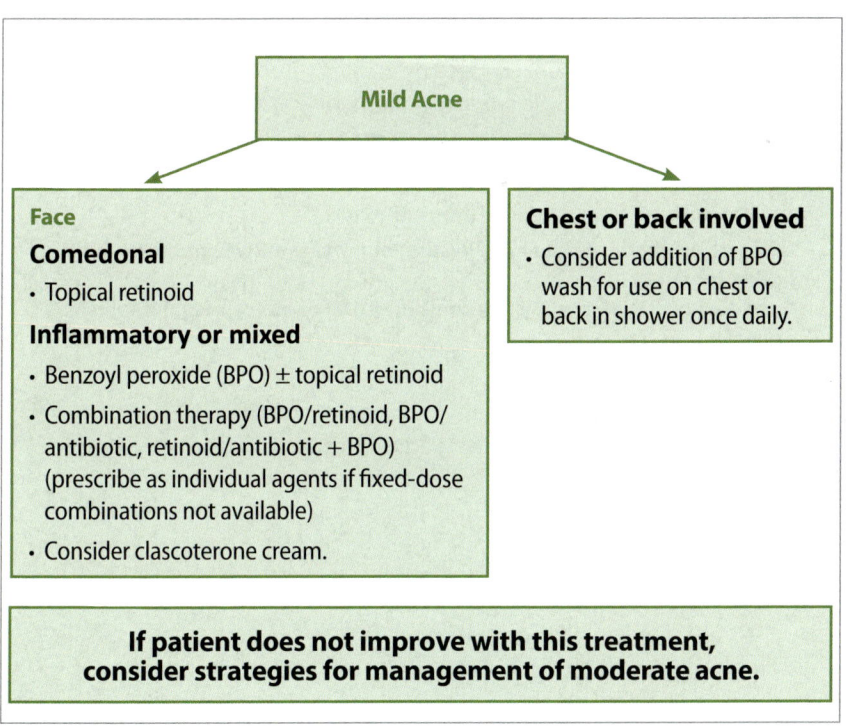

Figure 7.5. Treatment options for mild acne on the basis of lesion type.

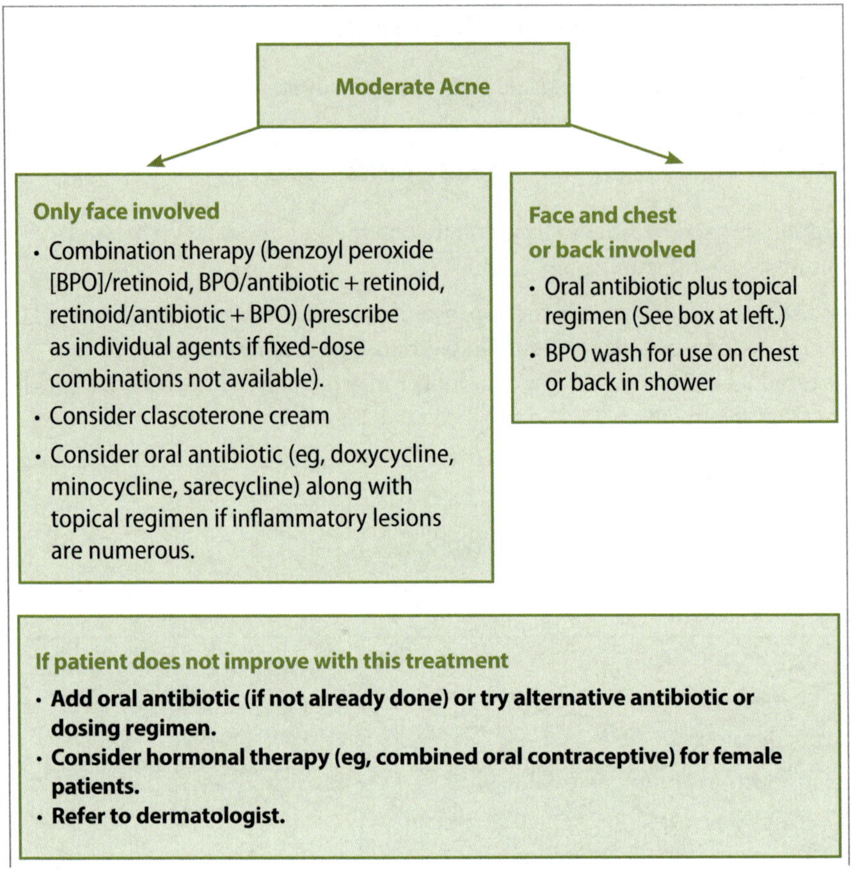

PEDIATRIC DERMATOLOGY

Moderate Acne

Only face involved
- Combination therapy (benzoyl peroxide [BPO]/retinoid, BPO/antibiotic + retinoid, retinoid/antibiotic + BPO) (prescribe as individual agents if fixed-dose combinations not available).
- Consider clascoterone cream
- Consider oral antibiotic (eg, doxycycline, minocycline, sarecycline) along with topical regimen if inflammatory lesions are numerous.

Face and chest or back involved
- Oral antibiotic plus topical regimen (See box at left.)
- BPO wash for use on chest or back in shower

If patient does not improve with this treatment
- **Add oral antibiotic (if not already done) or try alternative antibiotic or dosing regimen.**
- **Consider hormonal therapy (eg, combined oral contraceptive) for female patients.**
- **Refer to dermatologist.**

Figure 7.6. Treatment options for moderate acne on the basis of lesion type.

Chapter 7: Acne Vulgaris

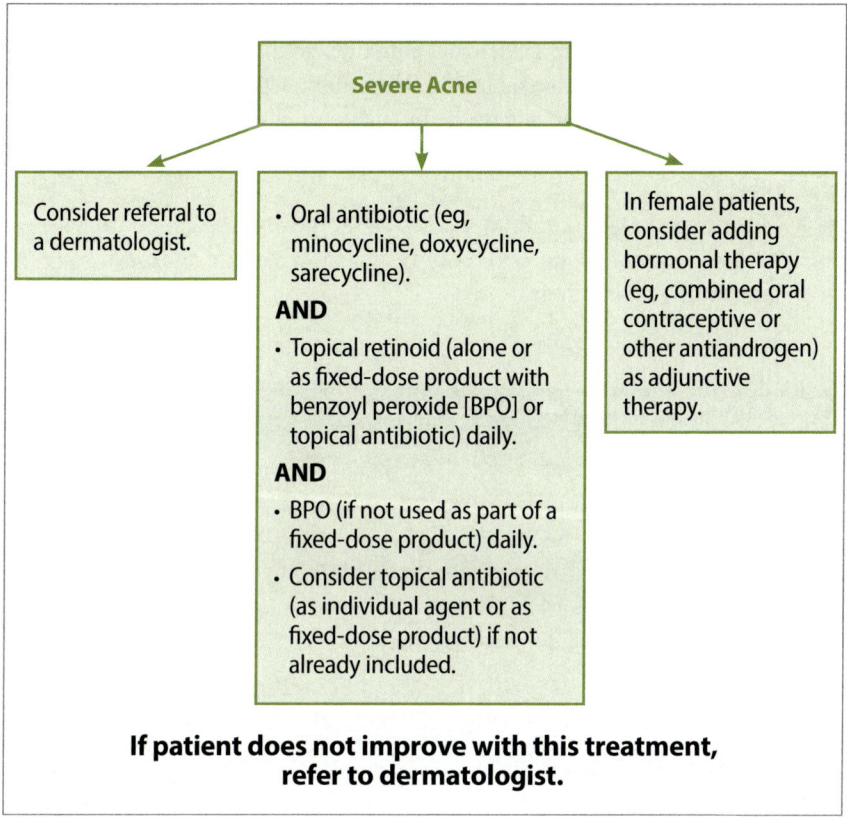

Figure 7.7. Treatment options for severe acne on the basis of lesion type.

- ▶ Acne treatment is facilitated by optimizing skin care and appropriate pharmacological intervention tailored to the lesion type and severity of disease.
  - Drying of the skin by therapeutic cleansers (eg, those containing salicylic acid) may be aggravated by prescription acne medications containing a retinoid (tretinoin, adapalene, tazarotene), benzoyl peroxide, and some antibiotic formulations. If these prescription products will be used, a mild cleanser should be recommended.
  - For those who develop dryness when using acne medications, judicious application of a noncomedogenic moisturizer may be useful.

- Therapy is in 1 of 4 categories:
  - Topical agents: retinoids, benzoyl peroxide, antibiotics, and fixed-dose combination products (Table 7.1) that combine 2 of these agents.
  - Oral antibiotics: minocycline, doxycycline, sarecycline, tetracycline, erythromycin (latter 2 used less often in the current era); occasionally others.
  - Hormonal therapy: combined oral contraceptives; oral antiandrogens, such as spironolactone; and recently developed topical androgen antagonist, clascoterone.
  - Isotretinoin.

Table 7.1. Topical Retinoids and Fixed-Dose Combination Products for Acne

Product Type/Active Ingredients	Recommended Dosing
Retinoids[a]	
Adapalene 0.1% cream, gel/0.3% gel	Daily at bedtime
Tretinoin 0.025% cream, gel/0.01% gel/0.04%, 0.06%, 0.08% 0.1% micro-gel/0.05% cream, gel/0.1% cream	Daily at bedtime
Tazarotene 0.05% cream, gel/0.1% cream, gel/0.045% lotion/0.1% foam	Daily at bedtime
Trifarotene 0.005% cream	Daily at bedtime
Antibiotic/BPO	
Clindamycin 1.2%/BPO 2.5% gel	Daily
Clindamycin 1.2%/BPO 3.75% gel	Daily
Clindamycin 1%/BPO 5% gel	Daily to twice daily
Erythromycin 3%/BPO 5% gel	Twice daily
Retinoid Containing	
Clindamycin 1.2%/tretinoin 0.025% gel	Daily at bedtime
Adapalene 0.1%/BPO 2.5% gel, 0.3%/BPO 2.5% gel	Daily at bedtime
Microencapsulated tretinoin 0.1%/BPO 3% cream	Daily at bedtime

Abbreviation: BPO, benzoyl peroxide.
[a] If prescribing a retinoid, consider beginning with adapalene 0.1% or tretinoin cream 0.025% to reduce the potential for drying or irritation.

- ▶ Treatment strategies are based on lesion type and severity of disease.
  - ▪ Mild acne: approximately one-fourth of the face is involved, lesions are comedones or a mixture of comedones and few to several papules or pustules, no nodules or scarring (Figure 7.2).
    - Topical retinoids or fixed-dose combination products containing a retinoid are ideal for comedonal and mild inflammatory acne, but correct use is essential to minimize problems of irritation. Benzoyl peroxide or fixed-dose combination products containing benzoyl peroxide are an alternative option.
    - Retinoid pearls.
      - Apply to a dry face.
      - Apply no more than a pea-sized amount for the entire face.
        1. If the entire face is to be treated, advise the patient to divide the pea-sized aliquot and dab equal amounts on each side of the forehead, each cheek, nose, and chin and then to rub it into the skin.
        2. Apply to all involved areas and zones rather than spot therapy (remember that topical retinoids play a preventive as well as a therapeutic role in acne).
      - Use a noncomedogenic moisturizer, if needed, to counteract extreme dryness associated with topical retinoid therapy.
    - Consider topical androgen antagonist (clascoterone).
  - ▪ Moderate acne: approximately one-half of the face is involved, there are several to many papules or pustules and a few to several nodules, a few scars may be present (Figures 7.3 and 7.4).
    - The initial combination of a retinoid, benzoyl peroxide, and an antibiotic is recommended for the synergy of addressing different aspects of disease pathogenesis. Retinoids are comedolytic and prevent development of comedones, antibiotics decrease *C acnes* and reduce inflammation, and benzoyl peroxide—a nonantibiotic antimicrobial—lowers the likelihood of developing antibiotic-resistant *C acnes*. The ultimate choice of products depends on disease severity, likelihood of patient adherence (fixed-dose combination products may increase adherence), and medication cost and access (branded fixed-dose combination products are more expensive).

- Examples of effective topical therapy for moderate acne include the following:
  - Fixed-dose topical combination product containing a retinoid and benzoyl peroxide.
  - Fixed-dose topical combination product containing a retinoid and an antibiotic, along with benzoyl peroxide (in the form of a wash or leave-on product).
  - Fixed-dose topical combination product containing benzoyl peroxide and an antibiotic, along with a topical retinoid.
  - Topical retinoid, antibiotic, and benzoyl peroxide prescribed as individual agents.
  - Consider topical androgen antagonist (clascoterone).
  - For inflammatory truncal acne, 2 antibiotic foams are available: clindamycin 1% and minocycline 4%.
- Oral antibiotics should be added if significant numbers of inflammatory lesions are present or the chest and back are significantly involved. Again, concomitant use of benzoyl peroxide is recommended because it appears to decrease the risk of developing antibiotic resistance. Systemic antibiotics are not recommended as monotherapy for acne. The duration of oral antibiotic use should be as short as feasible, with consideration for discontinuation at 3- to 6-month intervals.
- Female patients who have significant inflammatory acne, particularly those who have premenstrual or menstrual flares, may benefit from hormonal intervention, such as a combined oral contraceptive or spironolactone.
- Severe acne: approximately three-fourths or more of the face is involved; there are many papules, pustules, cysts, and nodules; scarring often is present (Figure 7.8).
  - Nodulocystic acne or the presence of scarring warrants prompt consideration for isotretinoin therapy (with referral to a dermatologist).
  - High-dose oral antibiotics in combination with topical therapy (eg, benzoyl peroxide and topical retinoid) are an option while considering isotretinoin.
  - In female patients, hormonal or antiandrogen therapies can also be considered; however, if they fail and the patient continues to have nodulocystic or scarring lesions, isotretinoin should be strongly considered.
- ▶ Topical retinoids or the combination of topical retinoids and benzoyl peroxide is recommended as maintenance therapy to minimize the likelihood of relapse.

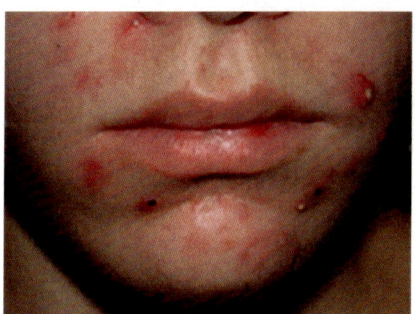

Figure 7.8. In severe acne, nodules and scarring are present.

Prognosis

▶ Acne vulgaris is often, but not always, self-limited and resolves by the late teenage or early adult years.

▶ Treatment is warranted during periods of disease activity to alleviate disfigurement, enhance well-being, and prevent permanent scarring.

▶ Management can be challenging because patient expectations are high, efficacy of treatment is variable, and potential medication side effects need to be weighed against benefits, with appropriate matching of therapeutic aggressiveness and severity of disease.

▶ Patients require periodic clinical assessments to evaluate response to therapy and provide ongoing support and encouragement.

When to Worry or Refer

▶ Failure of topical or oral therapies after 2 to 3 months of appropriate use.

▶ Severe acne with presence of nodules, cysts, or scarring.

▶ Early-onset acne at younger than 7 years (or other signs of androgen excess) warrants hormonal evaluation.

Resources for Families

- American Academy of Dermatology: Acne: tips for managing.
  https://www.aad.org/public/diseases/acne-and-rosacea/acne
- American Academy of Pediatrics: HealthyChildren.org.
  www.HealthyChildren.org/acne
- MedlinePlus: Information for patients and families (in English and Spanish) sponsored by the US National Library of Medicine and National Institutes of Health.
  https://www.nlm.nih.gov/medlineplus/acne.html
- Society for Pediatric Dermatology: Patient handout on acne.
  https://pedsderm.net/for-patients-families/patient-handouts/#Anchor-Acne
- Society for Pediatric Dermatology: Patient handout on isotretinoin.
  https://pedsderm.net/for-patients-families/patient-handouts/#Isotretinoin
- WebMD: Information for families is contained in Skin Problems and Treatments.
  www.webmd.com/skin-problems-and-treatments/acne/default.htm

CHAPTER
8

Neonatal and Infantile Acne

Introduction/Etiology/Epidemiology

Neonatal Acne

- Neonatal acne may present at birth but more commonly appears during the first 4 weeks after birth.
- More common in male neonates.
- Etiology may be related to elevated maternal and/or fetal androgens.
- The term *neonatal cephalic pustulosis* has been proposed to describe a more pustular presentation (Figure 8.1). In these patients, the etiology is thought to be due to a hypersensitivity response to resident yeast (eg, *Malassezia* [formerly *Pityrosporum*] species), given rapid response to topical antifungal therapy.

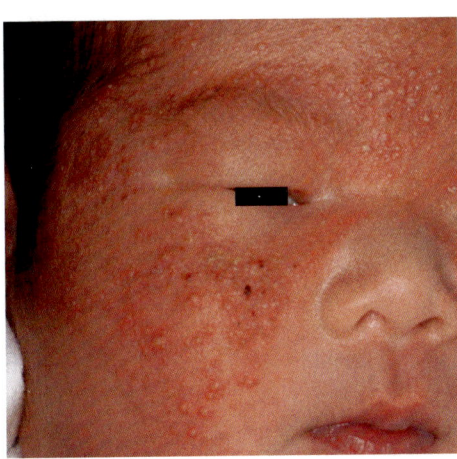

Figure 8.1. Numerous erythematous pustules on the forehead and cheeks in a newborn with neonatal cephalic pustulosis. The eruption cleared rapidly with topical antifungal therapy.

Infantile Acne

- Later onset than neonatal acne, between 1 and 12 months of life.
- Considered to be androgen driven with associated sebaceous gland hyperactivity.
- Spontaneously resolves between 6 and 12 months in most patients.
- Occasionally more persistent or more severe with the potential for scarring.

Signs and Symptoms

Neonatal Acne

- Inflammatory, erythematous papules and pustules (Figure 8.2).
- Primarily on the cheeks but also scattered on the entire face, extending into the scalp.
- Comedones typically absent; truncal involvement rare.

Infantile Acne

- Full range of typical acneiform lesions may be seen, including open and closed comedones; papules and pustules (Figure 8.3); and, rarely, nodules.
- Occurs most commonly on the face and may also have chest and back involvement.
- Scarring may be present.

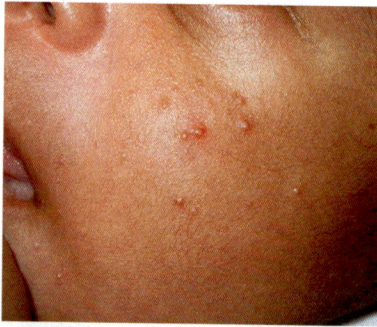

Figure 8.2. Papules and pustules on the cheek of a newborn who has neonatal acne; comedones are absent.

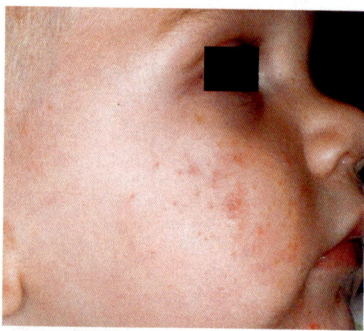

Figure 8.3. Erythematous papules and pustules on the cheek with some open comedones in infantile acne.

Look-alikes

Disorder	Differentiating Features
Neonatal Acne	
Miliaria rubra or pustulosa	• Erythematous papules (miliaria rubra) or pustules (miliaria pustulosa); may be difficult to differentiate from neonatal acne. • Often more widely distributed in areas prone to occlusion such as the back.
Milia	• Pinpoint to small white, superficial papules without surrounding erythema.
Sebaceous hyperplasia	• Yellow (not erythematous) papules, typically on the nose.
Seborrheic dermatitis	• Erythematous, scaling patches (typically lacks discrete papules).
Staphylococcal pustulosis	• Favors intertriginous areas and occluded skin (eg, diaper area). • Pustules may rupture easily, leaving small peripheral collarettes of scale. • Skin culture reveals growth of *Staphylococcus aureus*.
Infantile Acne	
Lesions that may mimic infantile acne include all of those listed for neonatal acne. The presence of typical acne lesions, especially comedones, helps confirm the diagnosis.	
Keratosis pilaris	• Inflammatory type may mimic acne lesions. • Papules have central keratotic plug. • Facial involvement typically limited to lateral aspect of the cheeks; similar lesions may be noted on extensor surfaces of upper arms and thighs. • Other atopic history may be present. • Often a positive family history.

Treatment

Neonatal Acne

▶ Neonatal acne often spontaneously resolves within the first 6 months; watchful waiting with gentle skin care is appropriate in mild cases.

▶ For more significant involvement, topical therapies such as 2.5% benzoyl peroxide, 2% erythromycin solution or gel, or 1% clindamycin lotion can be applied sparingly nightly or every other night until resolution is noted.

▶ If neonatal cephalic pustulosis is suspected, treatment with a topical antifungal cream (eg, econazole, clotrimazole, or ketoconazole) typically leads to rapid resolution.

Infantile Acne

- More severe or persistent infantile acne may lead to scarring, and treatment is often indicated.
- Topical 2.5% benzoyl peroxide, topical 2% erythromycin solution or gel, or topical 1% clindamycin lotion may be useful for inflammatory papules and pustules (these may be applied once or twice daily as tolerated).
- Topical retinoids (eg, tretinoin 0.025% cream, adapalene 0.1% cream) may be helpful for comedones as well as inflammatory lesions, but side effects of erythema and irritation can be problematic in some patients. Begin topical retinoid use with application every second or third night, progressing to nightly application, if tolerated, over 2 to 3 weeks.
- More severe variants of infantile acne may require oral antibiotics (typically erythromycin).
- In rare cases of severe nodulocystic disease in infants, isotretinoin has been used safely and successfully; such patients merit referral to a pediatric dermatologist.

Prognosis

- Neonatal acne is a self-limited disorder that typically results in no long-term sequelae.
- Infantile acne is also typically self-limited, but more persistent or severe disease may result in long-term scarring.
- The relationship of severe infantile acne to later risk of acne vulgaris is unclear, but some investigators believe it is a risk factor for more significant adolescent and adult acne.

When to Worry or Refer

- Unusually severe neonatal or infantile acne.
- Severe or unresponsive disease may require endocrine testing to assess for excess androgens.

Resource for Families

- Cleveland Clinic: Baby acne.
  https://my.clevelandclinic.org/health/diseases/17822-baby-acne

CHAPTER 9

Periorificial Dermatitis

Introduction/Etiology/Epidemiology

- Periorificial dermatitis (formerly known as perioral dermatitis) is an acneiform disorder of facial skin initially described in older teenagers and young adult women but also seen in younger children.
- Some consider this a pediatric form of acne rosacea, displaying a combination of acneiform papules and pustules along with varying degrees of erythema in a periorificial distribution.
- A granulomatous juvenile variant of classic periorificial dermatitis exists. It is sometimes referred to as *granulomatous periorificial dermatitis*.
- The cause is unknown, but it has been associated with chronic application of topical corticosteroids (or use of steroids in other forms, including inhaled), as well as bubble gum, oils, greases, and fluoridated toothpastes.
- Both male and female patients can be affected.

Signs and Symptoms

- Erythematous to flesh-colored monomorphous papules and papulopustules distributed around the mouth, with a narrow zone of sparing around the vermilion border (Figures 9.1 and 9.2).

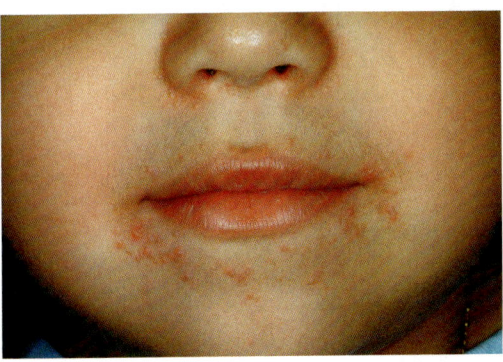

Figure 9.1. Periorificial dermatitis. Erythematous papules and papulopustules around the nares and mouth, with a rim of sparing around the vermilion border.

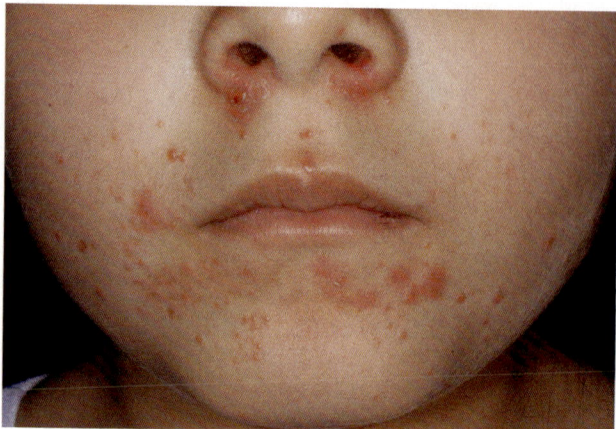

Figure 9.2. Periorificial dermatitis. Erythematous fine papules previously treated with topical corticosteroids around the nares and mouth in a young child.

- Scaling may be present.
- Comedones are absent.
- Other periorificial areas are commonly affected, including the peri-nasal and periorbital regions. There may be a history of recurrent chalazion and hordeolum (sty).
- The granulomatous variant presents in a similar fashion but with prominence of translucent, pink to flesh-colored or tan papules (Figure 9.3) and often a history of prior corticosteroid application.

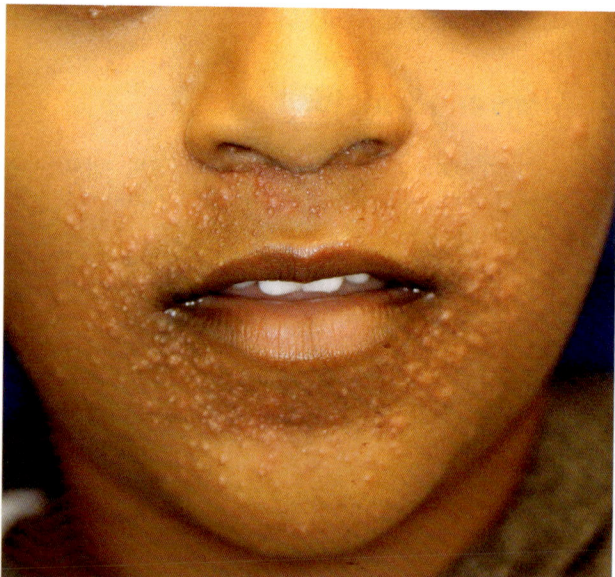

Figure 9.3. Granulomatous periorificial dermatitis. Flesh-colored to pink, translucent papules in the perioral and peri-nasal locations, with some lower periorbital involvement, in a child.

Look-alikes

Disorder	Differentiating Features
Atopic dermatitis	• Less papular and typically more scaly. • Other areas of body usually affected. • Pruritus usually present.
Acne vulgaris	• Distribution of early lesions more commonly in the T-zone (ie, forehead, nose, and chin). • Comedones present. • Onset rarely occurs between 1 and 7 years of age.
Allergic contact dermatitis	• Less papular and may be more geometric in distribution. • History of exposure to antigen may be present. • Pruritus usually present and significant.
Irritant contact dermatitis (eg, caused by lip licking or pacifier)	• Less papular and may be more geometric in distribution. • History of lip licking or pacifier use present. • Involved areas often have sharp geometric borders. Vermilion border is typically involved.
Flat warts	• Small, skin-colored to tan, flat-topped papules may coalesce into plaques. • Erythema typically absent. • May be present elsewhere on the body. • Koebnerization (ie, distribution of lesions in a linear fashion after skin trauma or scratching) may be evident.
Sarcoidosis	• When limited to face, may be difficult to distinguish from periorificial dermatitis. • Papules often reddish brown. • Often in other locations (eg, neck, upper trunk, extremities).
Benign cephalic histiocytosis	• Usually occurs in children 3 years or younger. • Papules may be erythematous, but often yellowish brown, and may simulate flat warts. • Typically not periorificial in distribution.

How to Make the Diagnosis

▶ The diagnosis is made clinically on the basis of lesion morphology and characteristic distribution.

▶ Skin biopsy may be useful in questionable cases but is rarely necessary.

Treatment

- Mild to moderate cases: topical calcineurin inhibitors (eg, pimecrolimus cream, tacrolimus ointment) or topical antibiotics, most commonly metronidazole or erythromycin, applied once to twice daily. Topical sulfacetamide with or without sulfur may also be useful.
- Severe cases: oral antibiotic therapy (eg, with erythromycin, azithromycin; in patients older than 8 years, doxycycline or minocycline) for a minimum of 6 to 8 weeks with gradual tapering to avoid rebound flaring.
- Treatment consideration: Topical corticosteroids lead to initial improvement in periorificial dermatitis, but rapid flaring is seen when they are discontinued. If the patient's condition has been treated with this agent, consider tapering the potency of the topical steroid gradually over weeks; another option is to substitute the topical steroid with a topical calcineurin inhibitor as monotherapy or concurrently with a systemic antibiotic (if more severe).

Prognosis

- The condition improves slowly (often requires 4–12 weeks) but steadily with appropriate therapy.
- Treatments should be used until clearing has occurred, with gradual tapering to prevent rebound.
- Postinflammatory hyperpigmentation or hypopigmentation may be seen and generally resolves over several months.

When to Worry or Refer

- Consider referral if the diagnosis is in question or the condition has not responded to appropriate therapy.

Resources for Families

- Society for Pediatric Dermatology: Patient handout on perioral dermatitis (also available in Spanish).
  https://pedsderm.net/for-patients-families/patient-handouts/#PerorialDermatitis
- WebMD: Information for families is contained in Skin Problems and Treatments.
  www.webmd.com/skin-problems-and-treatments/perioral-dermatitis

Skin Infections

Localized Viral Infections

CHAPTER 10 — **Herpes Simplex** 89

CHAPTER 11 — **Herpes Zoster** 99

CHAPTER 12 — **Molluscum Contagiosum** 105

CHAPTER 13 — **Warts**. 111

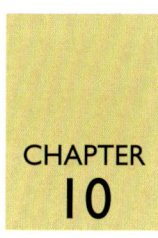

CHAPTER 10

Herpes Simplex

Introduction/Etiology/Epidemiology

- ► Herpes simplex virus (HSV) 1 (HSV-1) and HSV-2 are 2 members of the *Herpesviridae* family of viruses that also includes varicella-zoster virus (VZV); Epstein-Barr virus; cytomegalovirus; and human herpesviruses 6, 7, and 8.

- ► Primary HSV infection is generally a childhood disease involving the mouth (herpetic gingivostomatitis), lips, or eyes.
    - Serological evidence of HSV-1 infection increases steadily with age, and 18% to 35% of children are estimated to have infection by 5 years of age.
    - In many cases, acquisition of HSV infection does not cause symptoms.
    - If acquisition of infection is accompanied by clinical disease, it is characterized as primary clinical disease. Such syndromes (eg, primary HSV gingivostomatitis) are typically moderate to severe illnesses accompanied by fever, lymphadenopathy, constitutional symptoms, and more severe or prolonged cutaneous or mucocutaneous disease.

- ► HSV infections are characterized by the phenomenon of latency. After initial infection, individuals are prone to subsequent recurrences of localized cutaneous disease at the site of initial infection resulting from reactivation of latent virus in regional sensory or autonomic nerve ganglia. Recurrent HSV is generally a more limited clinical syndrome than primary HSV.

- ► Asymptomatic acquisition of primary HSV infection may subsequently lead to clinically recognized disease, often with features of recurrent HSV (ie, milder disease).

- ► HSV infections are typically transmitted by direct contact with skin lesions or infectious mucous membrane secretions.

- HSV-2 infection is most commonly acquired by sexual contact; however, HSV-1 prevalence in anogenital infections has been increasing.
  - Genital HSV-2 infection in prepubertal children should raise suspicion of child abuse.
  - HSV-2 is the most common cause of neonatal HSV infection globally. The yearly incidence of neonatal HSV has increased in the United States, occurring in as many as 5 per 10,000 deliveries in 2015.
- Neonatal HSV (Figure 10.1) most commonly occurs as a result of transmission during passage through the birth canal, less often via ascending infection. It is rarely caused by postnatal transmission from a caregiver.
  - Neonates born to mothers who have a primary genital infection are at the highest risk (25%–60%) of becoming infected.
  - Risk of transmission to newborns by mothers shedding HSV as the result of a reactivated infection is significantly lower (2%).
  - Approximately two-thirds of neonates with disseminated or central nervous system disease have skin lesions, but these lesions may not be present at onset of symptoms.

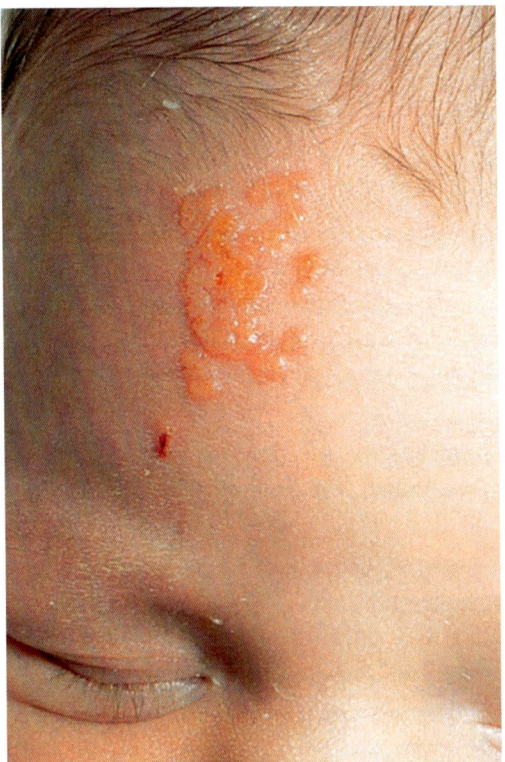

Figure 10.1. Clustered vesicles on an erythematous base in an infant with neonatal herpes simplex virus infection.

Signs and Symptoms

- Grouped 1- to 2-mm vesicles on an erythematous base are the classic lesions of HSV skin infection (Figure 10.1). In darker skin types, the erythematous base may appear more violaceous (Figure 10.2).
- Skin vesicles evolve to form pustules, erosions, and crusts.
- Mucosal vesicles in areas of friction (eg, mouth, vulvovaginal area, anorectal area) are rapidly unroofed and form small ulcers.
- Coalescent vesicles or erosions may appear as larger bullae or superficial ulcerations.
- Lesions may occur on any cutaneous or mucocutaneous site but are most common on the face.
- Skin lesions are sometimes pruritic but typically painful. Primary infection syndromes may cause severe pain.
- Regional lymphadenopathy is common, particularly with primary HSV infection.
- Recurrent HSV infection is often preceded by a characteristic brief prodrome of itching or dysesthesia at the site of impending recurrence.

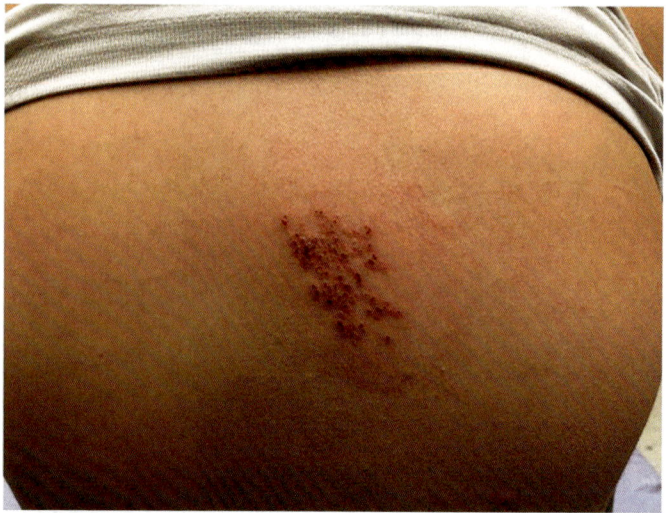

Figure 10.2. Grouped vesicles in herpes simplex virus infection with central heme crust and mild underlying violaceous color changes in a patient with skin of color.

- Distinctive regional distributions of HSV infection are recognized as the following clinical syndromes:
  - Primary HSV gingivostomatitis: Children who are affected develop ulcers on the buccal mucosae, tongue, gingivae, and perioral skin (Figure 10.3). These findings may be accompanied by fever, lymphadenopathy, and constitutional symptoms.
  - Herpes labialis (cold sore): Lesions occur on the lips, most often at the vermilion border; most common type of recurrent herpes infections overall (Figure 10.4).
  - Herpetic whitlow: Deep-seated painful vesicles on the distal portion of the finger; may be primary or recurrent HSV infection (Figure 10.5).
  - Genital HSV infection: In addition to mucocutaneous symptoms, secondary symptoms may include fever, swelling, and dysuria.
  - Ocular HSV infection: Corneal involvement may cause keratoconjunctivitis, which may be associated with pain, photophobia, and eye discharge.
  - Herpes gladiatorum: Typically seen in participants of contact sports, and characteristic lesions may affect the head, neck, and upper extremities. Rarely, the cutaneous findings may lack vesicles.

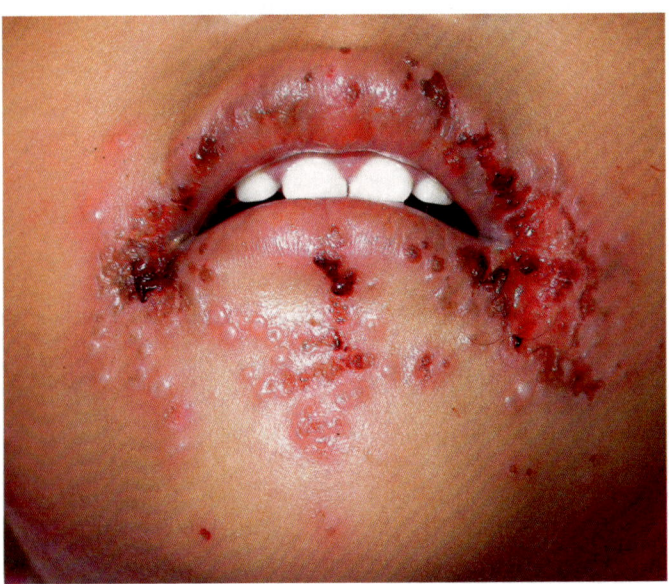

Figure 10.3. Grouped vesicles and ulcers affecting the perioral skin are observed in herpes simplex virus gingivostomatitis. Note that the periphery of grouped vesicles may form a scalloped appearance.

Chapter 10: Herpes Simplex

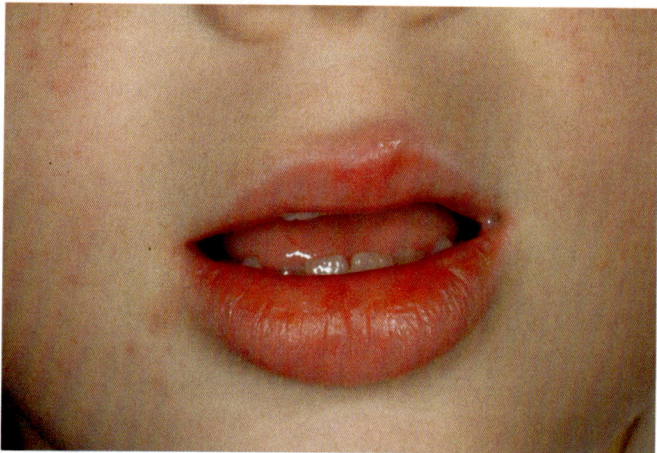

Figure 10.4. Herpes labialis (cold sore). Vesicles occur on the lips, most often at the vermilion border.

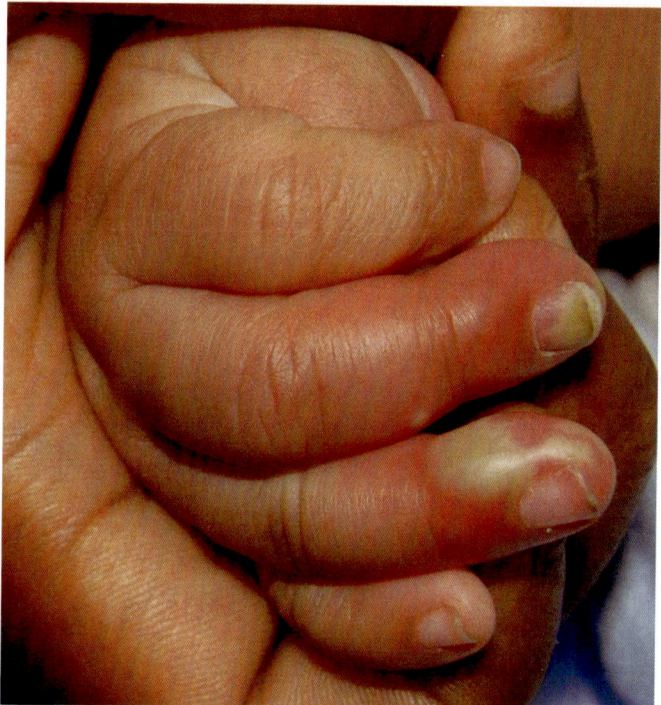

Figure 10.5. Deep-seated vesicles with surrounding erythema and swelling located on the finger are characteristic of herpetic whitlow.

- Eczema herpeticum: severe, widespread HSV infection in an individual with preexisting generalized skin disease, most often atopic dermatitis (Figure 10.6). Patients may present with fever, malaise, and numerous monomorphic vesicles and heme-crusted, punched-out erosions in areas of active underlying skin disease.
- Zosteriform herpes simplex: manifests as recurrent shingles.

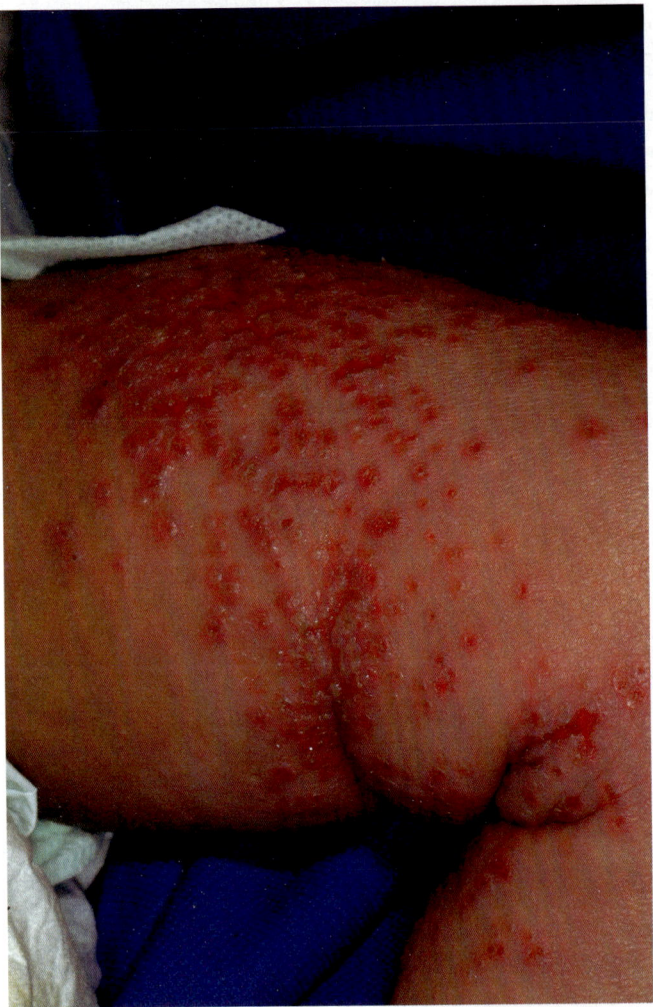

Figure 10.6. Eczema herpeticum is characterized by numerous vesicles and monomorphous erosions with a punched-out appearance, typically in areas of active dermatitis.

Look-alikes

Disorder	Differentiating Features
Herpes zoster	• Usually presents as multiple lesions in a dermatomal distribution. May be difficult to distinguish clinically from herpes simplex virus (HSV) infection if the dermatomal distribution is absent (ie, if there is only 1 group of vesicles).
Allergic contact dermatitis	• May appear in a geometric or linear distribution (if due to plants). • Pruritus a common feature.
Hand, foot, and mouth disease	• Individual (not grouped) vesicles. • Palm and sole involvement is a prominent feature. • Vesicles often oval. • With severe disease, larger bullae may be present. • In "eczema coxsackium," lesions may predominate in areas prone to atopic dermatitis, may be numerous, and may be clustered (ie, closely simulates eczema herpeticum).
Herpangina	• Vesicles and erosions primarily involve the palate, uvula, and tonsillar pillars. • No involvement of surrounding perioral skin or lips.
Aphthous stomatitis (canker sores)	• Single or multiple (usually ≤3) discrete, shallow ulcers, 3 to 6 mm in size, affecting the oral mucosa. • Lesions have grayish white membrane and sharp, slightly raised, red borders.
Bullous impetigo	• Flaccid bullae or round, superficial erosions with a rim of surrounding scale. • No deep-seated vesicles as seen in HSV infection. • Culture grows *Staphylococcus aureus*.
Blistering distal dactylitis	• May be difficult to distinguish clinically from herpetic whitlow. • Solitary bulla, whereas the lesions of HSV infection often are smaller vesicles. • Culture typically positive for *Streptococcus pyogenes*, less often *S aureus*.
Thermal burn	• May mimic herpetic whitlow, but history of injury usually is present.
Bullous mastocytoma	• Peau d'orange appearance of surface, often with hyperpigmentation. • History of localized blistering, which may become less likely after infancy. • Positive Darier sign (urtication after firm stroking of lesion).

How to Make the Diagnosis

▶ The diagnosis usually is made clinically on the basis of the classic clinical morphology and distribution of lesions, especially when supported by history of recurrence.

▶ Laboratory investigations can be useful when the diagnosis is uncertain.
- Viral culture is a reliable method for confirming the diagnosis and is considered the criterion standard, although, in many settings, it has been replaced by polymcrase chain reaction testing.
- Polymerase chain reaction testing, when available, is a highly sensitive and specific diagnostic test.
- Direct immunofluorescence examination of lesional swabs offers rapid diagnosis and can distinguish HSV and VZV infection with high sensitivity, but such testing may not be available in many office settings.
- Serological studies are less useful clinically.
- Tzanck test of a fresh vesicle can provide rapid information, but utility of the test is limited by experience or expertise of the clinician and hampered by suboptimal sensitivity and specificity (Figure 10.7). A positive Tzanck test result cannot distinguish between HSV and VZV infection.

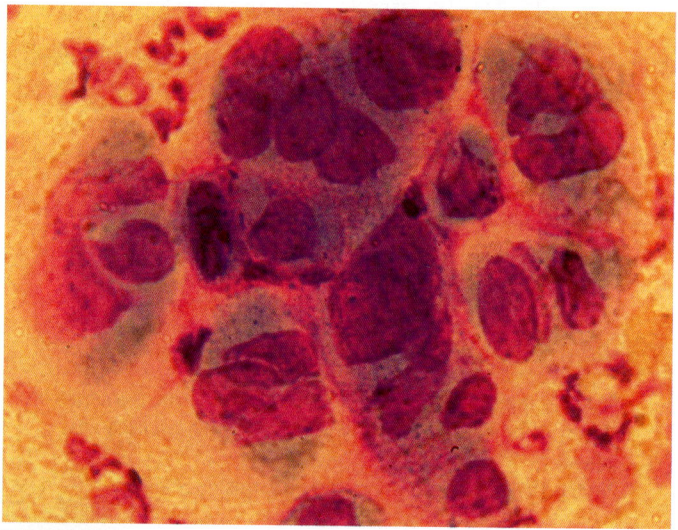

Figure 10.7. Tzanck test in herpes simplex virus infection; multinucleated giant cells are present.

Treatment

- Supportive therapy suffices in most cases, using simple cleansing and comfort measures, astringent gels, soothing moisturizers, or topical antibiotic ointments (to prevent secondary bacterial infection).
- Oral analgesics (eg, viscous lidocaine solution, benzocaine lozenges, compounded mouthwashes) may be useful for associated pain.
- Oral antiviral therapy is indicated for severe disease, frequently recurrent disease, and individuals who are immunosuppressed. Oral acyclovir, valacyclovir, or famciclovir may be used, depending on the patient's age. Treatment is more effective when started earlier (eg, in the first 48 hours) in the outbreak.
- Severe primary infections, infections in those who are immunocompromised, recurrences associated with erythema multiforme, and eczema herpeticum should be treated systemically (oral or intravenous, depending on severity and host risk factors); some of these patients may merit inpatient hospitalization.
- Neonatal HSV infection requires parenteral acyclovir therapy.
- The decision to treat less severe or recurrent outbreaks is based on the frequency and severity of the lesions and level of distress to the patient or family.
- Current treatment guidelines are summarized in the current edition of AAP *Red Book*®: *Report of the Committee on Infectious Diseases* (**https://redbook.solutions.aap.org**).

Prognosis

- In most individuals who are immunocompetent, HSV infections beyond the neonatal period are mild and self-limited and have an excellent prognosis.
- Circumstances in which disease may be more severe and require more aggressive therapy are discussed in the next section.

When to Worry or Refer

- Newborns and infants 6 weeks or younger who have evidence of HSV infection should be evaluated immediately and treated with intravenous acyclovir. Consultation with a pediatric infectious disease specialist is desirable.

- ▶ Widespread lesions over eczematous skin (ie, eczema herpeticum) or infection in a child who is immunocompromised can be severe, often requiring hospitalization and treatment with intravenous acyclovir.
- ▶ Widespread oral lesions (ie, HSV gingivostomatitis) with resulting mouth pain and dehydration require hydration, antiviral therapy, and analgesia.
- ▶ Patients who develop erythema multiforme or Stevens-Johnson syndrome after HSV infection should be referred to a dermatologist and often require suppressive antiviral therapy in an effort to prevent recurrences.
- ▶ Involvement in or around the eye should be immediately evaluated by an ophthalmologist.
- ▶ Evidence of central nervous system involvement (eg, seizures, behavioral changes, lethargy) warrants emergent evaluation.
- ▶ Sexual abuse should be suspected in children with anogenital herpes infection if there is no clear history of autoinoculation as the source of infection.

Resources for Families

- ▶ American Academy of Dermatology: Herpes simplex: diagnosis and treatment.
  https://www.aad.org/diseases/a-z/herpes-simplex-treatment
- ▶ American Academy of Pediatrics: HealthyChildren.org.
  healthychildren.org/English/health-issues/conditions/skin/Pages/Herpes-Simplex-Virus-Cold-Sores.aspx
- ▶ American Sexual Health Association: Nonprofit organization that provides information for patients in English and Spanish on sexually transmitted infections, including HSV infection. Website provides links to support groups for those who have genital HSV infection.
  www.ashasexualhealth.org/stdsstis/herpes
- ▶ MedlinePlus: Information for patients and families (in English and Spanish) sponsored by the US National Library of Medicine and National Institutes of Health.
  https://medlineplus.gov/herpessimplex.html
- ▶ WebMD: Information for families is contained in Skin Problems and Treatments.
  https://www.webmd.com/skin-problems-and-treatments/understanding-cold-sores-basics#1

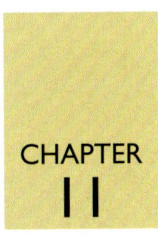

CHAPTER
11

Herpes Zoster

Introduction/Etiology/Epidemiology

- Herpes zoster (shingles) is reactivation of latent varicella-zoster virus (VZV) infection in the sensory nerve root ganglia, which persists after preceding varicella infection (chickenpox).
- May occur at any age, but incidence increases with age.
- Incidence in children is low; higher risk of herpes zoster exists in young children whose mothers had varicella during pregnancy or who themselves had early primary varicella (ie, within the first year after birth).
- Higher incidence in children with HIV infection, acute lymphocytic leukemia, or congenital (or other acquired) immunodeficiency disorders.
- May occur in children who have received past varicella vaccination but at lower rates than after wild-type primary VZV infection.
- Individuals who have active herpes zoster lesions may transmit VZV by direct contact to those without immunity. If infected, the nonimmune individual would develop varicella, not herpes zoster.

Signs and Symptoms

- Pain, itching, or paresthesia in a localized distribution may precede the skin eruption, but this is more common in adults than in children.
- Malaise, headache, and fever may precede or accompany the eruption, but mild itching is often the only associated symptom.
- The eruption is characteristically unilateral, with the distribution of 1 to 3 dermatomes (Figures 11.1 and 11.2).
- Thoracic dermatomes are most commonly involved in children, followed by the fifth and seventh cranial nerves.

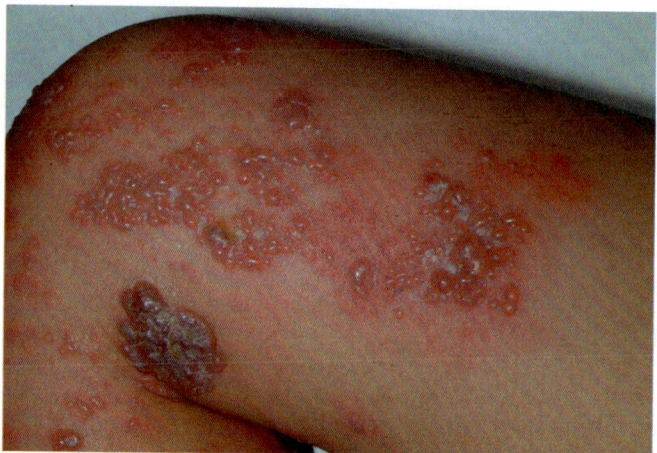

Figure 11.1. Herpes zoster is characterized by grouped vesicles in a dermatomal distribution with surrounding erythema.

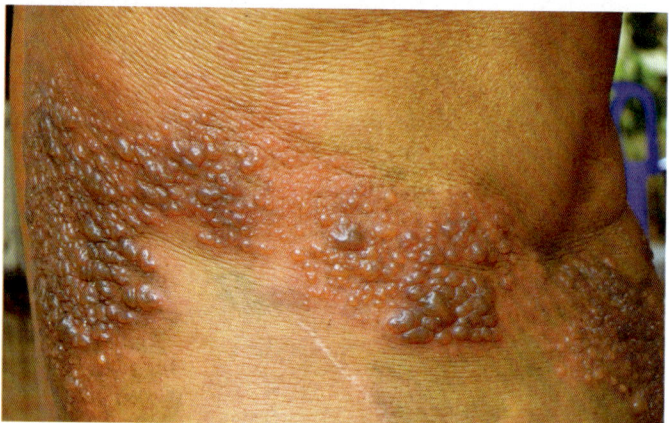

Figure 11.2. Herpes zoster in a patient with skin of color. Grouped vesicles and surrounding skin have a violaceous color. Reproduced with permission from Shutterstock.

- ▶ Nasal tip involvement implies involvement in the nasociliary branch of the ophthalmic branch of the trigeminal nerve (Hutchinson sign); this is a predictor of possible ocular disease (eg, keratitis, conjunctivitis, scleritis).
- ▶ Individual lesions may appear as grouped erythematous papules or circumscribed erythematous patches that evolve to discrete grouped vesicles on an erythematous base. Sequential crops of lesions within the dermatome may be noted after symptom onset.

- ▶ Vesicles may become cloudy pustules before rupturing and forming crusts (analogous to the evolution observed in varicella and herpes simplex virus [HSV] infections).
- ▶ The entire process lasts from 1 to 3 weeks.
- ▶ Severe symptoms, extensive disease (beyond the primary dermatomes), and scarring may occur in patients who are immunosuppressed. Such individuals also are at risk for viral dissemination and visceral complications.
- ▶ Postherpetic neuralgia is uncommon in children and is usually limited to those who have had severe disease in the setting of immunosuppression or ophthalmic involvement.

Look-alikes

Disorder	Differentiating Features
Herpes simplex virus infection	• Usually localized without dermatomal distribution. • Dermatomal herpes simplex virus infection tends to be recurrent (but may otherwise be very difficult to distinguish clinically).
Allergic contact dermatitis	• Not usually dermatomal in distribution. • Itch more prominent than pain.

How to Make the Diagnosis

- ▶ Clinical appearance of lesions, dermatomal distribution, and history usually provide sufficient information for accurate diagnosis.
- ▶ Laboratory investigations can be useful when the diagnosis is uncertain.
  - Polymerase chain reaction, when available, is a specific, sensitive, and useful diagnostic tool.
  - Direct immunofluorescence of lesional swabs offers rapid diagnosis and can distinguish HSV and VZV infection with high sensitivity, but such testing may not be available in many office settings.
  - Viral culture from skin lesions can be performed but is limited by difficulty in isolating VZV in cell culture.
  - Serological tests are of limited usefulness.
  - Tzanck test of a fresh vesicle can provide rapid information, but utility of the test is limited by experience or expertise of the clinician and hampered by suboptimal sensitivity and specificity. A positive Tzanck test result cannot distinguish between HSV and VZV infection.

- A history of recurrent zoster usually indicates the patient has HSV infection, not zoster.
- Attempts to elicit history of exposure to contact allergens, especially poison ivy, should be made to exclude the possibility of allergic contact dermatitis in patients in whom pruritus is the prominent symptom.

Treatment

- Specific therapy is unnecessary in children with mild symptoms and limited involvement.
- Topical antipruritics (eg, menthol and camphor lotions) and oral antihistamines are useful for relief of itching.
- Antiviral therapy with acyclovir (oral or intravenous) or other oral antiviral agents (eg, famciclovir, valacyclovir) should be considered in patients at high risk who have findings concerning for eye involvement, those who are immunosuppressed, or in any patient with more severe disease or significant symptoms.
- Aluminum acetate solution compresses may be soothing and help to speed drying and healing of blisters.

When to Worry or Refer

- Complicated infection in a patient who is immunocompromised may require hospitalization.
- Referral is indicated if the diagnosis is uncertain.
- An ophthalmologist should be consulted for zoster in the distribution of the ophthalmic branch (V_1) of the trigeminal nerve or if nasal tip involvement is present.

Resources for Families

- American Academy of Dermatology: Shingles: diagnosis and treatment.
  https://www.aad.org/public/diseases/contagious-skin-diseases/shingles
- Centers for Disease Control and Prevention: About shingles (herpes zoster).
  www.cdc.gov/shingles/about/index.html
- MedlinePlus: Information for patients and families (in English and Spanish) sponsored by the US National Library of Medicine and National Institutes of Health.
  https://www.nlm.nih.gov/medlineplus/shingles.html
- Society for Pediatric Dermatology: Patient handouts.
  https://pedsderm.net/for-patients-families/patient-handouts/#HerpesInfection
- WebMD: Skin problems and treatments: shingles resource center.
  www.webmd.com/skin-problems-and-treatments/shingles/default.htm

CHAPTER 12

Molluscum Contagiosum

Introduction/Etiology/Epidemiology

- Discrete papular eruption commonly seen in infants and children.
- Spread through skin-to-skin contact.
- Caused by a poxvirus.
- Although this infection is classically associated with immunodeficiency or sexual transmission in adults, it is not typically associated with this history in infants and children.
- May occur as a sexually transmitted infection in sexually active adolescents and young adults.

Signs and Symptoms

- Usually without symptoms.
- Lesions are 1- to 6-mm, discrete, skin-colored, pink (Figure 12.1) to pearly (Figure 12.2) papules that may mimic vesicles; some lesions are umbilicated (ie, have a central dell or depression) or a central hyperkeratotic core.
- Widespread or sometimes "giant" (8–15 mm) lesions may occur in individuals who are immunosuppressed.
- Extensive lesions often are observed in children with atopic dermatitis.
- Can occur on any cutaneous location but commonly seen on face, eyelids, neck, chest, axillae, folds of extremities, and genital region.
- Eyelid lesions may be associated with chronic conjunctivitis or keratitis.
- May be associated with a mild to moderate dermatitis occurring in the vicinity of the papules, known as molluscum dermatitis (Figure 12.3).
- Linear arrangement of lesions may be present due to autoinoculation (Koebner phenomenon) (Figure 12.4).

- Genital location most common when occurring as a sexually transmitted infection in sexually active adolescents or young adults but may also be seen in younger children.
- Enlargement of lesions with erythema is often noted in association with the host immune response against the virus (Figure 12.5) and often heralds involution of the lesions. This has been termed the *beginning of the end*, or *BOTE sign*.

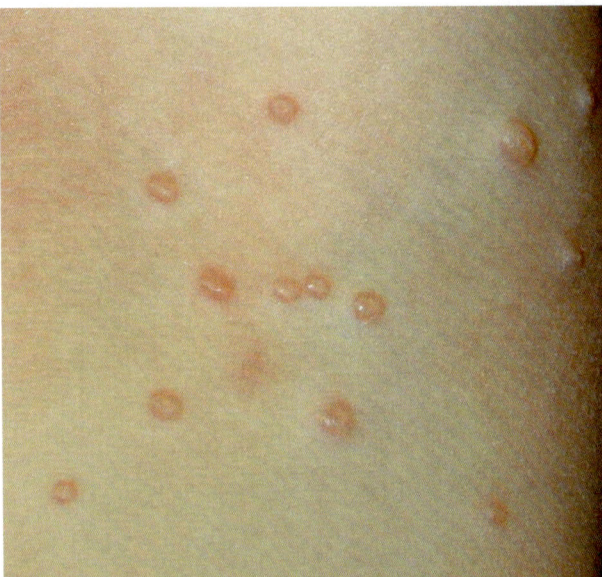

Figure 12.1. Skin-colored to pink translucent papules are typical of molluscum contagiosum. Note umbilication (ie, central depression) of larger lesions.

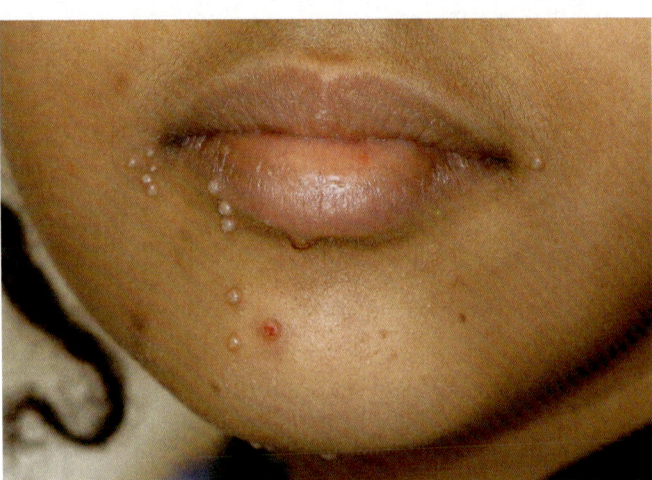

Figure 12.2. Pearly papules of molluscum contagiosum. Note the central hyperkeratotic core in some of the lesions.

Chapter 12: Molluscum Contagiosum 107

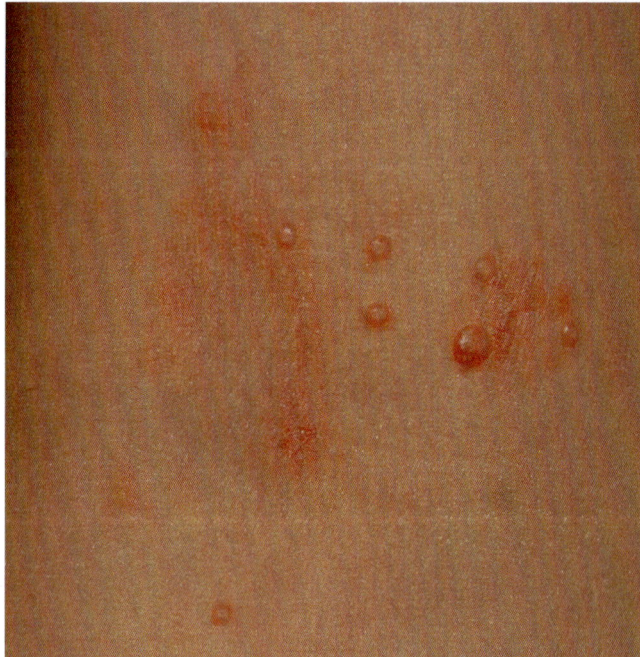

Figure 12.3. Molluscum dermatitis. Erythematous patches with scale surround lesions of molluscum contagiosum.

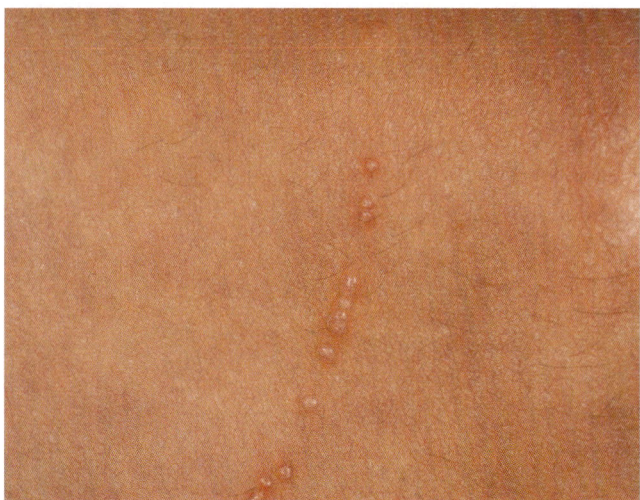

Figure 12.4. Molluscum contagiosum with koebnerization, manifested as several lesions in a linear distribution.

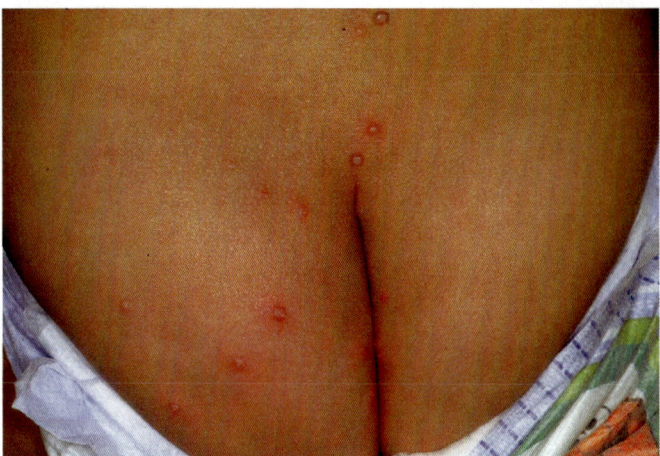

Figure 12.5. Molluscum lesions with enlargement and erythema, signifying the host immune response against the virus. These lesions resolved shortly thereafter.

Look-alikes

Disorder	Differentiating Features
Milia	• Small white papules that lack central umbilication. • Often limited to facial distribution.
Frictional lichenoid dermatitis	• Uniformly spaced, skin-colored to pink to hypopigmented papules on elbows, knees. • No central keratin plug or umbilication.
Closed comedones	• Small white papules that lack central umbilication. • Occur in older children or adolescents. • Most often limited to facial distribution.
Flat warts	• Flat-topped papules or small thin plaques. • Umbilication absent.
Cryptococcosis	• Molluscum-like lesions possible in patients who are immunocompromised. • May have systemic symptoms. • May have ulcers in addition to papules.
Histoplasmosis	• Molluscum-like lesions possible in patients who are immunocompromised. • May have systemic symptoms. • May have ulcers in addition to papules.

How to Make the Diagnosis

- The diagnosis is made clinically based on the appearance of lesions.
- A skin scraping of a characteristic papule can be used for a crush preparation and stained with Giemsa or methylene blue, revealing numerous characteristic molluscum (Henderson-Paterson) bodies at direct microscopy; this is rarely necessary.
- Skin biopsy occasionally is used for large or atypical lesions.

Treatment

- Lesions often resolve spontaneously over several months or years. In 1 study, the mean time to resolution was 13 months.
- Watchful waiting is an acceptable management plan, although treatment is often requested by parents.
- Application of cantharidin (blister beetle extract) is a painless and effective procedure; however, it must be performed by an experienced clinician and only in the office setting (not for home use). Although cantharidin had previously been an off-label therapy, the US Food and Drug Administration has now approved cantharidin 0.7% in a single-use device for the treatment of molluscum contagiosum in those aged 2 years or older. Blistering is an expected outcome of treatment with cantharidin and can be quite significant in some patients, although most patients tolerate the treatment quite well.
- Berdazimer 10.3% topical gel was also recently approved by the US Food and Drug Administration for patients aged 1 year or older. This nitric oxide–releasing agent is applied once daily to lesions and is approved for application at home by patients or caregivers.
- Curettage of individual lesions is effective, but limitations include pain, fear (in young children), and risks of spread and scarring.
- Lesions near the eyelid margin, causing chronic conjunctivitis, may require surgical excision.
- Cryotherapy with liquid nitrogen also is effective but may be traumatic for young children in whom it is poorly tolerated.

- Imiquimod cream is an off-label option for treatment. Although applied 3 times weekly for genital condylomata, treatment of molluscum generally requires daily application and may require many weeks of application; irritant contact dermatitis is a common limiting side effect of this therapy.
- Topical retinoids (eg, tretinoin) have been used, mainly for facial lesions; mechanism of action is probably induction of irritant dermatitis, which may be a limiting side effect. This is an off-label indication for retinoids.
- Immunotherapy using intralesional injection of skin test antigens (most often *Candida*) may be effective, but published data are limited, and the associated pain, anxiety, and need for repeated injections make this option less feasible for young children.

When to Worry or Refer

- When treatment is requested but is not available in your practice.
- When diagnosis is uncertain.
- When extensive disease is present.
- When molluscum is associated with poorly controlled atopic dermatitis.

Resources for Families

- American Academy of Dermatology: Molluscum contagiosum: overview.
  https://www.aad.org/diseases/a-z/molluscum-contagiosum-overview
- American Academy of Pediatrics: HealthyChildren.org.
  https://www.healthychildren.org/molluscumcontagiosum
- Society for Pediatric Dermatology: Patient handout on molluscum contagiosum.
  https://pedsderm.net/for-patients-families/patient-handouts/#Molluscum
- WebMD: Information for families is contained in Skin Problems and Treatments.
  www.webmd.com/skin-problems-and-treatments/molluscum-contagium

CHAPTER
13

Warts

Introduction/Etiology/Epidemiology

- Epithelial growths are induced by different subtypes of human papillomavirus (HPV).
- Clinical wart subtypes correlate with different HPV subtypes.
- Very common in children.
- Most spontaneously resolve over years.
- Often recalcitrant to multiple therapies.
- Transmission may occur person to person, from fomites, or from autoinoculation.
- Usually asymptomatic, but large or multiple plantar lesions may be associated with pain, limitation in activities.
- Can be disfiguring.
- In patients who have immunodeficiency (including HIV infection), lesions may be numerous and widespread.

Signs and Symptoms

- Common warts: discrete, skin-colored to hyperpigmented papules with characteristic verrucous surface (Figure 13.1). Sometimes, the surface is more mammillated (bumpy) (Figure 13.2). Lesions may exhibit tiny dark specks that are thrombosed capillaries. Some warts may have a filiform (stalklike) appearance (Figure 13.3).
- Plantar warts: rough or smooth papules and plaques localized to the plantar aspect of the feet, most often over weight-bearing surfaces. Lesions exhibit tiny dark specks that are thrombosed capillaries. Occasionally, several warts may coalesce and form larger mosaic warts (Figure 13.4).

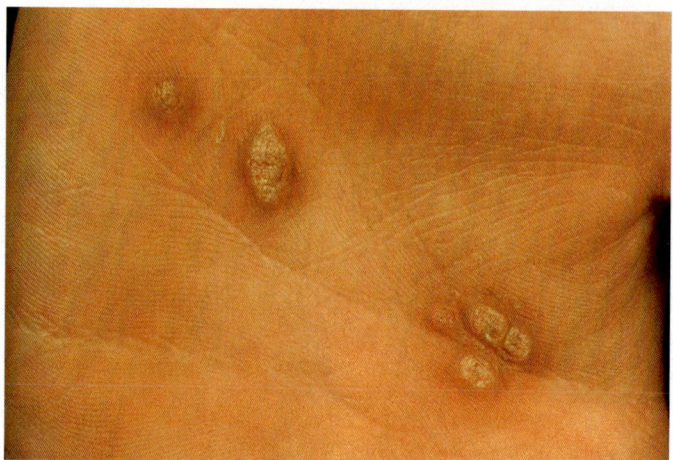

Figure 13.1. Common warts appear as rough (ie, verrucous) papules.

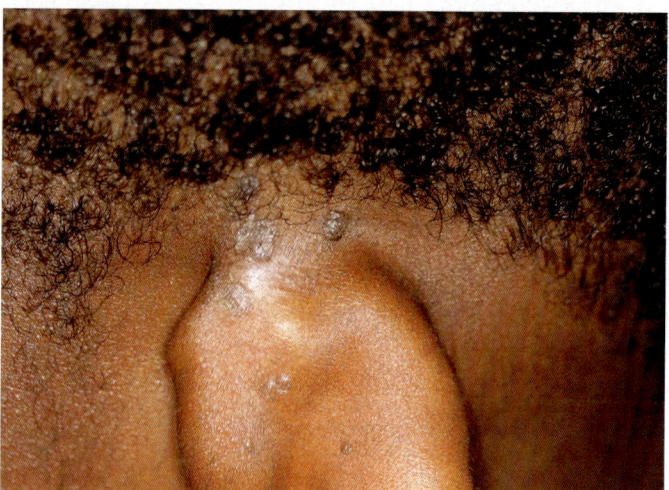

Figure 13.2. This child with skin of color had postauricular warts that were hyperpigmented, mammillated (rounded) papules.

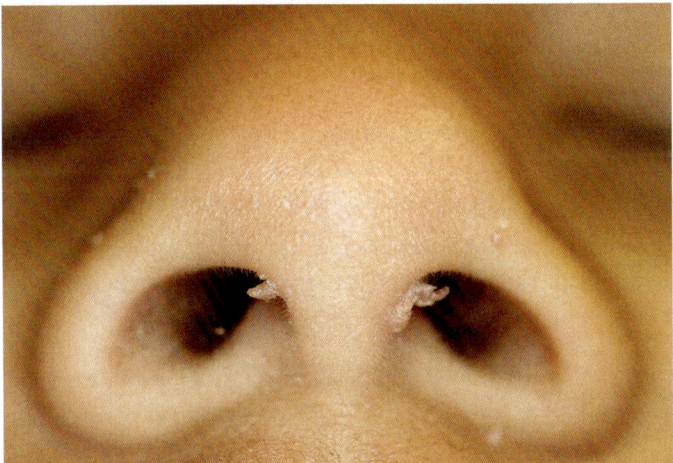

Figure 13.3. Verrucous papules with filiform (stalklike) appearance on the medial nares. Note the smaller smooth papules on the alar rims, which also were warts.

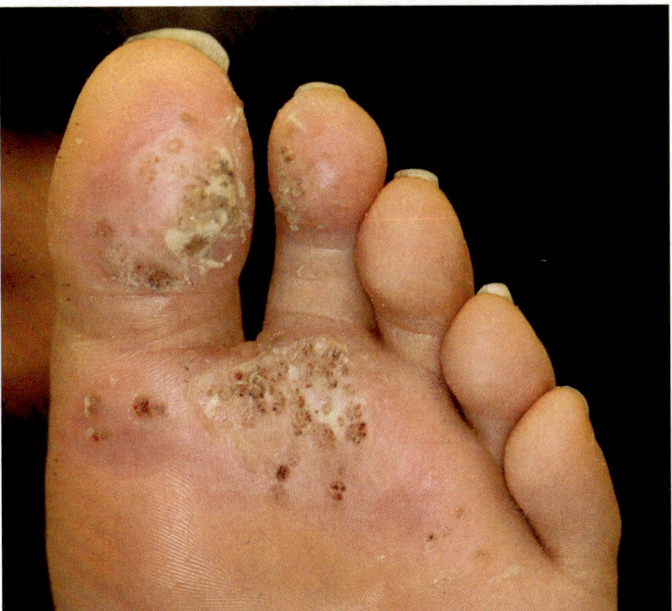

Figure 13.4. Multiple verrucous papules with pinpoint thrombosed vessels coalescing to form mosaic plantar warts. There is mild maceration surrounding some of the lesions and partial clearance due to treatment with salicylic acid.

- Flat warts: smooth, pink or skin-colored, flat-topped papules, 1 to 3 mm, typically seen on the face or legs, but may occur in other locations (Figure 13.5).
- Anogenital warts (ie, condylomata acuminata): discrete papules or confluent plaques; pink to red or skin colored; localized to genitalia or adjacent skin of inguinal, thigh, suprapubic, or perianal areas (Figure 13.6).
- Periungual warts: often occur in association with common warts; present as papules, confluent plaques, or nodules adjacent to nails, occasionally with destructive involvement of the proximal or lateral nail fold areas.

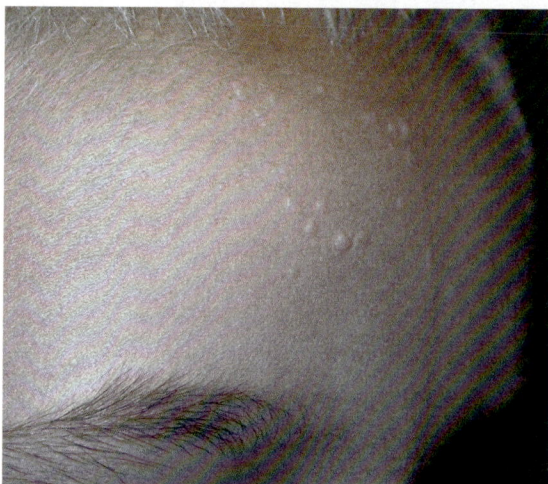

Figure 13.5. Flat warts are small, flat-topped papules.

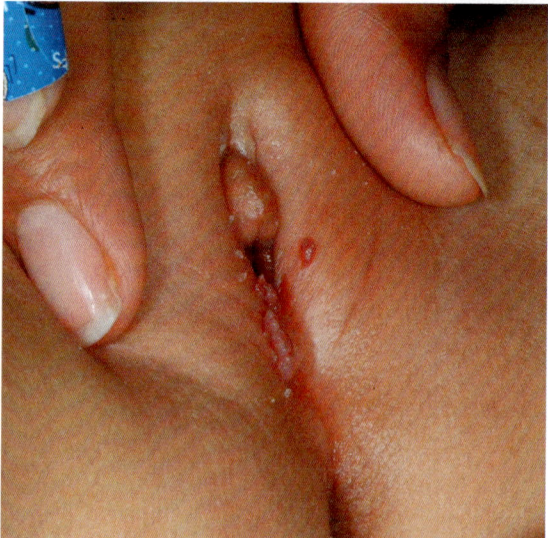

Figure 13.6. Condylomata acuminata appear as skin-colored papules and plaques.

Look-alikes

Disorder	Differentiating Features
Plantar Warts	
Callus	• Located over points of friction or pressure. • Lacks black specks (ie, thrombosed capillaries). • Dermatoglyphics often preserved.
Condylomata Acuminata	
Condylomata lata	• Appear as moist white plaques. • Associated with secondary syphilis.
Molluscum contagiosum	• White, pearly, or translucent papules that may have central umbilication.
Flat Warts	
Lichen planus	• Violaceous papules that may exhibit a white lacy pattern on the surface (Wickham striae). • White papules or lacy white plaques may be present on the buccal mucosa.
Lichen nitidus	• White or skin-colored, flat-topped tiny papules, often clustered together. • Atopic history common.
Molluscum contagiosum	• White, pearly, or translucent papules that may have central umbilication.
Benign cephalic histiocytosis	• May be difficult to differentiate from flat warts. • Limited to face; rarely involves other skin surfaces.
Common Warts	
Epidermal nevi	• Present since birth or shortly thereafter. • Linear or whorled distribution may be evident.
Granuloma annulare	• Annular (ringlike) papules or plaques with a smooth surface.
Knuckle pads	• Fibrous to hyperkeratotic plaques or papules overlying interphalangeal joints. • Rough (ie, verrucous) surface tends to be absent.

Treatment

- ▶ Warts are often self-limited, usually asymptomatic, and do not necessarily require treatment. None of the current treatments are uniformly effective, and patients and parents should understand the potential limitations of therapy.

- ▶ The risk-to-benefit ratio of therapy must be considered, and care should be exercised to avoid overly painful or traumatic treatments in young children.

- ▶ First-line therapy is usually a topical salicylic acid plaster or liquid, with or without duct tape occlusion (Box 13.1).

Box 13.1. Optimizing Use of Over-the-Counter Salicylic Acid Therapy for Warts
Apply 17% salicylic acid liquid to wart(s). • May use a plaster impregnated with salicylic acid if desired. • May use a higher concentration of salicylic acid for management of warts on the plantar surface of the foot.
Air-dry for 2 to 3 minutes (develops into a white film).
Occlude surface of wart with duct tape or similar adhesive tape.
Remove tape in the morning.
If further debridement is necessary, gently file tissue down with a disposable emery board to avoid autoinoculation.
Repeat nightly until wart is resolved.
Notes • This treatment is most effective for plantar warts. • Do not apply to facial, fold, or genital area warts. • If area becomes macerated or inflamed, withhold treatment for 1 to 3 nights, then resume. • May take up to 8 weeks to see improvement in the wart. Prolonged treatment is almost always necessary, particularly for plantar warts.

- ▶ A compounded cream of 5-fluorouracil and salicylic acid applied under tape occlusion nightly may be effective.

- ▶ Cryotherapy with spray or cotton swab application of liquid nitrogen or other cryogen is effective if used repeatedly (with treatments separated by 2–4 weeks) but should be reserved for motivated, older children who can tolerate painful procedures. In the interval between cryotherapy treatments, any remaining wart should be treated with topical salicylic acid as described previously.

- Topical imiquimod is approved for treatment of condylomata acuminata and is applied to lesions 3 times weekly on nonconsecutive days (and occasionally nightly) until resolved for up to 16 weeks.
- Off-label use of imiquimod may be beneficial for common warts when applied daily to warts; however, its efficacy is often limited by the hyperkeratosis found in common warts, and irritant dermatitis may be seen with its use.
- Cimetidine (30–40 mg/kg/d orally divided twice a day or 3 times a day) for 6 to 8 weeks or more may be effective in some children; not approved by the US Food and Drug Administration for this indication.
- Other treatment options for common warts include intralesional injection of skin test antigens (eg, *Candida*, *Trichophyton*), intralesional chemotherapy injections (eg, bleomycin), and topical immunotherapy with squaric acid; these therapies are not approved by the US Food and Drug Administration, and published data are limited.
- Other potential treatment options for condylomata acuminata include prescription therapies such as podofilox solution or gel, sinecatechins ointment, or in-office application of podophyllin or trichloroacetic acid.
- Treatments such as pulsed dye laser and surgical excision are occasionally considered but do not necessarily offer greater efficacy. Surgery entails a high risk of permanent scarring and potential for recurrence.

When to Worry or Refer

- Patients with symptomatic warts that have not responded to standard therapies should be referred for discussion of other treatment options.
- Patients who are immunosuppressed and have multiple lesions merit more aggressive therapy given the potential association between warts and an increased risk of cutaneous malignancy, as well as an increased likelihood of a more extensive and protracted course.
- Anogenital warts in children may be a marker for sexual abuse, although autoinoculation, vertical transmission (a consideration primarily in children <3 years), and benign (nonsexual) modes of transmission are also possible. If the history or physical examination raises concern, referral and thorough investigation are vital.

Resources for Families

- American Academy of Dermatology: Warts: diagnosis and treatment.
  https://www.aad.org/diseases/a-z/warts-treatment
- American Academy of Pediatrics: HealthyChildren.org.
  https://www.healthychildren.org/warts
- MedlinePlus: Information for patients and families (in English and Spanish) sponsored by the US National Library of Medicine and National Institutes of Health.
  https://www.nlm.nih.gov/medlineplus/warts.html
- Society for Pediatric Dermatology: Patient handout on warts.
  https://pedsderm.net/for-patients-families/patient-handouts/#Warts
- WebMD: Information for families is contained in Skin Problems and Treatments.
  https://www.webmd.com/skin-problems-and-treatments/warts#1

Skin Infections

Systemic Viral Infections

CHAPTER 14 — **Erythema Infectiosum/Human Parvovirus B19 Infection (Fifth Disease)** 121

CHAPTER 15 — **Gianotti-Crosti Syndrome** 127

CHAPTER 16 — **Hand, Foot, and Mouth Disease (HFMD) and Other Enteroviral Exanthems** 131

CHAPTER 17 — **Measles**. 141

CHAPTER 18 — **Papular-Purpuric Gloves-and-Socks Syndrome (PPGSS)**. 147

CHAPTER 19 — **Roseola Infantum (Exanthem Subitum)** 151

CHAPTER 20 — **Rubella** 155

CHAPTER 21 — **Unilateral Laterothoracic Exanthem (ULE)** 161

CHAPTER 22 — **Varicella** 165

CHAPTER 14

Erythema Infectiosum/ Human Parvovirus B19 Infection (Fifth Disease)

Introduction/Etiology/Epidemiology

- ▶ Caused by human parvovirus B19.
- ▶ Usually affects children between 4 and 10 years of age.
- ▶ Most common in the winter and spring, with endemic peaks every 6 to 9 years.
- ▶ Transmission is via respiratory droplets, blood and blood products, or vertically from mother to fetus.
- ▶ Incubation period is 4 to 14 days.
- ▶ Clearance of viremia precedes appearance of the erythema infectiosum rash by several days; thus, patients who have the skin eruption are not considered contagious.

Signs and Symptoms

- ▶ Up to 50% of infections may be subclinical.
- ▶ During the viremic stage, patients may develop prodromal symptoms of fever, malaise, myalgias, pharyngitis, and headache.
- ▶ After the viremic phase, the first stage of erythema infectiosum reveals the classic finding of a slapped cheek appearance with bright red erythema on the cheeks, typically sparing the perioral region (Figures 14.1 and 14.2).
- ▶ The second stage appears 1 to 4 days after the facial rash appears and is characterized as erythematous patches, papules, and plaques that partially clear, leaving a lacy, reticular pattern of erythema, especially on the flexor surfaces of the arms. This phase of the exanthem may wax and wane over the next 1 to 4 weeks (Figure 14.3).

- Pruritus is sometimes prominent.
- After the exanthem fades, it is commonly reactivated for several weeks to months by physical factors, including sunlight, physical activity, or hot baths.
- Arthralgia and arthritis may be the most common manifestation of parvovirus B19 infection in adolescents and adults, especially if female. However, this is less frequent in younger children. The joint symptoms are typically brief in duration, preferentially affecting larger joints, and may be pauciarticular or polyarticular. Rarely, the arthralgia may persist for months to years.
- Human parvovirus B19 exhibits tropism for erythroid progenitor cells, and individuals with predisposing hematologic conditions resulting in a shortened red blood cell half-life (eg, sickle cell disease, spherocytosis, thalassemia) are at risk for aplastic crises. These crises occur before and in the early periods of the exanthem.
- Pregnant women who are susceptible and become infected with human parvovirus B19 during the first half of their pregnancy may transmit the infection to their developing fetus, with subsequent risk of fetal anemia, nonimmune fetal hydrops, and fetal death in 2% to 6% of cases.

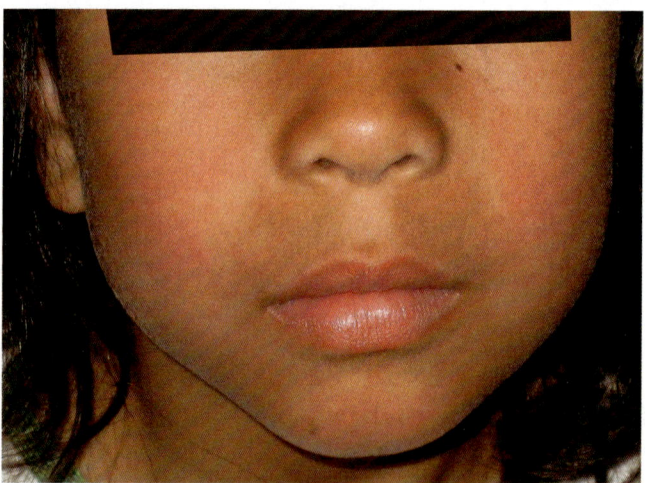

Figure 14.1. The first stage of erythema infectiosum in a child with skin of color. There are erythematous patches on the cheeks. From Redbook Visual Library. Courtesy of H. Cody Meissner, MD, FAAP.

Chapter 14: Erythema Infectiosum/Human Parvovirus B19 Infection

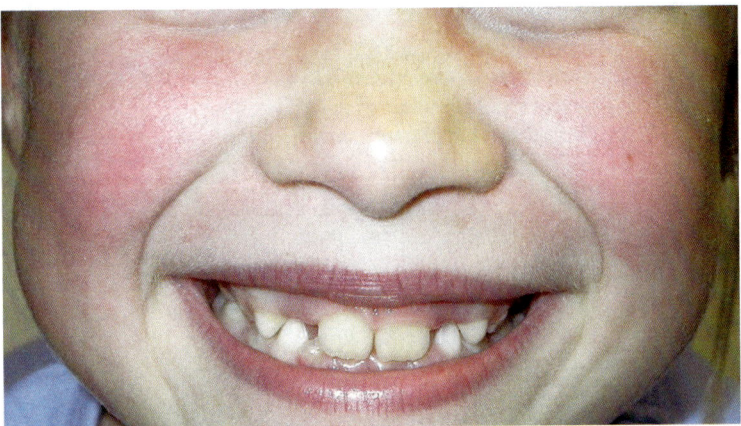

Figure 14.2. The first stage of erythema infectiosum exhibits erythematous cheeks (ie, a slapped cheek appearance).

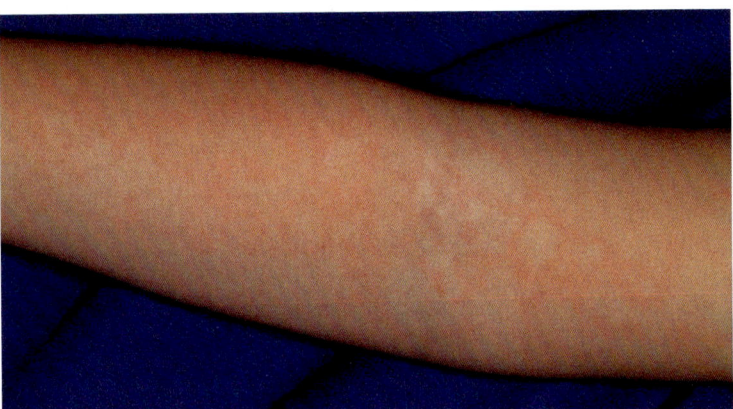

Figure 14.3. The second stage of erythema infectiosum produces an erythematous lacy, reticulated exanthem on the extremities.

Look-alikes

Disorder	Differentiating Features
Exanthematous drug eruption	• History of drug exposure elicited. • Slapped cheek appearance absent. • Typically presents with red macules and papules.
Nonspecific viral exanthem	• Fever or other symptoms may be present. • Slapped cheek appearance absent. • Typically presents with red macules and papules.
Livedo reticularis	• Typically a long-standing finding, not acutely acquired. • Slapped cheek appearance absent.
Exanthem of juvenile idiopathic arthritis	• Clinical features of juvenile idiopathic arthritis present. • Slapped cheek appearance absent. • Exanthem most apparent during febrile periods.
Scarlet fever	• Circumoral pallor may give slapped cheek appearance. • Generalized, sandpaper-like eruption. • Pharyngitis and lymphadenopathy usually present.
Urticaria	• Acute onset of pruritic and edematous papules, plaques, wheals. • Distribution usually generalized. • Dermatographism may be present. • Lesions last less than 24 hours and migrate to other areas.

How to Make the Diagnosis

▶ The diagnosis is most often made clinically on the basis of characteristic findings.

▶ Serological detection of immunoglobulin M directed against human parvovirus B19 can confirm the diagnosis when obtained within 30 days of illness onset.

Treatment

▶ No specific treatment is indicated.

▶ Children with the characteristic rash can return to school or child care, as they are no longer considered contagious.

▶ Nonsteroidal anti-inflammatory drugs may be used for arthritis.

▶ Hospitalization and red blood cell transfusion may be required in children with transient aplastic crises.

Prognosis

- Erythema infectiosum typically resolves without sequelae.
- Patients with parvovirus B19 infection who are immunodeficient may develop chronic bone marrow suppression, and intravenous immunoglobulin therapy has been used in this setting.
- Pregnant women who have been exposed should be advised to contact their obstetric health professional to discuss potential risks and be offered serological testing. If acute infection is confirmed, serial fetal ultrasonography should be considered to monitor for fetal hydrops, congestive heart failure, and intrauterine growth restriction.

When to Worry or Refer

- Referral may be indicated if atypical features are present or the diagnosis is in question.
- Pregnant women exposed to or infected with human parvovirus B19 should consult their obstetric health professional (as discussed previously).
- Patients who are immunocompromised and patients with predisposing blood disorders who are exposed to human parvovirus B19 should be monitored for signs and symptoms of aplastic crises.

Resources for Families

- American Academy of Pediatrics: HealthyChildren.org.
  https://www.healthychildren.org/FifthDisease
- Centers for Disease Control and Prevention: Alphabetical listing of diseases and conditions provides information for families.
  www.cdc.gov/parvovirusB19/index.html
- MedlinePlus: Information for patients and families (in English and Spanish) sponsored by the US National Library of Medicine and National Institutes of Health.
  https://www.nlm.nih.gov/medlineplus/fifthdisease.html

CHAPTER
15

Gianotti-Crosti Syndrome

Introduction/Etiology/Epidemiology

- Also known as papular acrodermatitis of childhood and papulovesicular acrolocated syndrome.
- Distinctive exanthem of childhood affecting face, buttocks, and extensor surfaces of extremities.
- Predominantly occurs in children between the ages of 1 to 6 years.
- Initially described in association with hepatitis B infection.
- Subsequently demonstrated also to occur in response to a variety of viral infections and vaccinations.
  - Epstein-Barr virus is probably the most common cause worldwide and in the United States.
  - Enteroviruses, hepatitis A and B, cytomegalovirus, adenovirus, rotavirus, parvovirus, human herpesvirus 6, rubella, respiratory syncytial virus, paramyxovirus, parainfluenza virus 2, and SARS-CoV-2 have all been associated.
  - Potential associations with some vaccines have also been reported.

Signs and Symptoms

- Abrupt onset of symmetrically distributed erythematous or skin-colored papules.
- May be lichenoid (ie, flat-topped) or firm, dome-shaped edematous papules.
- Symmetrically localized to the face (Figure 15.1), extensor surfaces of the extremities (Figure 15.2), and buttocks (largely sparing the trunk); occasionally, lesions will be most prominent on the distal surfaces of the extremities and buttocks.

- Lesions range in size from 1 to 10 mm and typically appear monomorphous within the individual patient.
- Confluence of papules may lead to the appearance of edematous plaques, especially on the elbows and knees.
- Pruritus is variable.
- Occasionally mild prodromal symptoms such as low-grade fever and upper respiratory symptoms may be reported; lymphadenopathy may be present at examination.
- Hepatomegaly and abnormal liver function study results may be present in hepatitis-associated cases.

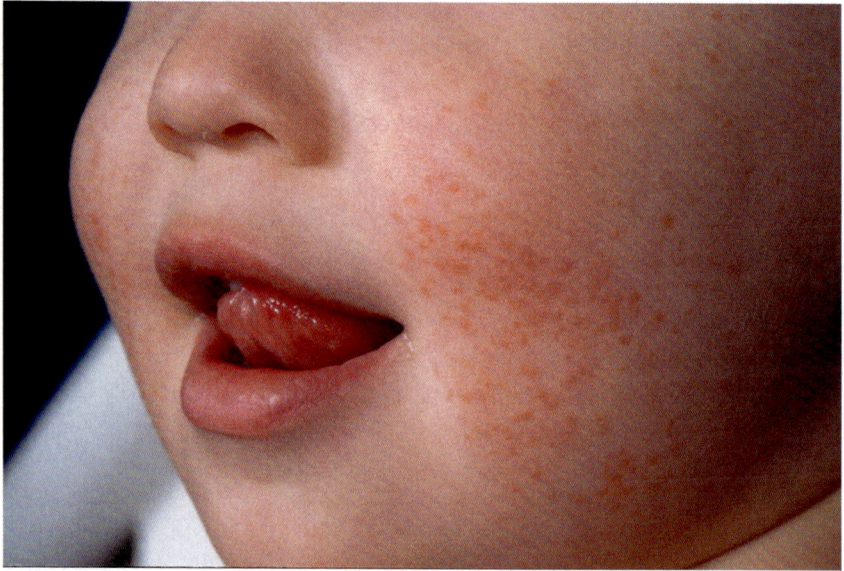

Figure 15.1. Erythematous papules distributed symmetrically on the face of a child with Gianotti-Crosti syndrome.

Chapter 15: Gianotti-Crosti Syndrome 129

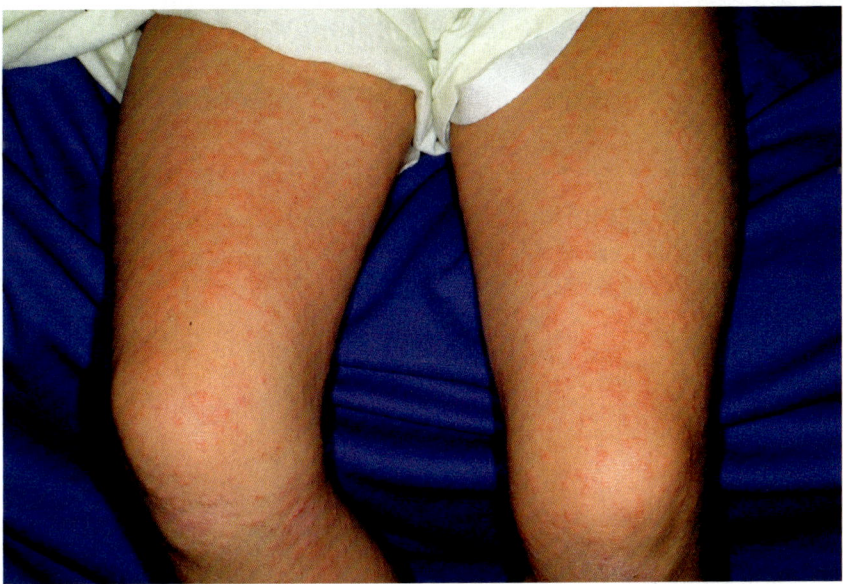

Figure 15.2. The papules of Gianotti-Crosti syndrome often are located symmetrically on the extensor surfaces of the lower extremities. This young child also had lesions on the face and extensor surfaces of the upper extremities.

Look-alikes

Disorder	Differentiating Features
Insect bites	• Not distributed symmetrically. • May exhibit a central punctum.
Papular atopic dermatitis	• More likely to present in a chronic, recurrent pattern. • Atopic history present.
Lichen planus	• Purple polygonal papules that may have fine, white reticulated scale on surface. • Most often distributed on volar surfaces of wrists, lower legs, and ankles. • White, reticulated patches often present on buccal mucosae.
Lichenoid drug eruption	• History of medication use. • Generalized, with truncal involvement as well.
Molluscum contagiosum	• Not distributed symmetrically. • Individual lesions are pearly and translucent and often contain a central punctum or depression. • Acute onset unusual; the number of lesions typically increases gradually over weeks to months. • Some reports in the literature suggest occasional coexistence of molluscum and a Gianotti-Crosti–type presentation, the latter likely representing an id-type reaction.

How to Make the Diagnosis

- The diagnosis is made clinically on the basis of the unique appearance and distribution of lesions.
- Skin biopsy may occasionally be useful in diagnosis but rarely is necessary.
- Routine serological evaluations for hepatitis B infection are not indicated; testing should be based on clinical suspicion and examination findings concerning for hepatitis.

Treatment

- Rarely necessary, aside from reassurance and education about the natural history.
- Oral antihistamines for pruritus.
- Topical steroids do not change the natural history of the skin eruption; may be helpful for treating pruritus.

Prognosis

- Self-limited, with eventual complete resolution (sometimes with postinflammatory pigmentary alteration).
- Lesions may persist for up to 8 to 12 weeks, in contrast to most other viral exanthems.

Resources for Families

- DermNet NZ: Papular acrodermatitis of childhood.
  https://www.dermnetnz.org/topics/papular-acrodermatitis-of-childhood
- National Organization for Rare Disorders: Information for patients and families.
  https://rarediseases.org/rare-diseases/gianotti-crosti-syndrome

Hand, Foot, and Mouth Disease (HFMD) and Other Enteroviral Exanthems

Introduction/Etiology/Epidemiology

Hand, Foot, and Mouth Disease
- The most distinctive enteroviral exanthem.
- Typical hand, foot, and mouth disease (HFMD) most often caused by coxsackievirus A16 but may be caused by coxsackieviruses A5, A7, A9, A10, B1, B2, B3, and B5 and enterovirus 71; more recently described atypical HFMD caused primarily by coxsackievirus A6.
- Most commonly occurs in the summer or fall.
- Classically seen in children younger than 5 years.
- Incubation period is 3 to 6 days.
- Highly contagious; may occur in epidemics.

Herpangina
- A characteristic enanthem that clinically overlaps with the enanthem of HFMD (without features of the exanthem).
- Most often caused by coxsackieviruses from groups A and B.
- Most commonly seen in children between 3 and 10 years of age.

Eruptive Pseudoangiomatosis
- An uncommon exanthem characterized by the sudden appearance of several small, angioma-like lesions in the setting of a viral prodrome or illness.

- Most often seen in infants and children, although reported in adults (often immunocompromised) as well.
- Associated with echovirus subtypes 25 and 32, although other viral etiologies such as cytomegalovirus have been suggested.

Signs and Symptoms

HFMD

- Brief prodrome of fever, malaise may occur.
- Cough, diarrhea noted infrequently.
- Cervical and submandibular lymphadenopathy occasionally observed.
- An enanthem precedes the characteristic exanthem.
- HFMD enanthem
  - Vesicles that erode to form ulcers on a red base; size ranges between 4 and 8 mm (Figure 16.1).
  - Most common on buccal mucosae and tongue.
  - May also involve palate, uvula, gingivae, and tonsillar pillars.
  - Lesions are often quite painful, sometimes severe enough to lead to anorexia, dehydration.
- HFMD exanthem
  - Deep-seated vesicopustules with grayish white color, 3 to 7 mm in size; often the vesicles are oval (Figures 16.2 and 16.3).
  - Vesicles often have surrounding erythema.
  - Typically, lesions are limited to the palms and soles but also may involve lateral surfaces of hands and feet; involvement of buttocks, elbows, knees, and perineum may also be seen in younger children.
- Atypical HFMD exanthem
  - In patients with atypical HFMD, vesicles are often larger and more numerous. The lesions may enlarge into bullae, become hemorrhagic, or present as erosions (Figure 16.4).
  - Distribution of lesions in atypical HFMD may be generalized but often with accentuation around the mouth (Figure 16.5), in the anogenital region, and on the extensor aspects of the extremities.
  - Lesions of atypical HFMD may have a predilection for areas of eczematous dermatitis, a presentation termed *eczema coxsackium,* as well as areas of prior skin injury, such as a sunburn (Figure 16.6).

Chapter 16: Hand, Foot, and Mouth Disease (HFMD) and Other Enteroviral Exanthems

▶ Temporary Beau lines (ie, transverse grooves in the nail plate) or nail shedding (onychomadesis) (Figure 16.7) may occur a few weeks to a few months after HFMD, presumably because of nail matrix arrest; these secondary changes are common after atypical HFMD.

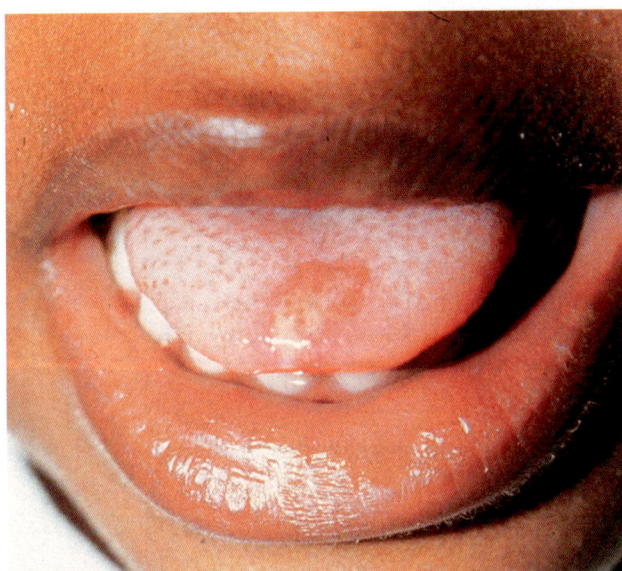

Figure 16.1. Ulcers may occur on the tongue or buccal mucosae in hand, foot, and mouth disease.

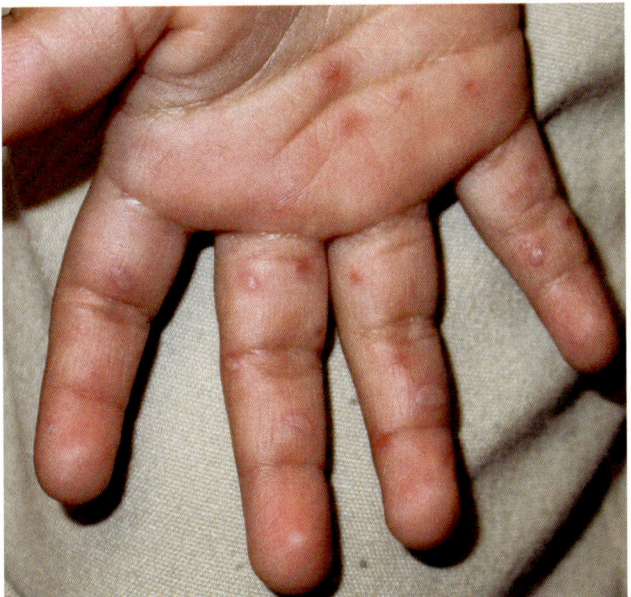

Figure 16.2. Oval vesicles with surrounding erythema on the hand of a child who has hand, foot, and mouth disease.

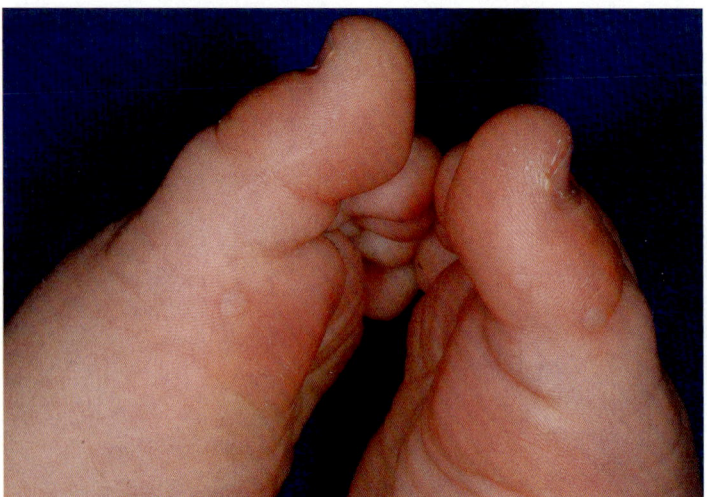

Figure 16.3. Hand, foot, and mouth disease. Oval vesicles with mild surrounding erythema.

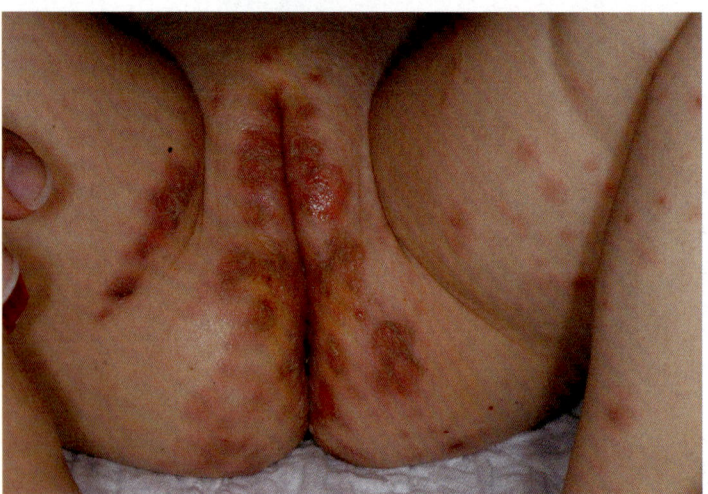

Figure 16.4. Ruptured bullae and large erosions in a young girl with atypical hand, foot, and mouth disease.

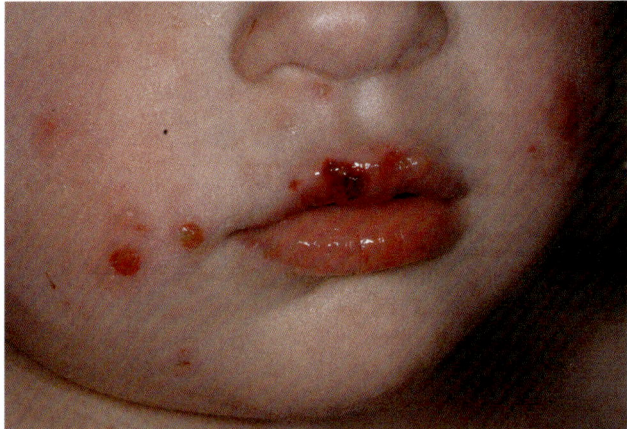

Figure 16.5. Perioral vesicles and erosions in a toddler with atypical hand, foot, and mouth disease.

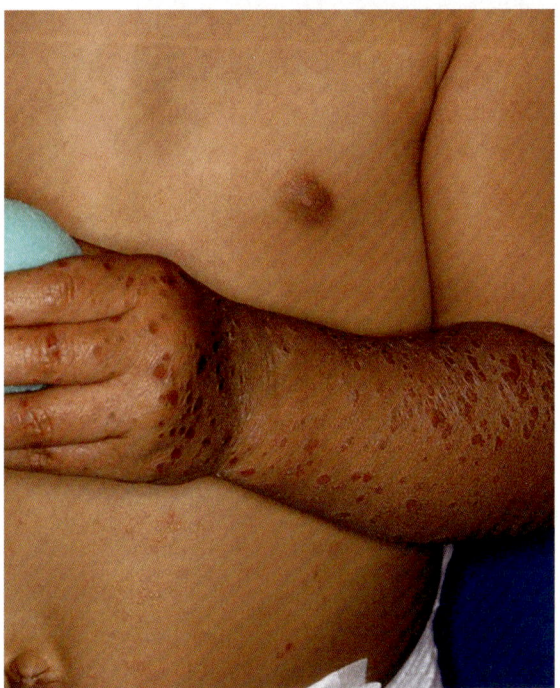

Figure 16.6. Eczema coxsackium. Crusted erosions and flattened vesicles overlying lichenified plaques of eczema on the left arm.

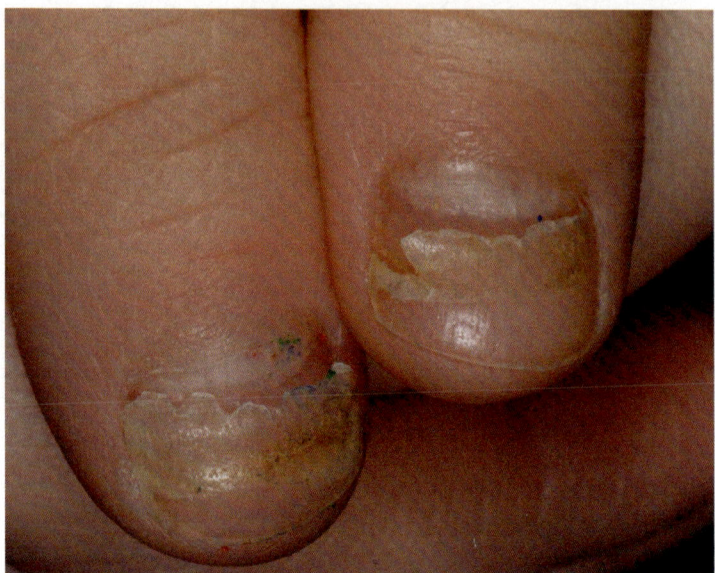

Figure 16.7. Onychomadesis (nail shedding) after hand, foot, and mouth disease in an otherwise healthy 4-year-old.

Herpangina

- Enanthem with painful tiny vesicles and punched-out erosions.
- Distributed on soft palate, uvula, tonsillar pillars, and posterior pharynx.
- Erosions typically have a rim of erythema and a yellowish gray coating.
- Fever and sore throat are common; 25% may have abdominal pain, vomiting.
- Erosions persist for approximately 7 days.

Eruptive Pseudoangiomatosis

- Acute onset of multiple, small (2–4 mm), bright red (hemangioma-like) papules with a rim of blanching.
- Lesions blanch with pressure.
- Preceding or concurrent fever, headache, upper respiratory symptoms may be present.
- Lesions resolve spontaneously over 1 to 2 weeks without treatment.

How to Make the Diagnosis

- Diagnosis of HFMD, herpangina, and eruptive pseudoangiomatosis is usually made clinically.
- Although rarely necessary, a specific diagnosis of enteroviral infections may be made with viral culture, serological testing, or polymerase chain reaction–based testing of lesional swabs, nasopharyngeal swabs, blood, stool, or urine.
- Viral polymerase chain reaction testing or direct fluorescent examination for herpes simplex virus is relatively rapid and may be clinically helpful to distinguish these infections from atypical HFMD, eczema coxsackium, or the oral erosions of herpangina.
- Skin biopsy may be necessary to distinguish eruptive pseudoangiomatosis from other vascular lesions if the process is not resolving spontaneously as expected.

Treatment

- Generally, simple supportive measures (ie, oral fluids, analgesics, and antipyretics) are adequate for HFMD and herpangina.
- Severe pain may require more aggressive pain management; hospitalization for intravenous hydration and narcotic analgesics occasionally is required.
- Eruptive pseudoangiomatosis usually requires no therapy.

Look-alikes

Disorder	Differentiating Features
Typical Hand, Foot, and Mouth Disease	
The typical appearance and distribution of lesions usually prevents confusion with other disorders.	
Atypical Hand, Foot, and Mouth Disease	
Eczema herpeticum	• Uniform, punched-out heme-crusted erosions in areas of atopic dermatitis predominate. • Viral test result positive for herpes simplex virus.
Varicella	• Less common in era of universal vaccination. • Crops of lesions in varying stages (papules, vesicles, crusts) are seen.
Bullous impetigo	• Flaccid blisters and superficial erosions with peripheral collarette of blister roof. • Honey-colored crusts may or may not be present. • Predominance of lesions around the nose, hands, diaper area. • Bacterial culture positive for *Staphylococcus aureus*.
Allergic contact dermatitis	• Localized erythema, papules, and vesicles in a geometric pattern consistent with an external cause. • Itch (often severe) very common.
Autoimmune blistering disorders	• Uncommon. • Progressive and unremitting without immunosuppressive therapy.
Herpangina	
Herpes gingivostomatitis	• Blisters and erosions commonly involve the perioral skin as well as oral mucosa.
Aphthous ulcer (canker sores)	• Usually a chronic or recurring problem. • Fever and other symptoms of herpangina typically lacking. • In severe disease (recurrent major aphthous ulcer), ulcers larger than 1 cm may develop.
Eruptive Pseudoangiomatosis	
Infantile hemangioma	• Appears in the first weeks to month after birth and gradually involutes over several years. • Typically solitary, although a diffuse pattern of numerous small lesions can occur.
Pyogenic granuloma	• Friable, red vascular papule that bleeds easily with minor trauma. • Typically solitary.
Bacillary angiomatosis	• Occurs in individuals who are immunocompromised, most often in the setting of HIV infection.

Prognosis

- The prognosis for HFMD, herpangina, and eruptive pseudoangiomatosis is excellent; all typically resolve without sequelae.
- Typical nail regrowth is the norm after enteroviral onychomadesis.

When to Worry or Refer

- If the diagnosis is in question or lesions are persistent or recurrent.
- Consider hospitalization if fluid intake is inadequate or dehydration is suspected or when pain control at home is inadequate.
- Because enteroviruses are a major cause of meningitis in summer and fall, neck stiffness, lethargy, or severe irritability should prompt a thorough evaluation.

Resources for Families

- American Academy of Pediatrics: HealthyChildren.org.
  https://www.healthychildren.org/HandFootMouth
- Centers for Disease Control and Prevention: Alphabetical listing of diseases and conditions provides information for families.
  www.cdc.gov/hand-foot-mouth/index.html

CHAPTER 17

Measles

Introduction/Etiology/Epidemiology

- Acute febrile illness caused by measles virus, an RNA virus of the genus *Morbillivirus* in the Paramyxoviridae family.
- Humans are the only natural host.
- Transmitted by direct contact with infectious droplets or, less commonly, by airborne spread.
- Immunization program in the United States, started in 1963, resulted in more than 99% decrease in reported incidence. Two vaccine doses are needed to ensure protection.
- Noteworthy increase in measles cases occurred in the United States from 1989 to 1991 as a result of low immunization rates in preschool-aged children, especially in urban areas.
- Indigenous cases became markedly less common until recently, when increasing numbers of cases began to be observed; 222 cases were reported to the Centers for Disease Control and Prevention in 2011, and 1,282 cases were reported in 2019. Case numbers decreased during the COVID-19 pandemic, likely related to decreased travel.
- Because of several significant outbreaks, the first 9 months of 2019 saw the highest number of measles cases in the United States recorded since 1992. Most cases occurred in persons who were unvaccinated.
- Vaccine failure occurs in up to 5% of children who receive a single dose of vaccine at 12 months or older.
- Patients are contagious from 1 to 2 days before the onset of symptoms (3–5 days before the rash) and up to 4 days after the appearance of the rash.
- Incubation period is 10 to 14 days from exposure to onset of symptoms.
- Classically occurs in the winter and spring; sporadic cases can occur year-round.

Signs and Symptoms

- Prodrome of high fever, cough, coryza, conjunctivitis, and enanthem precedes the exanthem by 2 to 4 days.
- Characteristic enanthem: Koplik spots.
  - Appear during the prodromal phase and fade 2 to 3 days after onset of exanthem.
  - White or bluish gray punctate papules superimposed on an erythematous base, located on buccal mucosa, often adjacent to molars (Figure 17.1).
- Exanthem begins behind the ears and at the scalp margin, rapidly spreading downward to involve most of the body (cephalocaudal spread).
- Discrete erythematous papules and macules appear and gradually become confluent (Figure 17.2).
- Pruritus is uncommon.
- Eruption lasts 4 to 7 days before fading, often with fine desquamation.
- Generalized adenopathy and splenomegaly may occur with the exanthem.
- *Modified measles* may occur in infants with residual maternal antibody or in individuals who were previously vaccinated.
  - Less severe illness.
  - Shortened prodrome.
  - Exanthem less confluent.
  - Koplik spots may be absent.
- *Atypical measles* previously occurred in those who received killed measles vaccine (which has not been used for many years) and then were exposed to wild-type measles virus. It presents as a syndrome with high fever; abdominal pain; nodular pulmonary lesions; severe headache; and an acral (ie, distal extremities, hands, feet) eruption with vesicular, vesiculopustular, or purpuric lesions.

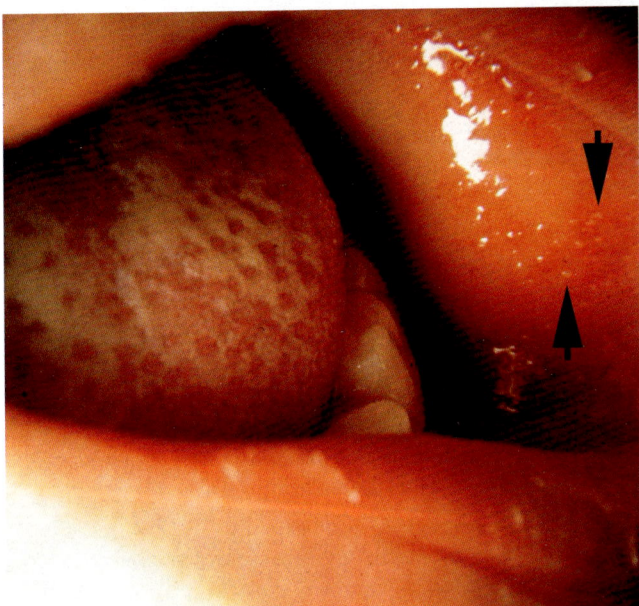

Figure 17.1. Koplik spots (arrows): punctate whitish gray papules on an erythematous base that appear on the buccal mucosa.

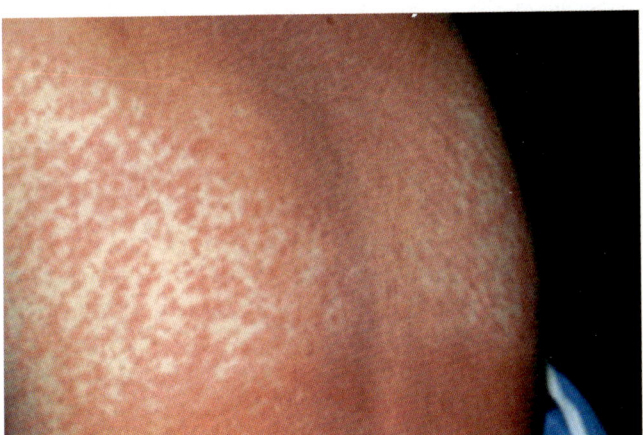

Figure 17.2. Measles produces an erythematous macular and papular eruption.

Look-alikes

A number of viral exanthems may mimic the rash of measles; however, the typical symptoms of measles are lacking.

Disorder	Differentiating Features
Exanthematous drug eruption	• History of drug exposure.
Rubella	• Patients generally well with slight fever, arthralgias, or arthritis. • Posterior cervical, suboccipital, or postauricular lymphadenopathy common. • Rash typically lighter in color.
Roseola	• Patients often appear well and lack typical symptoms of measles (ie, cough, conjunctivitis, and coryza). • Characteristic history of high fever followed by abrupt defervescence (which coincides with onset of exanthem).
Erythema infectiosum	• Patients appear well. • Slapped cheek appearance and presence of a lacy, reticulated erythematous eruption.
Infectious mononucleosis	• Patients exhibit sore throat and malaise; exudative pharyngitis noted at examination. • Conjunctivitis absent. • Exanthem classically exacerbated by receipt of antibiotics in the penicillin class.
Kawasaki disease	• Lymphadenopathy, fissuring of lips, and acral edema prominent. • Cough and coryza uncommon symptoms. • Exanthem (especially desquamation) often accentuated in perineum. • Bacille Calmette-Guérin vaccination site may develop edema, erythema, crusting.
Rocky Mountain spotted fever	• May mimic atypical measles. • Headache is a prominent symptom; history of a tick bite may be elicited. • Rash spreads centripetally.
Meningococcemia	• May mimic atypical measles. • Patients seriously ill. • Purpura widespread (not limited to acral areas).
Papular-purpuric gloves-and-socks syndrome	• May mimic atypical measles. • Characteristically petechial or purpuric erythema of palms and soles with sharp demarcation at wrists and ankles.
COVID-19	• Multiple possible rash morphologies, including morbilliform (measles-like), but also urticarial, vesicular, petechial, pseudo-chilblains, and vaso-occlusive or ischemic. • Other features of SARS-CoV-2 infection usually present; may be history of known exposure. • Antigen or polymerase chain reaction test results positive for SARS-CoV-2.

How to Make the Diagnosis

- The diagnosis is made clinically based on typical symptoms and physical findings (eg, Koplik spots).
- The diagnosis may be confirmed by any 1 of the following:
  - Measles immunoglobulin (Ig) M antibody.
  - Polymerase chain reaction–based assays (specifically reverse transcriptase polymerase chain reaction). This and measles IgM are the diagnostic methods of choice.
  - Fourfold or greater increase in measles IgG antibody titers in paired acute and convalescent specimens.
  - Isolation of measles virus in cell culture from urine, blood, or nasopharyngeal secretions.
  - All suspected or confirmed measles cases should be reported to local public health agencies.

Treatment

- No specific antiviral therapy is available. Ribavirin has been used in patients who are severely ill or immunocompromised.
- Vitamin A treatment in children with measles in resource-limited countries has been associated with decreased morbidity and mortality rates.
- In patients who are hospitalized, airborne isolation is recommended until 4 days after onset of the exanthem in children who are otherwise healthy and for the duration of illness in patients who are immunocompromised.

Prognosis

- Usually good with supportive care.
- Complications include bacterial otitis media, secondary bacterial pneumonia, laryngotracheobronchitis, thrombocytopenia, hepatitis, and diarrhea.
- Rare complications include encephalitis (including subacute sclerosing panencephalitis, which may occur years after infection), myocarditis, pericarditis, acute glomerulonephritis, and Stevens-Johnson syndrome.
- Young infants, children who are malnourished, children with immunodeficiencies, and pregnant patients are at highest risk of complications.

When to Worry or Refer

- Consultation with a pediatric infectious disease specialist is recommended if the diagnosis is in question.
- Pregnant patients exposed to measles should consult their obstetric health professional.

Resources for Families

- American Academy of Pediatrics: HealthyChildren.org.
  https://www.healthychildren.org/Measles
- Centers for Disease Control and Prevention: Alphabetical listing of diseases and conditions provides information for families in English and Spanish.
  www.cdc.gov/measles/index.html
- MedlinePlus: Information for patients and families (in English and Spanish) sponsored by the US National Library of Medicine and National Institutes of Health.
  https://www.nlm.nih.gov/medlineplus/measles.html

CHAPTER 18

Papular-Purpuric Gloves-and-Socks Syndrome (PPGSS)

Introduction/Etiology/Epidemiology

- Caused by any of multiple viral agents, although parvovirus B19 is the most common cause.
- Other reported etiologic associations include human herpesvirus 6, human herpesvirus 7, measles virus, and cytomegalovirus.
- Most often affects young adults but has occurred in children.
- Most common during the spring and summer.
- There appear to be epidemiologically relevant differences between the immune response to parvovirus B19 in papular-purpuric gloves-and-socks syndrome (PPGSS) compared with that in patients with erythema infectiosum.
  - Clearance of viremia correlates with appearance of the rash in erythema infectiosum, such that patients with the skin eruption are not considered contagious.
  - The eruption of PPGSS seems to coincide with viremia; therefore, patients with clinical findings should be considered potentially infectious.

Signs and Symptoms

- Rapidly progressive erythema and edema of the palms and soles (Figure 18.1), with progression to a petechial or purpuric appearance with sharp demarcation at the wrists and ankles.
- Lesions may also occur on the elbows, knees, buttocks, and dorsal surfaces of the hands and feet.
- Associated symptoms include low-grade fever, malaise, myalgias, anorexia, and joint pain.

- ► Patients often report pruritus, burning discomfort, or pain at sites of involvement.
- ► Associated enanthem presents as vesicles and small erosions on the palate, posterior pharynx, tongue, and mucosal surfaces of the lips.
- ► Lymphadenopathy occurs in 16% of patients.

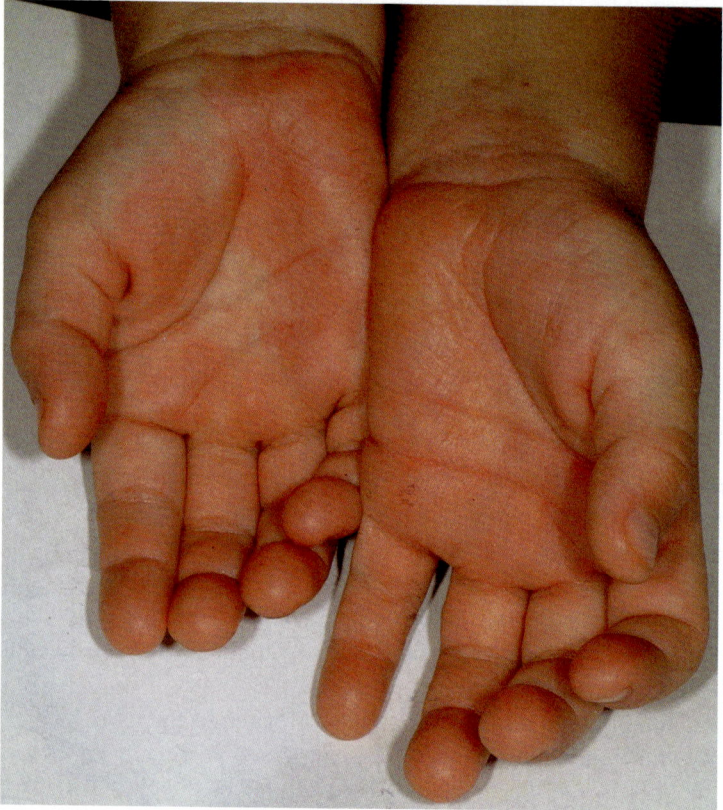

Figure 18.1. Erythema and edema of the palms early in the course of papular-purpuric gloves-and-socks syndrome.

Look-alikes

Disorder	Differentiating Features
Cutaneous vasculitis	• Purpuric papules or nodules (ie, palpable purpura). • Widespread, not typically limited to the hands and feet (although there may be preferential involvement of the lower extremities).
Rocky Mountain spotted fever	• Patients acutely ill with fever and severe headache. • Lesions spread centripetally to involve the arms, legs, and trunk (ie, do not remain limited to the hands and feet). • History of a tick bite may be elicited.
Meningococcemia	• Patients acutely ill with fever and malaise. • Purpura usually not limited to the hands and feet. • Areas of purpura may develop blistering and/or become necrotic.
Hand, foot, and mouth disease	• Round or oval deep-seated vesicles with surrounding erythema. • Petechiae and purpura absent.

How to Make the Diagnosis

▶ The diagnosis is made clinically based on the characteristic appearance and distribution of the eruption.

▶ Measurement of serum anti-parvovirus B19 immunoglobulin M and/or polymerase chain reaction studies may be useful in B19-associated cases if the diagnosis is in question.

Treatment

▶ Supportive care with symptom treatment for pruritus.
▶ No specific therapy is available.

Prognosis

▶ Spontaneous resolution usually occurs over 1 to 2 weeks.

▶ Exposed pregnant women should be advised to contact their obstetric health professional to discuss potential risks and be offered serological testing. If acute infection is confirmed, serial fetal ultrasonography should be considered to monitor for fetal hydrops, congestive heart failure, and intrauterine growth restriction.

When to Worry or Refer

- ▶ Consultation with a pediatric dermatologist or infectious disease specialist is indicated when the diagnosis is uncertain.
- ▶ Pregnant women exposed to or who have acquired human parvovirus B19 infection should consult their obstetric health professional (as discussed previously).

CHAPTER 19

Roseola Infantum (Exanthem Subitum)

Introduction/Etiology/Epidemiology

- Caused by human herpesvirus (HHV) 6 in most cases, occasionally HHV-7.
- Usually affects infants and children between 6 months and 3 years of age (peak age: 6–7 months).
- Occurs throughout the year but may be more common in the spring and fall.
- Transmission is airborne via respiratory droplets.
- Incubation period is 9 to 10 days.
- After primary infection, the virus becomes latent and may reactivate with weakened immune status.

Signs and Symptoms

- The hallmark finding is a high fever (38.3°C to 41.1°C [101°F to 106°F]) without a rash that lasts for 3 to 5 days in an otherwise well-appearing or sometimes irritable infant.
- The exanthem of roseola typically occurs within 1 to 2 days after defervescence.
- Rose pink macules and papules on the neck and trunk (Figure 19.1) are characteristic; the rash also may involve the extremities and face.
- A faint halo of blanching may be seen surrounding each individual lesion.
- An enanthem with red papules on the soft palate and uvula (referred to as *Nagayama spots* or *uvulopalatoglossal spots*) occurs in two-thirds of cases.
- Associated findings may include pharyngitis, tonsillitis, periorbital edema, and lymphadenopathy (occipital, postauricular, or posterior cervical).

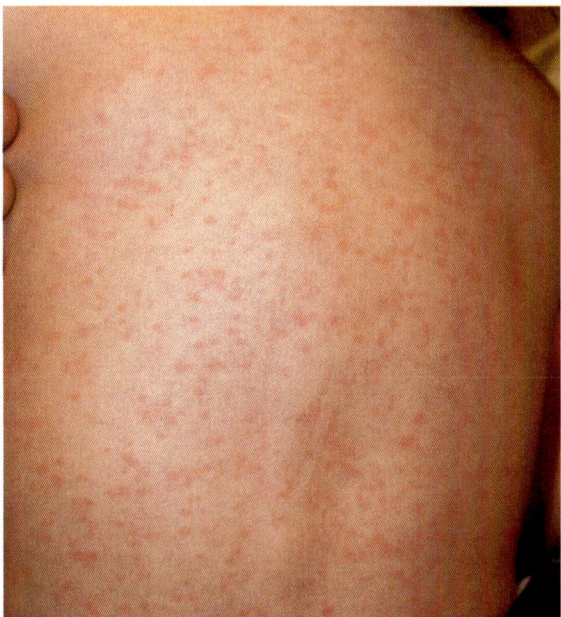

Figure 19.1. Roseola infantum. Erythematous macules and papules in an infant who developed the eruption after several days of high fever.

- Neurologic complications of HHV-6 or HHV-7 infection can occur, including febrile seizures and, rarely, encephalitis.
- Reactivation of disease in immunocompromised hosts may be asymptomatic or present with rash, fever, encephalitis, pneumonitis, hepatitis, and bone marrow suppression.

Look-alikes
- A variety of viral agents, including enteroviruses, adenoviruses, parvovirus B19, rubella, rotavirus, and parainfluenza virus, may cause a clinical picture similar in appearance to that of roseola. The appearance of the rash after defervescence is characteristic of roseola.
- Acute graft-versus-host disease in recipients of stem cell transplants may have a similar presentation.

How to Make the Diagnosis

- Characteristic clinical findings in the appropriate age group, with an exanthem after high fever, are highly suggestive of the diagnosis.
- Laboratory confirmation is usually unnecessary; in atypical or questionable cases in which it is indicated, specific serological and polymerase chain reaction testing are available.

Treatment

- Most cases require only supportive care.
- Patients who are immunocompromised may warrant consideration for antiviral therapy; ganciclovir, foscarnet, and cidofovir have been used. Referral to a pediatric infectious disease specialist is indicated in this setting.

Prognosis

- Roseola infantum typically resolves without sequelae.

When to Worry or Refer

- Consult a pediatric infectious disease specialist if patient is immunocompromised.

Resources for Families

- American Academy of Pediatrics: HealthyChildren.org.
  https://www.healthychildren.org/roseola
- WebMD: Information for families is contained in Skin Problems and Treatments.
  www.webmd.com/skin-problems-and-treatments/tc/roseola-topic-overview

- A characteristic (but not specific) enanthem, Forchheimer spots, may present with erythematous and petechial macules on the soft palate.
- Patient usually appears well, but associated pharyngitis and arthritis may be present; the latter may last for several months.
- Fever is usually absent in young children.
- Rare complications include encephalitis, myocarditis, pericarditis, hepatitis, anemia, thrombocytopenia, and neutropenia.

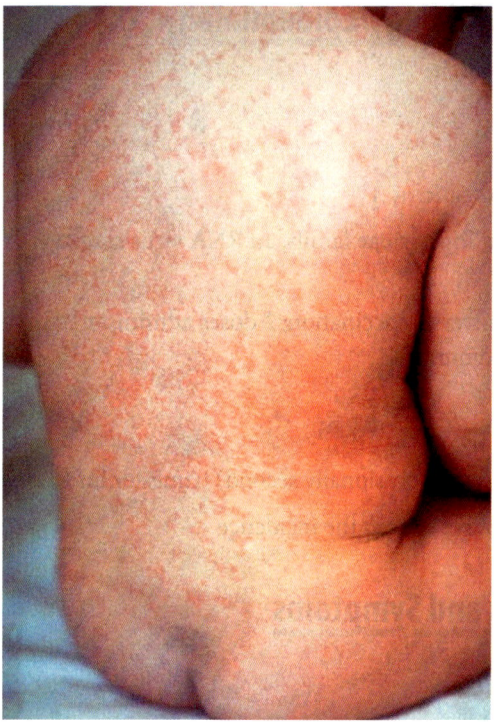

Figure 20.1. An erythematous macular eruption occurs in rubella.

Congenital Rubella

- Neonate may present with disseminated bluish purple papules and nodules ("blueberry muffin" rash) (Figure 20.2) and thrombocytopenia, typically within the first days of life.
- Neonatal hepatitis with jaundice can occur.
- Embryopathy: deafness, congenital heart defects, cataracts, pigmentary retinopathy, glaucoma, intrauterine growth restriction, and developmental delay.

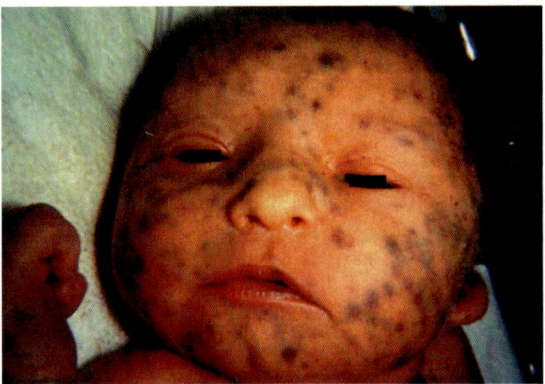

Figure 20.2. Bluish purple nodular eruption ("blueberry muffin" rash) in a newborn with congenital rubella infection.

Look-alikes

Disorder	Differentiating Features
Classic Rubella	
Measles (rubeola)	• Patients ill with fever, cough, coryza, and conjunctivitis. • Exanthem more intensely red.
Enteroviral infection	• May have characteristic clinical syndrome (eg, hand, foot, and mouth disease). • Eruption may have a petechial component. • Posterior cervical and suboccipital lymphadenopathy uncommon.
Infectious mononucleosis	• Patient ill with fever, pharyngitis, malaise.
Exanthematous drug eruption	• History of drug exposure. • Posterior cervical and suboccipital lymphadenopathy are typically absent.
Congenital Rubella	
Cytomegalovirus infection	• Cataracts (present in congenital rubella) absent.
Toxoplasmosis	• Infants often asymptomatic.
Congenital syphilis	• Infants have rhinorrhea (often bloody), condylomata lata (flat-topped papules and plaques located at mucocutaneous junctions, including the perineum and angles of the mouth), and scaly, copper-colored papules and plaques. • Exanthem may be vesiculobullous, often involves palms and soles.
Herpes simplex virus infection	• Typical skin lesions often present (eg, clustered vesicles on an erythematous base).
Congenital thrombocytopenia (eg, Wiskott-Aldrich syndrome, neonatal thrombocytopenia)	• Petechiae may be present, but hepatosplenomegaly, cataracts, intrauterine growth retardation, and other features of congenital rubella syndrome are absent.

How to Make the Diagnosis

- The rash of rubella is nonspecific; a clinical diagnosis of rubella cannot be confirmed.
- Congenital rubella syndrome should be considered in a newborn with "blueberry muffin" lesions and 1 or more characteristic findings of embryopathy, including congenital cataracts, deafness, cardiac defects, thrombocytopenia, hepatosplenomegaly, or microcephaly.
- Diagnostic tests available for rubella include
  - Viral culture from nasal mucosa swabs.
  - Viral culture from urine, cerebrospinal fluid, tissue, or nasopharyngeal swabs in congenital rubella.
  - Serological testing for rubella immunoglobulin (Ig) M antibodies or a fourfold or greater increase in IgG antibodies in paired acute and convalescent specimens may be helpful. On the day of rash onset, only 50% of patients will have positive rubella IgM results; more than 90% of cases will be IgM positive by 5 days after rash onset. In congenital rubella, IgM remains positive for several months.
  - Polymerase chain reaction–based assays available.

Treatment

- No specific therapy available.
- Supportive care includes use of nonsteroidal anti-inflammatory agents for arthritis.
- Children who are affected should avoid contact with pregnant women and should be excluded from school until 7 days after onset of the rash.
- Multidisciplinary care is recommended for congenital rubella (including ophthalmology, cardiology, and developmental pediatrics).

Prognosis

- Rubella is typically a self-limited illness.
- Arthritis may last for several months.
- The prognosis for congenital rubella syndrome is guarded and depends on the extent of involvement.

When to Worry or Refer

- ▶ Referral may be warranted if the diagnosis is in question.
- ▶ Pregnant women potentially exposed to rubella should consult an infectious disease specialist and their obstetric health professional.

Resources for Families

- ▶ American Academy of Pediatrics: HealthyChildren.org.
  https://www.healthychildren.org/rubella
- ▶ Centers for Disease Control and Prevention: Alphabetical listing of diseases and conditions provides information for families in English and Spanish.
  www.cdc.gov/rubella/index.html
- ▶ MedlinePlus: Information for patients and families (in English and Spanish) sponsored by the US National Library of Medicine and National Institutes of Health.
  https://www.nlm.nih.gov/medlineplus/rubella.html

CHAPTER 21

Unilateral Laterothoracic Exanthem (ULE)

Introduction/Etiology/Epidemiology

- An uncommon exanthem that was rediscovered in 1992 and 1993 and correlated with earlier published reports.
- Also known as asymmetric periflexural exanthem of childhood.
- Etiology unknown but seems most likely to be a viral exanthem.
- Mean age of reported patients is 2 years.

Signs and Symptoms

- Onset of the eruption often preceded by low-grade fever and mild gastrointestinal or upper respiratory symptoms.
- Most patients develop a unilateral red, patchy exanthem on the trunk with extension toward the axilla (Figure 21.1).
- In some, the rash may begin on the lower abdomen, in the inguinal region, or on an extremity (Figure 21.2).
- Lesional morphology is variable, including morbilliform, scarlatiniform, urticarial, vesicular, reticulated, and purpuric patterns.
- Pruritus is common, but secondary bacterial superinfection is rare.
- Exanthem often generalizes to bilateral involvement but usually maintains a unilateral predominance on initial side of involvement.
- Spontaneous resolution begins during the third week and can be associated with fine desquamation and postinflammatory pigmentary changes. The eruption may persist for up to 2 months before resolving.

162 PEDIATRIC DERMATOLOGY

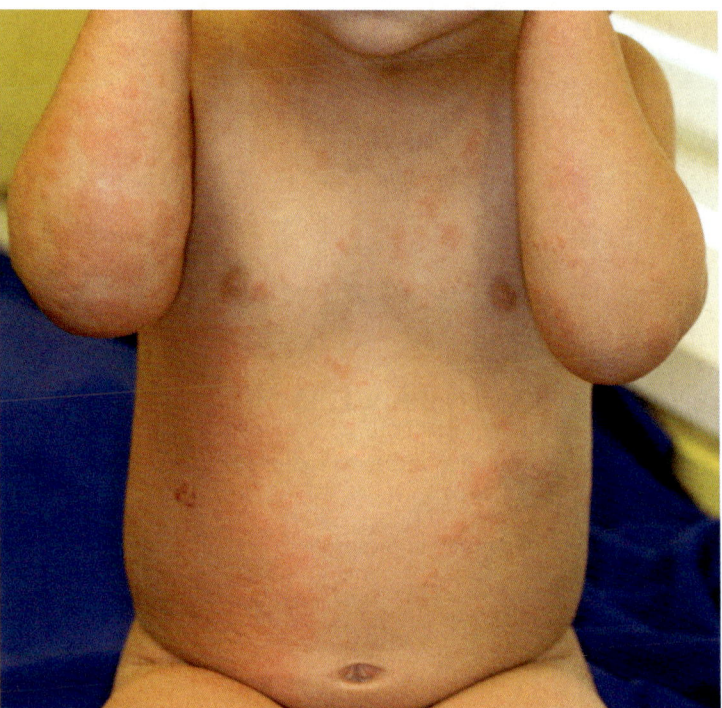

Figure 21.1. Unilateral laterothoracic exanthem. Erythematous papules coalescing into plaques on the trunk and upper extremities; note a predominance on the right side, which was the initial side of involvement.

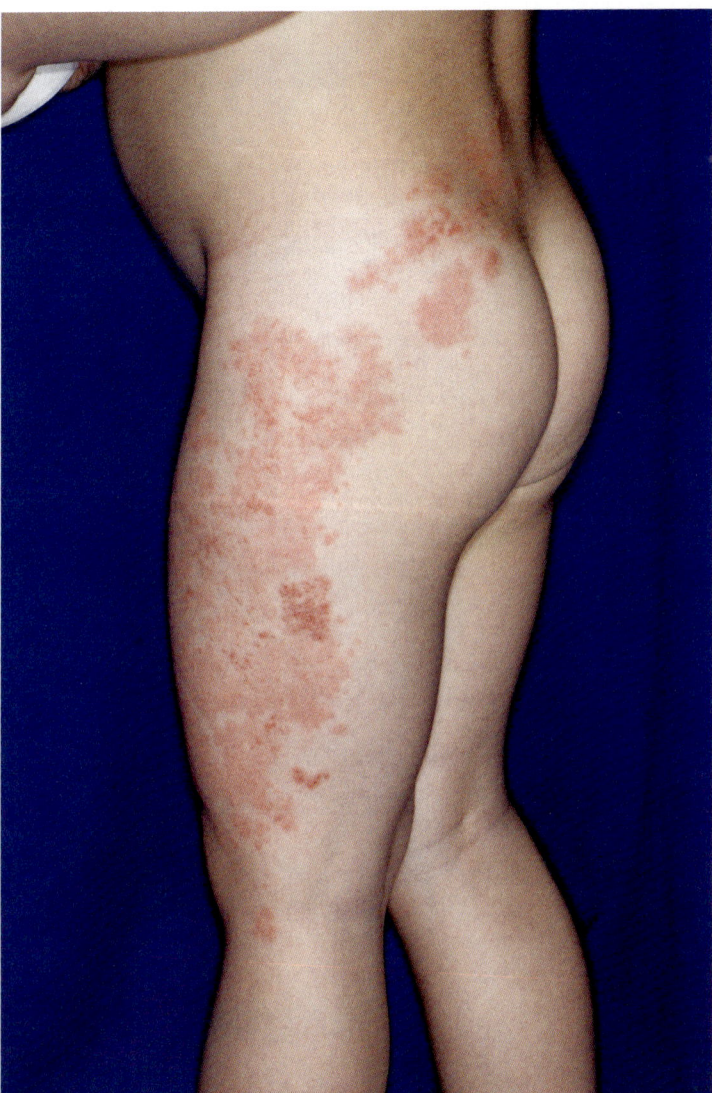

Figure 21.2. Unilateral laterothoracic exanthem. In this young child, the eruption began predominantly on the lower extremity, as seen here.

Look-alikes

Disorder	Differentiating Features
Contact dermatitis	• May be difficult to distinguish from early unilateral laterothoracic exanthem (ULE). • History of exposure to an allergen may be obtained. • Does not generalize as typically seen in ULE.
Papular eczema	• Eruption typically is symmetrically distributed (not unilateral) and often involves the extremities. • History of atopic dermatitis may be elicited.
Tinea corporis	• Annular papules and plaques that have an elevated, scaly border and central clearing. • Usually more localized than ULE.
Pityriasis rosea	• Eruption symmetrically distributed on the trunk (not unilateral). • Typical lesions are oval, thin plaques with long axes oriented parallel to lines of skin stress. • Trailing scale (free edge points inward) is present.
Gianotti-Crosti syndrome	• Concentrated on the cheeks, upper extremities, knees, and buttocks with relative sparing of the trunk.

How to Make the Diagnosis

▶ The diagnosis is made clinically on the basis of the unilateral clinical presentation (or history of unilateral onset), with eventual generalization and prolonged course.

Treatment

▶ Topical corticosteroids or oral antihistamines may be useful for pruritus but will not alter the natural history of the eruption.

Prognosis

▶ Spontaneous resolution (in 3–8 weeks) without sequelae is typical.

When to Worry or Refer

▶ Consider referral when the diagnosis is in question.

Resource for Families

▶ DermNet NZ: Laterothoracic exanthem.
https://www.dermnetnz.org/topics/laterothoracic-exanthem

CHAPTER
22

Varicella

Introduction/Etiology/Epidemiology

- Acute febrile illness caused by varicella-zoster virus, a double-stranded DNA virus of the Herpesviridae family.
- Humans are the only natural host of varicella-zoster virus.
- Highly contagious disease of childhood transmitted by person-to-person contact; airborne spread has been documented.
- Immunization with a live, attenuated virus vaccine has been available in the United States since 1995 and is highly effective. Incidence dropped dramatically since that time, but outbreaks still occur owing to undervaccination. Mild forms can also occur in those who have been vaccinated.
- Incubation period typically is 14 to 16 days (range, 10–21 days) from exposure to onset of symptoms.
- Infections usually occurred during the winter and spring in the pre-vaccine era; cases now may occur year-round without notable seasonality.

Signs and Symptoms

- Vesicular exanthem that usually begins on the scalp or trunk.
- Lesions may appear in crops and may first appear as red macules, which quickly develop a surface vesicle (Figure 22.1).
- Individual lesions appear as a clear vesicle on an erythematous base ("dewdrop on a rose petal").
- The lesions usually crust within hours to days and then begin to heal gradually.
- The exanthem spreads centrifugally, so fresh vesicles may be seen on the extremities, with older crusted lesions on the trunk. Lesions in varying stages of development are characteristic of varicella (Figure 22.2).

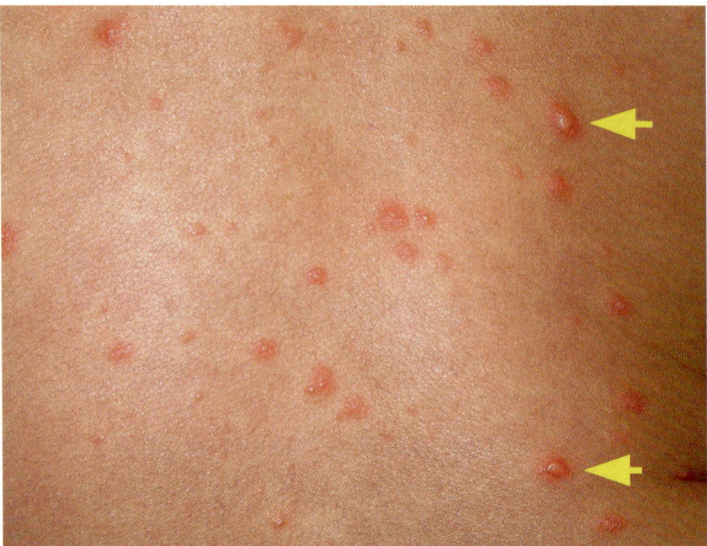

Figure 22.1. Varicella. Typical vesicles ("dewdrop on a rose petal") are present (arrows).

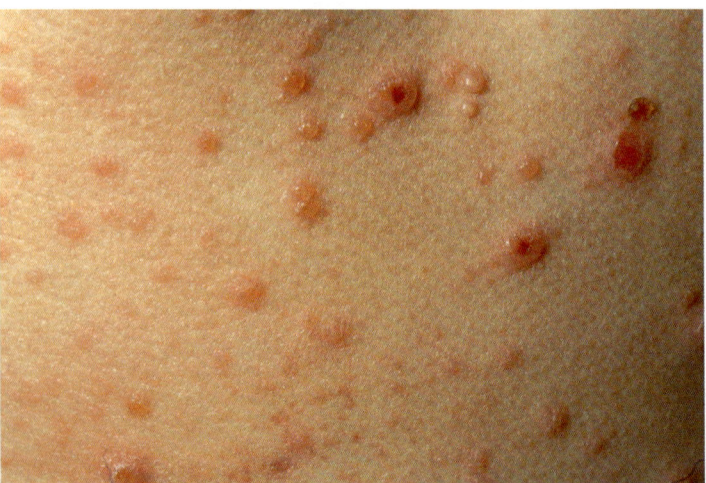

Figure 22.2. In varicella, lesions are in different stages of development. This patient demonstrates papules, vesicles, and crusts.

- Increased numbers of lesions may be seen in areas of skin injury or irritation (eg, atopic dermatitis sites, areas of sunburn).
- Low-grade fever and malaise are typical; more severe disease may occur in adolescents, adults, and individuals who are immunocompromised.
- Pruritus is common and sometimes severe.

▶ Complications include staphylococcal and streptococcal superinfection of skin lesions, pneumonia, encephalitis, and purpura fulminans. Streptococcal superinfection usually presents with a reappearance of fever in the patient who is several days into the illness. Reye syndrome (liver dysfunction and neurologic symptoms) may occur in children taking salicylates.

▶ Chickenpox occurring in a person who has previously received the varicella vaccine generally is a milder illness than in a child who is unvaccinated, with fewer lesions (<50), lower fever, and shorter disease duration.

Look-alikes

Disorder	Differentiating Features
Hand, foot, and mouth disease (HFMD)	• Eruption concentrated on the hands, feet, and buttocks (is not typically generalized, although in recent years a more severe and diffuse form of HFMD has been observed; see below). • Oval vesicles with a rim of erythema (classic appearance of "dewdrop on a rose petal") are lacking.
Other enteroviral exanthems	• Erythematous macules and papules that may mimic early varicella; petechiae may be present. • Severe form of HFMD may present with widespread vesicles or bullae; lesions tend to predominate on distal extremities, anogenital region, and face; in some instances, involvement may be concentrated at sites of preceding atopic dermatitis (so-called eczema coxsackium).
Herpes simplex virus infection	• Clustered (not single) vesicles on an erythematous base. • Eruption typically localized, not generalized.
Bullous insect bite reaction	• Eruption not generalized. • Lower extremities most often involved. • Constitutional symptoms absent.
Rickettsialpox	• Black eschar at site of primary mite bite. • Absence of vesicles with the appearance of a dewdrop on a rose petal.
Disseminated herpes zoster (shingles)	• Occurs in patients who are immunocompromised. • Reactivation of varicella-zoster virus may cause dissemination beyond dermatomal borders, with visceral involvement.
Smallpox (variola)	• Rash begins on face and rapidly spreads to the distal extremities; later involves the trunk (ie, centripetal distribution, unlike centrifugal distribution seen in varicella). • Vesicles and pustules are deep-seated and firm (not fragile as in varicella). • All lesions are simultaneously in the same stage of development.

How to Make the Diagnosis

- Characteristic clinical features of lesional morphology, distribution, and progression usually suggest the diagnosis of varicella.
- Laboratory testing is rarely necessary in uncomplicated disease. If testing is required, the following tests may be available:
  - Vesicular fluid or crusts sent for polymerase chain reaction (PCR) testing. This is the preferred method owing to superior sensitivity and specificity.
  - Scrapings of the base of intact vesicles with direct fluorescent antibody examination provide rapid diagnosis, but sensitivity is inferior to that of PCR.
  - Viral culture from skin lesions can be performed, but sensitivity is limited compared with that of PCR, and results may take several days.
  - Fourfold increase in titer in serum varicella immunoglobulin G antibody between acute and convalescent samples can confirm diagnosis retrospectively, but this method is seldom used or indicated.

Treatment

- In children who are immunocompetent, supportive care is directed at measures to reduce itching and prevent secondary bacterial skin infection.
- Antipruritic lotions with menthol, camphor, colloidal oatmeal, or calamine are helpful, as are antihistamines administered orally.
- Once- to twice-daily baths and trimming of fingernails will minimize trauma from scratching (and risk of secondary bacterial superinfection).
- Oral acyclovir can reduce the duration and severity of varicella in children who are otherwise healthy, if initiated within the first 24 hours of rash. It is not recommended for routine use in children who are otherwise healthy but is indicated for those at risk of serious disease, including those older than 12 years; with chronic cutaneous or pulmonary disease; receiving long-term salicylate therapy; and receiving short, intermittent, or aerosolized steroid therapy. Consult the current edition of *Red Book®: Report of the Committee on Infectious Diseases* **(https://redbook.solutions.aap.org)** for guidelines.
- Secondary bacterial infections, most often caused by *Staphylococcus aureus* or *Streptococcus pyogenes*, should be treated with a systemic antibiotic on the basis of local susceptibility patterns.

Prognosis

- Children who are healthy typically recover uneventfully, and scarring is rare.
- Children with uncomplicated chickenpox who have been excluded from school or child care may return when all lesions have crusted. Persons who are immunized who have not developed crusting may return when no new lesions have appeared in the last 24 hours.
- Permanent cutaneous scars are possible, especially in areas of secondary infection.

When to Worry or Refer

- Varicella lesions may become secondarily infected with *S aureus* or *S pyogenes*; these should be managed appropriately. Such infections may progress rapidly and require prompt treatment and close follow-up. Hospitalization is sometimes necessary.
- Individuals who are immunocompromised, infants, adolescents, adults, pregnant people, and individuals with chronic pulmonary or cutaneous conditions are at risk of severe disease. If exposed to varicella, they should be treated in consultation with a pediatric infectious disease specialist. Postexposure prophylaxis is available and effective if initiated promptly.

Resources for Families

- American Academy of Pediatrics: HealthyChildren.org.
  https://www.healthychildren.org/varicella
- Centers for Disease Control and Prevention: Alphabetical listing of diseases and conditions provides information for families in English and Spanish.
  www.cdc.gov/chickenpox/index.html
- MedlinePlus: Information for patients and families (in English and Spanish) sponsored by the US National Library of Medicine and National Institutes of Health.
  https://www.nlm.nih.gov/medlineplus/chickenpox.html

Skin Infections

Localized Bacterial Infections

CHAPTER 23 — **Acute Paronychia**............................ 173

CHAPTER 24 — **Blistering Distal Dactylitis**..................... 177

CHAPTER 25 — **Ecthyma** 181

CHAPTER 26 — **Folliculitis/Furunculosis/Carbunculosis** 185

CHAPTER 27 — **Impetigo** 191

CHAPTER 28 — **Perianal Bacterial Dermatitis** 197

CHAPTER 23

Acute Paronychia

Introduction/Etiology/Epidemiology

- Paronychia (ie, inflammation of the periungual nail folds) occurs when the cuticle becomes disrupted by maceration or injury and pathogens enter the space.

- Paronychia occurs more frequently in individuals who often have their hands in water or in children with a habit of finger sucking or nail-biting. In addition, trauma to the periungual folds is another risk factor for its development.

- *Staphylococcus aureus* is the agent primarily responsible for acute paronychia. Paronychia with a green discoloration may indicate the presence of *Pseudomonas*. *Candida* species most often result in chronic paronychia (Chapter 35C).

- Acute paronychia typically lasts less than 6 weeks, while chronic paronychia (Chapter 35C) refers to paronychia lasting more than 6 weeks.

- Some medications, including oral retinoids, epidermal growth factor receptor inhibitors, chemotherapy agents, and antiretrovirals, can increase the risk for paronychia.

Signs and Symptoms

- Periungual folds show erythema, swelling, and tenderness (Figures 23.1 and 23.2).

- Purulent drainage is commonly present.

- Although it is most common to have only 1 nail involved, multiple nail involvement can be seen, especially with medication-induced paronychia.

- Patients with chronic infections may have dermatitis of the surrounding areas (ie, fingers, hands).

▶ Paronychia of the toenails can be seen with ingrown toenails, retronychia (inward growth of the nail plate at the proximal nail fold), or congenital malalignment of the great toenails.

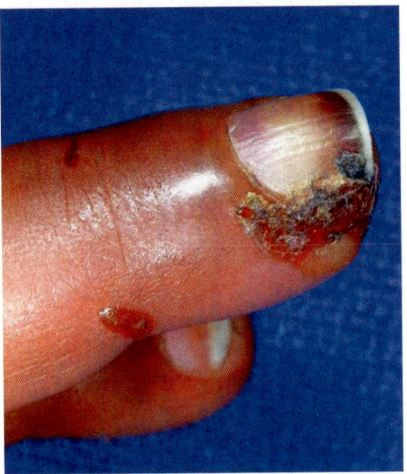

Figure 23.1. Acute paronychia with inflammation, pustule formation, and crusting of the periungual fold.

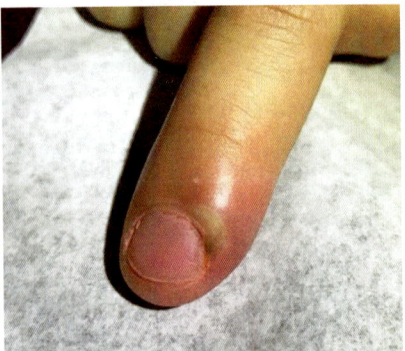

Figure 23.2. Acute paronychia with loculated pus and surrounding erythema.

Look-alikes

Disorder	Differentiating Features
Chronic paronychia	• Problem long-standing (not acute). • Usually without symptoms. • Swelling and erythema of proximal and lateral nail folds with loss of cuticle; purulent drainage absent. • May have associated nail dystrophy (eg, ridging, pitting).
Felon	• A bacterial infection of the digital pulp space of the finger (also typically caused by *Staphylococcus aureus*, less often by streptococci). • Characterized by severe pain, swelling, erythema in the pad of the distal fingertip.
Herpes simplex virus infection (ie, herpetic whitlow)	• Usually presents as discrete, deep-seated, often clustered vesicles with surrounding erythema. • Usually very painful. • Regional lymphadenopathy may be present. • Recurrent lesions can be associated with prodromal symptoms. • Viral culture or polymerase chain reaction testing will confirm herpes simplex virus.
Blistering distal dactylitis	• Usually presents as a tender, deep-seated blister on the volar surface of the distal finger pad. • Bacterial culture reveals group A β-hemolytic streptococci (or occasionally *S aureus*).
Psoriasis	• Pitting is most typical nail change in psoriasis. • Lateral onycholysis may result in disruption of the periungual folds; paronychia may eventually result.
Trauma	• History of trauma. • Absence of purulent discharge. • Cuticle usually healthy.

How to Make the Diagnosis

▶ The condition is often diagnosed based on the clinical features.

▶ Gram stain and culture of the drainage can identify the organisms.

▶ Bacterial culture usually reveals *S aureus*, although group A β-hemolytic streptococci and rarely other organisms may be etiologic.

Treatment

- An oral antistaphylococcal antibiotic (eg, cephalexin) usually is effective and also provides coverage against group A β-hemolytic streptococci. Failure of treatment may indicate presence of methicillin-resistant *S aureus*, and changing therapy to clindamycin, doxycycline (in children >8 years), trimethoprim-sulfamethoxazole, or another appropriate agent (based on bacterial culture and sensitivity testing) should be considered.
- Topical antibiotic ointment (eg, mupirocin, retapamulin) may be used in mild cases, but the condition often requires systemic therapy.
- Warm soaks may hasten resolution.
- Drainage and culture of purulent pockets occasionally is necessary.
- Preventive strategies include the following:
    - Institute drying measures, including minimizing exposure to water and wearing gloves for wet work.
    - Avoid trauma, when feasible.

Prognosis

- Acute paronychia usually resolves completely without long-term sequelae.
- Mechanical factors or exposures may result in recurrence.
- Permanent nail ridging or dystrophy may result with severe infections.

When to Worry or Refer

- Consider referral to a dermatologist or infectious disease specialist for patients who have severe or extensive involvement or in whom standard treatment does not work.

Resource for Families

- MedlinePlus: Information for patients and families (in English and Spanish) sponsored by the US National Library of Medicine and National Institutes of Health.
www.nlm.nih.gov/medlineplus/ency/article/001444.htm

CHAPTER 24

Blistering Distal Dactylitis

Introduction/Etiology/Epidemiology

- ▶ Blistering distal dactylitis is a bullous skin infection caused most often by group A β-hemolytic streptococci; other groups of β-hemolytic streptococci; and, less often, by *Staphylococcus aureus,* which occasionally can be methicillin-resistant *S aureus* (MRSA).
- ▶ The peak incidence is in school-aged children.

Signs and Symptoms

- ▶ Tender, superficial tense bullae occur on the distal volar (palmar surface) finger pads (Figure 24.1) or, less often, the plantar surface of the toes; erythema usually surrounds the bullae.
- ▶ May involve 1 or more digits.
- ▶ Larger bullae may extend around to involve the nail folds.
- ▶ There is generally an absence of systemic symptoms.

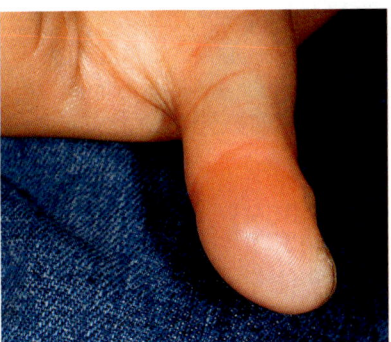

Figure 24.1. Blistering distal dactylitis. Note tense bulla of the thumb.

Look-alikes

Disorder	Differentiating Features
Herpes simplex virus infection (ie, herpetic whitlow)	• Deep-seated, clustered vesicles with surrounding erythema. • May have a history of recurrent lesions in the same sites. • Viral culture or polymerase chain reaction testing demonstrates herpes simplex virus. • Regional lymphadenopathy may be present.
Bullous impetigo	• Flaccid, thin-walled bullae or tender shallow erosions surrounded by a peripheral collarette, representing the remnant of the blister roof. • Usually multiple lesions present, can be clustered. • Does not typically occur on distal palmar fingertip; common locations include face, diaper region, and extremities.
Acute paronychia	• Erythema and swelling of lateral or proximal nail folds. • Discrete vesicles or bullae typically absent. • Bacterial culture most often demonstrates *Staphylococcus aureus*.
Hand, foot, and mouth disease	• Lesions tend to occur on the sides of the fingers or toes as well as palms and soles. • Blisters have an elliptical ("football") shape and are more deep-seated; may have a grayish white color. • Multiple, smaller blisters present. • Oral blisters or erosions (herpangina lesions) are characteristically present. • Fever, malaise often present.
Burn	• History may be confirmatory. • Clinical signs or historical information concerning for abuse or neglect may be present.
Epidermolysis bullosa	• Trauma-induced bullae occur recurrently. • Weber-Cockayne syndrome variant may be localized to the hands and feet; however, multifocal involvement usually seen (with multiple lesions) and not limited to distal digits. • Other forms of epidermolysis bullosa have additional lesions located on other areas of the body or mucosae.

How to Make the Diagnosis

▶ The diagnosis is usually made based on the clinical findings.

▶ Gram stain or bacterial culture of the blister fluid is often confirmatory; typically grows group A β-hemolytic streptococci, occasionally *S aureus*.

Treatment

- Drainage of the bullae can decrease pain if it is present; perform bacterial culture on fluid obtained to confirm the causative organism.
- Although oral penicillin or erythromycin for 10 days is usually effective, an antistaphylococcal antibiotic (eg, cephalexin) often is selected because some cases may be caused by *S aureus*.
- Failure of response may indicate presence of MRSA and suggests consideration for a change of therapy to clindamycin, doxycycline (traditionally limited to children >8 years, although recent *Red Book*® recommendations suggest that this medication can be safely used at any age for 21 days or fewer without concern for dental enamel staining), trimethoprim-sulfamethoxazole, or another appropriate agent (as based on bacterial culture and sensitivity testing).

Prognosis

- The prognosis for children with blistering distal dactylitis is excellent.
- Lesions heal completely without permanent sequelae.

When to Worry or Refer

- Consider referral to a dermatologist or infectious disease specialist for patients who have severe or extensive involvement, in whom there is a question about the diagnosis, or in whom standard treatment does not work.

Resource for Families

- Medscape: Nail disorders in children.
  https://www.medscape.com/viewarticle/718695_3

CHAPTER
25

Ecthyma

Introduction/Etiology/Epidemiology

- Ecthyma is a deep and ulcerative pyoderma (a deep cutaneous infection) that is most prevalent in tropical climates.
- The most common causative organisms are group A β-hemolytic streptococci (GABHS) and *Staphylococcus aureus*.
- Although the lesions may initially seem to be impetigo, the organisms progress to invade beyond the epidermis and deeper into the dermis.
- Ecthyma can develop at sites of previous skin disorders, such as insect bites or scabies.

Signs and Symptoms

- The extremities and buttocks are most often involved.
- Ecthyma lesions may be vesicopustules or crusted erosions; usually there is surrounding erythema. Often lesions will progress to become necrotic in appearance, with deep punched-out ulcers (Figure 25.1). The ulcer can be saucer shaped with a raised surrounding border.
- Lesions are often crusted, and removal of the crust reveals a deeper ulcer.
- Lesions are painful and often multifocal; they heal slowly over a few weeks, often with scar formation.

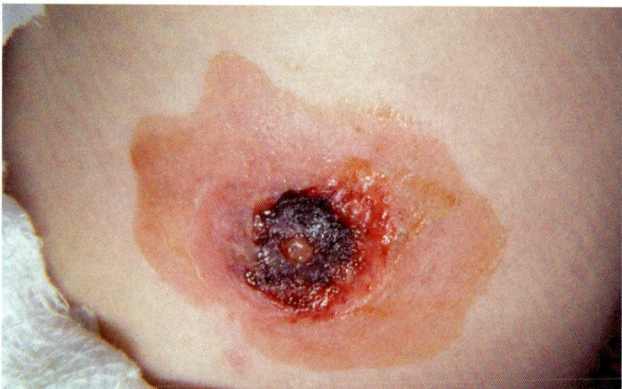

Figure 25.1. Ecthyma lesion with central necrotic crust.

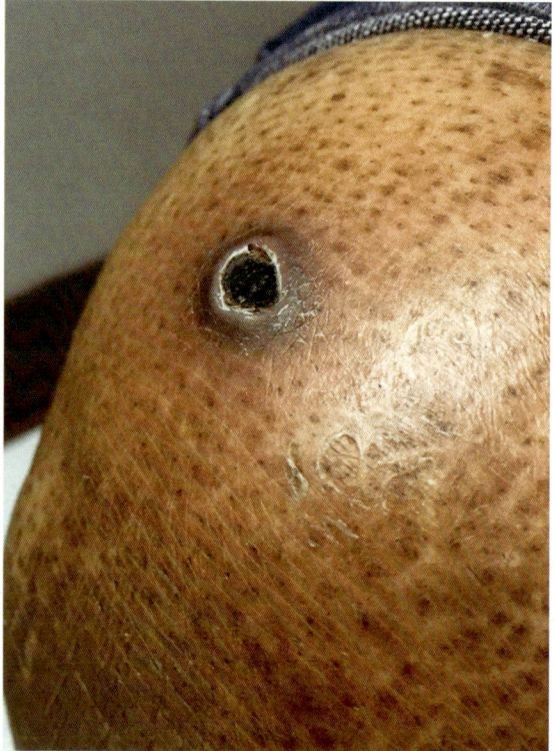

Figure 25.2. Ecthyma gangrenosum lesion in a patient with skin of color. Note the central crusted ulceration with surrounding faintly visible erythema. Reproduced with permission from Khoo T, Ford F, Lobo Z, Psevdos G. One thing after another: ecthyma gangrenosum. *Am J Med*. 2018;131(5):510-511.

Look-alikes

Disorder	Differentiating Features
Impetigo	**Non-bullous** • Superficial erosions with honey-colored crust. **Bullous** • Fragile bullae that rupture rapidly leaving round superficial erosions. • Periphery of lesions may exhibit a collarette of scale, which is the remnant of the bulla roof.
Brown recluse spider bite	• Timing of lesion appearance corresponds with exposure to spider. • Usually becomes painful after a few hours. • Usually a single location rather than a multifocal process. • Initial lesion noted to have central hemorrhagic area with surrounding edema and erythema; may produce the "red, white, and blue sign" (ie, rings of color surrounding the lesion). • Rapidly progresses, resulting in large necrotic plaque, commonly with eschar formation.
Ecthyma gangrenosum	• Localized septic vasculitis usually associated with *Pseudomonas aeruginosa* bacteremia. • Lesions initially present as hemorrhagic papules. • Subsequently progresses into deep ulcer with necrosis (Figure 25.2) and, occasionally, eschar formation. • Often accompanied by high fever, myalgias. • Most children who are affected are immunosuppressed.
Cutaneous anthrax	• Spores enter through a cut or an abrasion. • Initial lesion is a painless, pruritic papule that subsequently develops a central clear bulla. • When bulla ruptures, necrosis and an ulcer develop, surrounded by massive edema and multiple smaller lesions.
Vasculitis	• Many vasculitic processes can present with hemorrhagic papules with necrosis, including hypersensitivity vasculitis, Henoch-Schönlein purpura, and polyarteritis nodosa. • Associated symptoms (eg, fever) and other signs (eg, hematuria, hematochezia, arthritis) may assist in diagnosis and help to differentiate these disorders from ecthyma.
Cigarette burns	• History or findings during clinical examination often arouse suspicion for child abuse. • Lesions in various stages of healing commonly noted.

How to Make the Diagnosis

- The clinical findings usually lead to the correct diagnosis.
- Bacterial culture often reveals GABHS.
- Skin biopsy (usually unnecessary) shows an intense polymorphonuclear infiltrate and organisms on tissue Gram stain.

Treatment

- Systemic antibiotic therapy is the treatment of choice.
- The chosen antibiotic should have activity against GABHS and *S aureus* (because the latter is an occasional cause or may be present as a secondary infectious agent). Failure of therapy indicates the need to review culture and sensitivity results for presence of methicillin-resistant *S aureus* or to reconsider the diagnosis.

Prognosis

- Because of the penetration into the dermis, ecthyma lesions often heal with permanent scarring.
- Rapid healing usually occurs with appropriate antibiotic therapy.

When to Worry or Refer

- Consider referral to a dermatologist for patients who have severe or extensive disease or in whom standard treatment does not work.

Resource for Families

- MedlinePlus: Information for patients and families (in English and Spanish) sponsored by the US National Library of Medicine and National Institutes of Health.
  www.nlm.nih.gov/medlineplus/ency/article/000864.htm

CHAPTER 26

Folliculitis/Furunculosis/Carbunculosis

Introduction/Etiology/Epidemiology

- Definitions
  - Folliculitis: superficial inflammation surrounding a follicle.
  - Furuncle: bacterial folliculitis of a single follicle that involves a deeper portion of the follicle; also known as *boils*.
  - Carbuncle: bacterial folliculitis that involves the deeper portions of several contiguous and interconnected follicles, often draining at multiple points on the cutaneous surface.
- Types of folliculitis include the following:
  - Bacterial folliculitis (the most common type) is most often caused by *Staphylococcus aureus*. Although many of these isolates are still methicillin-sensitive *S aureus* (MSSA), some may be methicillin-resistant *S aureus* (MRSA).
  - *Pseudomonas* (hot tub) folliculitis is usually caused by gram-negative bacteria (most often *Pseudomonas aeruginosa*).
  - Gram-negative bacteria can also cause folliculitis in patients with acne who are receiving long-term antibiotic therapy.
  - *Malassezia* (formerly *Pityrosporum*), a yeast, may be a cause of folliculitis localized to the back, upper chest, shoulders, and upper arms.
  - *Demodex* (a skin mite) folliculitis presents as an erythematous, follicular papulopustular eruption on the face, usually in hosts who are immunocompromised (eg, children receiving chemotherapy for leukemia).
- Predisposing conditions for furuncles and carbuncles include obesity, diabetes, immunodeficiency, and malnutrition, as well as warm, humid climates.

Signs and Symptoms

▶ Folliculitis is characterized by discrete follicular-centered pustules with surrounding erythema (Figures 26.1 and 26.2).
  - The most common locations are the buttocks and thighs, especially in young children.
  - Occasionally, folliculitis can be seen in areas that are subject to occlusion and irritation from clothing.
  - Lesions are most often painless; however, they can be mildly tender and may be pruritic.
  - *Pseudomonas* folliculitis often presents with localization of lesions to areas covered by the bathing garment.

▶ Furuncles and carbuncles present as erythematous papulonodules or nodules, often with a central punctum (Figure 26.3).
  - The central area tends to be the point where fluctuance will develop.
  - Pain is common, and fever may be present.
  - Pain diminishes after drainage of the lesion.

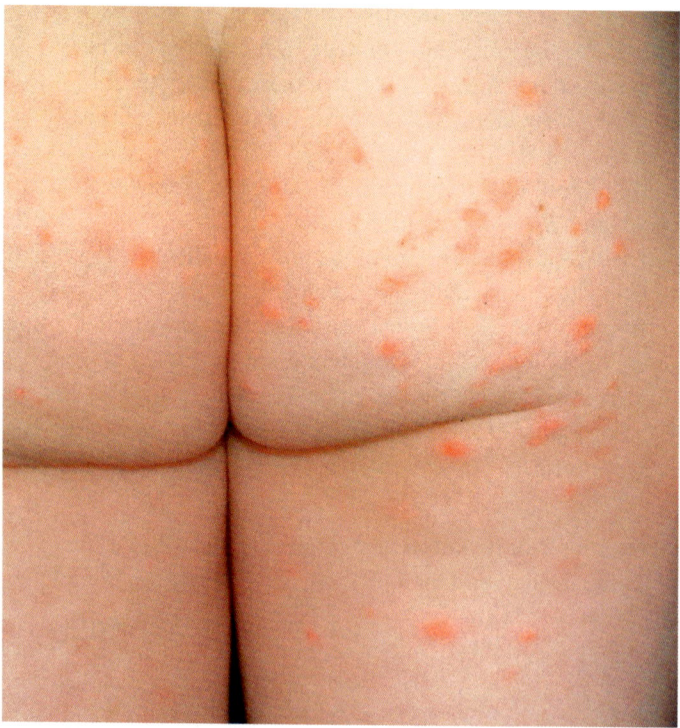

Figure 26.1. Folliculitis with erythematous papules and papulopustular eruption of the buttocks.

▶ Skin and soft-tissue infections due to community-acquired MRSA often present as furuncles and carbuncles.
  - Lesions typically are erythematous, fluctuant, and painful.
  - They may have purulent drainage.
  - Other family or household members may have (or previously have had) similar lesions.

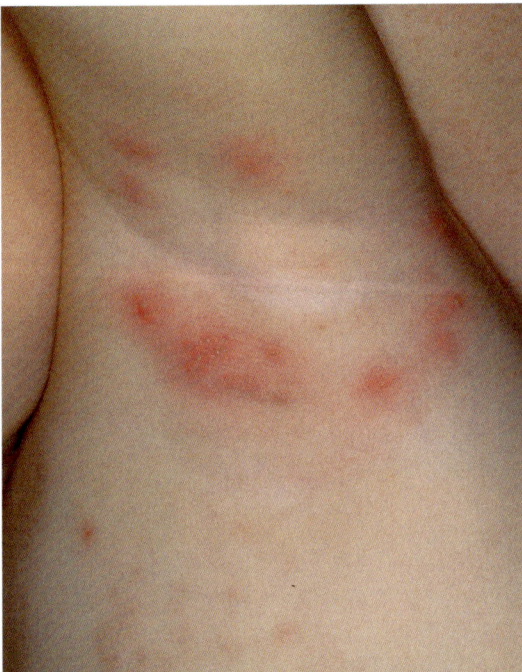

Figure 26.2. The lesions of folliculitis are erythematous papules and pustules centered around follicles.

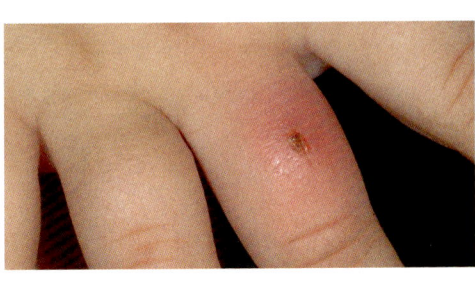
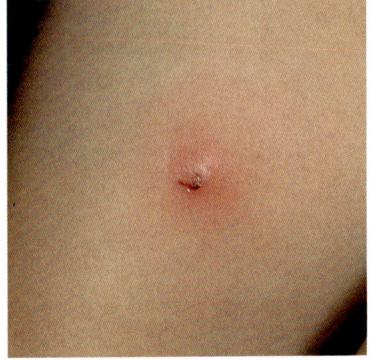

Figure 26.3. Furuncles. These nodular lesions may drain from the central portion.

Look-alikes

Disorder	Differentiating Features
Folliculitis from opportunistic organisms (especially in patients who are immunocompromised)	• Persistent despite appropriate therapy. • Patients with leukopenia may show less erythema than expected.
Viral exanthem	• Erythematous papules and macules. • Pustules usually lacking. • Lesions not centered around hair follicles. • Other symptoms (eg, upper respiratory, gastrointestinal) may be present.
Insect bites	• Usually have a central punctum present at close inspection. • Most often occur on exposed areas. • Extreme pruritus common. • May see linear groupings ("breakfast, lunch, and dinner" sign), especially with fleabites. • Pustules rare. • Lesions not centered around hair follicles.
Acne nodule	• May look very similar to a carbuncle, but typical acne lesions (ie, open and closed comedones) usually also present. • Lesions typically are limited to face, chest, shoulders, and back.
Hidradenitis suppurativa	• Recurrent papules, cysts, sinus tracts, and nodules that heal with scarring. • Typically located in axillary and inguinal regions; occasionally involve posterior auricular area.

How to Make the Diagnosis

▶ The diagnosis is usually made clinically.
▶ Skin swab for bacterial culture will usually reveal the causative agent.
▶ When furuncles or carbuncles are drained, a swab of the contents should be sent for bacterial culture and sensitivities.

Treatment

▶ Preventive measures include the following:
  - Avoid tight-fitting clothing.
  - Change clothing after activities with excessive sweating.
  - Lose weight (if applicable).

- Use antibacterial cleansers such as those that contain chlorhexidine (avoid ear canals), benzoyl peroxide, or sodium hypochlorite at least twice weekly.
- For nasal carriers of *S aureus,* intranasal mupirocin (for patient and family contacts) may diminish recurrences.
- Patients who are prone to frequent recurrences may benefit from dilute bleach baths: ¼ to ½ cup of sodium hypochlorite solution (liquid bleach) added to a full bathtub of water and used as a soak for 10 minutes twice weekly. Use of a sodium hypochlorite cleanser (as noted previously) is another option.

▶ Treatment for folliculitis
- Antibacterial skin cleansers, including chlorhexidine (avoid ears), benzoyl peroxide, or sodium hypochlorite.
- Topical antibiotic may suffice for mild cases (eg, clindamycin, mupirocin, retapamulin, ozenoxacin).
- Oral antistaphylococcal antibiotic (eg, cephalexin, dicloxacillin) for moderate to severe cases. A therapy duration of 5 to 7 days is typically recommended but should be tailored to the individual patient on the basis of resolution of signs and symptoms. If MRSA is suspected or isolated, use of clindamycin, doxycycline (traditionally limited to children >8 years, although recent *Red Book*® recommendations suggest that this medication can be safely used at any age for 21 days or fewer without concern for dental enamel staining), trimethoprim-sulfamethoxazole, or another appropriate agent (as determined with antibiotic susceptibility testing) is indicated.
- Culture of purulent material whenever possible.

▶ Treatment for furunculosis and carbunculosis
- Warm, moist compresses to promote or facilitate drainage.
- Incision and drainage may be necessary for larger or more fluctuant lesions or if the process is caused by MRSA. Incision and drainage are recommended as initial therapy for MRSA-associated furuncles and carbuncles, with or without antibiotics.
- Skin swab of pustular fluid should be sent for bacterial culture.
- Oral antistaphylococcal antibiotic (eg, cephalexin, dicloxacillin) for 5 to 7 days is typically recommended but should be tailored to the individual patient on the basis of resolution of signs and symptoms for MSSA; if MRSA is suspected or isolated, use of clindamycin, doxycycline (see age discussion earlier), trimethoprim-sulfamethoxazole, or another appropriate agent (as determined with antibiotic susceptibility testing) is indicated.

- Of note, in community-associated MRSA skin and soft-tissue infection, the *Red Book* highlights the utility of drainage in management; according to those guidelines, drainage plus systemic oral therapy are associated with better outcomes compared with drainage alone.
- Studies in adults with recurrent disease have shown the benefit of a 7-day course of oral rifampin and doxycycline in conjunction with nasal mupirocin.

Prognosis

▶ In children with typical immunity, the prognosis is excellent.

▶ Recurrence is common, especially in the continued presence of common risk factors.

▶ Individuals who are immunocompromised may have infections with unusual organisms that are more difficult to diagnose and treat.

When to Worry or Refer

▶ Consider referral to a dermatologist or infectious disease specialist for patients who have severe or extensive disease, do not respond to standard treatments, are immunocompromised, or have recurrent infections.

▶ If the patient develops a severe infection with MRSA that requires hospitalization, an infectious disease specialist should be consulted.

Resources for Families

▶ Centers for Disease Control and Prevention: Methicillin-resistant *Staphylococcus aureus* (MRSA) basics.
 www.cdc.gov/mrsa

▶ Centers for Disease Control and Prevention: Preventing hot tub rash. Patient information on *Pseudomonas* (hot tub) folliculitis.
 https://www.cdc.gov/healthy-swimming/prevention/preventing-hot-tub-rash.html?CDC_AAref_Val=https://www.cdc.gov/healthywater/swimming/swimmers/rwi/rashes.html

▶ MedlinePlus: Information for patients and families (in English and Spanish) sponsored by the US National Library of Medicine and National Institutes of Health.
 www.nlm.nih.gov/medlineplus/ency/article/000823.htm

CHAPTER
27

Impetigo

Introduction/Etiology/Epidemiology

- Impetigo is a superficial bacterial infection of the skin.
- In North America, the etiologic agent is primarily *Staphylococcus aureus*. In some cases, group A β-hemolytic streptococci may be cultured; however, it is most often present as a secondary agent. *Streptococcus* is the primary cause in only a small percentage of cases.
- Increased incidence in the summer is due to disruptions in the skin barrier from cuts, scrapes, and insect bites.
- Although impetigo can be seen across all age groups, it is most common among infants and children.
- There are 2 forms of impetigo: bullous and non-bullous (approximately 70% of cases).

Signs and Symptoms

- Non-bullous (ie, crusted or common) impetigo: Initial lesion is a superficial vesicle that ruptures easily; exudate dries to form a honey-colored crust (Figure 27.1).
- Bullous impetigo: A superficial fragile, flaccid, thin-walled bulla containing serous fluid or pus forms and then rapidly ruptures to form a round, erythematous erosion, often with a surrounding collarette of scale (remnant of the blister roof) (Figures 27.2, 27.3, and 27.4).
- Lesions tend to be located in exposed areas, especially the face and extremities.
- Diaper area involvement is common in infants.
- Lesions often spread via autoinoculation, from skin-to-skin contact, and less often via fomites (eg, towels, razors, clothing).

Look-alikes

Disorder	Differentiating Features
Herpes simplex virus infection	• Clustered vesicles with surrounding erythema (ie, appear as on an erythematous base). • After vesicles rupture, ulcers form (deeper than the erosions observed in impetigo). • May occur inside the mouth or on other mucous membranes and usually painful.
Varicella-zoster virus infection	**Primary (acute) varicella** • Individual vesicles with surrounding erythema. • Rash begins on the trunk and then spreads to the extremities. • Rash tends to have symmetric distribution. • Mucous membranes often involved. **Herpes zoster (shingles)** • Clustered vesicles with surrounding erythema located in a dermatomal distribution. • History of acute varicella or varicella vaccination.
Folliculitis	• Small follicular-centered pustules (1–2 mm) with rim of surrounding erythema. • Hair may be seen protruding from center of pustule (most easily visualized with side lighting).
Ecthyma	• Indurated, painful papules that have surrounding erythema. • Often presents as punched-out, crusted, ulcerated papules. • Usually caused by *Streptococcus pyogenes*.
Contact dermatitis	• May be papules, vesicles, or bullae. • Itching commonly reported (not typical in impetigo). • Location of lesions corresponds to exposure to the contact allergen. • Configuration of lesions may be unusual (eg, linear in plant dermatitis).
Inflicted cigarette burns	• Uniform lesion size (approximately 8 mm). • Often located on the hands and feet. • Usually heal with scarring. • Often deeper than impetigo.

How to Make the Diagnosis

- The diagnosis is most often made based on the clinical findings.
- Gram stain of the contents of a vesicle or bulla demonstrates gram-positive cocci.
- Bacterial culture can assist in identifying the specific etiologic agent and antibiotic sensitivities.

Treatment

- For milder, localized cases of non-bullous impetigo, topical mupirocin, retapamulin, or ozenoxacin can be applied 2 to 3 times daily for 5 to 7 days.
- When bullous impetigo is present or there is more widespread involvement in non-bullous impetigo, a 7- to 10-day course of a systemic antibiotic (eg, cephalexin) may be necessary, with attention to resistance patterns for each geographic location.
- Failure of response in 48 hours may be due to infection by methicillin-resistant *S aureus* and suggests the need for culture and a potential change of therapy to clindamycin, doxycycline (traditionally limited to children >8 years, although recent *Red Book*® recommendations suggest that this medication can be safely used at any age for ≤21 days without concern for dental enamel staining), trimethoprim-sulfamethoxazole, or another appropriate agent (as determined by results of antibiotic susceptibility testing).
- Warm water compresses can facilitate gentle debridement of the crusts.

Treating Associated Conditions

- Although uncommon, it is important to remember that if the impetigo is due to a nephritogenic strain of *Streptococcus pyogenes,* acute glomerulonephritis can be a sequela.

Prognosis

- The prognosis for children with simple impetigo is good, and complete resolution is typical.

When to Worry or Refer

▶ Consider referral to a dermatologist for patients who have severe or extensive disease in whom the diagnosis is in question or for those in whom standard treatment does not work.

Resources for Families

▶ American Academy of Pediatrics: HealthyChildren.org.
https://www.healthychildren.org/English/health-issues/ conditions/skin/Pages/Impetigo.aspx

▶ MedlinePlus: Information for patients and families (in English and Spanish) sponsored by the US National Library of Medicine and National Institutes of Health.
www.nlm.nih.gov/medlineplus/impetigo.html

▶ WebMD: Information for families is contained in Skin Problems and Treatments.
https://www.webmd.com/skin-problems-and-treatments/ understanding-impetigo-basics

CHAPTER 28

Perianal Bacterial Dermatitis

Introduction/Etiology/Epidemiology

- Perianal bacterial dermatitis (formerly known as perianal streptococcal dermatitis) is a distinctive superficial infection primarily caused by group A β-hemolytic streptococci. Less often it is caused by other groups of β-hemolytic streptococci or *Staphylococcus aureus*.
- There is a male predominance, and the condition has a peak incidence of 3 to 6 years of age.
- Other family members may be similarly affected (especially if there is a history of co-bathing), or patient may have concomitant streptococcal pharyngitis.

Signs and Symptoms

- The typical presentation is that of intense perianal erythema (Figure 28.1), often with associated pruritus, burning, or tenderness to touch.
- Maceration, exudate, fissuring, or desquamation may also be present.
- Sharply demarcated perianal erythema is present, with a distinct border between affected and unaffected skin.
- Balanoposthitis (Figure 28.2) or vulvovaginitis may also be present.
- Parents may report that the child has pain with defecation, stool holding, blood-tinged stools, or increased irritability.
- Fever is rare.

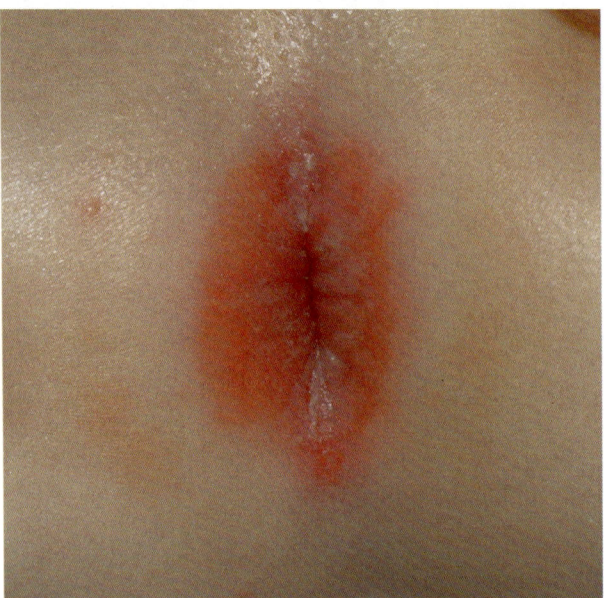

Figure 28.1. Perianal bacterial dermatitis is characterized by marked perianal erythema and purulent drainage.

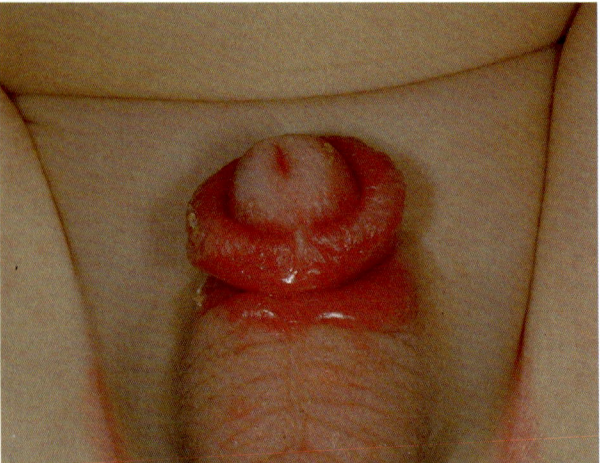

Figure 28.2. Streptococcal balanoposthitis (ie, inflammation of the glans penis and foreskin). This occurred in an infant who also had perianal bacterial dermatitis, and culture result was positive for group A β-hemolytic streptococci.

Look-alikes

In each of the conditions listed herein, a bacterial culture would fail to demonstrate group A β-hemolytic streptococci.

Disorder	Differentiating Features
Candidiasis	• Erythema primarily involves the fold areas. • Satellite papules or papular pustules often present. • Exudate is white, often "cheesy" rather than purulent. • Typically painless and associated symptoms (eg, painful defecation) usually absent.
Psoriasis	• Sharply demarcated scaly plaques. • Psoriasis lesions may be seen elsewhere (eg, umbilicus, scalp). • Family history may be positive for psoriasis. • Pitting of the nails may be present.
Seborrheic dermatitis	• Erythematous patches with greasy yellow scale. • Other sites (eg, scalp, umbilicus, anterior diaper area) often affected without localization to just the perianal area.
Irritant contact dermatitis	• May see lichenification from chronic scratching. • Not usually as intensely red as perianal bacterial dermatitis. • Usually lacks purulent drainage.
Pinworm infestation (*Enterobius vermicularis*)	• Pruritus is the prominent symptom, especially at night. • May see worms with flashlight after child is sleeping. • May coexist with perianal bacterial dermatitis.
Lichen sclerosus et atrophicus	• Presents as hypopigmentation with atrophy of genital area, primarily in female patients. • "Cigarette paper" wrinkling of the affected skin often present. • Tends to be distributed in an hourglass configuration (involving vulva, perineum, and perianal area). • Early disease may present with erythema, occasional bullae, or hemorrhage. • Dysuria may be reported.
Sexual abuse	• Lacerations may be evident, especially if the abuse was recent. • Bruising of the surrounding areas may be present. • Vulvovaginitis from gonococcal infection reveals drainage that is more greenish, usually malodorous.

How to Make the Diagnosis

- The diagnosis is suspected clinically and confirmed with bacterial skin culture.
- A specific request to the laboratory is usually necessary because routine processing of perianal swabs may involve inhibitors to the growth of group A β-hemolytic streptococci.
- *S aureus* may occasionally be the etiologic agent.

Treatment

- Oral penicillin or amoxicillin (erythromycin may be used if penicillin allergy) for 10 days, combined with topical antibiotics.
- Antistaphylococcal antibiotic may be necessary if caused by *S aureus*; the antibiotic selected should be guided by sensitivity testing results.

Treating Associated Conditions

- Vulvovaginitis or balanoposthitis, if present, usually responds to the same therapy.
- Guttate psoriasis may be associated with the condition and is treated with therapies typical for psoriasis. (See the Papulosquamous Diseases section [Chapters 47–54].)

Prognosis

- The prognosis is excellent, usually with complete healing after therapy.
- More than 1 course of treatment is occasionally required.

When to Worry or Refer

- Consider referral to a dermatologist when the diagnosis is in doubt or when disease is severe or extensive or does not respond to standard treatment.
- If the history or examination findings are concerning for abuse, appropriate evaluation and reporting to child protective services is indicated.

Resource for Families

▶ MedlinePlus: Information for patients and families (in English and Spanish) sponsored by the US National Library of Medicine and National Institutes of Health.
www.nlm.nih.gov/medlineplus/ency/article/001346.htm

Skin Infections

Systemic Bacterial, Rickettsial, or Spirochetal Infections With Skin Manifestations

CHAPTER 29 — **Lyme Disease** 205

CHAPTER 30 — **Meningococcemia** 211

CHAPTER 31 — **Rocky Mountain Spotted Fever (RMSF)** 217

CHAPTER 32 — **Scarlet Fever** 223

CHAPTER 33 — **Staphylococcal Scalded Skin Syndrome (SSSS)** 231

CHAPTER 34 — **Toxic Shock Syndrome (TSS)** 237

CHAPTER 29

Lyme Disease

Introduction/Etiology/Epidemiology

- Tick-borne illness caused by the spirochete *Borrelia burgdorferi*.
- Most common vector-borne disease in the United States.
- Three clinical stages: early localized, early disseminated, late.
- The infection most commonly occurs after a bite from a nymph tick. The most common tick vectors in the United States are:
  - *Ixodes scapularis* (deer or black-legged tick) in the east and Midwest.
  - *Ixodes pacificus* (western black-legged tick) in the west.
- More than 80% of cases occur in New England and the eastern mid-Atlantic states; less frequently occurs in the upper Midwest, especially Minnesota and Wisconsin.
- Incubation from tick bite to the appearance of first clinical manifestations of Lyme disease (ie, erythema migrans) ranges from 3 to 32 days (median, 11 days).

Signs and Symptoms

- Early localized stage begins 7 to 14 days after the tick bite (range, 3–32 days).
  - Erythema migrans typically is the first clinical manifestation of Lyme disease (occurs in 70% to 80% of patients).
    - Appears at the site of the tick bite as an erythematous macule or papule.
    - Typically non-pruritic.
    - Lesion expands rapidly to form a large (>5 cm), round erythematous patch often showing central clearing (ie, forming a ring) (Figure 29.1).
    - Bull's-eye appearance with concentric rings appears in a minority of cases.
  - Accompanying features include fever, malaise, headache, mild meningismus, myalgias, lymphadenopathy, and arthralgias.

- ▶ Early disseminated stage begins weeks to months after the tick bite.
  - Multiple smaller erythema migrans lesions are characteristic.
  - Low-grade fever may be present.
  - Intermittent migratory arthralgias and myalgias, headache (often severe), fatigue.
  - Neurologic manifestations, including peripheral and cranial neuropathy (most commonly seventh nerve or Bell palsy), lymphocytic meningitis.
  - Ophthalmologic manifestations, including uveitis, conjunctivitis, and optic neuritis, may occur.
  - Carditis leading to atrioventricular conduction defects occurs rarely in children.
- ▶ Late disease begins weeks to months after the tick bite in patients not treated at an earlier stage.
  - Arthritis, usually monoarticular or pauciarticular, particularly in large joints. Joint swelling often is out of proportion to the degree of pain or disability.
  - Encephalopathy, encephalomyelitis, peripheral neuropathy (occurs rarely).
  - Conjunctivitis, uveitis, or keratitis may occur.
  - Skin manifestations may include lymphocytoma cutis and acrodermatitis chronica atrophicans, although the latter is seen quite infrequently in the United States.

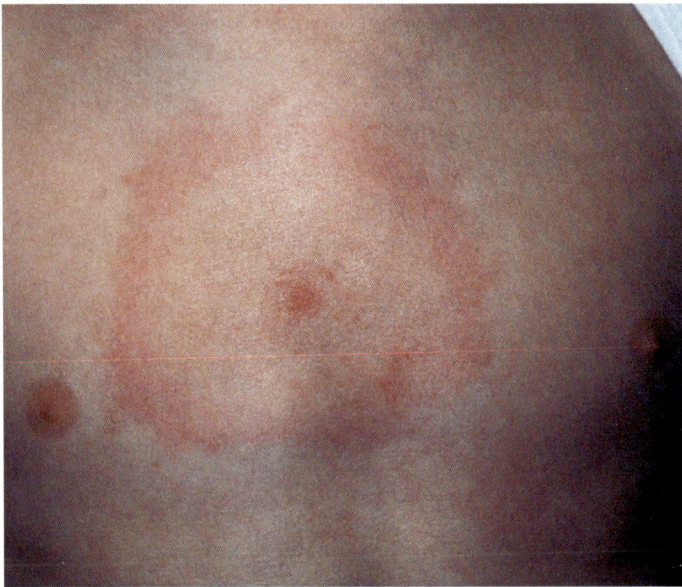

Figure 29.1. Annular erythema migrans lesion of early localized Lyme disease.

Chapter 29: Lyme Disease

Look-alikes

Disorder	Differentiating Features
Erythema multiforme	• Lesions are smaller than erythema migrans, and multiple target lesions present, especially on the extremities, palms, and soles. • Lesions may develop a dusky or vesicular center. • True target lesions are present (ie, central duskiness or blister, ring of pale edema, and outer rim of erythema).
Fixed drug eruption	• Often dusky purple to hyperpigmented patch or plaque. • Central erosion may be present. • Recur in same location with each exposure to offending agent.
Tinea corporis	• Presents as an annular red plaque (palpable), not patch. • Scale usually present.
Urticaria	• Multiple lesions nearly always present. • Lesions come and go quickly (usually within hours). • Presents as erythematous wheals, often arcuate or annular. • Usually pruritic.
Arthropod bites	• Multiple lesions often present. • Pruritus very common, often severe. • Edematous papules or papulovesicles, not rings. • Papules may be clustered in linear groupings ("breakfast, lunch, and dinner" sign).
Southern tick-associated rash illness (STARI)	• Seen in south and southeastern United States. • Not associated with infection from *Borrelia burgdorferi*. • After tick bite from *Amblyomma americanum* (Lone Star tick). • Erythema migrans lesion, similar to that of Lyme disease but without dissemination; primary extra-cutaneous symptoms limited to fever, fatigue, headache, and myalgia. • It is unknown whether therapy is indicated or beneficial, but most patients receive antibiotic therapy, given the clinical resemblance to early localized Lyme disease.

How to Make the Diagnosis

- The diagnosis of early localized Lyme disease is usually suggested clinically on the basis of the appearance of erythema migrans, especially when history of a tick bite is present or in those who have had a plausible geographic exposure.

- Recognition that a tick bite occurred is very uncommon because the nymphs are tiny.

- Testing uses a 2-tiered algorithm developed by the Centers for Disease Control and Prevention (https://www.cdc.gov/lyme/hcp/diagnosis-testing/index.html). The first step is testing using enzyme immunosorbent assay or immunofluorescent antibody assay with confirmation of equivocal or positive results with Western blotting (immunoglobulin G and/or M depending on the duration of symptoms) or the second tier enzyme immunosorbent assay.
  - However, antibody test results may be falsely negative in early localized disease (fewer than one-half of children with a solitary erythema migrans lesion will be seropositive). For this reason, testing is not recommended for children who have erythema migrans; they should be treated based on a clinical diagnosis.

Treatment

- Early localized disease is treated with doxycycline, amoxicillin, or cefuroxime. In those unable to take 1 of these drugs, azithromycin is an alternative. Treatment duration is 7 to 14 days, depending on the antibiotic. (Consult the current edition of *Red Book®: Report of the Committee on Infectious Diseases* [https://redbook.solutions.aap.org] for drug dose and treatment duration.)

- Early disseminated or late disease is treated with various agents and regimens depending on the clinical manifestations. (Consult an infectious disease specialist or the most recent edition of *Red Book®: Report of the Committee on Infectious Diseases* [https://redbook.solutions.aap.org] for assistance in management of these presentations.)

- Tick avoidance is important for prevention.

Treating Associated Conditions

- A subset of patients who are treated may continue to have arthralgia and fatigue, a condition known as posttreatment Lyme disease syndrome. The cause of this condition is unknown but has not been linked to ongoing infection, and long-term antibiotic therapy has not been effective.

Prognosis

- The prognosis for children with Lyme disease is excellent when it is diagnosed early and treated promptly.

When to Worry or Refer

- Consider referral to a dermatologist or infectious disease specialist for patients who have atypical or persistent findings or in whom standard treatment is not effective.
- Consider referral to a rheumatologist for patients with chronic joint involvement.

Resources for Families

- American Academy of Pediatrics: HealthyChildren.org.
  https://www.healthychildren.org/lymedisease
- American Lyme Disease Foundation: Provides information about Lyme and supports research into the disease.
  www.aldf.com
- Centers for Disease Control and Prevention: Lyme disease.
  www.cdc.gov/lyme/index.html
- MedlinePlus: Information for patients and families (in English and Spanish) sponsored by the US National Library of Medicine and National Institutes of Health.
  www.nlm.nih.gov/medlineplus/lymedisease.html

CHAPTER 30

Meningococcemia

Introduction/Etiology/Epidemiology

- Caused by *Neisseria meningitidis*.
- Leading cause of bacterial meningitis in children aged 11 to 17 years in the United States. However, annual incidence rates for invasive meningococcal disease have decreased since the early 2000s.
- Transmission via respiratory droplets, direct oral contact, or indirect close contact.
- Approximately two-thirds of patients with meningococcemia will develop cutaneous manifestations.
- Incubation period is 1 to 10 days.

Signs and Symptoms

- Symptoms
  - At the outset, symptoms may mimic a viral illness (eg, fever, myalgias, headache, malaise). Early findings in young children may include leg pain, cold hands and feet (including gray acrocyanosis), and atypical skin color (pallor, mottling).
  - May have associated meningitis with headache, photophobia, vomiting, and nuchal rigidity.
- Cutaneous findings
  - Early on there are erythematous, urticarial, or morbilliform eruptions of macules and papules.
  - Petechiae of skin and mucous membranes, pustules, and vesicles often develop.
  - Purpuric lesions with jagged or stellate edges (Figure 30.1) may occur; may progress to bullae, necrosis, ulcers, and eschar.
  - Conjunctivae and retinae may reveal petechiae.

- Patients may develop profound hypotension and shock with overwhelming meningococcemia.
- Disseminated intravascular coagulation (Figure 30.2) may occur and, when present along with purpuric and necrotic plaques, is termed *purpura fulminans*.
- Autoamputation due to digital ischemia can be a potential complication.

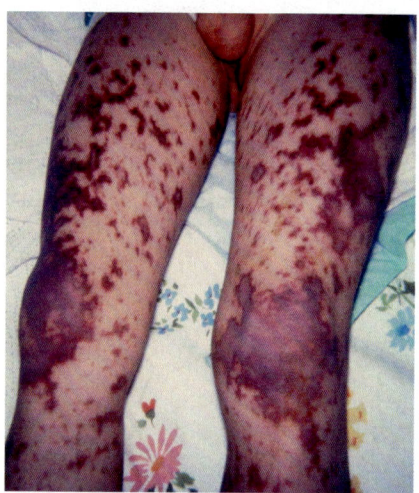

Figure 30.1. Meningococcemia. Purpuric plaques with jagged borders and early necrosis.

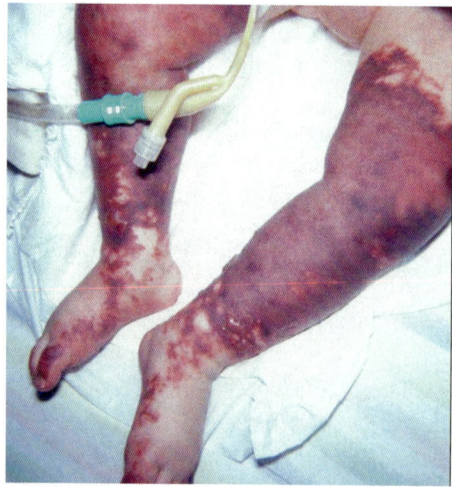

Figure 30.2. Meningococcemia. Disseminated intravascular coagulation.

Look-alikes

In each of the disorders listed herein, bacterial culture results will be negative or will not reveal *N meningitidis*.

Disorder	Differentiating Features
Gonococcemia	• May have petechiae or pustules, but they tend to be fewer in number than in meningococcemia. • Arthritis or arthralgias are present. • Patients usually appear less ill than with meningococcemia.
Rocky Mountain spotted fever	• History of tick bite may be elicited. • Patients initially appear less toxic than those who have meningococcemia. • Rash characteristically begins on the palms and soles as petechial macules and papules and then spreads centrally. • Severe headache common.
Henoch-Schönlein purpura	• Petechiae or palpable purpura most pronounced in dependent areas and areas under pressure (eg, waistband or sock line). • Edema common. • If fever present, usually low-grade. • Gastrointestinal and joint complaints common. • Nephritis may be present.
Other bacteremias (eg, *Streptococcus pneumoniae*, *Haemophilus influenzae* type b, gram-negative)	• Organisms seen on Gram stain of petechiae, buffy coat, or cerebrospinal fluid. • Positive blood culture results.

How to Make the Diagnosis

▶ Culture of the blood and/or cerebrospinal fluid are confirmatory.

▶ Antigen detection tests performed on cerebrospinal fluid are no longer used owing to low diagnostic sensitivity and specificity.

▶ Multiplex polymerase chain reaction assays are now widely available that detect multiple pathogens, including *N meningitidis*.

Treatment

- Supportive therapy, including fluids and vasoactive agents, as needed.
- Empiric therapy with ceftriaxone is recommended. Once a microbiological diagnosis is established, treatment options include ceftriaxone, penicillin G, and ampicillin (because organisms producing β-lactamase exist in the United States, reviewing susceptibilities is crucial before changing to penicillin or ampicillin). In a patient with life-threatening anaphylactic penicillin allergy, meropenem or ceftriaxone can be used, recognizing that the rate of cross-reactivity in adults allergic to penicillin is low. Consultation with a pediatric infectious disease specialist or the most recent edition of *Red Book®: Report of the Committee on Infectious Diseases* **(https://redbook.solutions.aap.org)** is recommended.
- Intermediate penicillin resistance is an increasing concern (especially in travelers from areas where penicillin resistance due to β-lactamase production has been reported); as a result, some recommend using ceftriaxone or (rarely) chloramphenicol until susceptibilities are available.
- Three quadrivalent conjugate meningococcal vaccines (MenACWY-CRM, MenACWY-D, MenACWY-TT) are available, and immunization is routinely recommended beginning at age 11 years. They can be used to prevent infection in high-risk groups from age 2 months (MenACWY-CRM), 9 months (MenACWY-D), or 2 years (MenACWY-TT) and older.
- A meningococcal B vaccine may be considered for those aged 16 to 23 years. For high-risk groups, individuals should receive the vaccine starting at 10 years of age.

Treating Associated Conditions

- If the patient develops disseminated intravascular coagulation, appropriate therapeutic measures should be instituted.
- Chemoprophylaxis is recommended for those who have had close contact with the index case in the 7 days before onset of illness (eg, household, child care, slept or ate in same dwelling). Consultation with a pediatric infectious disease specialist or the most recent edition of *Red Book®: Report of the Committee on Infectious Diseases* **(https://redbook.solutions.aap.org)** is recommended.

Prognosis

- The overall case fatality rate for invasive meningococcemia is 15%.
- Other potential sequelae (occurring in up to 19% of survivors) include hearing loss, neurologic variations, limb or digit amputations, and skin scarring.

When to Worry or Refer

- Patients with a presumed or confirmed diagnosis of meningococcemia should be evaluated in conjunction with an infectious disease specialist.

Resources for Families

- Centers for Disease Control and Prevention: Meningococcal disease. **www.cdc.gov/meningococcal**
- MedlinePlus: Information for patients and families (in English and Spanish) sponsored by the US National Library of Medicine and National Institutes of Health. **www.nlm.nih.gov/medlineplus/ency/article/001349.htm**
- National Meningitis Association: Site established by parents of children with a diagnosis of meningitis. Provides information about meningitis. **https://nmaus.org**

CHAPTER
31

Rocky Mountain Spotted Fever (RMSF)

Introduction/Etiology/Epidemiology

- The most common rickettsial infection in the United States.
- Caused by *Rickettsia rickettsii*, transmitted to humans by a tick bite. Infection results in a systemic small-vessel vasculitis.
- Tick vectors are dog ticks (*Dermacentor variabilis*) in the eastern and central United States and wood ticks (*Dermacentor andersoni*) in the northern and western United States. *Rhipicephalus sanguineus* (the brown dog tick) has more recently been confirmed as a possible vector in Arizona and Mexico.
- Transmission is highest in April to September, paralleling the tick season, but may occur throughout the year. The absence of a history of tick bite is common (about half of pediatric cases).
- Although it occurs in children, it is actually more common in adults because of occupational exposure (eg, forest rangers, outdoor workers).
- Incubation period is approximately 1 week (range, 3–12 days).
- Rapidly progressive (and potentially fatal) if not recognized, diagnosed, and treated early.

Signs and Symptoms

- Prodromal symptoms include
  - Malaise, myalgias (may be severe).
  - Headache (may be severe; prominent clinical feature).
  - Nausea and vomiting.
  - Photophobia.
- Subsequently, fever and rash develop.

- May present with prolonged capillary refill, weak pulses, or frank shock.
- Exanthem is present in approximately 80% to 90% of patients; usually appears around day 3 to 5 of illness.
  - Lesions are initially non-pruritic erythematous macules and papules occurring on the wrists and ankles and then spread distally to the palms and soles (Figure 31.1).
  - Lesions then spread centripetally (Figure 31.2).
  - The lesions evolve into petechial or purpuric macules and papules.
  - Larger areas of purpura or necrosis may occur.
  - In up to 10% of patients, the rash is completely absent (ie, "spotless Rocky Mountain spotted fever [RMSF]").
- Patients may develop multisystem disease (eg, central nervous system, cardiac, pulmonary, renal) and disseminated intravascular coagulation.

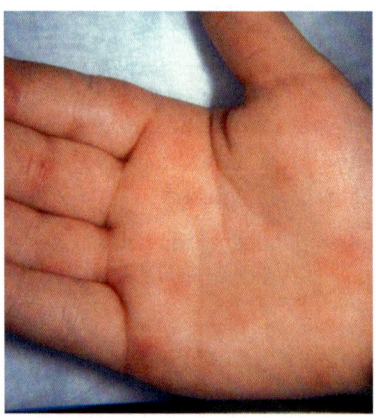

Figure 31.1. Rocky Mountain spotted fever. Note erythematous petechial macules on the palm.

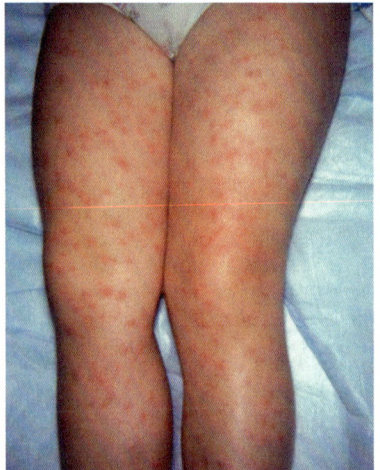

Figure 31.2. Rocky Mountain spotted fever with petechial lesions of the legs.

Chapter 31: Rocky Mountain Spotted Fever (RMSF)

Look-alikes

Note: History of tick bite would typically be absent in each of the following diagnoses (but RMSF should be diagnosed on the basis of clinical signs and symptoms and confirmed with diagnostic tests, whether history of a tick bite is present or absent).

Disorder	Differentiating Features
Meningococcemia	• Disease typically has abrupt onset with fever, myalgia, limb pain, prostration. • Papular, petechial, and purpuric lesions. • Meningeal signs may be present. • Hypotension, shock, disseminated intravascular coagulation may develop rapidly.
Henoch-Schönlein purpura	• Petechiae or palpable purpura most pronounced in dependent areas. • Lesions tend to be larger than those seen in Rocky Mountain spotted fever (RMSF). • Edema common. • If fever present, usually low-grade. • Gastrointestinal and joint complaints common. • Nephritis may be present.
Other bacteremias (eg, *Streptococcus pneumoniae*, *Haemophilus influenzae* type b, gram-negative)	• Organisms seen on Gram stain of petechiae, buffy coat, or cerebrospinal fluid. • Culture of organisms from a typically sterile site establishes the diagnosis.
Gonococcemia	• May have petechiae, but they tend to be fewer in number than in RMSF. • Arthritis or arthralgias are present. • Patients usually appear less ill than with RMSF.
Atypical measles	• Seen in individuals exposed to natural measles after receiving killed virus vaccinations. • High fever, headache, and myalgias; pneumonia and pleural effusions may also be present. • Hemorrhagic exanthem, which may be similar to that of RMSF.

How to Make the Diagnosis

- The diagnosis is made clinically (and treatment initiated based on clinical suspicion) and then confirmed with diagnostic testing.
  - Immunofluorescence antibody assay is the criterion standard serological test. However, a negative test result during the acute phase of the disease does not exclude RMSF because immunoglobulin (Ig) M and IgG antibodies begin to increase 7 to 10 days after the onset of symptoms.
  - Diagnosis may be confirmed with a fourfold or greater increase in IgG titer between acute- and convalescent-phase titers (obtained 2–4 weeks apart) obtained using immunofluorescence antibody assay or enzyme-linked immunosorbent assays.
  - Polymerase chain reaction assay of whole blood, tissue, or serum is also useful for diagnosis but may lack sensitivity.
- Biopsy specimen shows a mononuclear infiltrate with fibrin and thrombi; immunohistochemical stains may reveal the organism.
- Early laboratory findings may include thrombocytopenia, increased number of band forms (with expected or only slightly elevated white blood cell count), elevated liver transaminase levels, or hyponatremia.

Treatment

- Supportive therapy may be necessary, including fluids and vasoactive agents.
- Antibiotic treatment should be started as soon as the diagnosis is suspected (before diagnostic confirmation). It is most effective if initiated within the first 5 days of symptoms.
- Doxycycline is the drug of choice for all patients, including children of any age. Recent *Red Book* recommendations suggest that this medication can be safely used at any age for 21 days or fewer without concern for dental enamel staining.
- Treatment is administered until the patient has been afebrile for 3 days and has shown clinical improvement. The usual duration of therapy is 5 to 7 days but may be longer in severe cases.

Prognosis

- The prognosis for children with RMSF is good when diagnosed and treated early.

- Mortality rates (5%–10%) are highest in male patients, people older than 50 years, children younger than 10 years, and those with no history of a tick bite.

When to Worry or Refer

- Consultation with an infectious disease specialist should be considered for any patient with a presumed or confirmed diagnosis of RMSF, especially in children who are hospitalized.

Resources for Families

- Centers for Disease Control and Prevention: Alphabetical listing of diseases and conditions provides information for families in English and Spanish.
  www.cdc.gov/rmsf

- MedlinePlus: Information for patients and families (in English and Spanish) sponsored by the US National Library of Medicine and National Institutes of Health.
  www.nlm.nih.gov/medlineplus/ency/article/000654.htm

CHAPTER 32

Scarlet Fever

Introduction/Etiology/Epidemiology

- Scarlet fever (also known as scarlatina) is an exanthem (toxin-mediated) that generally occurs in association with group A β-hemolytic streptococcal (GABHS; ie, *Streptococcus pyogenes*) pharyngitis.
- Rarely, the eruption can be associated with a GABHS infection of a surgical wound, termed *surgical scarlet fever.*
- Prior exposure to GABHS results in a delayed skin reactivity exanthem to the pyrogenic A, B, C, and F exotoxins produced by *S pyogenes*.
- Age group most affected is 4 to 8 years.

Signs and Symptoms

- Fever.
- Incubation period is 2 to 5 days.
- Pharyngitis, including erythema of the posterior pharynx, tonsillar exudates, and soft palate petechiae.
- Tender anterior cervical lymphadenopathy.
- Headache and malaise are common.
- Skin eruption presents as diffuse blanchable erythema with numerous discrete pinpoint erythematous papules, sometimes likened to the consistency of sandpaper (sandpaper rash) (Figure 32.1). Rash involves the torso followed by the extremities, and, ultimately, it desquamates.
- Palms and soles are usually spared.
- Occasionally, tiny vesicles (miliaria crystallina or sudamina) may be seen on the abdomen, hands, and feet.
- Skin eruption is accentuated in skinfold areas. Linear and confluent petechiae in folds may also be present and are termed *Pastia lines* (Figure 32.2).

- Circumoral pallor is commonly present.
- The tongue initially has a white coating (white strawberry tongue) and later reveals prominent papillae and hyperemia (red strawberry tongue or raspberry tongue) (Figure 32.3).
- Desquamation is often noted in the perineal area during the acute infection, and peripheral desquamation (eg, affecting the hands and fingers) is seen 2 to 3 weeks after the onset of illness (Figure 32.4).
- A mild form of staphylococcal scalded skin syndrome (staphylococcal scarlet fever) may present with an identical rash, but the strawberry tongue and palatal enanthem of streptococcal scarlet fever are absent.

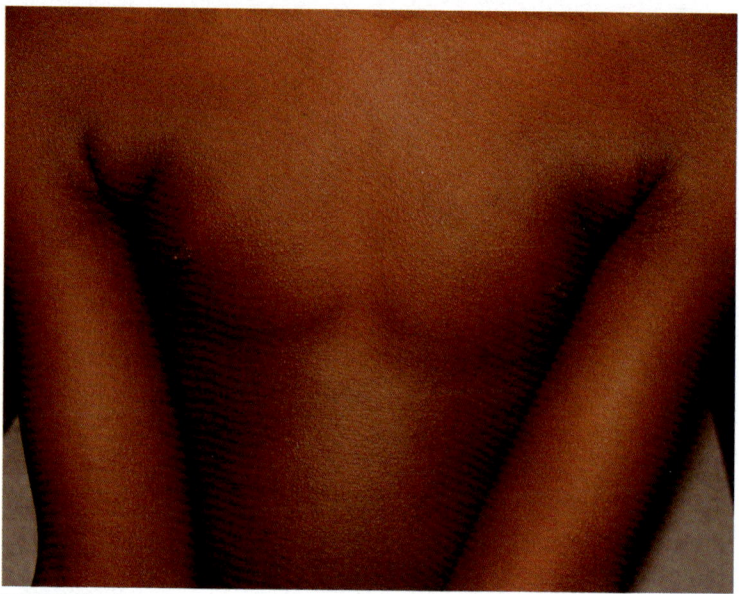

Figure 32.1. The rash of scarlet fever is composed of tiny papules, as seen in this young child. Note the subtle background erythema.

Chapter 32: Scarlet Fever 225

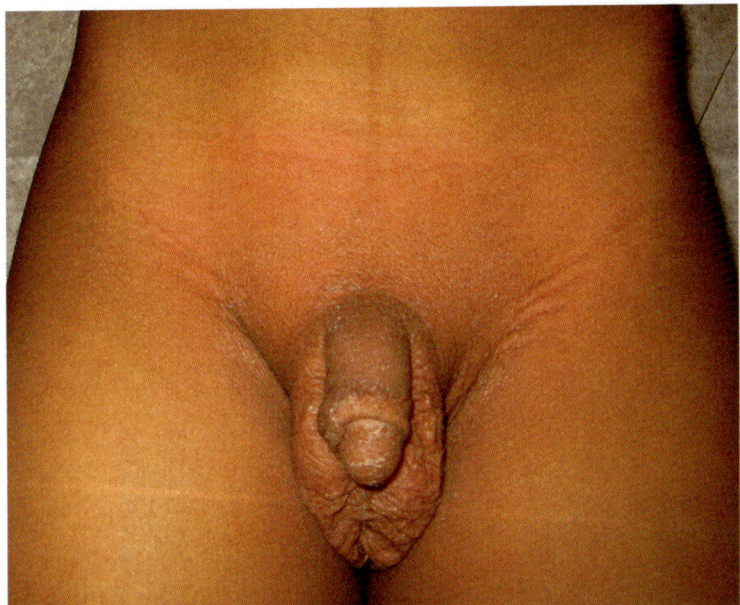

Figure 32.2. In scarlet fever, the rash often is accentuated in skinfolds.

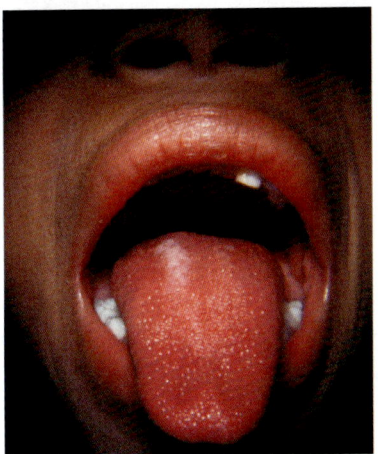

Figure 32.3. Scarlet fever. Red strawberry tongue or raspberry tongue.

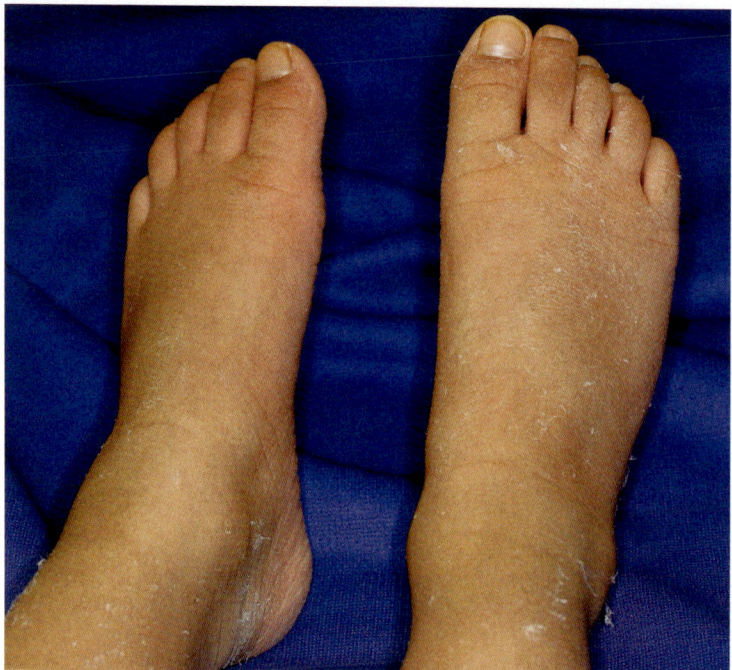

Figure 32.4. Scarlet fever with desquamation of the ankles and feet in a 5-year-old receiving antibiotic therapy.

Look-alikes

In each of the disorders listed as follows, test results for pharyngeal infection with *S pyogenes* would be negative.

Disorder	Differentiating Features
Staphylococcal scarlet fever	• Rash identical to that of streptococcal scarlet fever. • Strawberry tongue and palatal petechiae absent.
Staphylococcal scalded skin syndrome	• Erythema more widespread. • Bullae form, with subsequent rupture, peeling, and moist, denuded painful areas. • Oral mucous membranes usually spared.
Toxic shock syndrome	• Patients appear more ill. • Hypotension and multi-organ involvement present. • Conjunctival injection seen in toxic shock syndrome usually absent in scarlet fever.
Kawasaki disease	• Associated with prolonged high fever and classic constellation of clinical signs. • Skin eruption polymorphous but not typically sandpaper-like. • Oral changes consist primarily of hyperemia with lip fissuring; pharyngitis and pharyngeal symptoms absent. • Non-purulent conjunctival injection usually seen.
Infectious mononucleosis	• May be clinically similar to scarlet fever. • Reactive lymphocytosis often present. • Hepatosplenomegaly may be present. • Exanthem may appear or accentuate after administration of amoxicillin or ampicillin.
Arcanobacterium haemolyticum infection	• Similar clinical presentation to scarlet fever, but palatal petechiae and strawberry tongue are usually absent. • Typically affects teenagers or young adults. • If seeking diagnostic confirmation, laboratory should be notified to ensure throat swab specimen is plated on appropriate media.
Parvovirus B19 infection	• May mimic early scarlet fever. • Slapped cheek eruption may mimic circumoral pallor. • Pharyngitis mild or absent. • Eruption lacy and reticulated, not sandpaper-like.

How to Make the Diagnosis

▶ The diagnosis of scarlet fever is most often made clinically.

▶ A rapid streptococcal test or pharyngeal culture will confirm the diagnosis of streptococcal pharyngitis.

▶ When both results are negative with a typical clinical picture, consider staphylococcal scarlet fever, infectious mononucleosis, or *Arcanobacterium haemolyticum* infection (especially if in an adolescent).

Treatment

▶ The treatment of scarlet fever is the same as that for streptococcal pharyngitis (ie, penicillin V or amoxicillin divided 2 to 3 times daily for 10 days). However, oral amoxicillin administered as a single daily dose for 10 days is as effective as penicillin V given 3 times daily for 10 days.

▶ Azithromycin, clarithromycin, erythromycin, cephalexin, or clindamycin may be used in patients who are allergic to penicillin, but the choice will be governed by the nature of the penicillin allergy (ie, non-anaphylactic versus anaphylactic).

▶ Intramuscular penicillin G benzathine, administered in a single dose, is an appropriate alternative, particularly in children who are vomiting or in whom compliance is uncertain.

Treating Associated Conditions

▶ Acute rheumatic fever and acute glomerulonephritis are possible nonsuppurative sequelae of *S pyogenes* pharyngeal infections; the former is usually prevented with adequate treatment of the antecedent streptococcal infection.

▶ If a streptococcal strain associated with rheumatic fever has been detected in a community, patients should be observed for rheumatic fever symptoms.

- The terms *PANDAS* (Pediatric Autoimmune Neuropsychiatric Disorder Associated with Group A Streptococci) and *PANS* (Pediatric Acute-Onset Neuropsychiatric Syndrome) have been used (with some controversy) to describe a subset of children whose symptoms of obsessive-compulsive disorder or tic disorder are precipitated or exacerbated by group A streptococcal infection. However, data for such an association are based on the results of small studies that, at the time of this publication, have not been replicated. For additional information, please consult the current edition of the AAP *Red Book: Report of the Committee on Infectious Diseases*.

Prognosis

- The prognosis for scarlet fever is excellent, and most children who are treated recover fully without any long-term sequelae.

When to Worry or Refer

- Consider referral to a dermatologist for patients who have an exanthem with atypical features or in whom standard treatment does not work.

Resources for Families

- American Academy of Pediatrics: HealthyChildren.org.
  https://www.healthychildren.org/English/health-issues/conditions/skin/Pages/Scarlet-Fever.aspx

- MedlinePlus: Information for patients and families (in English and Spanish) sponsored by the US National Library of Medicine and National Institutes of Health.
  www.nlm.nih.gov/medlineplus/streptococcalinfections.html

- WebMD: Information for families is contained in the Health A-Z topics.
  www.webmd.com/a-to-z-guides/understanding-scarlet-fever-basics

CHAPTER
33

Staphylococcal Scalded Skin Syndrome (SSSS)

Introduction/Etiology/Epidemiology

- Caused by exfoliative toxins A and B produced by *Staphylococcus aureus*, most often from phage group 2.
- The toxin is spread hematogenously from the primary site of infection; it causes a cleavage in the granular layer of the epidermis that leads to formation of bullae.
- Most often seen in children younger than 5 years.
- When seen in older children, it is more often mild unless occurring in the setting of renal insufficiency or immunocompromise.

Signs and Symptoms

- Patients present with generalized erythema (often described as scarlatiniform or like a sunburn), tender skin, and irritability. Erythema often is more prominent in the skinfolds of the neck, axillae, and groin.
- Fever, malaise, lethargy, irritability can develop but are not always present.
- Flaccid bullae form, especially in intertriginous areas (Figure 33.1).
- Bullae rupture easily and produce large eroded areas surrounded by collarettes of skin (that are the remnants of the blister roof).
- Nikolsky sign is present (ie, lateral pressure on the skin causes a bulla to enlarge or an erosion to form).
- Crusting is present around the mouth, often with radial fissuring (ie, a sunburst appearance) (Figure 33.2).
- Common initial sites of infection include conjunctivae, nares, perioral area, and perineum and (in neonates) the umbilical region or an infected circumcision site.

- Oral mucous membrane changes are classically absent, but purulent conjunctivitis often is present.
- With healing, there is widespread desquamation.

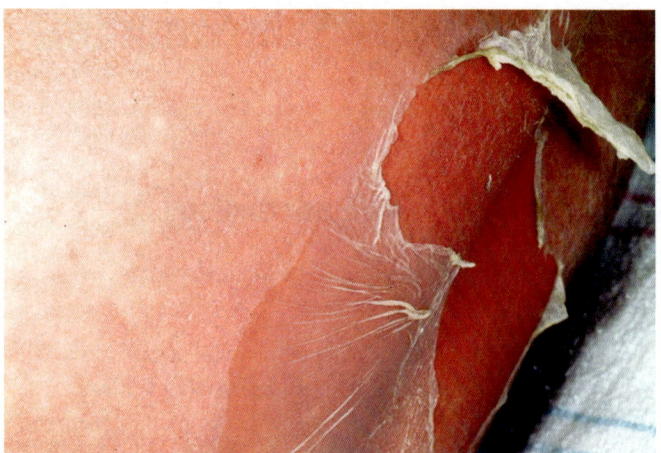

Figure 33.1. Staphylococcal scalded skin syndrome. Flaccid bullae form and rupture rapidly.

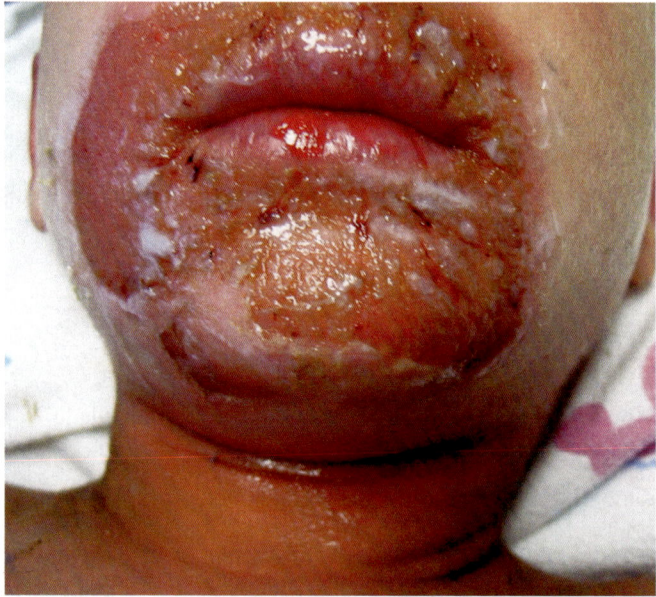

Figure 33.2. In staphylococcal scalded skin syndrome, erosions around the mouth often take on a "sunburst" appearance.

Look-alikes

Disorder	Differentiating Features
Streptococcal scarlet fever	• Eruption composed of fine papules (not diffuse macular erythema). • Blisters and erosions are absent.
Bullous impetigo	• Discrete and localized bullae and erythematous patches with peripheral collarettes. • Widespread erythema not present. • Patients appear well. • Fever usually absent.
Cellulitis	• Typically presents as ill-defined, localized indurated plaque (the remainder of the skin looks normal). • May be edematous, but blister formation rarely occurs.
Stevens-Johnson syndrome	• Blisters more tense and more discrete. • Typical target lesions may be present, with involvement of the palms and soles. • Erosions of the mucous membranes are present. • Widespread erosions unusual. • Frozen section of blister roof reveals full-thickness epidermis (only a few cell layers in staphylococcal scalded skin syndrome). • History of herpes simplex virus or *Mycoplasma* infection may be present.
Toxic shock syndrome	• Patients appear quite ill. • Hypotension and multi-organ involvement. • Skin blistering and denudation not typically seen. • Conjunctival injection present.
Kawasaki disease	• Associated with a prolonged high fever and classic constellation of clinical signs. • Erythema not usually as widespread. • Skin eruption polymorphous but not typically bullous or denuded. • Oral changes common, including hyperemia with lip fissuring. • Non-purulent conjunctival bulbar injection usually present.
Immersion burn	• Not generalized; buttocks or lower extremities usually involved. • Intertriginous areas spared. • History reported by caregiver(s) incompatible with child's development or examination findings.

How to Make the Diagnosis

- The diagnosis is often made clinically.
- A history of contact with an individual infected with *Staphylococcus*, especially in the setting of a community epidemic, may be present.
- Bullae are sterile, but culture from an initial site of infection (ie, perioral or peri-nasal areas, conjunctivae, or the umbilicus in neonates) or colonization may be positive for *S aureus*.
- Frozen section of a blister roof will confirm skin separation at the granular layer.
- Blood culture testing should be performed in any child who is seriously ill.

Treatment

- Oral systemic antistaphylococcal antibiotic for mild cases.
- Neonates and children with severe disease or who are toxic in appearance should receive parenteral therapy with antibiotics adequate to cover methicillin-resistant *S aureus* (eg, often a bactericidal agent like vancomycin or nafcillin combined with clindamycin [to reduce toxin production]).
- For those with severe disease and widespread erosions, closely monitor fluid and electrolyte status. Pain control should also be prescribed, as needed.

Treating Associated Conditions

- In patients with widespread denudation, fluid and electrolyte status should be closely monitored.
- If concomitant staphylococcal bacteremia is present, hospitalization with intravenous therapy is necessary. (See the Treatment section for details.)

Prognosis

- The prognosis for children with staphylococcal scalded skin syndrome is generally good.
- Skin generally heals without scarring within 2 weeks.
- Neonates have an increased risk of morbidity and mortality.

When to Worry or Refer

- Consider referral to a dermatologist or infectious disease specialist for patients who have an atypical presentation or in whom standard treatment does not work.
- Patients with severe or widespread disease and neonates with staphylococcal scalded skin syndrome should be hospitalized for observation, parenteral fluid administration, and antimicrobial therapy.

Resources for Families

- American Academy of Pediatrics: HealthyChildren.org.
  healthychildren.org/English/health-issues/conditions/infections/Pages/Staphylococcal-Infections.aspx
- Mayo Clinic: Staph infections.
  https://www.mayoclinic.org/diseases-conditions/staph-infections/symptoms-causes/syc-20356221

CHAPTER 34

Toxic Shock Syndrome (TSS)

Introduction/Etiology/Epidemiology

- A constellation of symptoms including acute fever, rash, malaise, myalgias, hypotension (or orthostatic hypotension or syncope), and multi-organ dysfunction.
- Caused by toxin-producing *Staphylococcus aureus* or *Streptococcus pyogenes*.
- Staphylococcal toxic shock syndrome (TSS) is most often caused by TSS toxin-1, a superantigen that stimulates production of tumor necrosis factor and other inflammatory mediators.
- Streptococcal TSS is caused by 1 of several exotoxins (see Look-alikes for discussion of streptococcal TSS).
- Toxin is produced by organisms particularly in suppurative sites, such as surgical wound infections or skin and soft-tissue infections. In the 1980s, staphylococcal TSS was associated with the use of superabsorbent tampons. The site of primary infection may not be immediately evident.

Signs and Symptoms

- The case definitions for staphylococcal and streptococcal TSS are presented in Table 34.1.
- Mucocutaneous findings in TSS
    - Generalized macular erythroderma (Figure 34.1)
    - Conjunctival injection
    - Necrolysis (necrosis with exfoliation)
    - Multiple pustules
    - Desquamation (seen 1–2 weeks after the onset of disease)

Table 34.1. Diagnostic Criteria for Staphylococcal and Streptococcal Toxic Shock Syndrome

Staphylococcal Toxic Shock Syndrome	Streptococcal Toxic Shock Syndrome

Clinical Findings
• Fever: temperature ≥38.9°C (102°F).
• Rash: diffuse macular erythroderma.
• Desquamation: 1–2 weeks after onset (especially palms, soles, fingers, toes).
• Hypotension: systolic blood pressure ≤90 mm Hg for adults and <5th percentile for age for children <16 years.
• Involvement of 3 or more of the following systems:
  – Gastrointestinal: vomiting or diarrhea at onset of illness.
  – Muscular: severe myalgia or creatine phosphokinase concentration greater than twice the upper limit appropriate.
  – Mucous membrane (vaginal, oropharyngeal, conjunctival) hyperemia.
  – Renal: serum urea nitrogen or serum creatinine concentration >2 times upper limit appropriate or urinary sediment with ≥5 white blood cells per high-power field in absence of urinary tract infection.
  – Hepatic: total bilirubin, aspartate aminotransferase, or alanine aminotransferase concentration greater than twice the upper limit appropriate.
  – Hematologic: platelet count ≤100,000/mm³
  – Central nervous system: disorientation, altered consciousness without focal neurologic signs.
	I. Isolation of group A streptococci
	  A. From a typically sterile site (eg, blood; cerebrospinal fluid; peritoneal fluid; joint, pleural, or pericardial fluid).
	  B. From a non-sterile site (eg, throat, sputum, vagina, open surgical wound, superficial skin lesion).
	II. Clinical signs of severity
	  A. Hypotension: systolic blood pressure ≤90 mm Hg for adults and <5th percentile for age for children <16 years.
	AND
	  B. Two or more of the following signs:
	  • Renal impairment: creatinine concentration ≥2 mg/dL for adults or at least 2 times the upper limit of reference for age.
	  • Coagulopathy: platelet count ≤100,000/mm³ and/or disseminated intravascular coagulation.
	  • Hepatic involvement: total bilirubin, aspartate aminotransferase, or alanine aminotransferase concentration at least twice the upper limit of reference for age.
	  • Adult respiratory distress syndrome (acute onset of diffuse pulmonary infiltrates and hypoxemia in absence of cardiac failure or by evidence of diffuse capillary leak).
	  • Generalized erythematous macular rash that may desquamate.
	  • Soft-tissue necrosis, including necrotizing fasciitis or myositis, or gangrene.

Table 34.1 (continued)

Staphylococcal Toxic Shock Syndrome	Streptococcal Toxic Shock Syndrome
Laboratory Criteria • Negative results on the following tests if performed: – Blood, throat, or cerebrospinal fluid cultures; however, blood culture result may be positive in select cases for *Staphylococcus aureus*. – Serological tests for Rocky Mountain spotted fever, leptospirosis, or measles.	**Laboratory Criteria** • As previously noted.
Case Classification • Confirmed: Case meets laboratory criteria and all 5 clinical findings, including desquamation (unless the patient dies before desquamation appears), are present. • Probable: Case meets laboratory criteria, and 4 of 5 clinical findings are present.	**Case Classification** • Confirmed: Case fulfills criteria IA, IIA, and IIB. • Probable: Case fulfills criteria IB, IIA, and IIB (if no other cause for the illness is identified).

Adapted with permission from American Academy of Pediatrics. *Staphylococcus aureus*. In: Kimberlin DW, Banerjee R, Barnett ED, Lynfield R, et al, eds. *Red Book: 2024–2027 Report of the Committee on Infectious Diseases*. 33rd ed. American Academy of Pediatrics; 2024:766–782, and Group A streptococcal infections. In: Kimberlin DW, Banerjee R, Barnett ED, Lynfield R, et al, eds. *Red Book: 2024–2027 Report of the Committee on Infectious Diseases*. 33rd ed. American Academy of Pediatrics; 2024:785–798.

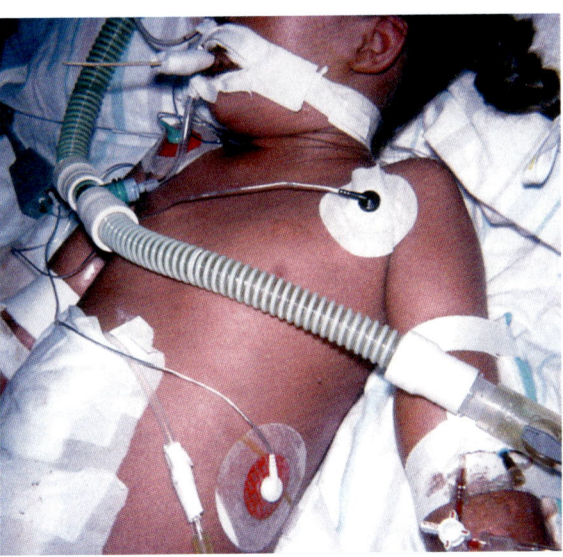

Figure 34.1. Toxic shock syndrome. This patient had widespread erythema, adult respiratory distress–like syndrome, and renal failure.

Look-alikes

Disorder	Differentiating Features
Staphylococcal scalded skin syndrome	• Crusting may be noted in perioral, peri-nasal regions. • Hypotension not typically present. • Bullae form, with subsequent rupture, peeling, and appearance of moist denuded, painful areas. • Multi-organ involvement usually absent.
Streptococcal scarlet fever	• Eruption composed of fine papules (not diffuse macular erythema). • Multi-organ involvement absent.
Staphylococcal scarlet fever	• Eruption composed of fine papules (not diffuse macular erythema). • Multi-organ involvement absent.
Stevens-Johnson syndrome	• Presents with tense, discrete blisters. • Typical target lesions may be present. • Erosions of the mucous membranes present. • Hypotension absent. • Multi-organ involvement not typically present.
Kawasaki disease	• Associated with prolonged high fever and classic constellation of clinical signs (see case definition in the current edition of *Red Book*®). • Diffuse erythroderma not typical. • Hypotension not typically present. • Prominent cervical lymphadenopathy often present.

How to Make the Diagnosis

▶ Diagnosis is confirmed by meeting the diagnostic criteria as detailed (or referenced) previously.

▶ In staphylococcal TSS, a positive culture result is not required to make the diagnosis.

▶ In streptococcal TSS, isolation of group A streptococci may be from blood; cerebrospinal fluid; peritoneal fluid; joint, pleural, or pericardial fluid (confirmed case when other criteria present); or throat, sputum, vagina, open surgical wound, or superficial skin lesion (probable case when other criteria present).

Treatment

- Supportive therapy, including maintaining fluid status and use of vasoactive agents as necessary. Anticipate multisystem organ failure.
- Perform a thorough search for and adequate drainage of suppurative sites. For streptococcal TSS with necrotizing fasciitis, emergent surgical debridement is needed.
- Specific therapy with antistaphylococcal antibiotic with activity against methicillin-resistant *S aureus* (eg, vancomycin, linezolid).
- Clindamycin (which inhibits toxin synthesis in susceptible isolates of *S aureus* and *S pyogenes*) often is recommended.
- Use of intravenous immunoglobulin may be considered for children who are critically ill, though its use is based on limited data.

Treating Associated Conditions

- Because multi-organ involvement is the norm, affected patients need appropriate monitoring and supportive care in a critical care setting.

Prognosis

- Mortality associated with staphylococcal TSS is approximately 3% to 10%. Pediatric mortality associated with streptococcal TSS is higher, especially when necrotizing fasciitis is present.
- Recovery time is shortened and mortality is lowered with use of appropriate antibiotics and eradication of the toxin-producing organisms from colonized sites.

When to Worry or Refer

- Consult an infectious disease specialist for patients who have an atypical presentation or who do not respond to standard treatment. Most or all patients with suspected or confirmed TSS require intensive care.
- Early consultation with surgical services for drainage or debridement of identified suppurative foci may be lifesaving.

Resources for Families

- American Academy of Pediatrics: HealthyChildren.org.
  healthychildren.org/English/health-issues/conditions/infections/Pages/Toxic-Shock-Syndrome.aspx
- MedlinePlus: Information for patients and families (in English and Spanish) sponsored by the US National Library of Medicine and National Institutes of Health.
  https://www.nlm.nih.gov/medlineplus/ency/article/000653.htm
- Toxic Shock Syndrome Information Service: An industry-sponsored site in the United Kingdom that provides information about TSS.
  www.toxicshock.com
- WebMD: Information for families is contained in Women's Health.
  www.webmd.com/women/guide/understanding-toxic-shock-syndrome-basics

Fungal and Yeast Infections

CHAPTER 35 — *Candida* 245

CHAPTER 35A — Angular Cheilitis/Perlèche 247

CHAPTER 35B — Candidal Diaper Dermatitis 251

CHAPTER 35C — Chronic Paronychia 255

CHAPTER 35D — Neonatal/Congenital Candidiasis 259

CHAPTER 35E — Thrush 263

CHAPTER 36 — Onychomycosis 267

CHAPTER 37 — Tinea Capitis 271

CHAPTER 38 — Tinea Corporis 281

CHAPTER 39 — Tinea Cruris 287

CHAPTER 40 — Tinea Pedis 291

CHAPTER 41 — Tinea Versicolor 297

CHAPTER
35

Candida

Introduction/Etiology/Epidemiology

- *Candida* species are ubiquitous and typically are noninvasive.
- *Candida* species exist as common flora in the gastrointestinal tract and mucocutaneous surfaces of humans.
- In immunocompromised hosts, *Candida albicans* is the most frequent species that may invade mucous membranes or moist or macerated cutaneous surfaces.
- Note: The next 5 chapters (35A–35E) outline various candidal disorders.

Resources for Families

- American Academy of Pediatrics: HealthyChildren.org.
  https://www.healthychildren.org/candida
- MedlinePlus: Information for patients and families (in English and Spanish) sponsored by the US National Library of Medicine and National Institutes of Health.
  https://www.nlm.nih.gov/medlineplus/ency/article/000880.htm

CHAPTER 35A

Angular Cheilitis/Perlèche

Introduction/Etiology/Epidemiology

- Inflammation and maceration of the angles of the mouth (ie, angular cheilitis or perlèche) can result from repeated licking, excessive salivation, or drooling.
- *Candida* species may then secondarily infect the areas directly or by extension of oral thrush.
- Perlèche is frequently observed in children with neurologic deficits who have difficulty managing oral secretions. It may also be seen with increased frequency in children who have increased drooling related to the presence of orthodontic appliances or immunocompromise.

Signs and Symptoms

- Erythema and fissuring of the angles of the mouth (Figure 35A.1).
- Exudate may be present.

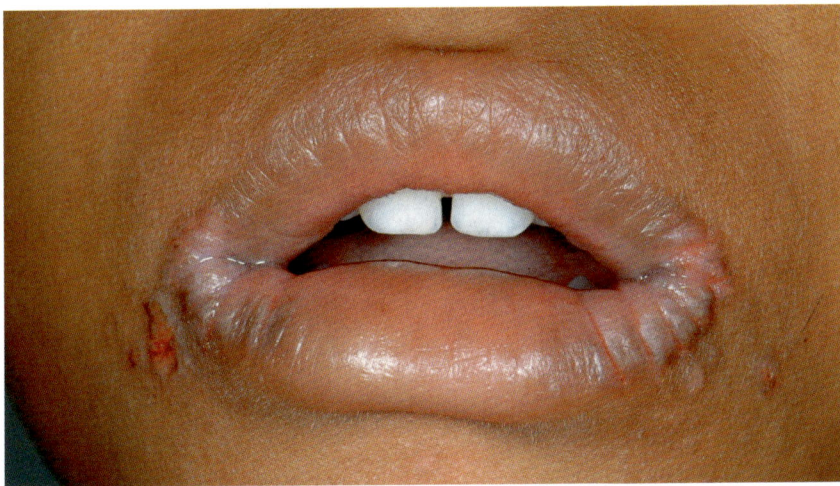

Figure 35A.1. Erythema, maceration, and fissuring of the corners of the mouth are observed in angular cheilitis.

Look-alikes

Disorder	Differentiating Features
Localized trauma	• Historical information suggesting trauma (eg, frequent and aggressive dental flossing).
Contact dermatitis	• Historical information suggesting exposure to an allergen.
Lip-licking dermatitis	• Historical information suggesting lip licking. • Well-defined erythematous patch surrounding mouth. • Occasionally may have associated angular cheilitis.
Secondary syphilis (mucous patch)	• A mucous patch may be located at the angle of the mouth, but patients generally have additional labial and intraoral lesions and rash elsewhere. • Patients often have systemic symptoms, including fever, malaise, or arthralgias, and generalized lymphadenopathy.

How to Make the Diagnosis

▶ The diagnosis is usually made clinically.

▶ If uncertainty exists, the diagnosis may be confirmed by microscopic observation of budding yeast or pseudohyphae in a potassium hydroxide preparation performed on scrapings of lesions or fungal culture (Figure 35A.2).

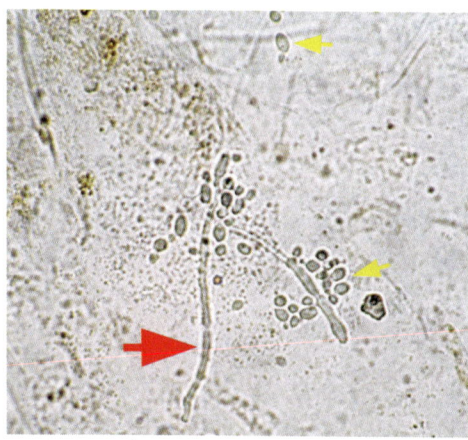

Figure 35A.2. A potassium hydroxide preparation reveals pseudohyphae (red arrow) and spores (yellow arrows) of *Candida* species.

Treatment

- Treatment focuses on the control or elimination of the inflammatory component with a low-potency topical steroid or topical calcineurin inhibitor, often in combination with the application of a topical antifungal agent (eg, nystatin, miconazole, clotrimazole) if secondary *Candida* infection is suspected.
- A combination antifungal-corticosteroid preparation (eg, nystatin in 0.1% triamcinolone ointment) is effective for short-term use, applied twice daily to the mouth angles until improved. If long-term use is required, a lower potency topical steroid is preferred.
- Minimize predisposing factors such as lip licking, thumb-sucking, and vigorous flossing.
- Persistent or repeated infection suggests a need for consideration of bacterial infection (*Staphylococcus aureus* or *Streptococcus pyogenes*) or immunodeficiency.

Treating Associated Conditions

- Identify and eliminate exposure to triggers responsible for irritant or allergic contact dermatitis.

Prognosis

- The prognosis for patients with angular cheilitis is excellent, but underlying predisposing conditions may lead to recurrences.

When to Worry or Refer

- Consider consultation with a dermatologist when the diagnosis is in doubt or lesions fail to respond to appropriate therapy.
- When confronting treatment-resistant cases, consider contact dermatitis, diabetes mellitus, or other immunosuppression.

Resource for Families

- DermNet NZ: Angular cheilitis.
  https://dermnetnz.org/topics/angular-cheilitis

CHAPTER 35B

Candidal Diaper Dermatitis

Introduction/Etiology/Epidemiology

- Common infection often precipitated by compromise of the cutaneous barrier (eg, by irritant diaper dermatitis).

Signs and Symptoms

- Confluent, beefy red patch that involves the creases; satellite lesions (eg, papules, pustules) are present beyond the advancing border (Figures 35B.1 and 35B.2).
- Often complicates noninfectious forms of diaper dermatitis (eg, irritant diaper dermatitis) and may occur as an adverse effect of oral antibiotic treatment.

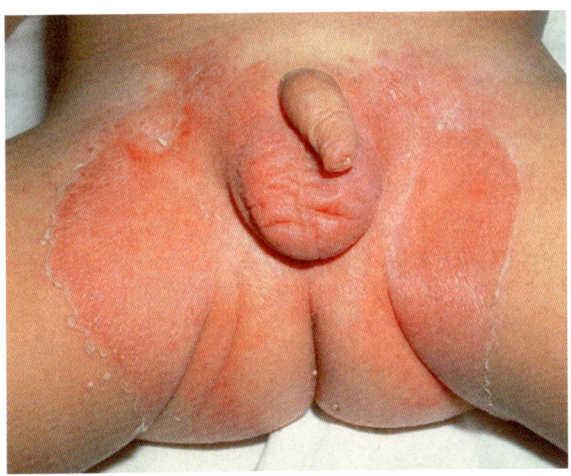

Figure 35B.1. Bright red patches that involve the creases and convexities are observed in candidal diaper dermatitis. Satellite lesions and scale are present.

Look-alikes (See also Chapter 101, Diaper Dermatitis.)

Disorder	Differentiating Features
Irritant dermatitis	• Erythematous patches involve the lower abdomen, buttocks, and thighs. • Convex surfaces involved. • Inguinal folds often spared.
Seborrheic dermatitis	• Salmon-pink patches with greasy scale that involve convexities and inguinal creases. • Involvement of scalp, face, postauricular creases, umbilicus, or chest may be present.
Intertrigo	• Erythema and superficial erosions located in skinfolds (eg, the inguinal creases). • May become secondarily infected with *Candida* species or *Streptococcus pyogenes*.
Psoriasis	• Erythematous scaling papules or plaques (scaling of the scalp and umbilicus may be present). • Lesions in the diaper area often lack scale characteristic of lesions elsewhere.
Acrodermatitis enteropathica	• Often begins when infants are weaned from human milk to cow milk formula. • Scaling erythematous eruption located around mouth and in diaper area. • Infants may have sparse hair, diarrhea, or failure to gain weight.
Langerhans cell histiocytosis	• Vesicles or pustules (often with a hemorrhagic crust); erythematous, orange, or yellow-brown papules or nodules; petechiae; erosions (especially in the diaper area, axillae, neck folds). • May have associated lymphadenopathy, bone swelling, diabetes insipidus. • Resistant to standard therapies.

How to Make the Diagnosis

▶ The diagnosis is usually made clinically.

▶ If diagnostic uncertainty exists, a potassium hydroxide preparation examination performed on scales from a skin scraping will reveal pseudohyphae or spores (Figure 35A.2). Fungal culture can also be considered.

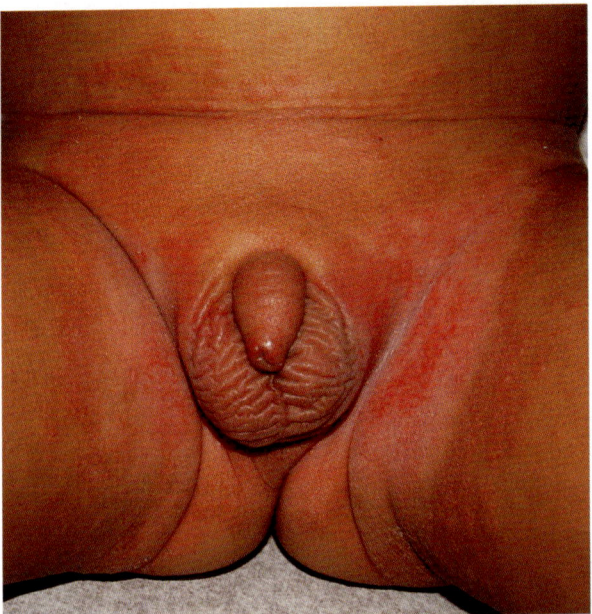

Figure 35B.2. Candidal diaper dermatitis in an infant with skin of color. There are erythematous patches involving the convexities and skinfolds and satellite papules. Postinflammatory hypopigmentation is present on the medial thighs.

Treatment

- Topical anti-candidal agent (eg, nystatin, miconazole, clotrimazole).
- When severe, a short course of oral fluconazole may be used.
- Concomitant use of a thick barrier cream or ointment is helpful (and should be applied over the topical antifungal agent).

Treating Associated Conditions

- If thrush is present, treat with oral nystatin or fluconazole.

Prognosis

- The prognosis for infants is excellent.

When to Worry or Refer

- Failure to respond to appropriate anti-candidal therapy warrants careful reconsideration of the diagnosis. However, repeated episodes are not uncommon in healthy infants.
- Persistent or recurrent episodes of candidal infection may suggest immunodeficiency, including HIV infection. However, repeated episodes without additional symptoms are not uncommon in healthy infants.

Resources for Families

- American Academy of Pediatrics: HealthyChildren.org. www.healthychildren.org/English/ages-stages/baby/diapers-clothing/Pages/Diaper-Rash.aspx
- Cleveland Clinic: Yeast diaper rash. https://my.clevelandclinic.org/health/diseases/22307-yeast-diaper-rash#:~:text=Diaper%20rashes%20are%20the%20result,known%20as%20Candida%20diaper%20dermatitis

CHAPTER 35C

Chronic Paronychia

Introduction/Etiology/Epidemiology

- Chronic paronychia is common among children who are thumb-suckers, nail-biters, or nail pickers.
- *Candida* species usually are responsible.

Signs and Symptoms

- Non-tender erythematous swelling of the skin surrounding the nail (Figure 35C.1).
- Loss of the cuticle in affected digits is common.
- Associated nail dystrophy may be present, most often presenting as pits or transverse ridges; yellow debris and separation of the nail plate from the nail bed may be present (Figure 35C.2).

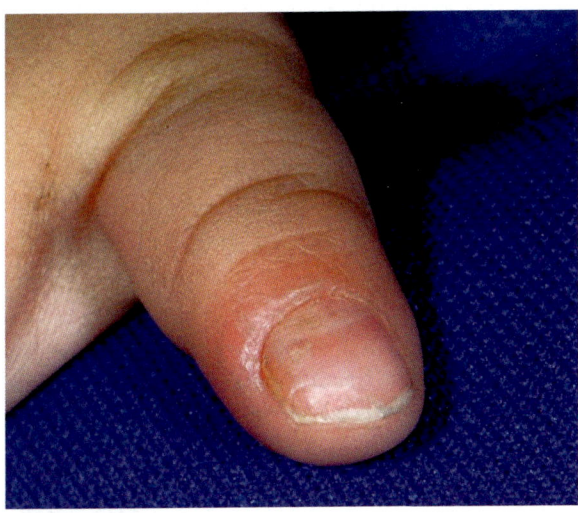

Figure 35C.1. Chronic paronychia caused by *Candida*. There is periungual erythema and loss of the cuticle.

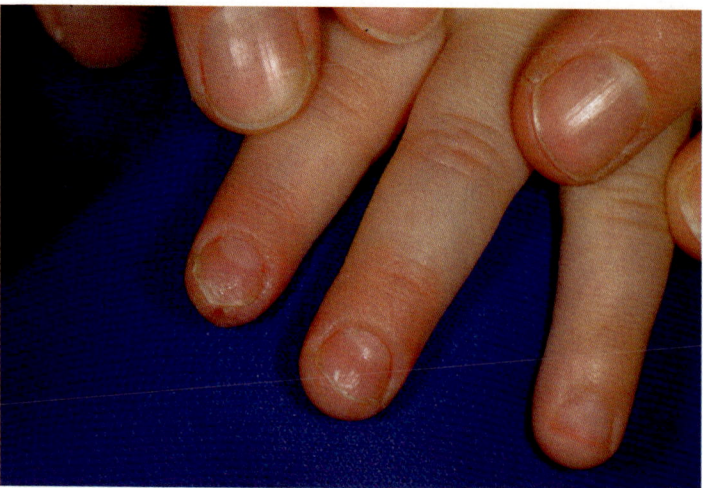

Figure 35C.2. Chronic paronychia caused by *Candida*. In addition to periungual erythema and cuticle loss, note the dystrophy of the nail plates.

Look-alikes

Disorder	Differentiating Features
Acute paronychia	• Acute onset with painful swelling, erythema, and purulent exudate. • Culture often positive for *Staphylococcus aureus*.
Tinea unguium (onychomycosis)	• Skin surrounding nail usually typical. • When toenails infected, usually evidence of associated tinea pedis (eg, fissuring, scaling, maceration between the digits). • Nail usually thickened and white to yellow, with debris under the nail plate.
Herpetic whitlow	• Acute onset of painful clustered vesicles or a bulla on an erythematous base. • May be located on a digit but seldom limited to proximal and lateral nail folds.
Blistering dactylitis	• Acute onset of a bulla affecting distal portion of a digit. • Located on digit but not limited to proximal or lateral nail folds. • Culture of blister fluid often yields group A β-hemolytic streptococci or *S aureus*.
Chronic mucocutaneous candidiasis	• Multiple digits involved. • Associated recurrent candidal mucocutaneous infections. • May have associated immunologic or endocrinologic variations.

How to Make the Diagnosis

- The diagnosis is usually made clinically.
- If uncertainty exists, the diagnosis may be confirmed by microscopic observation of budding yeast or pseudohyphae in a potassium hydroxide preparation performed on scrapings of the affected area, or by fungal culture (see Figure 35A.2).

Treatment

- Treatment is complicated by predisposing behaviors that cause trauma or moisture (eg, nail-biting, thumb-sucking). When possible, these factors should be addressed.
- Topical nystatin or an imidazole antifungal agent applied during the day and under occlusion at night (care must be taken to secure occlusive dressings to prevent aspiration by young patients).
- Oral fluconazole (or other appropriate agent) may be indicated in severe or persistent cases.

Treating Associated Conditions

- Provide positive feedback for substitute behaviors.
- Use of noxious agents to control thumb-sucking should be considered second-line therapy.

Prognosis

- Long-term prognosis is excellent (once predisposing factors have been eliminated).

When to Worry or Refer

▶ Involvement of multiple nails along with recurrent mucosal or skin infection may indicate the presence of chronic mucocutaneous candidiasis.

Resource for Families

▶ DermNet NZ: Paronychia. https://dermnetnz.org/topics/paronychia

CHAPTER 35D

Neonatal/Congenital Candidiasis

Introduction/Etiology/Epidemiology

- Uncommon infection that may be observed at birth or within a week of delivery.
- *Candida albicans* (occasionally a non-*albicans Candida* species) is acquired during passage through a colonized birth canal or by ascending infection before delivery.

Signs and Symptoms

- Eruption presents as papules and pustules superimposed on an erythematous base (Figure 35D.1) or as diffuse erythema with scaling (Figure 35D.2).
- Presence of papules and pustules on the palms and soles is characteristic.
- Nail dystrophy with yellow discoloration may be present (Figure 35D.3).
- Any body surface may be involved.
- Most full-term neonates experience a benign course, but very low-birth-weight neonates are at higher risk for invasive disease.

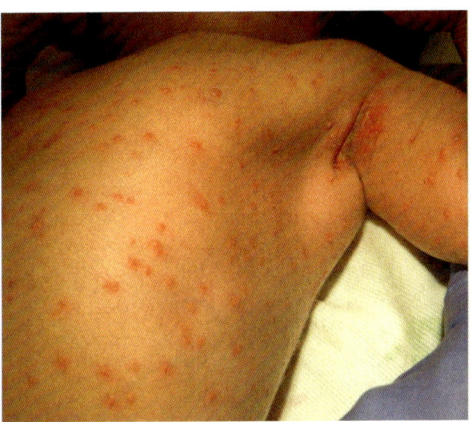

Figure 35D.1. Congenital candidiasis is characterized by erythematous papules, pustules, and scaling.

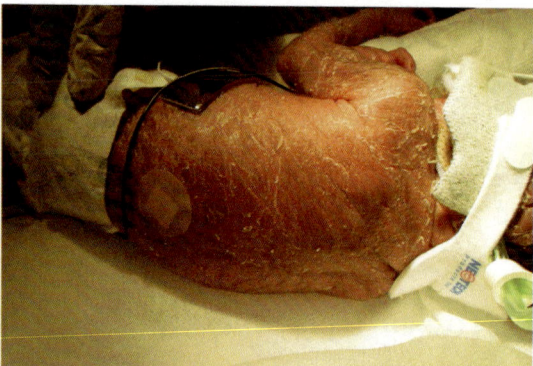

Figure 35D.2. Congenital candidiasis in a preterm neonate with skin of color. Note diffuse faint erythema with marked scaling and hyperkeratosis. Such preterm neonates have a higher risk for systemic dissemination of the fungal infection. Reproduced from Jani S, Ariss R, Chawla S. A preterm infant with a characteristic erythematous and scaly rash after birth. *Neoreviews.* 2020;21(7):e495–e498.

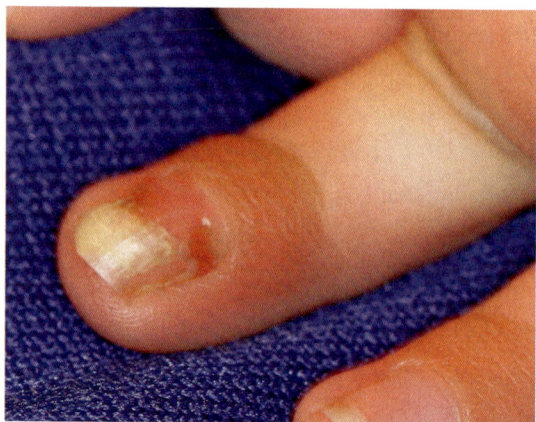

Figure 35D.3. Nail dystrophy in congenital candidiasis. There is yellow discoloration, onycholysis, and mild surrounding paronychia (ie, inflammation of proximal and lateral nail folds).

Look-alikes

In each of the disorders listed herein, a potassium hydroxide preparation would fail to demonstrate the pseudohyphae and spores that would be observed in candidal infection.

Disorder	Differentiating Features
Erythema toxicum	• Discrete, blotchy, erythematous macules or patches, each with a central papule, vesicle, or pustule. • Typically not present at birth. • Vesicular/pustular fluid contains eosinophils.
Transient neonatal pustular melanosis	• Pustules (without erythema) or ruptured pustules, which appear as small freckle-like hyperpigmented macules surrounded by a rim of scale. • Pustular fluid contains neutrophils.
Miliaria rubra	• Erythematous papules and papulopustules, often located in occluded areas and skinfolds.
Neonatal cephalic pustulosis (neonatal acne)	• Papules and pustules typically limited to face.
Staphylococcal folliculitis	• White to slightly yellow pustules with surrounding rim of erythema. • Gram stain or bacterial culture will reveal *Staphylococcus aureus*.
Scabies	• Occurs rarely during first month after birth. • Generalized eruption; may have vesicles but usually will be accompanied by erythematous papules or nodules and burrows. • Mineral oil preparation of scrapings of lesions will reveal mites, eggs, or fecal material.
Neonatal herpes simplex virus infection	• Typically clustered vesicles on an erythematous base (although solitary vesicles occasionally occur). • Lesions concentrated on head, particularly at sites of trauma (eg, those caused by a scalp electrode). • Neonates may have signs of sepsis (in disseminated disease) or seizures or coma (in central nervous system disease). • Direct fluorescent examination, viral culture, or polymerase chain reaction (skin lesions, cerebrospinal fluid) will confirm diagnosis.
Infantile acropustulosis	• Usually begins in first months (not in first days) after birth. • Vesicles or pustules that are limited to the hands and feet, including the palms and soles, wrists, and ankles. • Eruption lasts for 5 to 10 days and reappears every 2 to 4 weeks.
Incontinentia pigmenti	• Vesicles on an erythematous base appear at birth or within the first 2 weeks after birth. • Lesions arranged in a linear fashion on the extremities or in a swirled pattern on the trunk (along the Blaschko lines).
Eosinophilic pustular folliculitis	• Papules and pustules typically located on the scalp. • Exhibits a chronic, intermittent course. • Severe pruritus is usually present.

How to Make the Diagnosis

- The diagnosis is made by performing a potassium hydroxide preparation on skin scrapings (see Figure 35A.2) and fungal culture of specimens from the skin, placenta, or umbilical cord.

Treatment

- Topical application of an antifungal agent such as nystatin or clotrimazole.
- In neonates with diffuse skin involvement, oral fluconazole may accelerate resolution.
- In the rare patient who has evidence of (or risk factors for) systemic infection, complete evaluation for this possibility and parenteral antifungal therapy are required.

Prognosis

- The prognosis for term neonates with cutaneous congenital candidiasis is excellent.
- Low-birth-weight neonates (or those born to mothers with a history of an indwelling device [eg, cervical cerclage, intrauterine device]) are at increased risk for systemic involvement (eg, infection of blood, lungs, central nervous system, urinary tract).

When to Worry or Refer

- Consider consultation by a dermatologist when the diagnosis is in doubt or lesions fail to respond to appropriate therapy.
- When systemic disease is likely, immediate consultation with a pediatric infectious disease specialist is warranted.

Resource for Families

- American Academy of Pediatrics: HealthyChildren.org. **healthychildren.org/English/health-issues/conditions/infections/pages/Thrush-and-Other-Candida-Infections.aspx**

CHAPTER 35E

Thrush

Introduction/Etiology/Epidemiology

- Common condition among young infants.
- Antibiotic therapy that disrupts the typical oral flora may be a predisposing factor.
- Recurrent or persistent thrush, especially in an infant with other signs or symptoms or in older children, should raise concern about immunocompromised conditions (eg, HIV infection, another immunodeficiency disorder).

Signs and Symptoms

- Presents with discrete white plaques overlying an erythematous base that involve the buccal mucosa or tongue (Figures 35E.1 and 35E.2).
- Infants with thrush may be irritable and feed poorly.

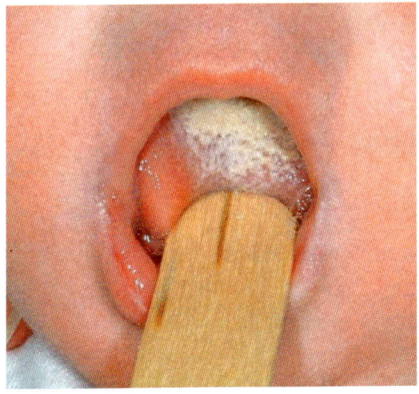

Figure 35E.1. White patches on the tongue or buccal mucosa are characteristic of thrush.

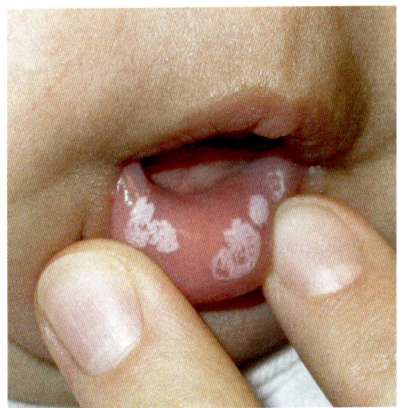

Figure 35E.2. White plaques on the lips of an infant who has thrush.

Look-alikes

Disorder	Differentiating Features
Retained food or formula	• White patches easily removed with a tongue depressor or gauze.
Geographic tongue	• Well-defined, sometimes annular patches that may appear to be erosions located on tongue. • Pattern of involvement changes daily.
Herpetic gingivostomatitis	• Multiple painful vesicles and ulcers located on buccal mucosa, tongue, or gingivae. • Perioral skin often reveals similar lesions. • Children febrile, appear ill, and at risk for dehydration.
Herpangina	• Small vesicles or shallow ulcers typically located on tonsillar pillars, soft palate, tonsils, and uvula. • Associated with fever, sore throat, or dysphagia.
Koplik spots of measles	• Gray-white dots often with surrounding erythema (appear before the exanthem). • Typically located on buccal mucosa adjacent to mandibular molars. • Patients generally appear ill with fever, cough, coryza, and conjunctivitis.

How to Make the Diagnosis

▶ The diagnosis usually is made based on clinical findings.

▶ If uncertainty exists, a potassium hydroxide preparation performed on a sample obtained from the mouth (by scraping the affected area with a tongue depressor) will demonstrate pseudohyphae or budding yeast (see Figure 35A.2). Fungal culture can also be considered.

Treatment

▶ Oral nystatin, miconazole, or fluconazole for the infant.

▶ Minimize predisposing factors such as contaminated pacifiers and nipples.

▶ If the infant is breastfeeding, assess for possible maternal candidal infection of the breast and treat accordingly.

▶ Persistent or frequently recurrent infections, especially in the presence of other signs and symptoms of systemic illness, should prompt consideration for immunodeficiency.

Prognosis

- The prognosis for infants who have thrush is excellent, and the course is usually benign.

When to Worry or Refer

- When the diagnosis is in doubt or lesions fail to respond to appropriate therapy, consultation with an immunologist or pediatric infectious disease specialist is warranted.

Resources for Families

- DermNet NZ: Oral candidiasis.
 https://dermnetnz.org/topics/oral-candidiasis
- Healthy Children: Thrush and other *Candida* infections.
 https://www.healthychildren.org/English/health-issues/conditions/infections/Pages/Thrush-and-Other-Candida-Infections.aspx

CHAPTER 36

Onychomycosis

Introduction/Etiology/Epidemiology

- Dermatophyte infection of nails usually caused by *Trichophyton rubrum*, *Trichophyton mentagrophytes*, or *Epidermophyton floccosum* (occasionally, molds may cause onychomycosis).
- Common in adolescents and adults; less common in children.
- In most pediatric cases, there is a family history of tinea pedis or onychomycosis.

Signs and Symptoms

- Toenails are more frequently involved than fingernails.
- Two forms are recognized.
  - Subungual onychomycosis: thickening of the nail with yellow discoloration distally or laterally that indicates separation of the nail from the nail bed (ie, distal and lateral subungual onychomycosis, respectively) (Figure 36.1).
  - Superficial white onychomycosis: white discoloration with a fine, powdery scale (Figure 36.2).
- One or multiple nails may be involved, but "skip nails" (with no involvement) are commonly seen.
- Most patients have evidence of coexisting tinea pedis.

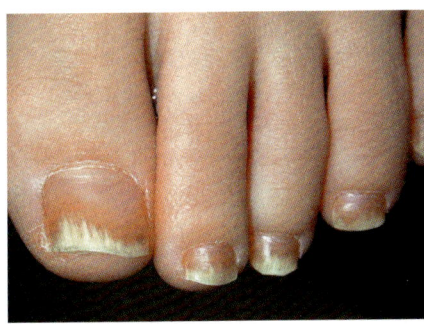

Figure 36.1. Thickening and yellowing of the nail and separation of the nail plate from the bed occur in subungual onychomycosis.

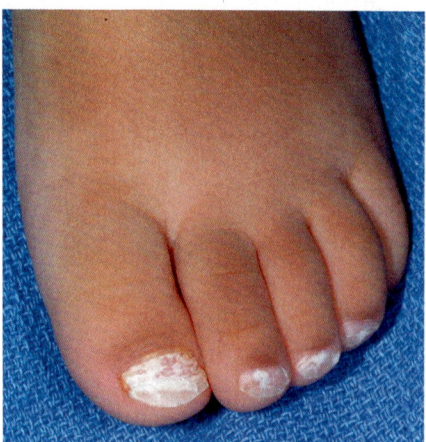

Figure 36.2. In superficial white onychomycosis, the surface of the nail appears white and has fine scale.

Look-alikes

In each of the conditions listed herein, a potassium hydroxide preparation or fungal culture would fail to confirm the presence of dermatophyte infection. Performance of these procedures often is necessary to assist in differential diagnosis.

Disorder	Differentiating Features
Psoriasis	• Nail pitting often present. • Typical psoriatic skin lesions may be present elsewhere.
Trachyonychia (20-nail dystrophy)	• Nails appear rough due to longitudinal ridging and pitting and are thin rather than thickened. • Pitting also commonly present.
Candidiasis	• Usually involves fingernails. • Erythema and edema of proximal nail fold present. • Loss of cuticle. • Typically occurs in young children who suck their fingers.
Pachyonychia congenita	• May be difficult to differentiate clinically from onychomycosis. • Thickening, tenting, and discoloration of fingernails and toenails. • Yellow or brown material accumulates beneath nail. • May have associated thickening of skin on palms and soles (ie, keratoderma). • Positive family history for similar changes is common.
Lichen planus	• Typical skin lesions usually present (ie, purple, polygonal papules and plaques). • Nails thin, have longitudinal striations or ridges, may split.

How to Make the Diagnosis

▶ The diagnosis usually is suspected clinically and may be confirmed by performing a potassium hydroxide preparation or fungal culture (eg, dermatophyte test medium, other fungal culture medium) on debris scraped from beneath the distal nail or nail clipping (distal or lateral subungual onychomycosis) or from the surface of the nail (superficial white onychomycosis).

Treatment

▶ Distal or lateral subungual onychomycosis (toenails).
  - Adolescents and adults: Oral therapy generally is required. (Be aware of potential drug interactions, adverse effects, and need for laboratory monitoring.)
    – Terbinafine 250 mg daily for 3 to 4 months.
    – Itraconazole 200 mg daily for 12 weeks, or 200 mg twice daily for 7 days once monthly for 3 to 4 months (courses should be separated by 21 days).
    – Fluconazole: preferred by some but not US Food and Drug Administration (FDA) approved for the treatment of onychomycosis.
    – Griseofulvin: poor cure rate, requires prolonged treatment course.
  - Children: Mild cases may respond to topical therapy (eg, ciclopirox [FDA approved for those 12 years and older], efinaconazole [6 years and older], tavaborole [6 years and older]). Disadvantages of topical therapy are the potential expense, diminished efficacy (compared to oral agents), and need for prolonged treatment (up to 48 weeks in adults). If oral therapy is prescribed, select dose based on weight. Terbinafine is FDA approved for onychomycosis in patients 2 years and older. (Note: Itraconazole and fluconazole are not specifically FDA approved for use in the treatment of onychomycosis in children, so treatment with these agents for this indication is considered off-label.)
▶ Superficial white onychomycosis may respond to topical therapy (eg, ciclopirox, efinaconazole) but may also require systemic therapy.

Prognosis

- The prognosis for successful eradication and cure is guarded. Cure rates as high as 80% have been reported with oral therapy, but recurrences are common.
- To prevent recurrences, advise the patient to dry feet carefully after bathing or showering, wear protective footwear in public showers, wear absorbent socks, and apply an absorbent powder containing an antifungal agent (eg, Zeasorb AF, Tinactin, Desenex, Lotrimin AF).

When to Worry or Refer

- Consider consultation when the diagnosis is in doubt or when appropriate therapy fails.

Resources for Families

- Society for Pediatric Dermatology: Patient handout on tinea infections.
  https://pedsderm.net/for-patients-families/patient-handouts/#Tinea
- WebMD: Information for families is contained in Skin Problems and Treatments.
  https://www.webmd.com/skin-problems-and-treatments/medical-reference/default.htm

CHAPTER 37

Tinea Capitis

Introduction/Etiology/Epidemiology

- Common dermatophyte infection of the scalp; in the United States, *Trichophyton tonsurans, Microsporum canis,* and *Microsporum audouinii* are responsible for most cases.
- *T tonsurans* is responsible for more than 90% of US infections.
- For reasons unknown, Black children are disproportionately affected.

Signs and Symptoms

Three patterns of infection may be observed.
- Alopecia
  - One or more round or oval patches of partial to complete alopecia with associated scaling (Figure 37.1).
  - Infections caused by *T tonsurans* cause hairs to break at the scalp, resulting in black dot hairs (the remnants of hairs remaining within the follicle) (see Figure 37.1).
  - Infections caused by *Microsporum* species cause hairs to break further from the scalp, resulting in incomplete alopecia; black dot hairs are absent.
- Seborrheic
  - Mimics seborrheic dermatitis (ie, dandruff) with patchy or diffuse whitish to gray scale (Figure 37.2).
  - Alopecia may be subtle.
- Inflammatory: When an inflammatory response to the infecting agent occurs, patients may develop
  - Papules, pustules, and crusting that may mimic bacterial folliculitis.
  - A tender, boggy mass known as a *kerion* (Figure 37.3).
- All forms of tinea capitis, but particularly inflammatory forms, may produce suboccipital or posterior cervical lymphadenopathy.

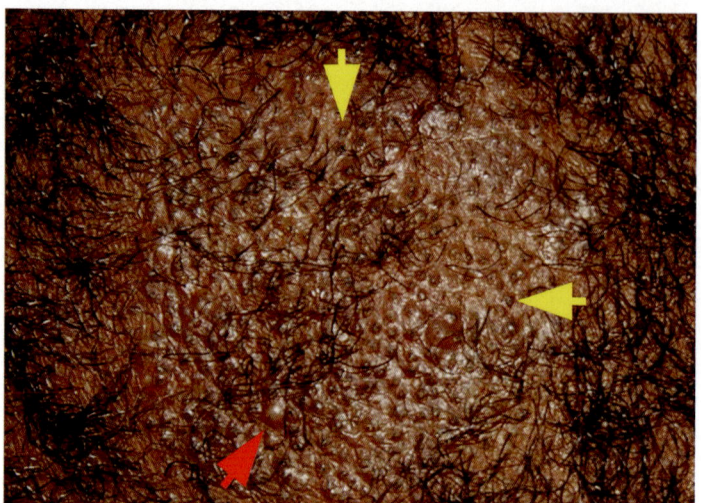

Figure 37.1. Tinea capitis. A well-defined patch of alopecia within which are scale, black dot hairs (yellow arrows), and pustules (red arrow).

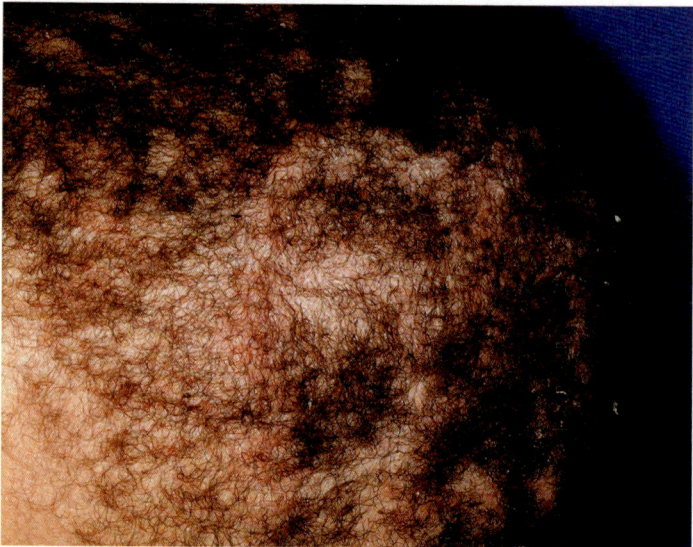

Figure 37.2. Diffuse scaling of the scalp is observed in the seborrheic form of tinea capitis.

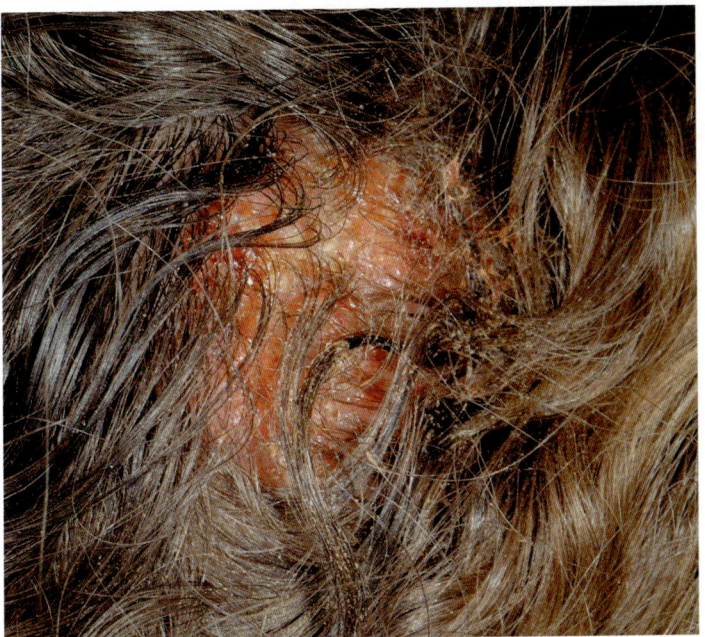

Figure 37.3. A kerion is a tender, boggy mass located on the scalp.

Look-alikes

In each of the conditions listed herein, a potassium hydroxide preparation or fungal culture would fail to confirm the presence of fungal infection.

Disorder	Differentiating Features
Alopecia areata	• Round or oval patches of alopecia that lack scaling, inflammation, or black dot hairs. • Nail pitting often present.
Trichotillomania	• Often ill-defined patches of alopecia within which hairs are of differing lengths. • Petechiae or hemorrhagic crusts may be present if hairs pulled from the scalp. • Scaling and black dot hairs absent. • History of hair manipulation may be offered by family (but not always).
Bacterial folliculitis	• Alopecia and scaling absent. • Culture positive for *Staphylococcus aureus*. • Note: In patients who have tinea capitis, *S aureus* often can be cultured from the scalp (although the pustules themselves may be sterile).
Bacterial abscess	• Less likely to produce alopecia than a kerion. • Scaling absent. • Culture of contents usually reveals *S aureus* or other bacterial organisms. • Note: In patients who have tinea capitis, *S aureus* often can be cultured from the scalp (although the pustules themselves may be sterile).
Traction alopecia	• Traction on hair may produce alopecia localized to areas where hair is parted. • Folliculitis may occur, but scaling and black dot hairs absent. • History of tight braids or ponytails often present, with hair thinning in peripheral zones.
Seborrheic dermatitis	• Typically does not produce alopecia. • Unlikely to occur in children (most often affects infants and those at or beyond puberty).

How to Make the Diagnosis

- ▶ The diagnosis usually is made clinically and supported by laboratory testing.
  - The presence of occipital lymphadenopathy and alopecia, or lymphadenopathy and scaling, are highly predictive of tinea capitis.
- ▶ A potassium hydroxide preparation performed on infected hairs will reveal spores within the hair shaft (ie, endothrix infection as caused by *T tonsurans*) (Figure 37.4) or on the surface of hairs (ie, ectothrix infection as caused by *Microsporum* species).
- ▶ Culture (the criterion standard for diagnosis) of scale or hair fragments on dermatophyte test medium (or other suitable medium) confirms the diagnosis (Figure 37.5). Consider performing a culture when diagnostic uncertainty exists; some also use culture to confirm a mycological cure prior to discontinuation of therapy.
  - Specimens for culture may be obtained with a Cytobrush, toothbrush, or premoistened cotton-tipped applicator.
  - Sensitivity of culture is high, even with delay in inoculation of medium due to transportation of specimen to laboratory.
- ▶ Wood lamp examination is useful only in ectothrix infections (ie, those caused by *Microsporum* species). In such cases, infected hairs will fluoresce. Infections caused by *T tonsurans* (>90% of infections) do not fluoresce.

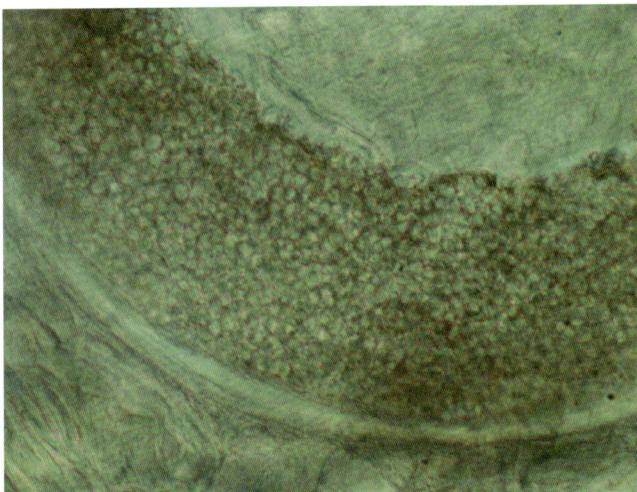

Figure 37.4. Tinea capitis caused by *Trichophyton tonsurans* produces an endothrix infection. The infected black dot hair is filled with arthrospores, the spherical objects shown here.

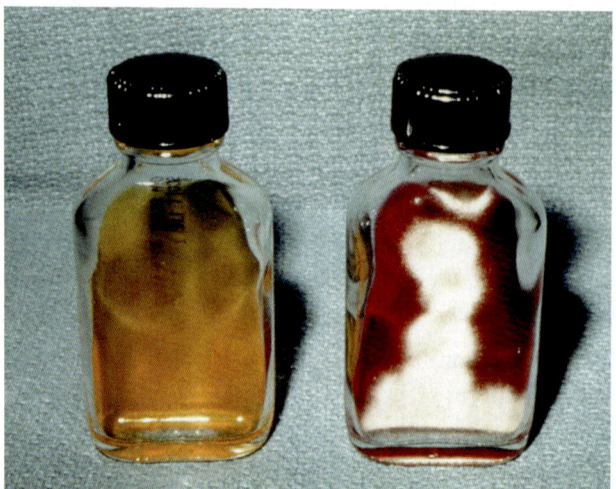

Figure 37.5. The diagnosis of tinea capitis may be confirmed by performing a fungal culture. Uninoculated medium is yellow (left). Within 2 weeks of inoculation with scale or black dot hairs scraped from the scalp, there is fungal growth and the medium turns red (right).

Treatment

▶ Oral therapy is required. A summary of treatment options is provided in Table 37.1.
  ▪ For many years, griseofulvin was considered the drug of choice for the treatment of tinea capitis. However, when compared with newer agents discussed as follows, it requires longer therapy and offers lower efficacy. Griseofulvin is administered at a dose of 20 to 25 mg/kg/d of the micro-sized preparation or 15 mg/kg/d of the ultramicro-sized preparation. Patients should be treated for 6 to 8 weeks minimum. Laboratory monitoring is not necessary.

- Terbinafine, fluconazole, and itraconazole have proven effective in treating tinea capitis (terbinafine is US Food and Drug Administration approved for tinea capitis in patients 4 years or older, while both fluconazole and itraconazole are not approved for this indication). Laboratory monitoring is considered with the use of these antifungal therapies.
  - These agents (particularly terbinafine) often are used to treat patients in whom griseofulvin fails. Many practitioners consider terbinafine as first-line therapy.
  - Terbinafine is less effective than griseofulvin in the treatment of tinea capitis caused by *Microsporum* species.
  - Fluconazole is the only systemic antifungal agent approved for use in patients younger than 2 years, although not specifically for tinea capitis.
- The use of an adjunctive antifungal shampoo containing selenium sulfide (1% or 2.5%) or ketoconazole 2% twice weekly will kill surface spores and, possibly, reduce spread of infection to others. The agent should be used for at least 2 weeks.
- Some authors recommend the addition of oral prednisone (eg, for 1–3 weeks) to the treatment regimen in patients who have severe inflammatory tinea capitis (ie, a kerion).
- Incision and drainage of a kerion is not indicated.
- Patients should be seen in follow-up 1 to 2 months after beginning therapy to assess response.
- Children should not be excluded from school once therapy is begun. Some experts recommend that asymptomatic family members use an antifungal shampoo, although evidence is lacking regarding the efficacy of this strategy. If a dog or cat is suspected to be the source of infection, the animal should be evaluated and treated if appropriate.

Table 37.1. Recommended Therapy for Tinea Capitis

Drug	Dosage	Duration
Griseofulvin microsize (liquid 125 mg/5 mL)	15–25 mg/kg/d (max 1 g/d)	6–8 wk; continue until clinically clear FDA approved for children ≥2 y
Griseofulvin ultramicrosize (tablets of varying size)	10–15 mg/kg/d (max 750 mg/d)	6–8 wk; continue until clinically clear FDA approved for children ≥2 y
Terbinafine tablets (250 mg)[a]	4–6 mg/kg/d (max 250 mg); or 10–20 kg: 62.5 mg 20–40 kg: 125 mg >40 kg: 250 mg	*Trichophyton tonsurans:* 4–6 wk *Microsporum canis:* 8–12 wk Not FDA approved for the treatment of tinea capitis in children
Terbinafine granules (125 mg and 187.5 mg)[b]	<25 kg: 125 mg 25–35 kg: 187.5 mg >35 kg: 250 mg	*Trichophyton tonsurans:* 4–6 wk *Microsporum canis:* 8–12 wk FDA approved for children ≥4 y
Fluconazole[c] (liquid 10 mg/mL, 40 mg/mL; tablet 50 mg, 100 mg, 150 mg, and 200 mg)	6 mg/kg/d (max 400 mg/d)	3–6 wk depending on severity Not FDA approved for the treatment of tinea capitis in children
Itraconazole solution[c] (10 mg/mL)	3 mg/kg/d (max 600 mg/d)	2–4 wk or longer, depending on severity Not FDA approved for the treatment of tinea capitis in children
Itraconazole capsule (65 mg, 100 mg)	5 mg/kg/d (max 600 mg/d)	2–4 wk or longer, depending on severity Not FDA approved for the treatment of tinea capitis in children

Abbreviations: FDA, US Food and Drug Administration; max, maximum.
[a] Some experts use "higher" dosing listed for terbinafine granules instead.
[b] Terbinafine granules have been discontinued in the in the United States.
[c] See *Red Book: 2024–2027 Report of the Committee on Infectious Diseases* Antifungal Drugs for Systemic Fungal Infections and Recommended Doses of Parenteral and Oral Antifungal Drugs, for adverse reactions and therapeutic drug monitoring recommendations.
From American Academy of Pediatrics. Tinea capitis. In: Kimberlin DW, Banerjee R, Barnett ED, et al, eds. *Red Book: 2024–2027 Report of the Committee on Infectious Diseases.* 33rd. American Academy of Pediatrics; 2024:854–858.

Treating Associated Conditions

- Although *Staphylococcus aureus* may be cultured from the scalp of children who have tinea capitis, antibiotic treatment usually is unnecessary.
- If clinical evidence of secondary bacterial infection is present, an antistaphylococcal antibiotic should be prescribed.

Prognosis

- The prognosis is excellent. With treatment, alopecia resolves in nearly all patients (those who have a large kerion occasionally will experience permanent alopecia).
- Reinfection is common in children who share potential fomites (eg, hats, scarves, headgear, earphones, combs, brushes) or those who are reexposed to infection (from children or pets).

When to Worry or Refer

- Refer patients if the diagnosis is in doubt or there is a failure to respond to therapy.

Resources for Families

- American Academy of Pediatrics: HealthyChildren.org. [also available in Spanish] **http://www.healthychildren.org/tinea**
- MedlinePlus: Information for patients and families (in English and Spanish) sponsored by the US National Library of Medicine and National Institutes of Health.
  https://www.nlm.nih.gov/medlineplus/ency/article/000878.htm
- Society for Pediatric Dermatology: Patient handout on tinea infections.
  https://pedsderm.net/for-patients-families/patient-handouts/#Tinea

CHAPTER 38

Tinea Corporis

Introduction/Etiology/Epidemiology

- Common fungal infection caused by the dermatophytes *Trichophyton tonsurans, Microsporum canis, Trichophyton mentagrophytes,* and *Trichophyton rubrum.*

Signs and Symptoms

- Small lesions appear as erythematous scaling plaques.
  - As a lesion enlarges, it becomes annular (ie, ringlike) with a raised, advancing, erythematous border and central clearing (Figure 38.1).
  - Atypical lesions may be present (eg, large rings, incomplete rings) (Figure 38.2).
- Lesions are variably pruritic and may be single or multiple (Figure 38.3).
- Application of a topical corticosteroid (due to misdiagnosis) may alter the typical appearance of lesions (eg, lesions may lack scale or an annular appearance).
- Multiple or disseminated lesions often present in athletes with prolonged skin-to-skin contact (ie, wrestlers, when it has been termed "tinea gladiatorum") or in immunocompromised patients.
- Especially in hair-bearing areas (eg, in young patients who shave their legs), tinea corporis can manifest as a deep-seated infection referred to as *trichophytic (Majocchi) granuloma.* This variant is a granulomatous folliculitis or perifolliculitis. Trichophytic granuloma may also occur when tinea corporis is inadvertently treated with a topical corticosteroid (Figure 38.4).

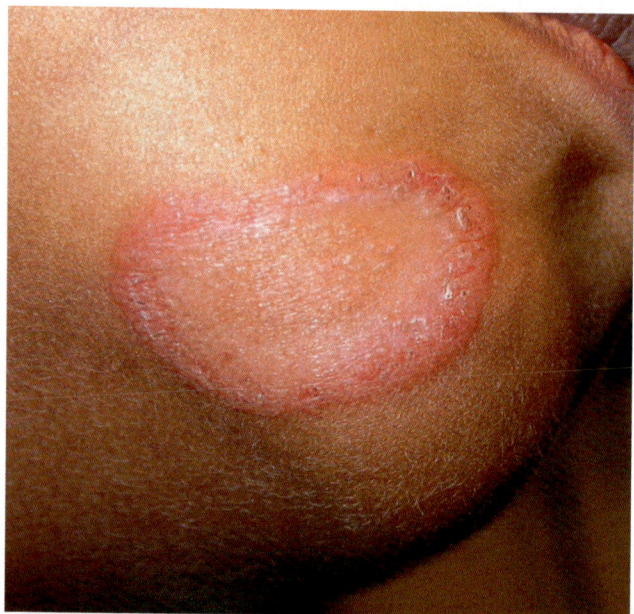

Figure 38.1. Lesions of tinea corporis are rings (ie, annuli) that have an elevated, erythematous, scaling border and central clearing.

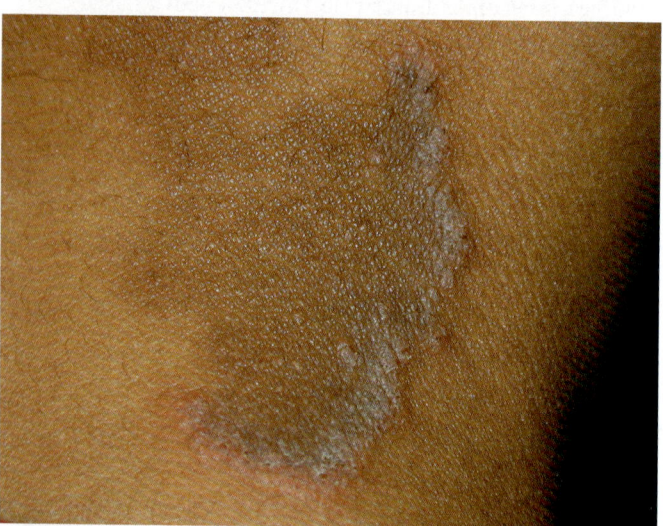

Figure 38.2. Occasionally, the lesions of tinea corporis may be atypical in their appearance. In this patient, there is an incomplete ring; however, the border is erythematous, elevated, and scaling. There is postinflammatory hyperpigmentation.

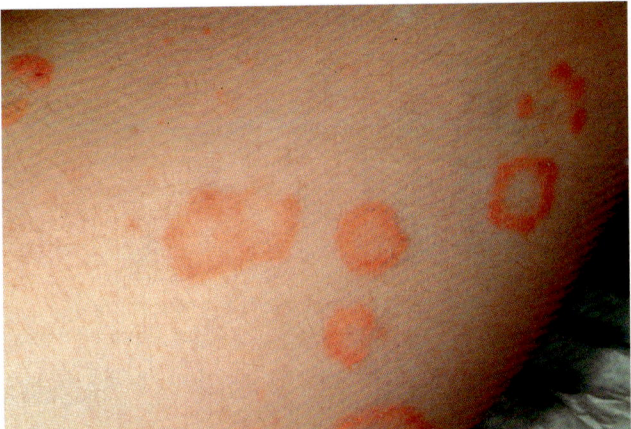

Figure 38.3. Lesions of tinea corporis may be multiple.

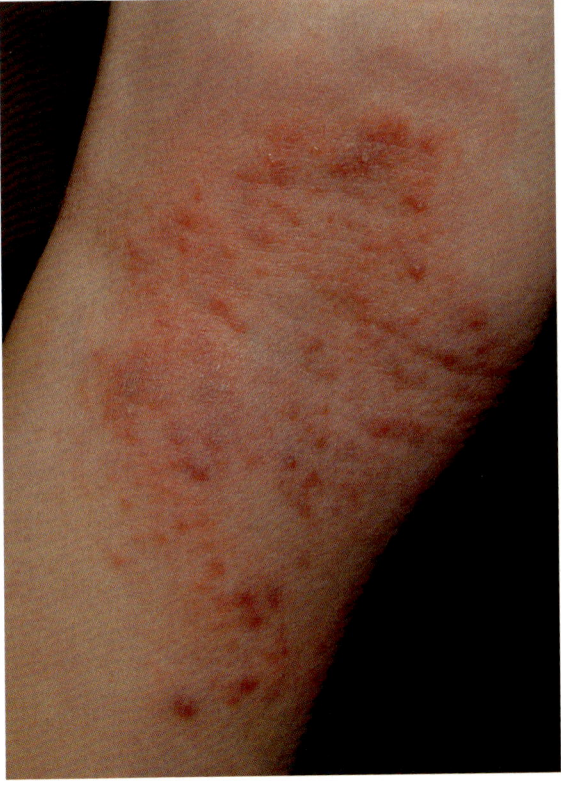

Figure 38.4. This child developed trichophytic (Majocchi) granuloma after a lesion of tinea corporis (initially thought to represent nummular eczema) was treated with a topical corticosteroid. Note the presence of follicular-based papules and pustules.

Look-alikes

In each of the conditions listed herein, a potassium hydroxide preparation or fungal culture would fail to confirm the presence of fungal infection.

Disorder	Differentiating Features
Pityriasis rosea	• Herald patch of pityriasis rosea may be confused with tinea corporis; however, often lacks elevated border. • Later appearance of the generalized eruption assists in diagnosis of pityriasis rosea. • Scaling lags behind the red border and has its free edge pointing inward ("trailing scale"), as opposed to leading edge scale seen in tinea.
Granuloma annulare	• Papules or nodules coalesce to form rings or incomplete rings. • Lesions often have violaceous, not erythematous, color. • Scaling absent.
Nummular eczema	• Lesions are round but lack central clearing. • Crust (not scale) usually present; lesions lack an elevated border. • History of atopic dermatitis may be present.
Psoriasis	• Erythematous papules or plaques that typically lack central clearing. • Scale of psoriatic lesions thick, unlike finer scale of tinea corporis. • Removal of scale causes pinpoint bleeding (Auspitz sign).
Ecthyma	• Lesions have thick crust, not scale, with surrounding erythema and induration. • Central clearing absent.

How to Make the Diagnosis

▶ The diagnosis usually is made clinically but can be confirmed by the presence of branching hyphae in a potassium hydroxide preparation performed on scale obtained from the border of a lesion (Figure 38.5) or culture (rarely necessary).

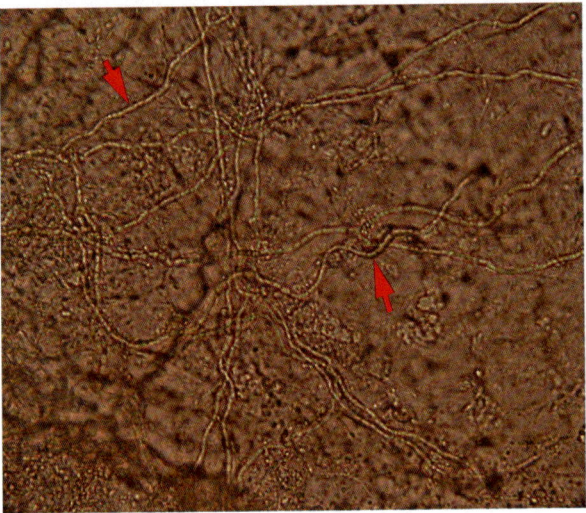

Figure 38.5. A potassium hydroxide preparation in tinea corporis; branching hyphae are seen (arrows).

Treatment

- Apply a topical antifungal agent, such as an imidazole (eg, clotrimazole, miconazole, ketoconazole), allylamine (eg, terbinafine, naftifine), or tolnaftate. The agent is applied to the entire lesion, including the area immediately beyond the border. Treatment should be continued until the lesion resolves, typically within 2 weeks. Some experts recommend treating for several weeks beyond the time when clinical resolution is observed.

- Oral antifungal agents (eg, griseofulvin, fluconazole, terbinafine) are reserved for patients with multiple or very large lesions (eg, as might occur in immunosuppressed individuals). Longer courses with oral antifungal agents may be required for deeper-seated tinea infections, such as trichophytic granuloma.

Prognosis

- Prognosis is excellent, although recurrences are common when children are continually exposed to infected pets or farm animals.

When to Worry or Refer

▶ Refer patients in whom the diagnosis is in doubt or the lesion(s) fails to respond to appropriate therapy.

Resources for Families

▶ American Academy of Pediatrics: HealthyChildren.org.
  https://www.healthychildren.org/tinea

▶ MedlinePlus: Information for patients and families (in English and Spanish) sponsored by the US National Library of Medicine and National Institutes of Health.
  https://www.nlm.nih.gov/medlineplus/ency/article/000877.htm

▶ Society for Pediatric Dermatology: Patient handout on tinea infections.
  https://pedsderm.net/for-patients-families/patient-handouts/#Tinea

▶ WebMD: Information for families is contained in Skin Problems and Treatments.
  https://www.webmd.com/skin-problems-and-treatments/what-you-should-know-about-ringworm#1

CHAPTER 39

Tinea Cruris

Introduction/Etiology/Epidemiology

- Dermatophyte infection of the skin of the groin; usually caused by *Trichophyton mentagrophytes* or *Epidermophyton floccosum*.
- More common in men; rare before puberty.
- Especially prevalent in warm, humid conditions.
- May occur in epidemics among athletic teams or military recruits.
- Infection may be transmitted via fomites (eg, athletic gear, clothing, towels).

Signs and Symptoms

- Characterized by an erythematous patch on the inner thigh and inguinal crease (may be unilateral or bilateral) (Figure 39.1).
- Borders of lesions are elevated and exhibit scale.
- May be intensely pruritic; scratching leads to erosions, inflammation, and lichenification.
- Scrotum is usually spared, although scratching may produce lichenification.

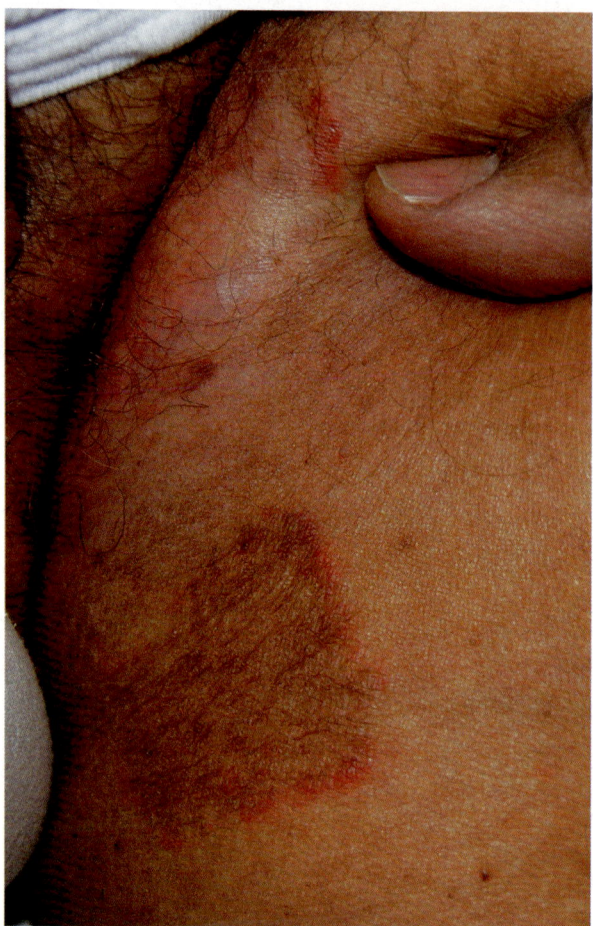

Figure 39.1. Tinea cruris is characterized by an erythematous or hyperpigmented patch with an elevated scaling border.

Look-alikes

In each of the conditions listed herein, a potassium hydroxide preparation or fungal culture would fail to confirm the presence of dermatophyte infection.

Disorder	Differentiating Features
Intertrigo	• Maceration caused by rubbing of apposing skin surfaces. • Borders poorly defined; scaling absent.
Candidiasis	• "Beefy" red patch. • Satellite lesions (papules, papulopustules) present. • Scrotum often involved.
Erythrasma	• Often red-brown or brown. • Elevated border and scaling absent. • Wood lamp examination will reveal coral red fluorescence.

How to Make the Diagnosis

▶ The diagnosis is made clinically and may be confirmed by performing a potassium hydroxide preparation on scale obtained from the border of the lesion (that will reveal branching hyphae). Fungal culture can also be considered.

Treatment

▶ Topical application of an antifungal agent, such as an imidazole (eg, clotrimazole, miconazole, ketoconazole), allylamine (eg, terbinafine, naftifine), or tolnaftate. The agent is applied until the eruption resolves, typically within 3 to 4 weeks.

▶ Advise patients to avoid tight-fitting clothing, dry carefully after bathing or showering, and apply an absorbent powder.

▶ If patients experience frequent recurrences, recommend the regular use of an absorbent powder containing an antifungal agent (eg, Zeasorb AF, Tinactin, Desenex, Lotrimin AF).

▶ Oral antifungal therapy rarely is necessary and is reserved for patients who have severe or recalcitrant disease.

Prognosis

- The prognosis is excellent.
- Reinfection may occur unless the predisposing environmental conditions are altered.

When to Worry or Refer

- Consider consultation when the diagnosis is in doubt or when appropriate therapy fails.

Resources for Families

- American Academy of Pediatrics: HealthyChildren.org.
  https://www.healthychildren.org/tinea
- Society for Pediatric Dermatology: Patient handout on tinea infections.
  https://pedsderm.net/for-patients-families/patient-handouts/#Tinea
- WebMD: Information on tinea cruris.
  https://www.webmd.com/men/causes-and-prevent-jock-itch#1

CHAPTER 40

Tinea Pedis

Introduction/Etiology/Epidemiology

- Dermatophyte infection of the feet; organisms responsible are *Trichophyton rubrum, Trichophyton mentagrophytes,* and *Epidermophyton floccosum.*
- Common in adolescents and adults; less common in childhood.
- Warm, moist environment of occlusive footwear predisposes to fungal infection.

Signs and Symptoms

Three forms of infection are recognized: interdigital, vesicular, and moccasin.

- Interdigital
  - Typically caused by *T rubrum* or *E floccosum.*
  - Pruritus, erythema, fissuring, scaling, and maceration occur in the interdigital spaces (Figure 40.1).
- Vesicular
  - Typically caused by *T mentagrophytes.*
  - Vesicles, bullae, and erosions appear on the instep of the foot or dorsal aspect of the foot or between the toes (Figure 40.2).
- Moccasin
  - Typically caused by *T rubrum* or *E floccosum.*
  - Erythema and scaling involve much of or all the plantar surface and sides of the feet (Figure 40.3).
- Rarely, a dermatophytid (id) or autosensitization reaction occurs that produces a widespread eczematous-appearing eruption composed of papules or deep-seated vesicles.

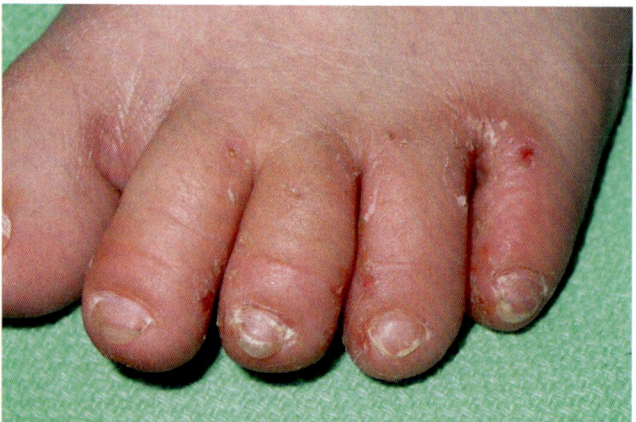

Figure 40.1. Erythema, scaling, fissuring, and erosions between the toes are seen in the interdigital form of tinea pedis.

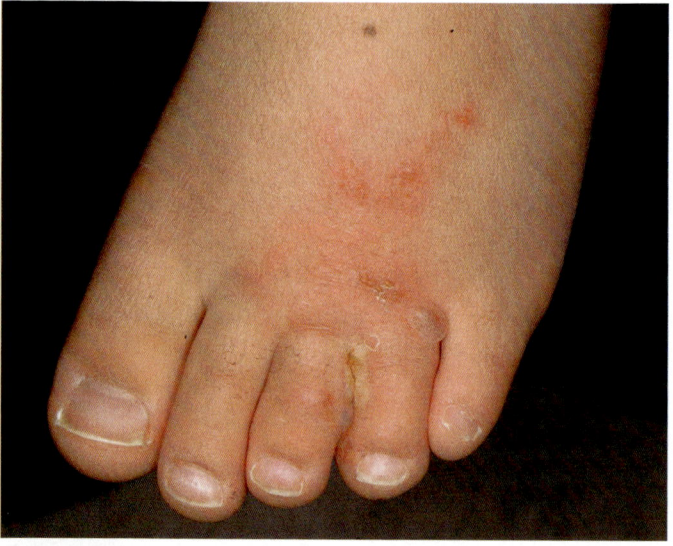

Figure 40.2. Erythematous plaques, maceration, and toe web bullae in a child with vesicular tinea pedis.

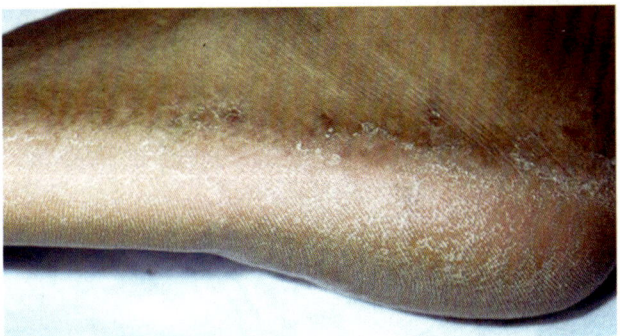

Figure 40.3. Moccasin form of tinea pedis with erythema and scaling involving the plantar surface and side of the left foot. Reproduced with permission from Ely JW, Rosenfeld S, Seabury Stone M. Diagnosis and management of tinea infections. *Am Fam Physician.* 2014;90(10):702–710.

Look-alikes

In each of the conditions listed herein, a potassium hydroxide preparation or fungal culture would fail to confirm the presence of fungal infection.

Disorder	Differentiating Features
Contact dermatitis	• Involves dorsum of feet; interdigital spaces spared.
Erythrasma	• Often red-brown or brown; involves interdigital spaces. • Elevated border and scaling absent. • Wood lamp examination reveals coral red fluorescence.
Juvenile plantar dermatosis	• Intense erythema with fissuring on the plantar surface of the foot, most typically the ball and heel, often with sparing of arch. • History of hyperhidrosis common. • Interdigital spaces spared. • History of atopic dermatitis often present.
Pitted keratolysis	• Small pits that may coalesce into larger, very superficial erosions present on plantar surface of foot. • Hyperhidrosis and malodor often present. • Interdigital spaces spared.

How to Make the Diagnosis

▶ The diagnosis is made clinically.
▶ If uncertainty exists, a potassium hydroxide preparation (revealing branching hyphae) or fungal culture (eg, dermatophyte test medium) may be performed (see Figure 37.5).

Treatment

- For typical infections, application of a topical antifungal agent, such as an imidazole (eg, clotrimazole, miconazole, ketoconazole), allylamine (eg, terbinafine, naftifine), or tolnaftate, is appropriate. The agent is applied until the eruption clears, typically within 3 to 4 weeks.
- Widespread, resistant, or severe infections may require oral therapy with griseofulvin or another antifungal agent.
- Advise patients to keep their feet dry and, if possible, to wear well-ventilated shoes or sandals.
- For patients who experience recurrences, recommend the regular use of an absorbent powder containing an antifungal agent (eg, Zeasorb AF, Micatin, Tinactin, Desenex, Lotrimin AF, and others).

Treating Associated Conditions

- If treatment of concomitant nail infection (ie, onychomycosis) is desired, oral therapy with terbinafine or itraconazole will be required.

Prognosis

- The prognosis is excellent.
- To prevent recurrences, advise patients to dry carefully after bathing or showering, wear protective footwear in public showers, wear well-ventilated shoes or sandals, and regularly apply an absorbent powder containing an antifungal agent (eg, Zeasorb AF, Micatin, Tinactin, Desenex, Lotrimin AF, and others).

When to Worry or Refer

- Consider consultation with a dermatologist when the diagnosis is in doubt or when appropriate therapy fails.

Resources for Families

- American Academy of Pediatrics: HealthyChildren.org.
  https://www.healthychildren.org/tinea
- MedlinePlus: Information for patients and families (in English and Spanish) sponsored by the US National Library of Medicine and National Institutes of Health.
  https://www.nlm.nih.gov/medlineplus/athletesfoot.html
- Society for Pediatric Dermatology: Patient handout on tinea infections.
  https://pedsderm.net/for-patients-families/patient-handouts/#Tinea
- WebMD: Information for families is contained in Skin Problems and Treatments.
  https://www.webmd.com/skin-problems-and-treatments/understanding-athletes-foot-basics

CHAPTER 41

Tinea Versicolor

Introduction/Etiology/Epidemiology

- Tinea versicolor (also known as pityriasis versicolor) is a common fungal infection that occurs in adolescents and adults; it rarely occurs in children.
- Causative organism is *Malassezia* (formerly *Pityrosporum*) species, which invades the stratum corneum.
  - The organism is a common inhabitant of the skin. When it enters a mycelial phase, clinical disease results.
  - The organism thrives in hot, humid environments and is lipophilic, thriving on skin with available lipid.

Signs and Symptoms

- Characteristic lesions are small, hypopigmented or hyperpigmented, round or oval macules located on the trunk, proximal extremities, and neck (Figures 41.1 and 41.2). Rarely, lesions may occur on the face.
  - Lesions have well-defined borders.
  - Individual lesions may coalesce into large patches.
  - Fine scaling may be present.
- In individuals with lighter skin tones who have hypopigmented lesions, sun exposure accentuates the appearance of the disorder, as surrounding uninfected skin darkens while infected skin does not.
- Lesions are generally asymptomatic (although pruritus may be present) but may cause considerable concern due to their appearance.

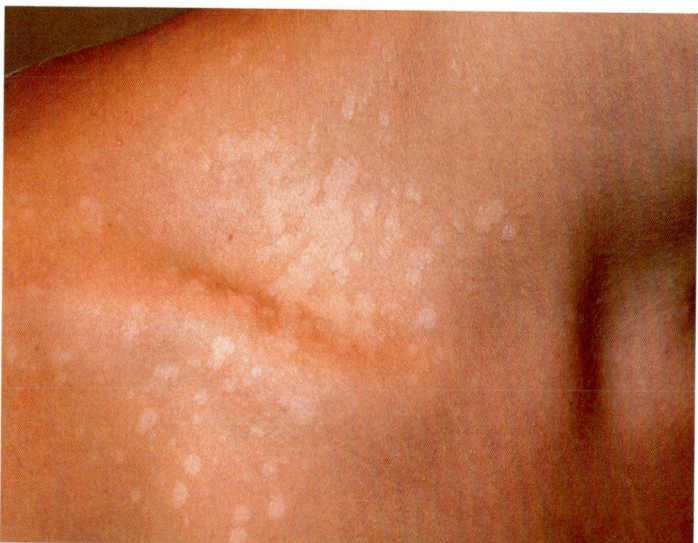

Figure 41.1. Well-defined hypopigmented scaling macules in tinea versicolor.

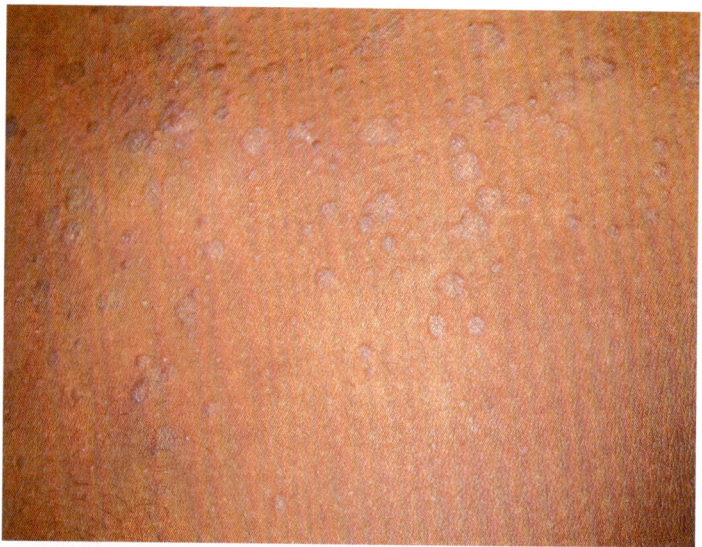

Figure 41.2. Well-defined hyperpigmented scaling macules in tinea versicolor.

Look-alikes

In each of the conditions listed herein, a potassium hydroxide preparation would fail to confirm the presence of spores and hyphae observed in tinea versicolor.

Disorder	Differentiating Features
Vitiligo	• Lesions of vitiligo depigmented so appear completely white. • Wood lamp examination reveals marked accentuation of depigmentation.
Pityriasis alba	• Lesions with indistinct borders. • Most often occurs on the face.
Pityriasis rosea	• Lesions elevated and inflammatory. • Lesions arranged with long axes parallel to lines of skin tension.
Confluent and reticulated papillomatosis (also known as Gougerot-Carteaud syndrome)	• May sometimes resemble hyperpigmented form of tinea versicolor. • Thin hyperpigmented papules that are confluent centrally and reticulated peripherally. • Lesions form rough-feeling thin plaques typically distributed on the chest, intermammary region, and/or upper back.

How to Make the Diagnosis

▶ The diagnosis usually is made clinically.

▶ If uncertainty exists, a potassium hydroxide preparation performed on scale from lesions will reveal short hyphae and spores (ie, "spaghetti and meatballs") (Figure 41.3).

▶ Examination of the skin with a Wood lamp in a darkened room may reveal a yellow-orange or blue-white fluorescence of affected areas.

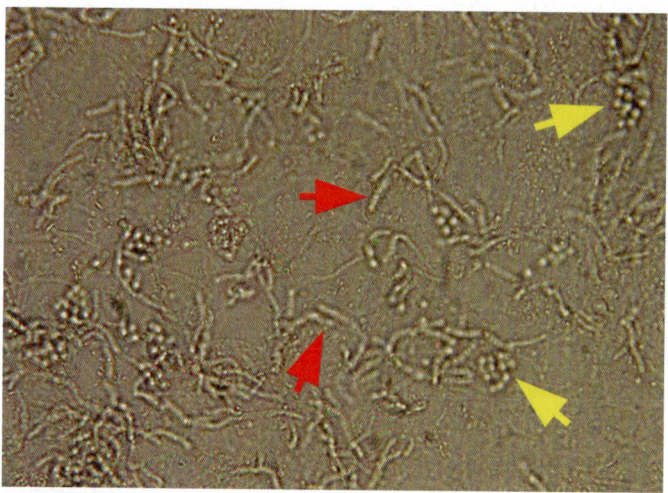

Figure 41.3. In tinea versicolor, potassium hydroxide preparation on scale obtained from a lesion demonstrates short hyphae (red arrows) and spores (yellow arrows) (ie, "spaghetti and meatballs").

Treatment

- ▶ Topical
  - If infection is very localized, topical antifungal agents (eg, imidazoles) are effective.
  - If infection is widespread (most patients), options include
    - Selenium sulfide 1% shampoo or 2.5% lotion.
      - Apply to entire affected area 10 minutes daily for 7 days.
      - Apply for 8 to 12 hours once each month for 3 months thereafter (to prevent recurrence).
    - Ketoconazole shampoo
      - Apply for 5 minutes daily for 1 to 3 days (will need to use this agent or selenium sulfide for prophylaxis as described previously).
    - Terbinafine 1% spray
      - Apply 1 to 2 times daily for 2 to 4 weeks.

- Systemic (off-label)
  - Usually reserved for persistent or recurrent infections or for patients who cannot use topical therapy.
  - Options include fluconazole (400 mg once, or 300 mg once and repeated in 1 week) or itraconazole (400 mg once or 200 mg/d for 7 days). Oral ketoconazole is no longer recommended owing to rare but possible risks, including severe liver injury and harmful interactions with other medications.
  - Advising physical activity after a dose promotes delivery of the drug to the skin surface via sweat and may enhance efficacy.
  - Prophylactic maintenance with selenium sulfide or ketoconazole shampoo (as previously described) may be helpful.

Prognosis

- The prognosis is excellent, but recurrences are very common.
- Advise patients that months may be required for pigmentation to return to its typical appearance after effective treatment.

When to Worry or Refer

- Consider consultation when the diagnosis is in doubt or when appropriate therapy fails.

Resources for Families

- American Academy of Dermatology: Tinea versicolor: diagnosis and treatment.
  https://www.aad.org/public/diseases/color-problems/tinea-versicolor
- American Academy of Pediatrics: HealthyChildren.org.
  https://www.healthychildren.org/tinea
- MedlinePlus: Information for patients and families (in English and Spanish) sponsored by the US National Library of Medicine and National Institutes of Health.
  https://www.nlm.nih.gov/medlineplus/ency/article/001465.htm

Infestations and Bites

CHAPTER 42 — **Cutaneous Larva Migrans** 305

CHAPTER 43 — **Head Lice** 309

CHAPTER 44 — **Insect Bites and Papular Urticaria** 315

CHAPTER 45 — **Scabies** 325

CHAPTER 46 — **Cercarial Dermatitis (Swimmer's Itch)** 333

CHAPTER 42

Cutaneous Larva Migrans

Introduction/Etiology/Epidemiology

- Also known as creeping eruption, larva migrans.
- A self-limited skin eruption caused by accidental penetration of the human host by the dog hookworm (*Ancylostoma caninum*) and cat hookworm (*Ancylostoma braziliense*). *Uncinaria stenocephala,* a hookworm that affects dogs and cats, has also been implicated in some cases. Other skin-penetrating nematodes may occasionally cause disease.
- Usually noted after travel to tropical and subtropical regions, including southeastern United States (especially Florida and Georgia), Central and South America, Africa, and the Caribbean.
- May occur in epidemics in high-income countries and in tourists.
- Adult hookworms release eggs in host animal's intestines, and eggs pass with feces into sandy, warm soil.
- Eggs hatch, releasing larvae that penetrate human skin and wander arbitrarily, producing serpiginous tracts.

Signs and Symptoms

- Erythematous, serpiginous plaques develop on skin (Figure 42.1).
- Incubation period is typically days but may last for several weeks in some patients.
- Lesions may "advance" up to 20 mm per day.
- Most common locations include feet (Figure 42.2), buttocks, and genitalia.
- May be intensely pruritic.
- Blisters may rarely occur.
- Eosinophilic pneumonitis (Löffler syndrome) may rarely occur and presents with fever, malaise, and cough.
- Peripheral blood eosinophilia may occur.
- Rarely, the larvae travel to the intestines, causing eosinophilic enteritis.

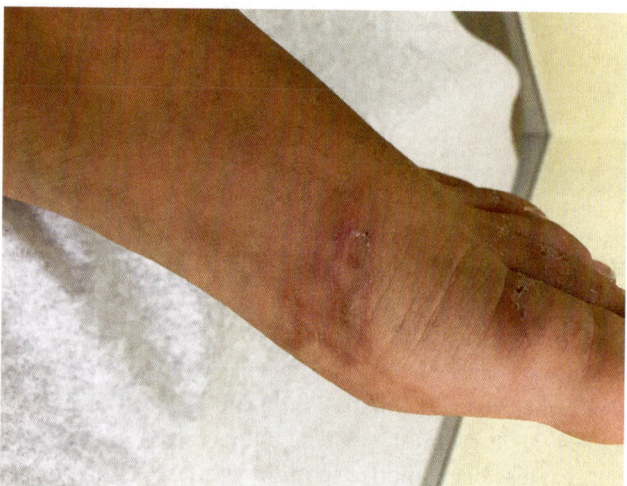

Figure 42.1. Cutaneous larva migrans. Serpiginous tracts on the dorsomedial aspect of the of a school-aged child.

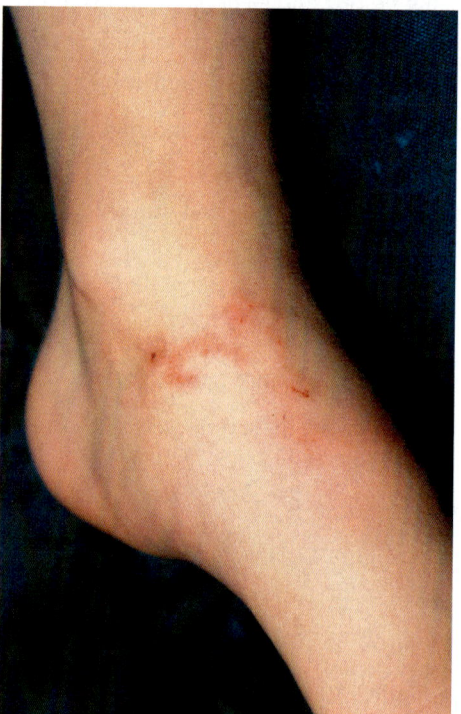

Figure 42.2. Cutaneous larva migrans. Note the serpiginous erythematous tracts on the dorsal aspect of the ankle and proximal aspect of the foot.

Look-alikes

Disorder	Differentiating Features
Scabies	• Burrows short (up to a few millimeters), do not migrate. • Widespread distribution, favoring folds, wrists, ankles, genitals, palms, and soles.
Tinea corporis	• Annular plaques enlarge in a centrifugal pattern. • Scale commonly present. • Pruritus less significant than in cutaneous larva migrans.
Other nematode infestations	• Variety of systemic manifestations depending on nematode; may include *Strongyloides stercoralis* and *Gnathostoma spinigerum*. • The serpiginous rash of larva currens (hypersensitivity reaction seen in some patients with strongyloidiasis) progresses at a faster rate, up to 10 cm per day.
Allergic contact dermatitis	• Bizarre patterning may be present. • Vesicles and bullae common. • History may be useful.
Phytophotodermatitis	• Erythematous eruption, which also usually develops after outdoor activities. • Patches correspond to sites of contact with offending photosensitizer (including lime or lemon juice, dill, parsley, parsnips, figs, celery); may present as linear streaks and "drip marks." • In addition to erythematous patches, vesicles and bullae are often present. • Heals with marked hyperpigmentation.

How to Make the Diagnosis

▶ Clinical examination findings combined with extreme pruritus and exposure history are usually confirmatory.

▶ Skin biopsy (rarely necessary) typically reveals intense eosinophilic infiltrate.

Treatment

- Process is self-limited, but symptoms usually necessitate therapy.
- Oral albendazole and ivermectin are both effective.
  - Albendazole: age older than 2 years: pediatric dose 15 mg/kg/d (maximum 400 mg/d) once daily for 3 days.
  - Ivermectin: 200 mcg/kg given orally once daily for 1 day. Safety in young infants (<15 kg) and in pregnant women is not established.
- Cryotherapy (traditional treatment) is rarely effective and is traumatic for young children; it should be avoided.

Treating Associated Conditions

- Secondary bacterial infection should be treated with an appropriate systemic antibiotic.

Prognosis

- Cutaneous larva migrans resolves completely without permanent sequelae.

When to Worry or Refer

- Referral to a dermatologist should be considered for patients in whom the diagnosis is in question or for whom conventional therapy is unsuccessful.

Resources for Families

- Centers for Disease Control and Prevention: Clinical features of zoonotic hookworm
  https://www.cdc.gov/zoonotic-hookworm/hcp/clinical-features/?CDC_AAref_Val=https://www.cdc.gov/parasites/zoonotichookworm/gen_info/faqs.html
- DermNet NZ: Cutaneous larva migrans.
  www.dermnetnz.org/arthropods/larva-migrans.html

CHAPTER 43

Head Lice

Introduction/Etiology/Epidemiology

- Infestation occurs commonly in children attending child care or school.
- Caused by *Pediculus humanus capitis,* the human head louse.
- Less commonly seen in Black children, in relation to diameter and nature and shape of their hair shafts.
- Transmission mainly via head-to-head contact; less commonly through fomites (eg, combs, hairbrushes, hats, towels, hooded jackets); prevention of spread is best focused on reducing active infestations and minimizing direct head-to-head contact.
- Affects all socioeconomic groups.
- Head louse (unlike body louse) does not transmit disease.
- Head lice are specific to humans and are not spread between humans and pets.

Signs and Symptoms

- Pruritus is the most common symptom, although many children may be asymptomatic, especially during the first weeks of a primary infestation.
- Secondary excoriation and bacterial infection may be present.
- Evidence of infestation (eg, live lice, nits, excoriations) is often most apparent behind the ears and at the nape of the neck.
- Regional (eg, cervical, suboccipital) lymphadenopathy is common if there is secondary bacterial infection.
- Live lice may be seen and are 2 to 4 mm in length.
- Nits (eggs) present as 0.5- to 0.8-mm, tan-brown concretions firmly affixed to hair shafts (Figure 43.1).
- Hatched (nonviable) nits are usually white.

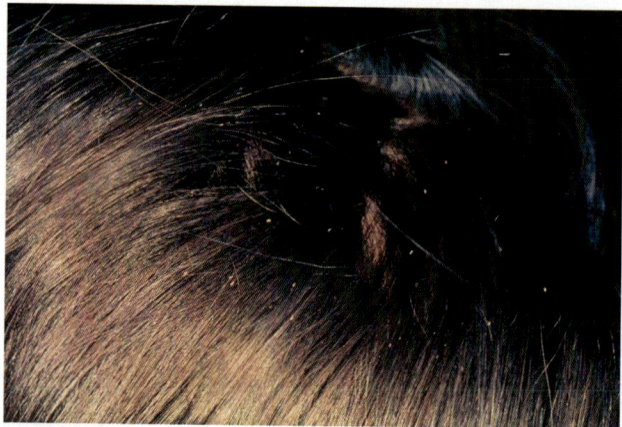

Figure 43.1. Head lice. Note numerous nits attached to hair shafts.

Look-alikes

Disorder	Differentiating Features
Seborrheic dermatitis	• Erythematous patches with greasy yellow scale. • Absence of live lice or nits. • White "dandruff" easily removed from hair shaft, unlike firmly affixed nits.
Psoriasis	• Well-demarcated, erythematous, scaly papules and plaques. • May note involvement in other regions (eg, elbows, knees, sacrum). • Absence of live lice or nits.
Hair casts	• Easily removed from hair shaft.
Piedra	• Loosely adherent, soft nodules of hair shaft. • Causes hair breakage. • May be black or white. • May also involve axillary, pubic hair.
Hair products	• Topically applied products (eg, hair spray, gel, mousse) may leave debris in hair that may mimic nits.

How to Make the Diagnosis

- Clinical examination: Identification of live lice is the criterion standard for diagnosis but can be difficult. The presence of viable nits on hairs (within 1 cm of the scalp) is highly suggestive of active infestation.
- Viability of nits can be assessed by mounting affected hairs on a glass slide and performing low-power microscopic examination; viable nits have an intact operculum (cap) at the nonattached end, whereas this cap is missing in hatched (nonviable) nits (Figure 43.2).

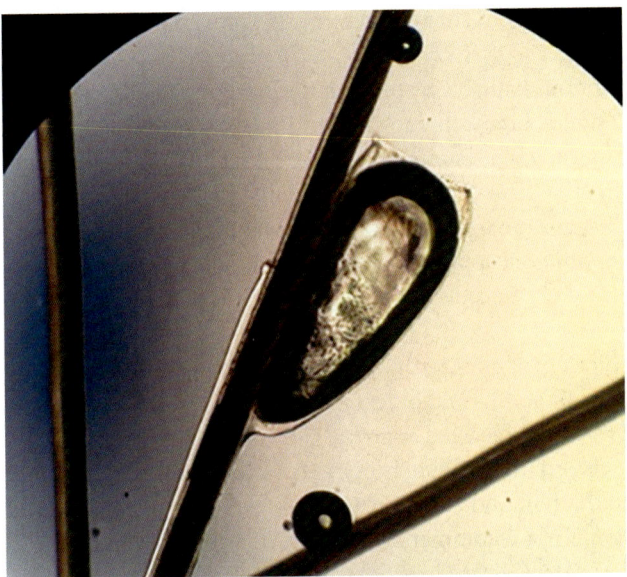

Figure 43.2. Head lice. Low-power microscopy reveals a hatched nit. Note the cement-like substance adhering the nit to the hair shaft. The flat surface (reflecting loss of the cap, or operculum) and absence of a developing louse within the egg confirms the hatched nature of this nit.

Treatment

- ▶ Pediculicides are the treatment of choice and include
  - Permethrin 1% cream rinse, available over the counter; first-line therapy; applied to hair that has been shampooed and towel dried; left on for 10 minutes and then rinsed; repeat treatment in 7 to 10 days; approved in infants 2 months and older.
  - Synergized pyrethrins (pyrethrin + piperonyl butoxide), available in a variety of over-the-counter products; applied to dry hair; also used for 10 minutes; repeat treatment in 7 to 10 days; should not be used in individuals with allergy to chrysanthemums; approved in children 2 years and older.
  - Malathion 0.5% lotion, available by prescription; applied to dry hair and rinsed in 8 to 12 hours; repeat therapy in 7 to 10 days if needed; approved in children 6 years and older (some endorse use down to 2 years of age); product is flammable.
  - Spinosad 0.9% suspension, a fermentation product of the soil bacterium *Saccharopolyspora spinosa*; applied to dry hair and rinsed in 10 minutes; repeat therapy in 7 days if needed; approved in infants 6 months and older.
  - Ivermectin 0.5% lotion; applied to dry hair and rinsed in 10 minutes; approved in infants 6 months and older.
  - Abametapir 0.74% lotion received approval (for infants 6 months and older) but at the time of this writing is not yet available in the United States; applied to dry hair and rinsed in 10 minutes.
  - Lindane 1% lotion is not recommended by the American Academy of Pediatrics (AAP) or the Centers for Disease Control and Prevention given concerns over neurotoxicity.
- ▶ Repeat topical therapy (7–10 days after the initial treatment) is usually recommended to ensure killing of any eggs that hatch after first treatment but may vary by product (see earlier list).
- ▶ Oral ivermectin (200 or 400 mcg/kg single dose) has been used off-label for children older than 2 years who weigh 15 kg or more with resistant disease; it is typically repeated in 9 to 10 days.
- ▶ Alternative off-label therapies include trimethoprim-sulfamethoxazole and "suffocation" therapies (eg, petroleum jelly, mayonnaise, olive oil); problem with latter is ability of human head louse to close respiratory spiracles temporarily, reopening them after removal of the occlusive agent.

- Before pediculicidal resistance is suggested, consider other causes of therapeutic failure, like misdiagnosis, repeat infestation, or treatment noncompliance.
- Manual removal of lice and nits with nit combing of wet hair is possible for those who prefer not to use a pediculicide.
- There now exist multiple lice-removal salons that offer manual nit removal and non-pediculicidal topical therapies; some also offer hot-air therapy.
- Close contacts should be examined and treated (if necessary), and bedding and clothing should be machine washed and dried on a high-heat setting. Necessary shared headgear (eg, batting helmets, computer headphones) can be wiped with a damp cloth between uses.
- "No-nit" policies, which prevent children with nits from attending child care or school, are not effective and can lead to academic and social struggles for children. The AAP recommends against no-nit policies and discourages routine classroom or school-wide screening for lice. No healthy child should be excluded from or allowed to miss schooltime because of head lice.

Treating Associated Conditions

- Secondary bacterial infection should be treated with an appropriate systemic antibiotic.
- Scalp dermatitis can be treated with topical corticosteroid solution (eg, fluocinolone 0.01% scalp solution, mometasone 0.1% solution).
- Severe pruritus may necessitate oral antihistamine therapy.

Prognosis

- Most patients with head lice respond well to therapy, and there are no permanent sequelae.

When to Worry or Refer

- Consider referral to a dermatologist for patients with disease that seems to be resistant to standard therapy (after considering misdiagnosis, reinfestation, or treatment noncompliance).
- An updated head lice clinical report is available at **https://publications.aap.org/pediatrics/article/150/4/e2022059282/189566/Head-Lice**.

Resources for Families

- American Academy of Pediatrics: HealthyChildren.org. **https://www.healthychildren.org/English/health-issues/conditions/from-insects-animals/Pages/Signs-of-Lice.aspx**
- Centers for Disease Control and Prevention: About head lice. **https://www.cdc.gov/lice/about/head-lice.html?CDC_AAref_Val=https://www.cdc.gov/parasites/lice/head**
- MedlinePlus: Information for patients and families (in English and Spanish) sponsored by the US National Library of Medicine and National Institutes of Health. **https://www.nlm.nih.gov/medlineplus/ency/article/000840.htm**
- National Pediculosis Association: Welcome to HeadLice.org. **www.headlice.org**

CHAPTER 44

Insect Bites and Papular Urticaria

Introduction/Etiology/Epidemiology

- ▶ Insect and arachnid bites occur throughout the world and may show seasonal variation.
- ▶ Some of dermatologic significance include 8-legged arachnids (ie, mites, ticks, spiders, scorpions) and 6-legged insects (ie, lice, flies, mosquitoes, fleas, bugs, bees, wasps, ants, caterpillars, and beetles).
- ▶ Some of these arthropods may be vectors for significant diseases.
- ▶ Protection against bites is a vital step in prevention of these reactions.
- ▶ Host reaction is an immune response against proteins found in arthropod saliva.
- ▶ This discussion includes mosquitoes, fleas, mites, bedbugs, ticks, and papular urticaria.

Signs and Symptoms

- ▶ Mosquitoes
  - Most common bite reactions in infants and children in the United States.
  - May serve worldwide as vectors for disease (eg, encephalitis [including West Nile encephalitis], yellow fever, malaria, dengue, filariasis, chikungunya, Zika virus).
  - Carbon dioxide (from breath and skin) serves as long-range attractant for mosquitoes.
  - Classically present as edematous, erythematous papules and urticarial wheals (Figure 44.1).
  - Small central crust or punctum may be visible at site of bite.
  - Vesicles, bullae, or hemorrhage may occur.
  - Excoriation may lead to secondary eczematous changes and impetiginization.
  - Systemic hypersensitivity reactions/anaphylaxis rarely are present.

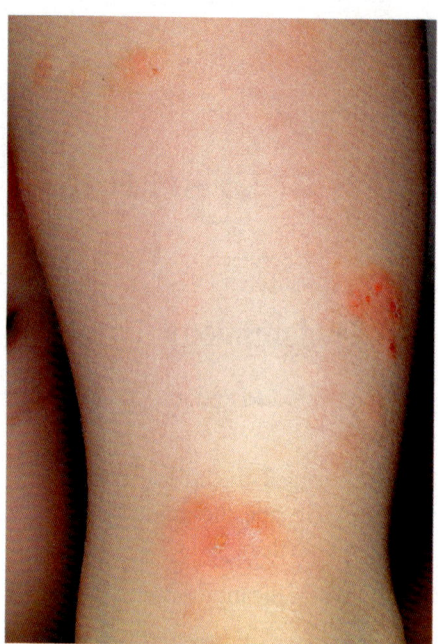

Figure 44.1. Mosquito bites.

▶ Fleas
- Ubiquitous insects with little host specificity.
- Common fleas in the United States include human flea (*Pulex irritans*), cat flea (*Ctenocephalides felis*), and dog flea (*Ctenocephalides canis*).
- May be vectors for cat scratch disease, endemic typhus, and plague.
- In addition to animal (pet) carriers, fleas may be found in carpets, floors, sandboxes, beaches, and grassy areas.
- Bites result in extremely pruritic papules or urticarial wheals, often with a central punctum.
- Reactions may evolve into large bullae (Figure 44.2).
- Most common location is the lower extremities; upper extremities and areas covered by tight clothing also common.
- Because fleas jump but cannot fly, bite reactions are often clustered in a linear configuration ("breakfast, lunch, and dinner" sign [Figure 44.3]).
- The sand flea, *Tunga penetrans* (chigoe or jigger flea), causes tungiasis, a painful condition presenting as an inflammatory nodule, usually on the toes or periungual skin; in this case the female flea burrows into the dermis and gradually enlarges. This disease is not endemic to the United States; it occurs mainly in Central and South America.

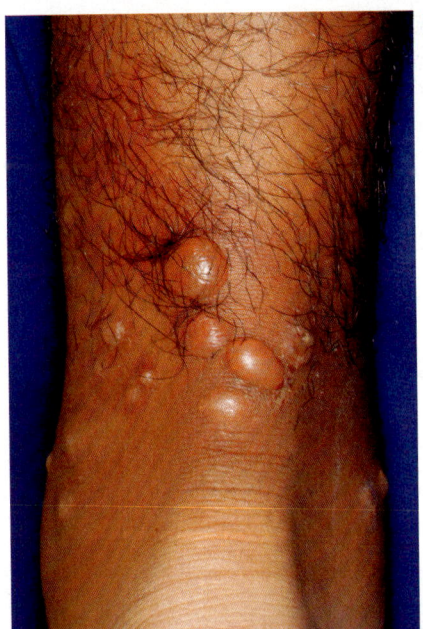

Figure 44.2. Bullous fleabite reaction.

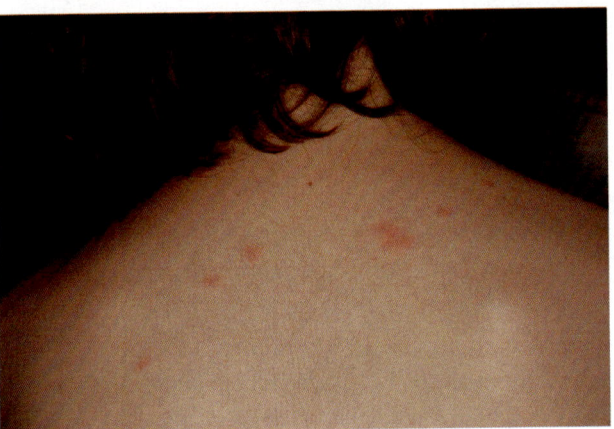

Figure 44.3. Fleabites. Note the "breakfast, lunch, and dinner" sign.

▶ Mites
- Small (0.1–2.0 mm) arachnids with numerous species, many of which live as parasites on animals or plants.
- Bites result in local reactions, and some may serve as vectors for disease.
- Mites of significance to humans include harvest mite (chiggers), grain mite, house mouse mite (vector for rickettsialpox), wheat mite, avian mite, dust mite, snake mite, rat/fowl mites, scrub mite (vector for scrub typhus), and mold mite.

- Clinically present as pruritic, erythematous urticarial 1- to 2-mm papules, occasionally with a visible central punctum or hemorrhage; lesions often are multiple (Figure 44.4).
- "Summer penile syndrome" is an acute hypersensitivity to chigger bites, presenting with intense penile swelling and pruritus.
- *Cheyletiella*, which are non-burrowing animal-specific mites (eg, cats, dogs, rabbits), may bite humans, resulting in grouped, pruritic papules. In infested pets, patches of fine powdery scale ("walking dandruff") are present.

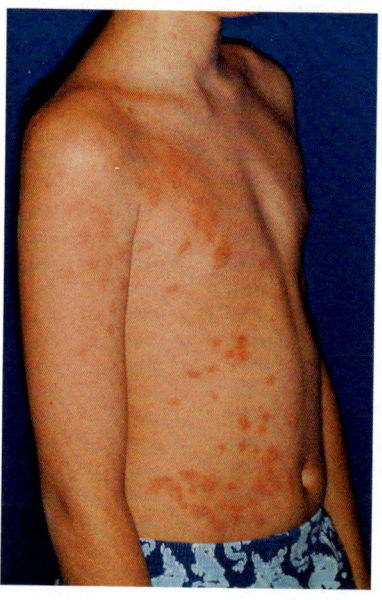

Figure 44.4. Mite bites. Multiple, clustered, edematous red papules and plaques.

▶ Bedbugs
- *Cimex lectularius* most common species to parasitize humans.
- Nocturnal insects that reside in cracks and crevices, mattress and wallpaper seams, and linens and come out to feed at night.
- Three to 7 mm in size, with flattened oval bodies (Figure 44.5).
- Bite reactions are erythematous papules with occasional bullous component.
- Linear clustering of reactions may be present (similar to "breakfast, lunch, and dinner" sign seen with fleabites).
- Potential vectors for blood-borne pathogens; methicillin-resistant *Staphylococcus aureus* and vancomycin-resistant *Enterococcus faecium* have also been recovered from some bedbugs.

- Resurgence in bedbugs has been noted in recent years, especially in hotels, hostels, and travel vessels (eg, aircraft, trains, cruise ships).
- Presence of eggs and fecal matter, or blood spots from the bugs (especially on background of white sheets or mattresses), may allow for easy identification.

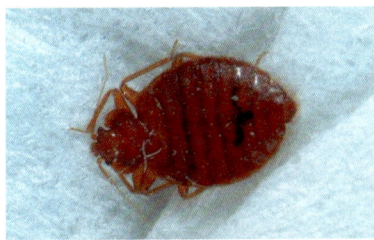

Figure 44.5. Bedbug. Note the flattened, oval body of this bug, which was brought into the clinic by the patient's mother.

► Ticks
- See Chapter 29 for a discussion of Lyme disease.
- Important vectors for disease, including Lyme disease, relapsing fever, Rocky Mountain spotted fever, boutonneuse fever (Mediterranean spotted fever), Q fever, ehrlichiosis, babesiosis, Colorado tick fever, and tularemia.
- Acute and chronic dermatoses may result from bites.
- Acute reaction may include erythematous, papular, nodular, bullous, or necrotic lesions.
- Chronic changes include persistent nodules (may have lymphoma-like characteristics on histologic examination), granulomas ("tick bite granuloma"), alopecia ("tick bite alopecia"; believed to be caused by a vigorous host immune response to tick saliva).
- Tick paralysis consists of ascending motor weakness and paralysis, resulting from neurotoxin that is injected while tick is engorged; it is reversible on removal of tick. It has been noted more commonly in young girls, possibly owing to longer hair, which may make tick identification more challenging.
- Immunoglobulin E antibody response against α-gal (oligosaccharide) may be associated with delayed urticarial response or anaphylaxis to ingestion of red meat.
- Tick removal is best accomplished by grasping the tick close to the skin with forceps and using gentle but steady traction, with care to avoid twisting, crushing, or severing the arachnid. Several commercial devices are available.

- Papular urticaria
    - Common, chronic condition of recurrent papules as a result of hypersensitivity to arthropod bites.
    - Fleabites are the most common cause.
    - Most common in late spring and summer.
    - Lesions are erythematous to hyperpigmented, urticarial pruritic papules (Figure 44.6).
    - May be generalized or erupt only at sites of past bite reactions.
    - Excoriation and secondary bacterial superinfection are common.
    - Lesions often heal with postinflammatory hyperpigmentation; recurrence is common.

A.

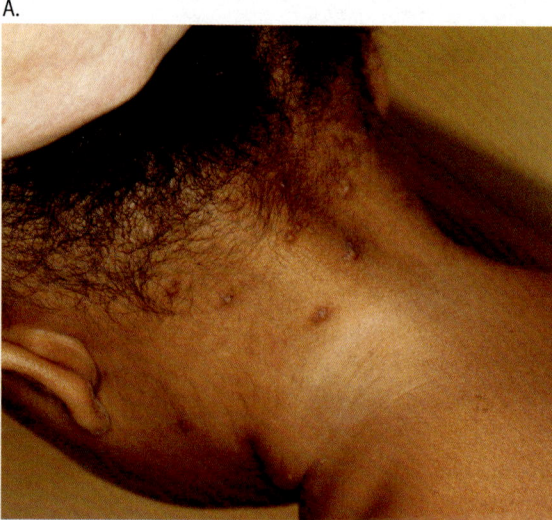

Figure 44.6. Papular urticaria. Edematous, pruritic pink and hyperpigmented papules intermittently flared at sites of prior fleabites on the neck and cheek (A). Another patient with persistent pink pruritic papules on the forearm after prior bite reactions (B).

B.

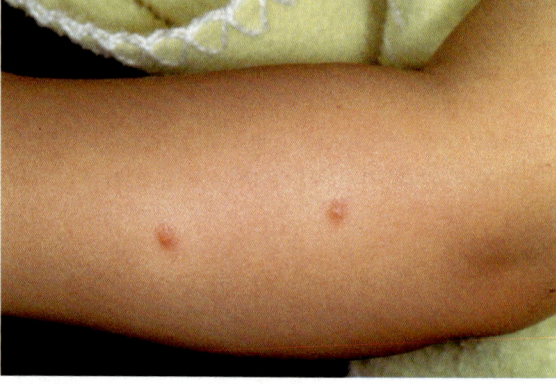

Look-alikes

Disorder	Differentiating Features
Pityriasis lichenoides	• Scaly or necrotic papules and plaques. • Diffuse distribution. • Usually non-pruritic. • Erupt in recurrent, cyclical fashion.
Lymphomatoid papulosis	• Red-brown papules and nodules. • Usually non-pruritic. • Histologic evaluation reveals lymphoma-like changes.
Bullous pemphigoid	• Unusual in children. • Widespread, tense bullae and vesicles. • Occasional mucosal involvement.
Urticaria	• Transient, with individual lesions resolving over hours. • Puncta, crusting, vesicles, bullae absent.
Bullous impetigo	• Fragile bullae that rupture easily. • Moist, erosive surface with peripheral collarette of scale. • Painful rather than pruritic.
Gianotti-Crosti syndrome	• Edematous, erythematous papules lacking central puncta. • Symmetric distribution on extensor upper and lower extremities, cheeks, and buttocks.

How to Make the Diagnosis

▶ Clinical examination, revealing edematous, pruritic papules and plaques with central puncta, crusting, vesicles, hemorrhage, or bullae.

▶ Environmental exposure history may be helpful (eg, exposure to infested pets in a child suspected of having fleabites).

▶ Skin biopsy (rarely necessary) reveals dermal and epidermal edema and numerous eosinophils.

Treatment

- Oral antihistamines
- Cool compresses
- Topical antipruritic agents, including calamine, camphor, and menthol lotions. Parents should be cautioned to secure camphor-containing agents to avoid inadvertent ingestion, which could be dangerous.
- For severe or more symptomatic lesions, use topical corticosteroid ointments or creams.
  - In younger children: mild- to mid-strength preparations.
  - In older children, teens, and adults: class I to II products often necessary (for non-facial, non-fold, nongenital regions only).
  - Applied once to twice daily.
  - Consider occlusion for severe reactions.
- Prevention includes avoidance of high-risk activities or exposure times, use of protective clothing, and use of insect repellents.
  - Most effective repellent is N,N-diethyl-3-methylbenzamide or DEET.
    - DEET is a broad-spectrum repellent with activity against mosquitoes, fleas, biting flies, and ticks.
    - Available in a variety of concentrations and vehicles.
    - Products with 20% to 30% concentration of DEET will provide adequate protection in most circumstances (around 2–5 hours of protection, depending on the concentration used).
    - DEET should not be used in infants younger than 2 months.
    - Repellent should be applied lightly and evenly (avoid skin saturation) on exposed skin, with caution not to apply near the eyes, mouth, or hands of young children.
    - DEET should not be applied to open wounds or inflamed areas.
    - Combination DEET and sunscreen preparations are not recommended because the need for frequent sunscreen application will result in unnecessary DEET exposure and potential toxicity.
    - Once indoors, all areas of application should be washed with soap and water.
    - Although there are rare reports of neurologic toxicity after DEET exposure, this is believed to be very rare and, in many reported events, the product was overapplied or orally ingested.
  - Other options for most insects include picaridin (used in a concentration up to 20%; reported efficacy similar to that of DEET), oil of lemon eucalyptus (para-menthane-3,8-diol or PMD; this agent should not be used in patients younger than 3 years), and 2-undecanone.

- Citronella, the active ingredient in many "natural" repellents, including oils, torch fuels, and candles, is not as effective as DEET or picaridin and should not be relied on as sole repellent in high-risk settings.
- Other essential oils that have been advocated include cedar, eucalyptus, lemongrass, and soybean; none have demonstrated effectiveness comparable with that of DEET or picaridin.
- Permethrin 0.5% spray is useful when applied to clothing, tents, and sleeping bags (it is not intended for application to the skin); this agent has activity against ticks, mosquitoes, flies, and chiggers.
- Some properties of infant and toddler skin may differ from those of adult skin until children are at least 2 years old. Because studies suggest the possibility that young skin may absorb more chemicals, DEET should be applied sparingly when needed, weighing the risks of exposure to potentially life-threatening insect-borne illnesses to the possible risks of absorbing chemicals into the body. Parents should be especially cautious when using DEET and other chemicals on newborns and preterm infants.

▶ For mosquitoes: Efforts to reduce insect populations (individual and community) are helpful.

▶ For fleas: Treatment of suspected animal hosts and cleaning of fomites (eg, carpets, floors, furniture) should be considered.

▶ For bedbugs: Consultation with a professional pest control service or cooperative extension is recommended. Although a variety of eradication strategies may be used (eg, insecticides, steam treatment), heat treatment has become increasingly popular and is effective. In this procedure, conducted by professional pest control services, the air temperature in a room or house is raised to greater than 48.9 °C (120 °F) for several hours, killing bedbugs and their eggs. Clothing and bedding should be washed in hot water and dried at high temperature.

Treating Associated Conditions

▶ Secondary bacterial infection of bite reactions should be treated with an appropriate systemic antibiotic.

▶ Tick bite granulomas may require treatment with intralesional corticosteroid injection or surgical excision.

▶ For patients with suspected tick bite, see also Chapter 29, Lyme Disease.

Prognosis

- Typical, uncomplicated bite reactions resolve completely without permanent sequelae.
- Papular urticaria may persist for months, rarely years, requiring intermittent therapy as necessary.

When to Worry or Refer

- Referral to a dermatologist should be considered for "bite reactions" that do not resolve or have atypical features.

Resources for Families

- eMedicineHealth: Insect bites and stings.
  https://www.emedicinehealth.com/insect_bites/article_em.htm
- MedicineNet: Bedbug bites.
  https://www.medicinenet.com/bed_bugs/article.htm
- Society for Pediatric Dermatology: Patient handout on papular urticaria.
  https://pedsderm.net/for-patients-families/patient-handouts/#PapularUrticaria
- WebMD: Bug bites directory.
  https://www.webmd.com/search?query=bug+bites+directory

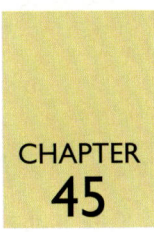

CHAPTER
45

Scabies

Introduction/Etiology/Epidemiology

- A worldwide problem affecting all ages, races, ethnicities, and socioeconomic strata.
- Caused by *Sarcoptes scabiei* variety *hominis*, the human scabies mite.
- Higher incidence in situations of overcrowding.
- Transmission occurs via direct skin-to-skin contact; acquisition from fomites (eg, bedding, clothing) is less common.
- Incubation period is approximately 3 weeks but shorter with reinfestation.
- Female mite lays eggs in skin burrows, which propagates the infestation.

Signs and Symptoms

- Pruritus (often most intense at night) may be severe and present before clinical lesions are apparent.
- Papules, burrows (white-gray threadlike lines), vesicopustules common (Figures 45.1 and 45.2).
- Nodules, which are seen primarily in infants and toddlers, may persist for months and indicate a vigorous host immune response (Figures 45.3 and 45.4).
- Common locations include interdigital spaces, wrists, ankles, axillae, waist, groin/genitalia, palms, and soles.
- Scalp involvement may be seen in infants.
- Secondary superinfection (usually *Staphylococcus aureus* or *Streptococcus pyogenes*) may occur.

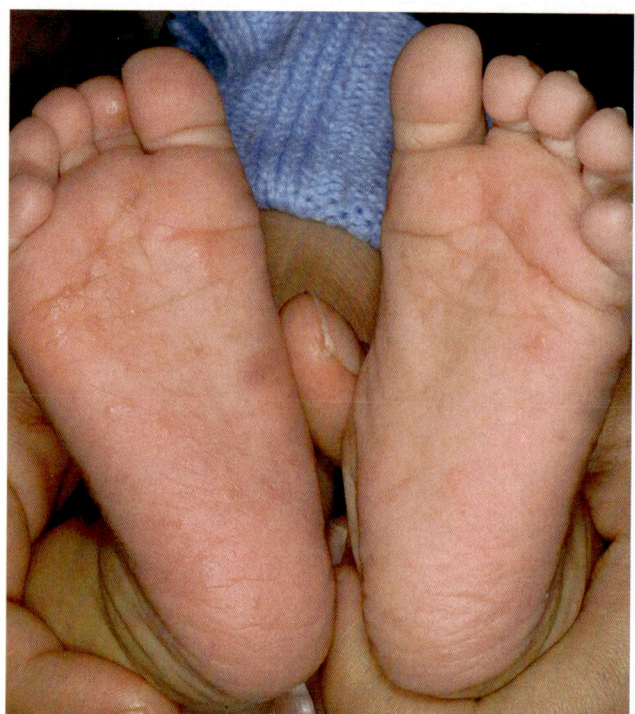

Figure 45.1. Scabies. Note papules, pustules, and linear burrows on the plantar surfaces of this infant.

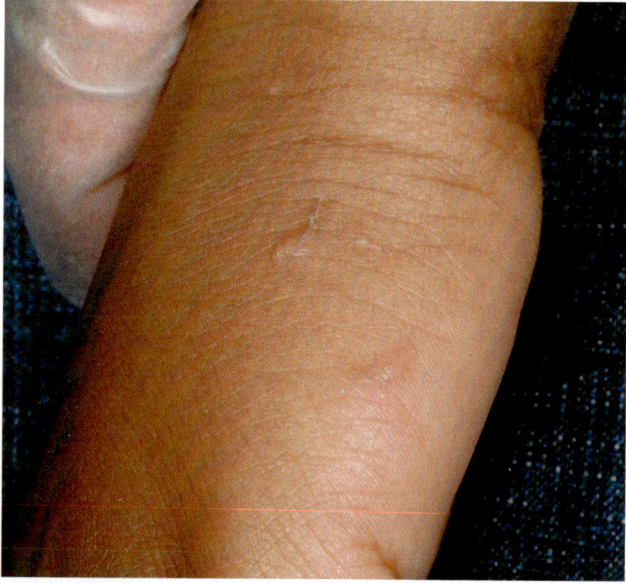

Figure 45.2. Scabies. Note linear burrows.

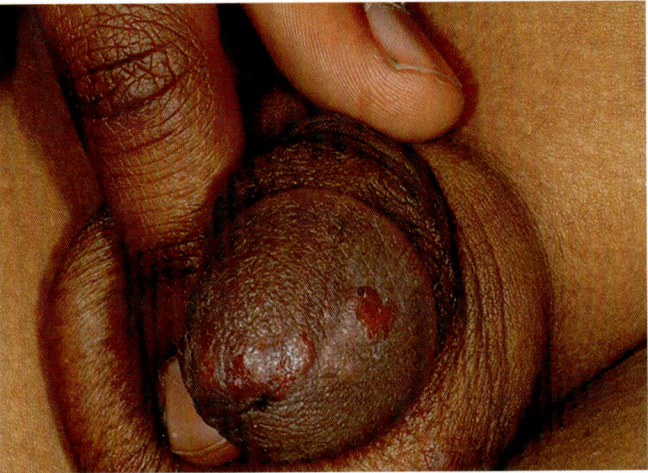

Figure 45.3. Scabies nodules in a young boy. Note papules and papulonodules on the glans penis.

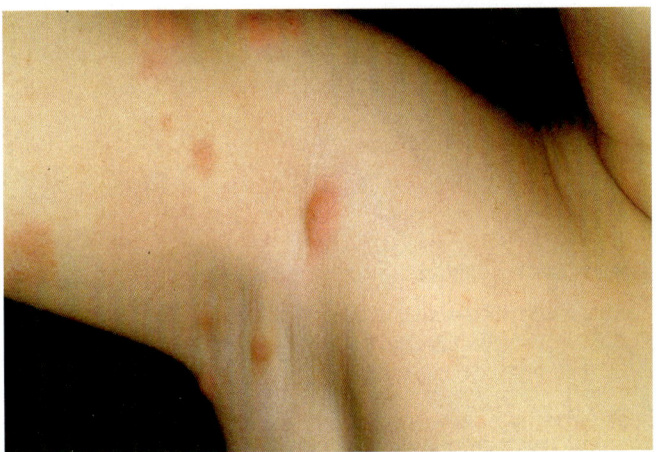

Figure 45.4. Scabies nodules. Papules and nodules in the axilla of a 2-year-old, 2 months after treatment for scabies infestation.

- ▶ Crusted (Norwegian) scabies.
  - Occurs in patients who are immunocompromised, especially those infected with HIV, or individuals with debilitation.
  - Presents as scaly, erythematous, hyperkeratotic plaques with excoriation.
  - May mimic eczema, psoriasis, or warts.
  - Frequently misdiagnosed and mismanaged given nondescript presentation.
  - Extremely contagious given the high number of mites that are present.

Look-alikes

Disorder	Differentiating Features
Acropustulosis of infancy	• Vesicopustules of wrists, palms, ankles, and aspects of the plantar feet occur in cyclical fashion, every 2 to 4 weeks. • Does not respond to permethrin therapy. • Lacks burrows. • May represent a post-scabies hypersensitivity response.
Arthropod bites	• Tend to be more discrete and fewer in number. • Palms and soles usually spared. • May be clustered in linear fashion. • Lack burrows.
Atopic dermatitis	• Atopic history common. • Characteristic distribution by age. • Diaper area/genitals usually spared in infants. • Lichenification often present, burrows absent.
Contact dermatitis	• Discrete patterning may be evident at sites of contact. • Less often papular, burrows absent. • Vesicles or bullae may be present.
Impetigo (crusted)	• Usually more focal. • Most common on the face, especially areas around the nose and mouth. • Burrows absent.
Langerhans cell histiocytosis	• Prominence of erythema and erosions in folds, burrows absent. • Lymphadenopathy common. • May have petechial or purpuric component. • Associated bone lesions or other organ involvement.
Papular urticaria	• Recurrent erythematous urticarial papules. • Burrows, vesicopustules absent.
Psoriasis	• Characteristic distribution, including scalp, elbows, knees, and sacral area. • Sharply demarcated papulosquamous lesions (scaling papules and plaques). • Lacks burrows.
Seborrheic dermatitis	• Erythema with greasy scaling. • Favors scalp, postauricular creases, skinfolds, groin, and umbilicus. • Lacks burrows, papules.
Viral exanthem	• Erythematous macules and papules. • Vesicopustules, burrows typically absent. • Associated symptoms/signs of viral illness may be present.

How to Make the Diagnosis

- Clinical features usually suggest the diagnosis.
- Confirmation made by mineral oil examination (see Chapter 2, Diagnostic Techniques), with microscopic identification of mites, eggs, or feces (scybala) (Figure 45.5).
- Skin biopsy rarely is necessary.

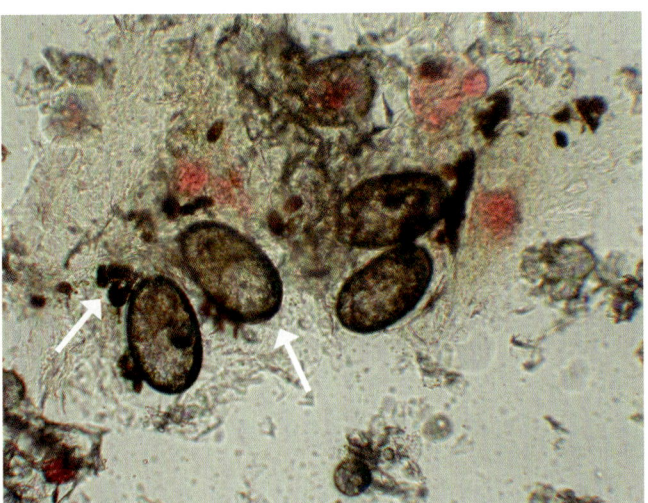

Figure 45.5. Mineral oil preparation in scabies (40× magnification). Note dark brown fecal pellets (scybala) (left arrow) and larger, oval-shaped eggs (right arrow).

Treatment

- Traditional treatment of choice is 5% permethrin cream, applied from neck to feet (head to feet in infants) and left on for 8 to 14 hours prior to rinsing.
- Permethrin should be thoroughly applied in a thin, even coat, and application should include web spaces, umbilicus, genitals, and gluteal cleft.
- Second treatment with permethrin 1 week after the initial treatment is recommended by some experts.
- Signs and symptoms of scabies may persist for several weeks after therapy and may be treated with topical antipruritics/anti-inflammatories and oral antihistamines as necessary.
- All close contacts should be treated.

- Alternative therapies include
  - Spinosad 0.9% topical suspension (approved in patients 4 years and older) applied and left on skin for a minimum of 6 hours prior to rinsing.
  - 5% to 10% sulfur in petrolatum.
  - Crotamiton 10% cream or lotion (high failure rate).
  - Benzyl benzoate 12.5% to 25% emulsion is applied nightly or every other night for 3 applications (but varying treatment regimens exist). This agent is not available in the United States.
  - Lindane lotion 1%; used extensively in the past but because of safety concerns should no longer be used.
  - Single-dose ivermectin (200 mcg/kg per dose) has been used (off-label) for crusted scabies or disease in immunocompromised patients; its safety in children weighing less than 15 kg has not been established. Topical ivermectin is reportedly effective.
- Environmental decontamination important: Machine wash clothing, bed linens, and towels in hot water and dry on high-heat setting.
- Prophylactic therapy of household members and other close contacts should be performed at the time the index case is treated initially.

Treating Associated Conditions

- Secondary bacterial infection: Treat with appropriate systemic antibiotic therapy.
- Scabies nodules: May be treated with topical or intralesional corticosteroids.

Prognosis

- Scabies usually responds well to therapy, and there are no permanent sequelae.
- Patients with crusted (Norwegian) scabies may be more resistant to treatment and may require multimodal or repeat therapy.

When to Worry or Refer

- Consider referral to a dermatologist if the diagnosis is in question, for patients who have severe or extensive disease, or for those in whom standard treatment is not effective.

Resources for Families

- American Academy of Dermatology: Scabies: diagnosis and treatment.
  https://www.aad.org/public/diseases/contagious-skin-diseases/scabies
- American Academy of Pediatrics: HealthyChildren.org.
  https://www.healthychildren.org/scabies
- MedlinePlus: Information for patients and families (in English and Spanish) sponsored by the US National Library of Medicine and National Institutes of Health.
  https://www.nlm.nih.gov/medlineplus/ency/article/000830.htm
- Society for Pediatric Dermatology: Patient handout on scabies.
  https://pedsderm.net/for-patients-families/patient-handouts/#Scabies

CHAPTER 46

Cercarial Dermatitis (Swimmer's Itch)

Introduction/Etiology/Epidemiology

- Also known as swimmer's itch, sawah itch, koganbyo.
- An inflammatory disorder caused by nonhuman schistosome parasites that penetrate human skin.
- Occurs most often in midwestern and southwestern United States, after swimming or wading in freshwater lakes; less commonly acquired in ocean waters.
- Most common species implicated is *Trichobilharzia*.
- Adult schistosome resides in mesenteric vasculature of birds or mammals and passes to intestine, and then eggs deposited into water with host feces; miracidia then hatch and penetrate snails (intermediate hosts), where they mature into cercariae (multicellular larvae) that reside in upper levels of water.
- Humans (accidental hosts) become infested when exposed to these waters and develop lesions that are classically limited to exposed areas of skin; skin lesions are the result of host immune response against dead cercariae.

Signs and Symptoms

- Nonspecific erythematous papules and papulovesicles on exposed skin (Figure 46.1).
- Pruritus common.
- Secondary excoriation and/or bacterial superinfection may occur.
- Postinflammatory pigmentary alteration is common and fades over time.

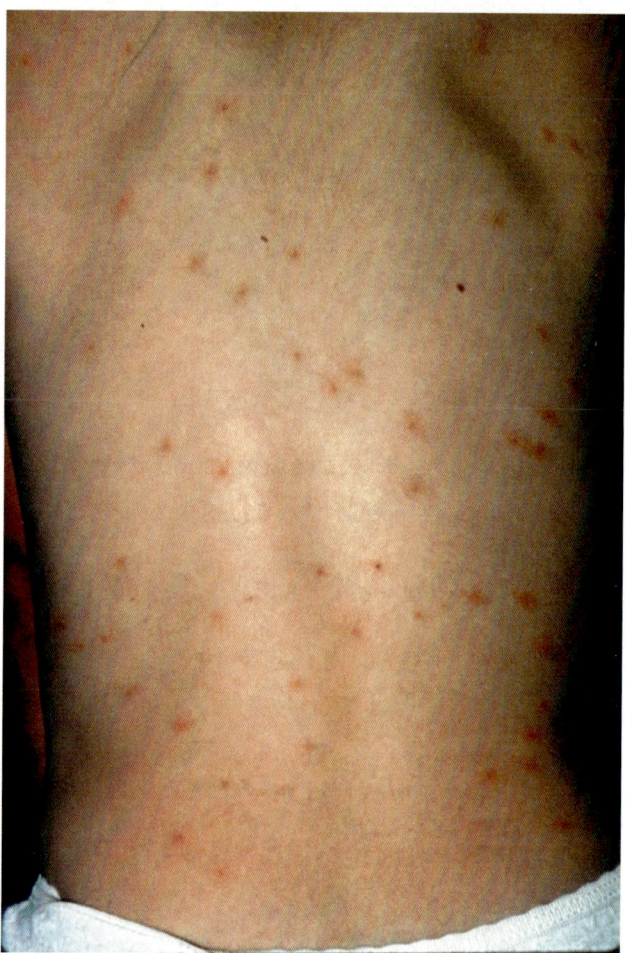

Figure 46.1. Cercarial dermatitis. There are erythematous papules on the patient's back.

Look-alikes

Disorder	Differentiating Features
Seabathers eruption (also known as sea lice)	• Not a true parasitic infestation; rather, a hypersensitivity reaction to the stinging nematocysts of cnidarian larvae, which include jellyfish, Portuguese man-of-war, sea anemone, and fire coral. • Usually associated with exposure to salt waters off Florida, in the Gulf of Mexico, or in the Caribbean. • Lesions typically limited to covered areas of skin (ie, by the swimming garment), as swimwear acts as filter and maintains contact between larvae and skin (Figure 46.2). • Pruritus often severe. • Other symptoms may be present: fever, chills, headache, fatigue, abdominal pain, nausea, diarrhea.
Pseudomonas (hot tub) folliculitis	• Caused by cutaneous infection with *Pseudomonas aeruginosa*. • Follows exposure to poorly chlorinated hot tubs or swimming pools. • Skin lesions composed of erythematous papules and pustules. • May occur diffusely but especially at sites covered by swimming garment (Figure 46.3). • Mild constitutional symptoms may be present: fever, malaise, headache, arthralgias.
Arthropod bite reactions	• History more consistent with potential exposures to arthropods (not typically water activities). • Edematous papules and plaques, often with central punctum, vesicle, or crust. • Lesions may be concentrated on lower legs (if caused by fleabites); may occasionally be bullous.
Allergic contact dermatitis	• History of exposure to potential contact allergen. • Lesions haphazardly distributed at sites that were in contact with the allergen. • Papules and papulovesicles typically become confluent into plaques, often with linear patterning.
Nonspecific viral exanthem	• Diffuse distribution (typically covered and uncovered areas of skin). • Morphology varies, including macules, papules, and plaques. • May present in morbilliform or urticarial patterns. • Fever, respiratory, or gastrointestinal symptoms may also be present. • Pruritus often mild or absent.

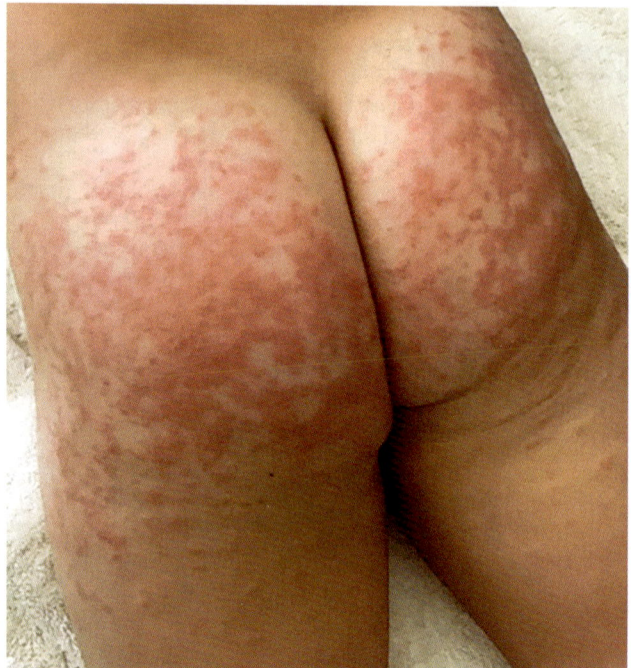

Figure 46.2. Seabathers eruption, a look-alike of cercarial dermatitis, usually appears after saltwater exposure and is located under garments worn while swimming. This 7-year-old boy developed itchy papules and plaques on areas covered by his swimsuit after swimming in the Bahamas.

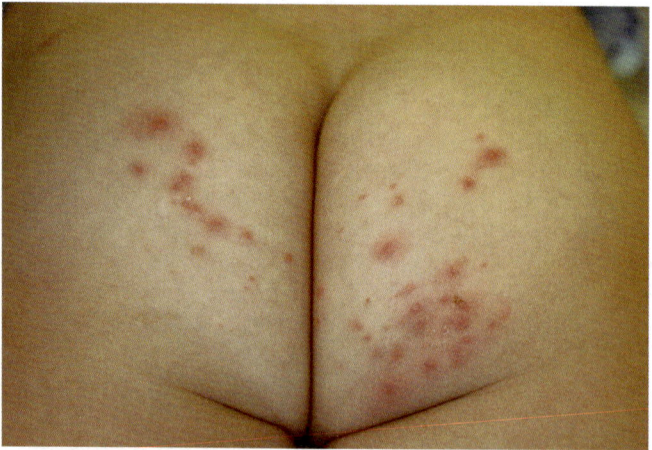

Figure 46.3. *Pseudomonas* (hot tub) folliculitis. Tender, erythematous papules and pustules clustered on the buttocks of a school-aged patient who had spent time in a hot tub.

How to Make the Diagnosis

- The distribution of skin lesions combined with the history of exposure to a freshwater lake will typically suggest the diagnosis of cercarial dermatitis.
- No diagnostic test is available; analysis via filtration and polymerase chain reaction study of water samples may be performed if confirmation of an outbreak is required.

Treatment

- Treatment is of symptoms and may include topical corticosteroids or antipruritic agents and oral antihistamines.
- Systemic corticosteroids are rarely indicated for severe cases.

Treating Associated Conditions

- Secondary bacterial superinfection should be treated with the appropriate systemic antibiotic.

Prognosis

- Cercarial dermatitis resolves completely over time, without permanent sequelae.

When to Worry or Refer

- Referral to a dermatologist should be considered for patients in whom the diagnosis is in question or for whom conventional therapy is unsuccessful.

Resources for Families

- American Academy of Pediatrics: HealthyChildren.org.
  https://www.healthychildren.org/English/tips-tools/symptom-checker/Pages/symptomviewer.aspx?symptom=Swimmer%27s+Itch+-+Lakes+and+Oceans

- Centers for Disease Control and Prevention: Parasites—about swimmer's itch.
  https://www.cdc.gov/swimmers-itch/about/?CDC_AAref_Val=https://www.cdc.gov/parasites/swimmersitch/index.html

- Healthline: What are the symptoms of swimmer's itch?
  https://www.healthline.com/health/cercarial-dermatitis#symptoms

Papulosquamous Diseases

CHAPTER 47 — **Lichen Nitidus** 341

CHAPTER 48 — **Lichen Planus (LP)** 345

CHAPTER 49 — **Lichen Striatus** 349

CHAPTER 50 — **Pityriasis Lichenoides** 353

CHAPTER 51 — **Pityriasis Rosea** 359

CHAPTER 52 — **Psoriasis** 363

CHAPTER 53 — **Pityriasis Rubra Pilaris (PRP)** 373

CHAPTER 54 — **Seborrheic Dermatitis** 377

CHAPTER 47

Lichen Nitidus

Introduction/Etiology/Epidemiology

- Lichen nitidus is a benign asymptomatic chronic eruption of unknown cause.
- Onset occurs in late childhood or adolescence.

Signs and Symptoms

- Patients present with an asymptomatic or mildly pruritic eruption composed of minute (1–2 mm), flat-topped skin-colored (Figure 47.1) or white (Figure 47.2) papules.
- Lesions often are clustered into circular plaques and may appear at any location.
- Papules may be arranged in a linear distribution at sites of trauma due to scratching (ie, the Koebner phenomenon) (see Figure 47.2).
- Lichen nitidus is a self-limited disorder.

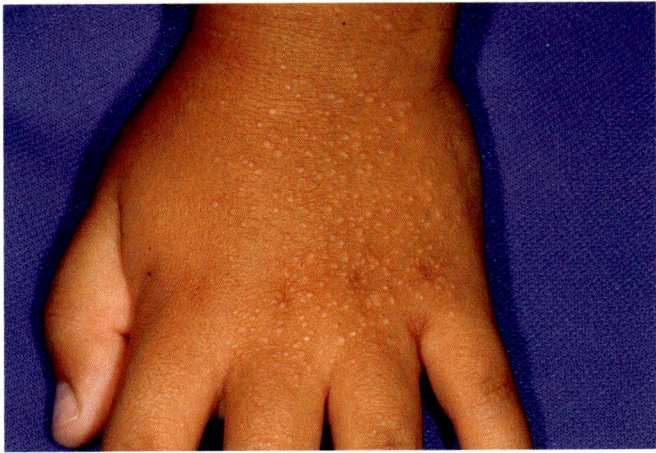

Figure 47.1. Flesh-colored, flat-topped papules clustered on the dorsal aspect of the hand of a young patient.

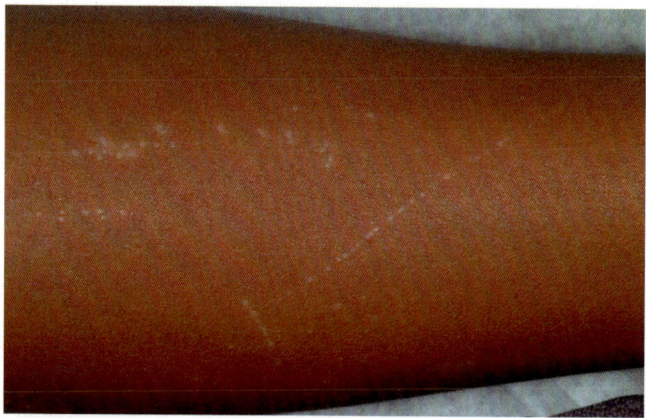

Figure 47.2. White, flat-topped papules, some in a linear arrangement, are characteristic of lichen nitidus.

Look-alikes

Disorder	Differentiating Features
Molluscum contagiosum	• Papules often vary in size. • Larger lesions exhibit umbilication. • Lesions pearlier and more translucent in quality.
Flat warts	• Variably sized verrucous, flat-topped papules. • Clustering into circular plaques not usually seen.
Papular atopic dermatitis	• Lesions are pruritic and skin-colored. • Evidence of atopic dermatitis elsewhere on the body. • Koebner phenomenon not observed.
Keratosis pilaris	• Skin-colored, keratotic (not flat-topped) papules centered about follicles. • Koebner phenomenon not observed. • Bilaterally symmetric distribution on cheeks, upper lateral aspects of the arms, and thighs.
Lichen planus	• Papules larger. • Papules pruritic, purple, polygonal (ie, have angulated borders), and often involve the penis.
Lichen spinulosus	• Clustered, skin-colored, keratotic (not flat-topped) papules centered about follicles. • Koebner phenomenon not observed.

How to Make the Diagnosis

- The diagnosis is made clinically.

Treatment

- No therapy is required.
- For patients who experience pruritus, a topical corticosteroid or topical calcineurin inhibitor may be applied or an oral antihistamine prescribed.

Prognosis

- The prognosis is excellent, with spontaneous resolution usually occurring within 12 months.

When to Worry or Refer

- Consider consultation if the diagnosis is uncertain or if the disease is widespread and symptomatic (eg, there is severe pruritus).

Resource for Families

- DermNet NZ: Lichen nitidus.
  https://dermnetnz.org/topics/lichen-nitidus

CHAPTER 48

Lichen Planus (LP)

Introduction/Etiology/Epidemiology

- Lichen planus (LP) is a distinctive papulosquamous eruption.
- The cause of LP is unknown; however, there is inflammatory damage to the cells of the basal layer of the epidermis.
  - LP may occur in association with autoimmune diseases as well as various infections, especially viral infections such as hepatitis C.
  - Reactions to drugs may cause an LP-like eruption.

Signs and Symptoms

- The lesions of LP are described as papules that are planar (flat-topped), pruritic, purple, and polygonal (angulated borders) and often involve the penis (the Ps of LP) (Figures 48.1 and 48.2).
  - Individual papules may coalesce into plaques, form rings, or be distributed in a linear fashion.
  - The surface of lesions may exhibit a network of fine white lines (ie, Wickham striae).
  - The flexor surfaces of the forearms and wrists, anterior portion of the legs, penis, and presacral areas most often are affected.
  - Papules may be distributed in a linear array at sites of trauma due to scratching (ie, the Koebner phenomenon).
- The oral mucosae often exhibit a white, lacy, or reticulated appearance (Figure 48.3); erosions may be present.
- Other findings include nail dystrophy or scarring alopecia.
- Pruritus typically is severe.
- Lesions range from asymptomatic to mildly pruritic.

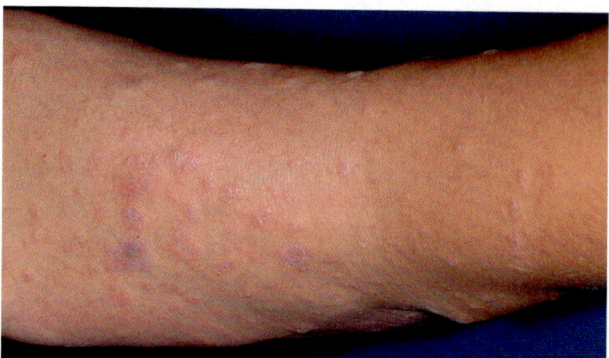

Figure 48.1. Violaceous, flat-topped papules are observed in lichen planus.

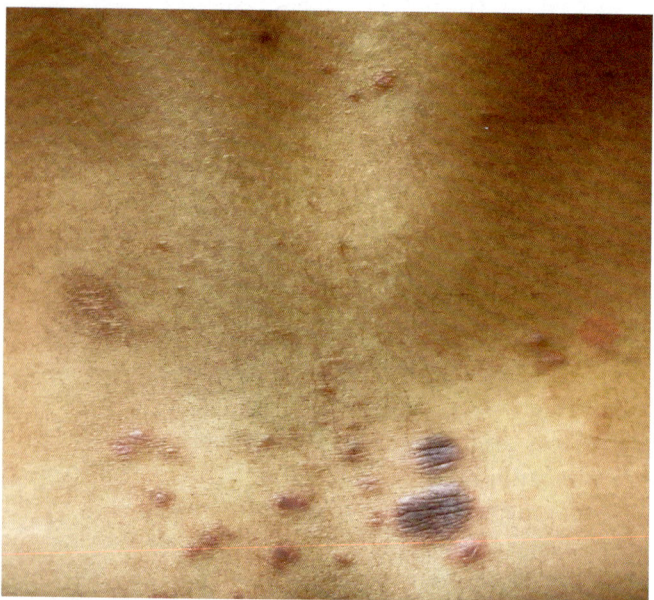

Figure 48.2. Lichen planus; violaceous and hyperpigmented papules and plaques on the lower back in a patient with skin of color.

Chapter 48: Lichen Planus (LP)

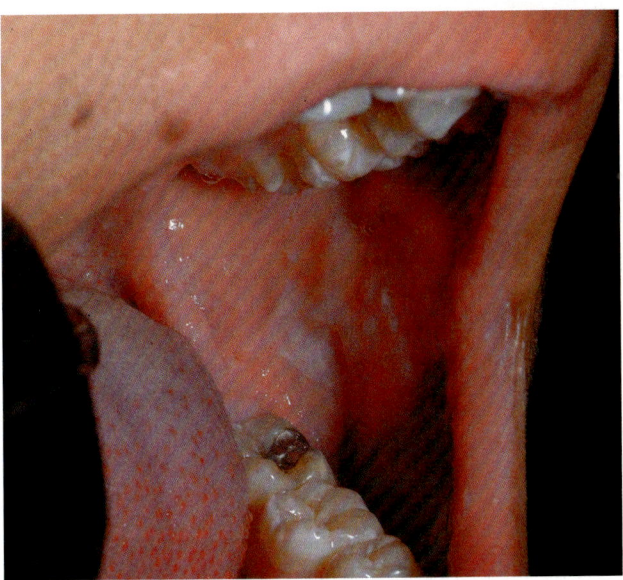

Figure 48.3. White, lacy, or reticulated plaques often are observed on the buccal mucosa of patients who have lichen planus.

Look-alikes

Disorder	Differentiating Features
Psoriasis	• Erythematous and covered by thick, adherent scale.
Keratosis pilaris	• Rough, keratotic papules centered about follicles. • Skin-colored or slightly erythematous. • Bilaterally symmetric distribution on cheeks, upper lateral arms, and thighs.
Lichen nitidus	• Small (1–2 mm), white, flat-topped papules that often are grouped.
Lichen striatus	• May be difficult to distinguish from linear lichen planus. • Process localized (lesions in a linear arrangement) and not present elsewhere. • Associated hypopigmentation common.

How to Make the Diagnosis

▶ The diagnosis is suspected clinically and may be confirmed by skin biopsy.

Treatment

▸ Mid-potency or stronger topical corticosteroids are used to control pruritus and hasten the resolution of lesions; topical calcineurin inhibitors may also be helpful.

▸ Oral lesions may be treated with a potent topical corticosteroid applied 3 to 4 times daily as needed.

▸ In children with more severe, widespread disease, a short course of oral corticosteroids can be effective. Additionally, UV-B phototherapy can be beneficial. Very severe, recalcitrant cases may require consideration of an oral retinoid or methotrexate.

Prognosis

▸ The prognosis is good; most pediatric patients experience a resolution of disease within 6 to 12 months of beginning therapy.

▸ Recurrences of LP are uncommon.

When to Worry or Refer

▸ Most patients who have LP will benefit from consultation with a pediatric dermatologist.

▸ Refer patients if the diagnosis is in doubt, when therapy fails, or when the disease is severe or widespread.

Resources for Families

▸ American Academy of Dermatology: Lichen planus: diagnosis and treatment.
https://www.aad.org/public/diseases/rashes/lichen-planus

▸ MedlinePlus: Information for patients and families (in English and Spanish) sponsored by the US National Library of Medicine and National Institutes of Health.
https://www.nlm.nih.gov/medlineplus/ency/article/000867.htm

▸ WebMD: Information for families is contained in Skin Problems and Treatments.
www.webmd.com/skin-problems-and-treatments/guide/common-rashes

CHAPTER 49

Lichen Striatus

Introduction/Etiology/Epidemiology

- Lichen striatus is a self-limited papulosquamous inflammatory disease of unknown cause.
- It most often occurs in young children (median age of onset is 2–3 years); female patients are affected more often than male patients.

Signs and Symptoms

- Lesions are small, erythematous or violaceous papules that typically begin on a proximal extremity and then extend down the extremity (although lesions may appear on the trunk and, less commonly, the face) (Figures 49.1 and 49.2).
  - The lesions follow Blaschko lines (ie, the paths of embryonic neural crest cell migration).
  - Distal extension of lesions may involve a nail, creating dystrophy.
  - Within 1 to 2 years, the papules resolve, leaving hypopigmentation that ultimately resolves.
- Lesions range from asymptomatic to mildly pruritic.

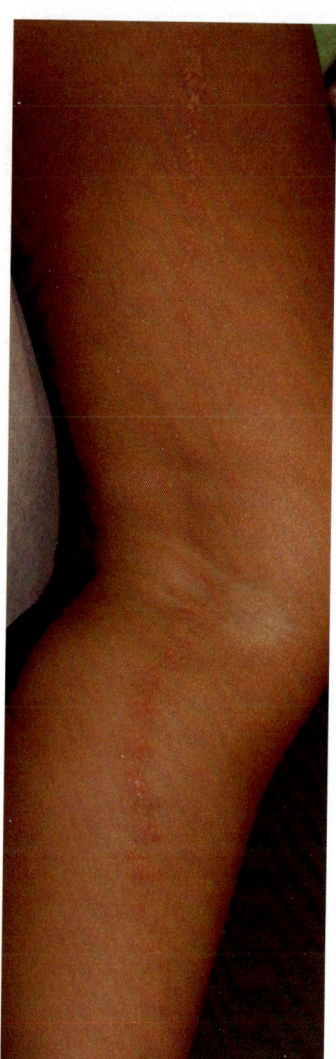

Figure 49.1. Linear arrangement of papules on the posterior thigh and leg in lichen striatus.

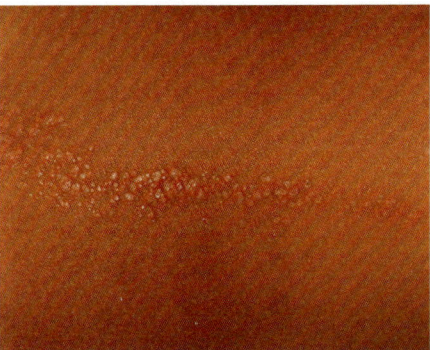

Figure 49.2. Close-up view of the patient in Figure 49.1. Note that in lichen striatus, the papules are flat-topped (ie, lichenoid).

Look-alikes

Disorder	Differentiating Features
Psoriasis	• Koebner phenomenon may cause some lesions to occur in linear arrangement, but typical lesions will be present elsewhere. • Lesions have thick adherent scale; if scale is removed, pinpoint bleeding may occur (Auspitz sign).
Lichen planus	• Koebner phenomenon may cause some lesions to occur in a linear arrangement, but typical lesions will be present elsewhere.
Lichen nitidus	• Koebner phenomenon may cause some lesions to occur in a linear arrangement, but typical lesions will be present elsewhere. • Small (1–2 mm), white papules.
Linear epidermal nevus	• Hyperpigmented plaque often with a rough surface. • Often present at birth. • Does not resolve spontaneously.

How to Make the Diagnosis

▶ The diagnosis is made clinically.

Treatment

▶ No treatment is necessary.
▶ The application of a mid-potency topical corticosteroid may be of some benefit when inflammatory lesions (ie, erythematous papules) are present.

Prognosis

- The prognosis is excellent, with spontaneous resolution occurring within 1 to 3 years.
- Recurrences are uncommon.

When to Worry or Refer

- Refer patients in whom the diagnosis is uncertain.

Resource for Families

- American Osteopathic College of Dermatology: Lichen striatus. **www.aocd.org/?page=LichenStriatus**

CHAPTER 50

Pityriasis Lichenoides

Introduction/Etiology/Epidemiology

- Pityriasis lichenoides is an uncommon papulosquamous eruption seen in children and young adults.
- Etiology is unclear, and most cases are idiopathic.
  - Some consider this condition to be a self-limited, cutaneous lymphoproliferative disorder.
- Pityriasis lichenoides is often considered a disease spectrum with acute and chronic forms. Clinical overlap between the 2 types often exists.
  - Pityriasis lichenoides et varioliformis acuta (PLEVA): characterized by the acute onset of crops of red or red-brown macules and papules that become vesicular or necrotic or form crust or scale.
  - Pityriasis lichenoides chronica (PLC): characterized by the gradual onset of crops of scaling papules and small plaques that resolve and recur over a period of several months to years, often healing with postinflammatory dyspigmentation.
- *Mucha-Habermann disease* is an older term that has traditionally been applied to PLEVA, but many consider this term broadly within the entire spectrum of disease.

Signs and Symptoms

- PLEVA
  - Abrupt onset of red to red-brown macules or papules (2–5 mm in diameter). Lesions may become vesicular, necrotic, hemorrhagic, or purpuric and may develop crust or scale (Figure 50.1).
  - An important clue is the presence of lesions in various stages of development.
  - As the condition evolves, lesions may become hemorrhagic, crusted, and necrotic, sometimes resulting in varioliform (chickenpox-like) scars and dyspigmentation.

- Most patients with PLEVA are asymptomatic, but some experience pruritus or systemic symptoms, such as fever, lymphadenopathy, and malaise.
- A rare subtype of PLEVA (febrile ulceronecrotic Mucha-Habermann disease) causes more widespread involvement with large necrotic and ulcerative nodules and plaques. Constitutional symptoms and high fever are often present.

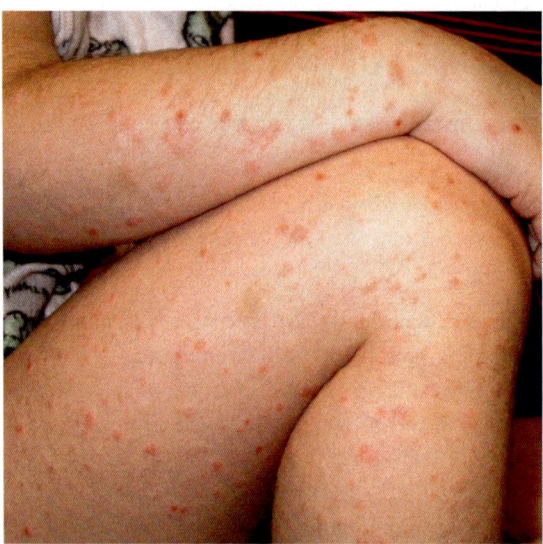

Figure 50.1. Erythematous crusted papules of pityriasis lichenoides et varioliformis acuta are seen in this child.

- PLC
  - Gradual onset of red-brown papules, often with an overlying scale or crust.
  - Lesions often appear, subside, and reappear in crops over weeks to months (sometimes years). Lesions are typically at various stages and morphologies (Figure 50.2). Postinflammatory dyspigmentation is often seen.
  - Constitutional symptoms are not typically seen in PLC, and lesions are usually asymptomatic.
- A widespread distribution is typically seen in PLEVA and PLC, with most lesions appearing on the trunk, buttocks, and extremities.
  - Involvement of the proximal extremities is typical; the palms and soles are usually spared.
  - Facial involvement is uncommon but may occur in darker skin types.
  - Clinical overlap often occurs between PLEVA and PLC.

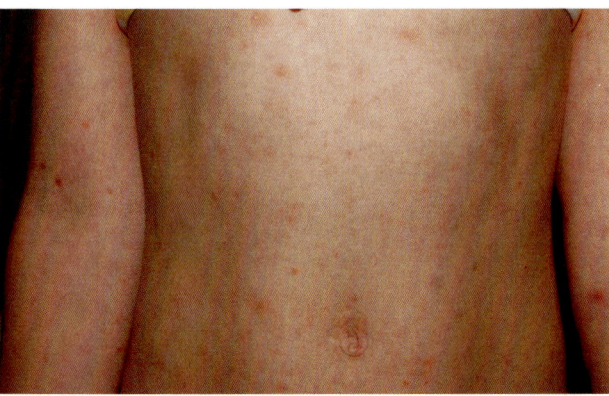

Figure 50.2. Crops of scaling papules are seen in this patient with pityriasis lichenoides chronica.

Look-alikes

Disorder	Differentiating Features
Pityriasis rosea	• Small, thin oval plaques with long axes parallel to lines of skin tension. • Typically lacks crusting, necrosis, blistering; hemorrhage only occasionally present. • Lesions covered by thin, fine "trailing scale" (lags behind advancing red border, and free edge of scale points inward toward center of plaque). • Course is typically less prolonged.
Guttate psoriasis	• Lesions covered with a thick, adherent silvery scale. • Lesions not usually present in differing stages. • Crusted, hemorrhagic, vesicular, and necrotic lesions absent.
Lichen planus	• Purple, polygonal papules and small plaques. • Fine scale (not thick adherent scale) is present. • Oral involvement common, with thin, white, elevated linear lesions forming a lacy, reticulated appearance. • Pruritus is common. • Crusted, hemorrhagic, vesicular, and necrotic lesions usually absent.
Varicella	• May resemble pityriasis lichenoides et varioliformis acuta (PLEVA) (when PLEVA is characterized by papules and vesicles). • More rapid progression of lesions, with more extensive involvement of face, scalp, and mucous membranes. • Distribution is classically centripetal, with most lesions on the trunk and fewer on the distal extremities. • Patient more often ill with fever and other systemic symptoms. • Shorter duration of disease than pityriasis lichenoides. • Markedly decreased incidence in era of universal varicella vaccination.
Gianotti-Crosti syndrome	• Symmetric, predominantly facial, buttock, and extensor extremity distribution with minimal involvement of the trunk. • Lesions are monomorphic, lack mica scale, and usually do not appear in recurrent crops. • Duration is typically less prolonged than pityriasis lichenoides.
Secondary syphilis	• Patients often ill with fever and lymphadenopathy. • Lesions often present on the palms and soles. • Lesions typically do not appear in recurrent crops.

How to Make the Diagnosis

▶ The diagnosis is usually made clinically based on the appearance and distribution of the lesions. If the diagnosis is in doubt, skin biopsy may be performed.

Treatment

▶ Treatment is often dependent on symptoms, and not all cases of pityriasis lichenoides require therapy.
▶ UV therapy, particularly UV-B, has been demonstrated to be a safe, effective treatment option. Natural UV exposure is also beneficial for patients.
▶ While topical steroids and oral antihistamines may be effective in patients with associated pruritus, neither have been shown to alter the disease course.
▶ Oral antibiotics (eg, erythromycin, azithromycin, tetracyclines [for those older than 8 years]), perhaps owing to their anti-inflammatory effect, have been shown to be effective in some patients. Patients typically are treated for several months. If a response is achieved, the dose may then be tapered and the drug ultimately discontinued.
▶ In occasional instances, methotrexate has been used but typically limited to the context of severe, refractory cases failing to respond to conservative measures.

Prognosis

▶ Prognosis is favorable, as pityriasis lichenoides is usually a self-limited disorder.
▶ The duration of pityriasis lichenoides is often unpredictable and variable, with some cases lasting weeks to months, while others may last for years.
▶ PLEVA typically has a shorter duration, but some cases may evolve into PLC. Flares and remissions over a period of months to years is typically seen in patients with PLC.
▶ Generally, there is a tendency toward improvement during the summer months, which is most likely related to natural UV exposure.

When to Worry or Refer

- If the diagnosis is in doubt, consider dermatology consultation or possible histopathologic confirmation.

Resources for Families

- American Osteopathic College of Dermatology: Pityriasis lichenoides.
  https://www.aocd.org/page/PityriasisLichenoid
- DermNet NZ: Pityriasis lichenoides.
  https://dermnetnz.org/topics/pityriasis-lichenoides
- Medscape: Pityriasis lichenoides.
  http://emedicine.medscape.com/article/1099078-overview

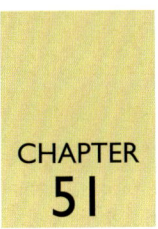

CHAPTER
51

Pityriasis Rosea

Introduction/Etiology/Epidemiology

- Pityriasis rosea is a benign, self-limited eruption of characteristic scaly papules and plaques in children and young adults.
- Etiology is unknown.
  - Seasonal incidence and clustering of cases suggest an infectious agent.
  - Some evidence supports a role for human herpesvirus 6 and 7.

Signs and Symptoms

- The initial lesion in as many as 80% of patients is the herald patch, a round or oval erythematous patch with a scaling border and central clearing that may be mistaken for tinea corporis or nummular eczema (Figure 51.1).
- Within 2 weeks, a generalized, sometimes pruritic eruption appears; individual lesions are erythematous papules and small (5–10 mm), thin, oval plaques with scale.
  - The plaques are oriented with their long axes parallel to lines of skin tension.
  - Lesions are concentrated on the trunk; on the back, the alignment of lesions may mimic the boughs of a fir (ie, the "Christmas tree" distribution) (Figure 51.2).
    - In "inverse" pityriasis rosea, lesions are concentrated on the neck, proximal extremities, groin, and axillae; there may be relative sparing of the trunk (Figure 51.3).
  - "Trailing scale" is present: Scale lags behind the advancing red border, with the free edge pointing inward toward the center of the plaque.
  - In persons with skin of color, the appearance of the eruption may differ.
    - The eruption may appear papular with few plaques (Figure 51.4).
    - The erythematous nature of the eruption may be more difficult to appreciate.
- New lesions appear for 2 to 3 weeks, and the eruption resolves typically over several weeks to months.

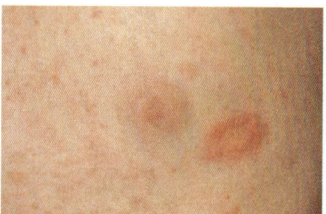

Figure 51.1. The herald patch is a round or oval erythematous patch that may be mistaken for tinea corporis.

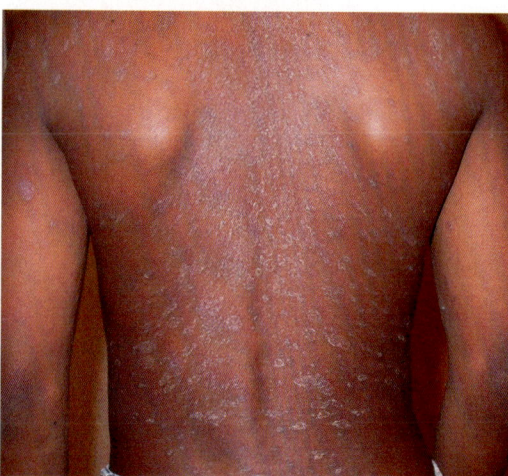

Figure 51.2. On the back, the alignment of lesions along lines of skin tension may mimic the appearance of the boughs of a fir tree (ie, the "Christmas tree" appearance).

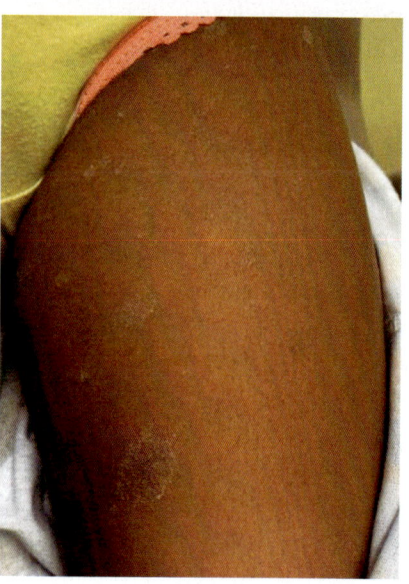

Figure 51.3. This patient with inverse pityriasis rosea has characteristic oval thin scaling plaques on the proximal thighs and inguinal folds, as well as in the axillae.

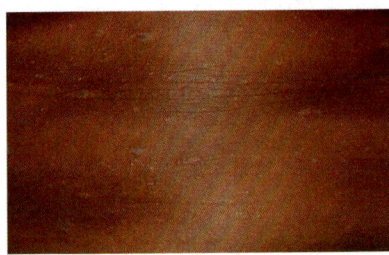

Figure 51.4. In patients with darker skin tones, erythema may be more difficult to appreciate in the papules and plaques of pityriasis rosea.

Look-alikes

Disorder	Differentiating Features
Tinea corporis	• May be confused with herald patch of pityriasis rosea. • Border often more elevated. • Potassium hydroxide preparation performed on scale from lesion reveals hyphae. • Generalized eruption not usually seen. • Trailing scale is absent.
Nummular eczema	• May be confused with herald patch of pityriasis rosea. • Covered with crust, as well as scale. • Pruritus may be present (but less common than with typical eczema). • Generalized eruption not typically seen. • Trailing scale is absent.
Secondary syphilis	• Patients often ill with fever and lymphadenopathy. • Lesions often present on the palms and soles.
Guttate psoriasis	• Lesions not oriented along lines of skin tension. • Lesions covered with a thick, adherent scale.
Pityriasis lichenoides chronica	• Often involves the extremities as well as the trunk. • Buttock involvement common. • Lesions not classically oriented along lines of skin tension. • Course more prolonged than that of pityriasis rosea.

How to Make the Diagnosis

▶ The diagnosis is made clinically.

Treatment

- Most children with pityriasis rosea require no therapy.
- If pruritus is present, an emollient containing menthol or phenol may be applied as needed (acts as a counterirritant that masks the sensation of pruritus) or a sedating antihistamine prescribed.
- Judicious sun exposure may reduce pruritus and hasten the resolution of the eruption. Medical phototherapy is occasionally prescribed for severe cases; tanning beds are now classified as group 1 carcinogens and are not recommended for this purpose.
- Counsel the patient and family about the prolonged course of the eruption.

Prognosis

- Prognosis is excellent, although the prolonged time required for resolution may be frustrating to patients and families.

When to Worry or Refer

- Consider consultation when the diagnosis is in doubt.
- If patient exhibits signs of secondary syphilis (eg, oral or genital mucosal lesions, lesions on the palms or soles), perform appropriate testing (ie, rapid plasma reagin or VDRL test).
- If lesions persist for longer than 3 months, consider referral to a pediatric dermatologist to assess for pityriasis lichenoides chronica, a disorder that (in its early stages) may mimic pityriasis rosea.

Resources for Families

- American Academy of Pediatrics: HealthyChildren.org.
  https://www.healthychildren.org/pityriasisrosea
- American Academy of Dermatology: Pityriasis rosea: diagnosis and treatment.
  https://www.aad.org/public/diseases/rashes/pityriasis-rosea

CHAPTER 52

Psoriasis

Introduction/Etiology/Epidemiology

- Papulosquamous (ie, elevated lesions with scale) condition with a tendency to persist or recur for years.
- Characterized by inflammation and hyperproliferation of the epidermis.
- Likely results from both a genetic predisposition (family history often is positive) and an environmental trigger (eg, stress, infection, trauma).
- Recent literature links psoriasis to other systemic comorbidities, in particular a higher prevalence of metabolic syndrome (ie, obesity, dyslipidemia, hypertension, and elevated blood glucose levels) and cardiovascular disease in children and adults. Psoriasis may occur in some children with juvenile idiopathic arthritis. Typically, this occurs within 2 years of diagnosis of juvenile idiopathic arthritis.

Signs and Symptoms

- Appearance of lesions
  - Lesions are well-defined papules, patches, and plaques that are pink to deep red and have an adherent white to silvery "micaceous" scale (Figure 52.1).
    - Removal of scale produces pinpoint bleeding points (Auspitz sign) due to dilated dermal capillaries (Figure 52.2).
    - Scale may be absent or less prominent in moist, intertriginous areas (eg, diaper area, axillae) (Figure 52.3).
  - Variants
    - Infantile psoriasis: may appear as generalized erythroderma or as sharply demarcated erythema (with minimal scale) in diaper region (Figure 52.4), axillae, and umbilicus.
    - Guttate psoriasis: Often precipitated by pharyngeal or perianal *Streptococcus pyogenes* infection; begins as generalized erythematous macules and papules (that may mimic a viral exanthem); later, characteristic scale appears (Figure 52.5).

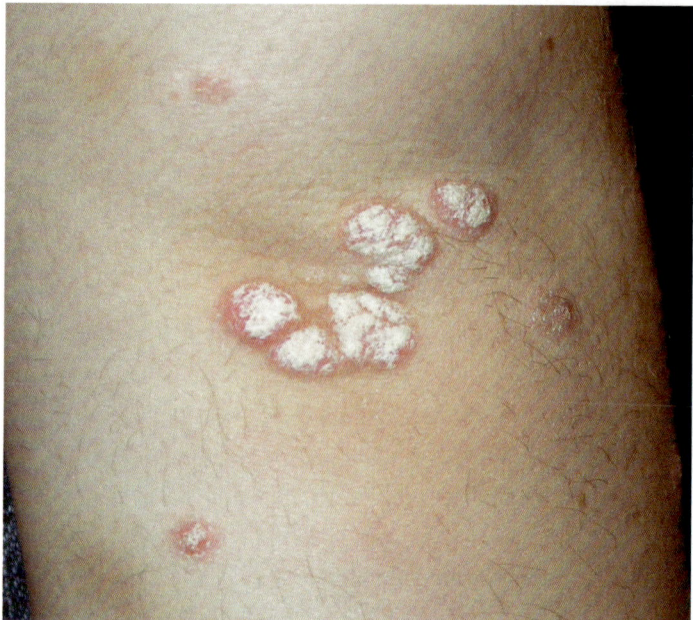

Figure 52.1. Typical lesions of psoriasis are erythematous papules and plaques that have a thick adherent scale.

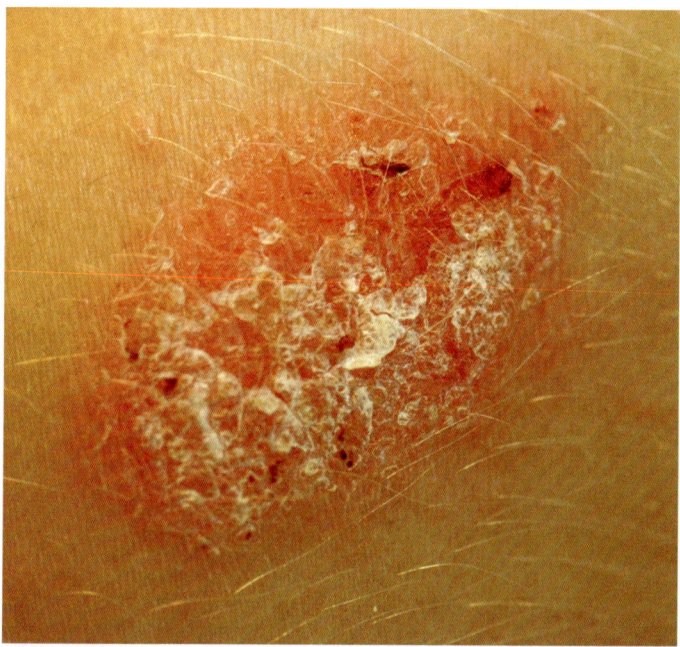

Figure 52.2. Plaque of psoriasis with Auspitz sign (pinpoint bleeding in areas of removed scale).

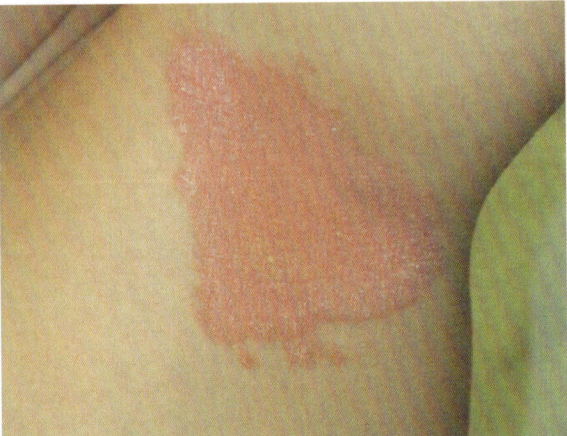

Figure 52.3. In occluded areas, such as the axilla, the lesions of psoriasis may lack scale.

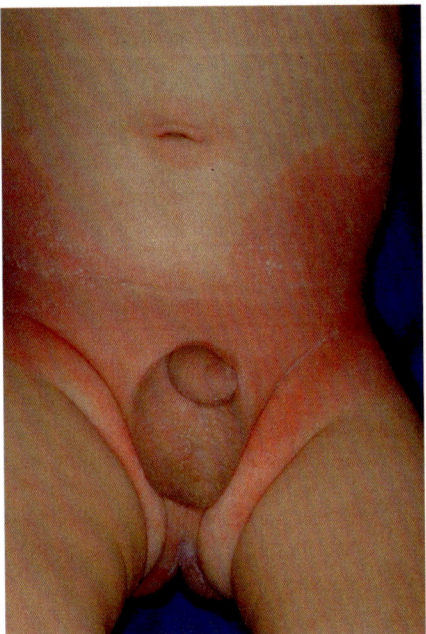

Figure 52.4. In infants, psoriasis may involve the diaper area, appearing as sharply defined erythematous patches with little scale. Also note involvement of the umbilicus, a common finding in psoriasis.

- Pustular psoriasis: small pustules studded over the surface of deep red plaques (Figure 52.6).
- Inverse psoriasis: lesions located predominantly in the axillae (Figure 52.7) and groin.

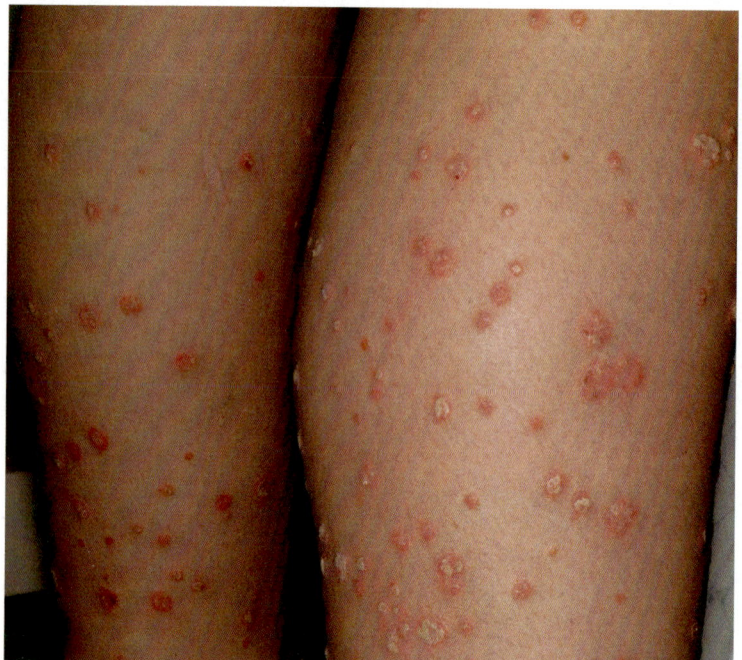

Figure 52.5. Guttate psoriasis is characterized by an eruption composed of widespread macules or papules that may mimic a viral exanthem. Over time, the lesions develop thick scale.

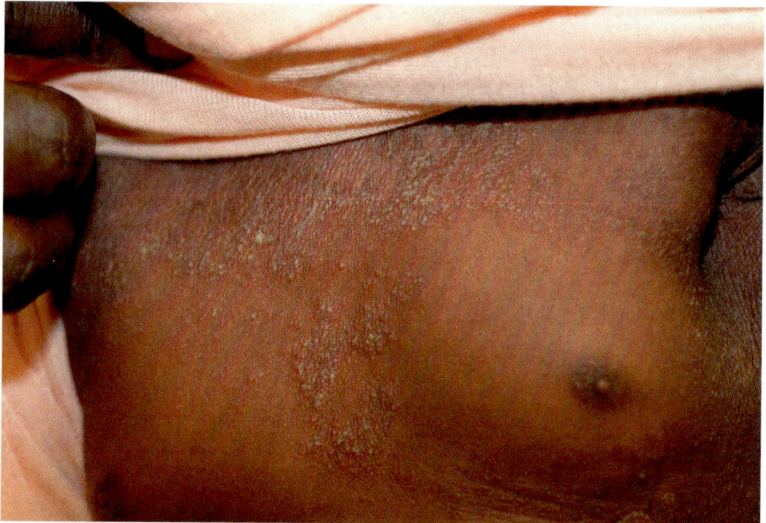

Figure 52.6. Pustular psoriasis. This patient presented with numerous pustules overlying red plaques.

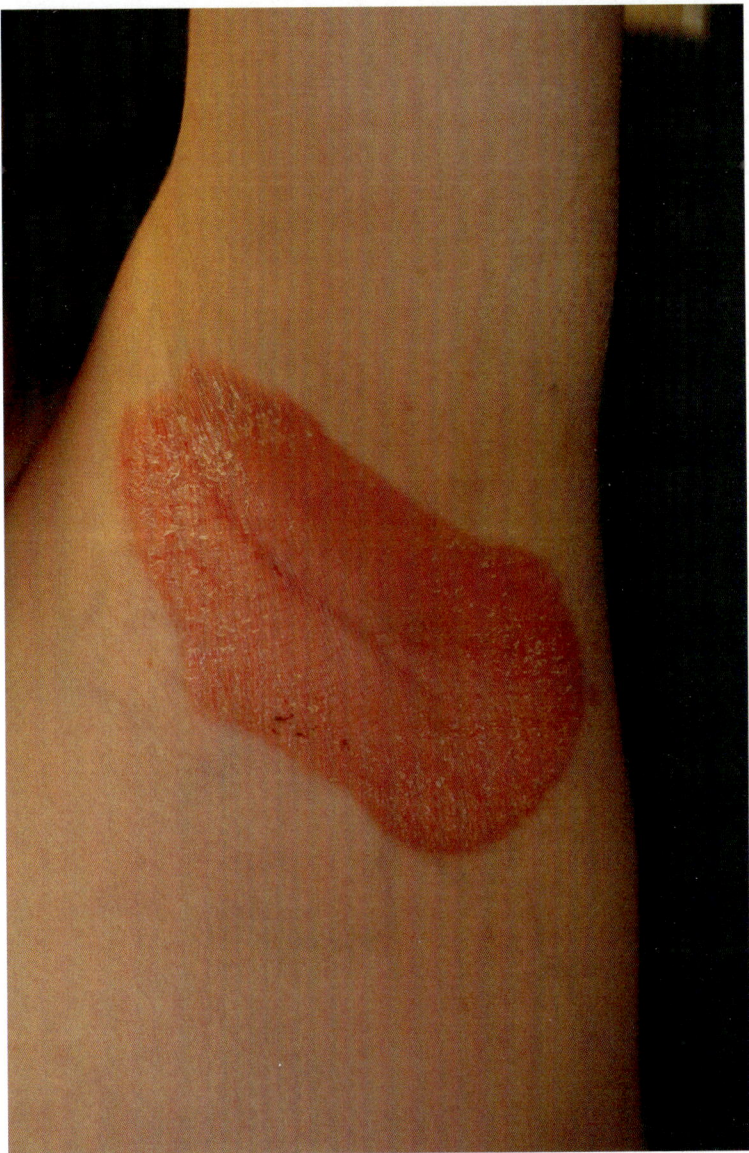

Figure 52.7. Left axillary vault with a plaque of inverse psoriasis (note reduced scaling due to intertriginous location).

- Distribution
  - Scalp (scaling and erythema) (Figure 52.8), posterior auricular regions, elbows (Figure 52.9), knees (Figure 52.10), umbilicus, and gluteal cleft; however, any body region may be affected.
  - Lesions appear in areas of trauma (ie, Koebner phenomenon), explaining involvement of the extensor surfaces of the extremities.
  - Nail involvement is common, consisting of pitting or thickening and yellowing.

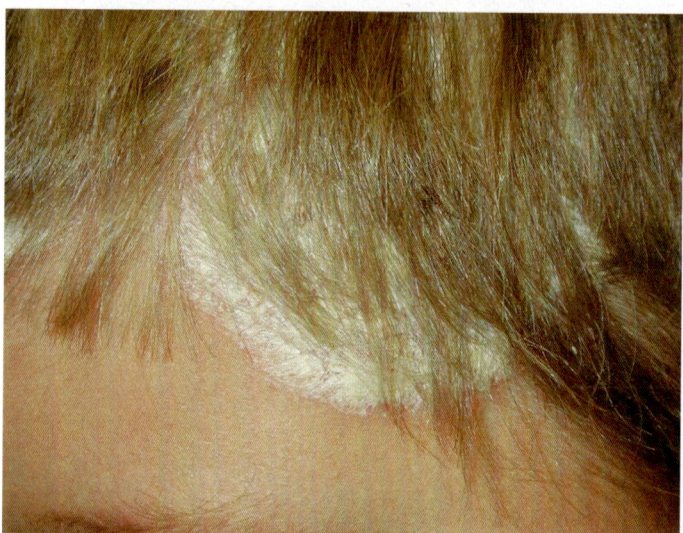

Figure 52.8. On the scalp, psoriasis causes erythema and thick scale.

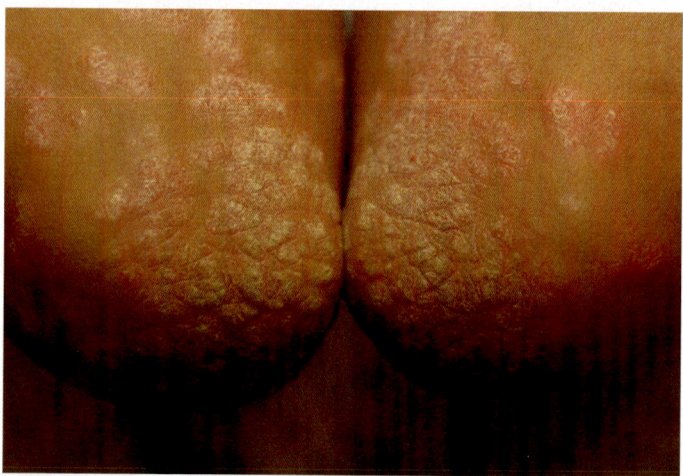

Figure 52.9. Psoriatic papules coalescing into plaques on the elbows of an affected teen.

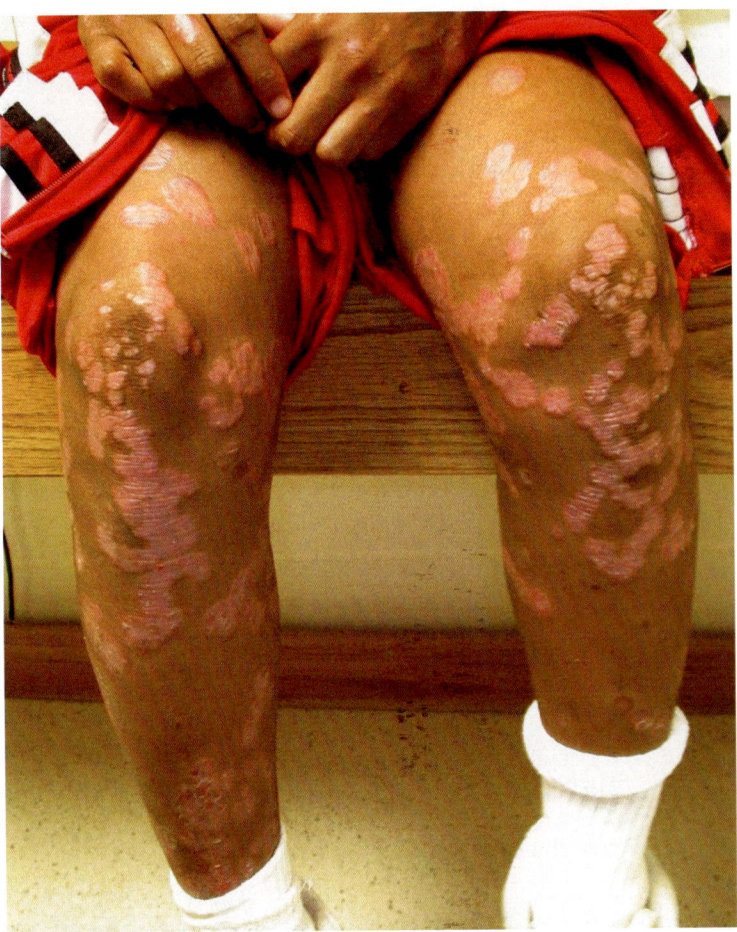

Figure 52.10. Patient with psoriasis of the knees and shins.

Look-alikes

Disorder	Differentiating Features
Lichen planus	• Purple or pink polygonal papules and small plaques. • Fine scale (not thick adherent scale) is present. • Oral involvement common, with thin, white, elevated linear lesions forming a lacy, reticulated appearance.
Dermatomyositis	• Patients may exhibit muscle weakness. • Characteristic cutaneous findings include heliotrope rash and Gottron papules (ie, erythematous papules located over the dorsal surfaces of interphalangeal joints of the fingers). • Lesional scaling is typically minimal.
Pityriasis rosea	• May be confused with guttate psoriasis. • Many patients first develop a herald patch followed by small, thin oval plaques with long axes parallel to lines of skin tension. • Lesions covered by thin, fine "trailing scale" (lags behind advancing red border, and free edge of scale points inward toward center of plaque).
Seborrheic dermatitis	• May be difficult to distinguish from psoriasis when only the scalp and face are involved. • Typical lesions have greasy, yellow/tan scales. • Auspitz sign absent. • In infants, seborrheic dermatitis and psoriasis may be indistinguishable.

How to Make the Diagnosis

▶ The diagnosis is made clinically based on the appearance and distribution of lesions.

▶ Observation of Auspitz sign strongly suggests a diagnosis of psoriasis.

▶ Skin biopsy can be helpful if the clinical presentation is not diagnostic.

Treatment

▶ Therapy is directed at reducing inflammation and normalizing epidermal proliferation.

- Topical therapy (first line): Treatment often involves more than 1 agent.
  - Mid-potency (or, occasionally, high-potency) topical glucocorticoids (often used in conjunction with calcipotriene).
  - Calcipotriene (vitamin D derivative): Normalizes epidermal proliferation; may be used as monotherapy or in conjunction with topical corticosteroids; may cause hypercalcemia in infants or small children if applied over large surface areas.
  - Others: anthralin or liquor carbonis detergens (also known as LCD, a tar derivative), topical phosphodiesterase-4 inhibitors, and topical retinoids occasionally used.
  - Moisturization is recommended to help maintain skin integrity.
- Phototherapy or photochemotherapy: UV-B or UV-A (alone or combined with psoralen, when known as PUVA) therapy may be used for patients with severe disease in whom topical therapy fails.
- Systemic therapy: Methotrexate, cyclosporine A, or acitretin may be used for patients with severe disease in whom topical therapy fails. Biologic agents (that target tumor necrosis factor-α, interleukin [IL]-12, IL-17, and/or IL-23) are increasingly used, with pediatric approval (for psoriasis) down to 6 years of age for ustekinumab, secukinumab, and ixekizumab and down to 4 years of age for etanercept.

Treating Associated Conditions

- When guttate psoriasis is suspected, test for pharyngeal (or perianal if the physical examination is suggestive) S pyogenes infection and treat if infection is confirmed.

Prognosis

- Psoriasis is a chronic disease, and recurrences may be anticipated.

When to Worry or Refer

- For patients with significant disease, consult with or refer to a pediatric dermatologist to optimize therapy.
- Refer patients in whom the diagnosis is uncertain, those in whom appropriate therapy does not work, or those in whom pustular disease develops.
- If there is clinical concern for possible psoriatic arthritis, refer to a pediatric rheumatologist.

Resources for Families

- American Academy of Dermatology: Psoriasis resource center.
  https://www.aad.org/public/diseases/scaly-skin/psoriasis

- American Academy of Pediatrics: HealthyChildren.org.
  https://www.healthychildren.org/English/health-issues/conditions/ skin/Pages/Psoriasis-Not-Eczema-Not-Allergy.aspx?_gl=1*rys8l4* _ga*MTgzMDQyODM3My4xNjg3ODgxNzUy*_ga_FD9D3XZVQQ* MTcwOTEzNDQ3NS40MDAuMS4xNzA5MTM3MDE1LjAuMC4w

- MedlinePlus: Information for patients and families (in English and Spanish) sponsored by the US National Library of Medicine and National Institutes of Health.
  https://www.nlm.nih.gov/medlineplus/ency/article/000434.htm

- National Psoriasis Foundation: Provides extensive information (in English and Spanish) about the disease and its treatment.
  https://www.psoriasis.org

- Society for Pediatric Dermatology: Patient handout on psoriasis.
  https://pedsderm.net/for-patients-families/patient-handouts/ #Psoriasis

Pityriasis Rubra Pilaris (PRP)

Introduction/Etiology/Epidemiology

- Rare inflammatory skin disorder of unknown etiology.
  - *CARD14* pathogenetic variants identified in a subset of patients with hereditary autosomal dominant form.
- Affects patients of all ages with 2 peaks of onset: 1 in the first decade after birth and another in adulthood. Although most pediatric patients develop symptoms in the teenage years, the disorder can also be seen during the first couple years of life.
- Most common differential diagnosis: psoriasis.
- Clinical presentation can be further subdivided into adult onset (classic or atypical) and childhood onset (classic juvenile, circumscribed juvenile, and atypical juvenile). The features of childhood onset pityriasis rubra pilaris (PRP) are summarized in Table 53.1.
- Circumscribed juvenile PRP is the most common subtype seen in children.

Signs and Symptoms

- Hyperkeratotic papules and plaques, often surrounding the hair follicles and demonstrating a salmon-colored hue.
- Palmoplantar involvement, characterized as thick waxy, erythematous plaques on the palms and soles, is common (Figures 53.1 and 53.2).
- Head and neck involvement is frequent in pediatric patients with PRP and is seen in up to 40%.
- Nails may be dystrophic, with thickening, onycholysis (ie, separation of nail plate from nail bed), transverse ridges.
- Pruritus may be present or absent.
- Involvement is symmetric in most patients.

Table 53.1. Features of Childhood Onset Pityriasis Rubra Pilaris (PRP)

Juvenile PRP Type	Frequency	Clinical Features
Classic juvenile (type III PRP)	14%–35%	• Generalized pattern. • Follicular keratotic papules. • Patients with extensive disease may demonstrate islands of uninvolved skin. • Palm and sole involvement common.
Circumscribed juvenile (type IV PRP)	Most common subtype in children	• Focal hyperkeratotic papules and plaques on the extensor surfaces of elbows, knees (Figure 53.3). • Palmoplantar lesions common.
Atypical juvenile (type V PRP)	Rare; may be familial and can have younger age of onset	• Follicular hyperkeratosis. • Ichthyosiform scaling. • Sclerodermatous changes can be seen on the palms and soles.

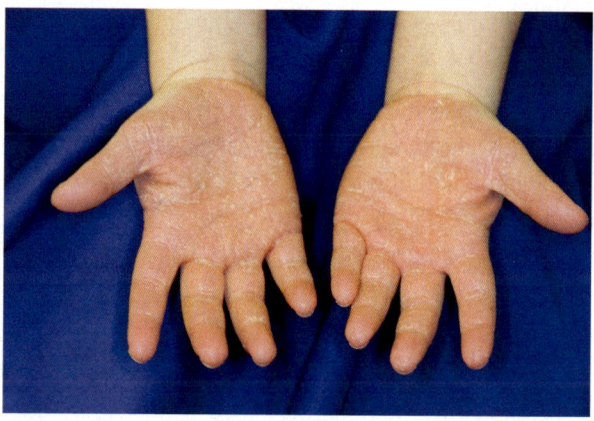

Figure 53.1. Palmar involvement in pityriasis rubra pilaris. Note symmetric, well-demarcated erythema, thickening of the skin, and scaling.

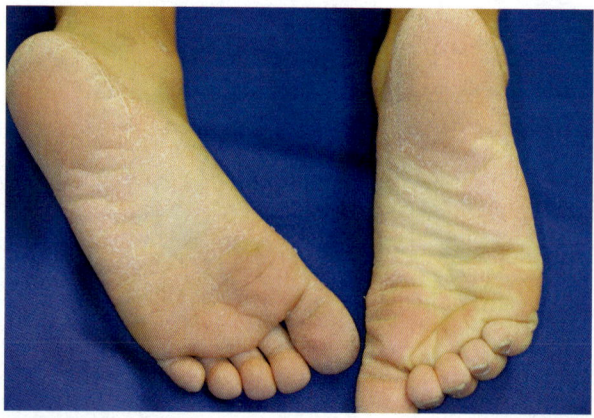

Figure 53.2. Plantar involvement in pityriasis rubra pilaris. Well-demarcated thickening of the soles with mild scaling and erythema in a child with juvenile circumscribed pityriasis rubra pilaris.

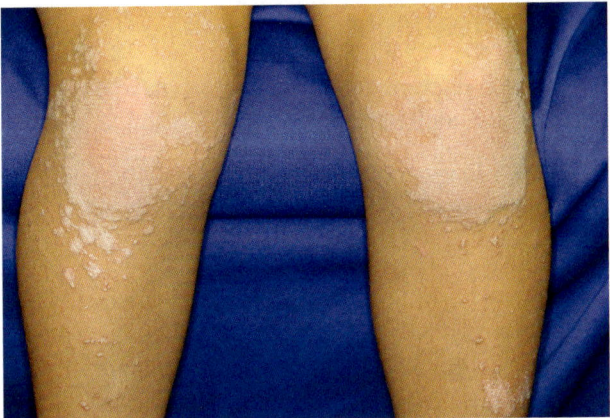

Figure 53.3. Well-demarcated erythematous scaling plaques with follicular prominence in a young child with pityriasis rubra pilaris.

Look-alikes

Disorder	Differentiating Features
Psoriasis	• Characteristic body sites often involved (eg, scalp, postauricular skin, genitalia, extensor surfaces, periumbilical skin), although there is some overlap, as pityriasis rubra pilaris may involve similar areas. • May have associated joint pain, swelling (ie, psoriatic arthritis). • Thick, adherent silvery scales are characteristic.
Pityriasis rosea	• Acute onset of thin scaly plaques, often in a Christmas tree configuration on trunk. • Larger plaque (herald patch) precedes development of smaller plaques. • Lacks palmar and plantar involvement.
Atopic dermatitis	• Pruritic, scaly papules and plaques. • Personal or family history of atopic diseases common. • Characteristic body sites involved (eg, flexural surfaces in children; extensor involvement typically limited to infants). • Typically lacks palmar and plantar involvement.

How to Make the Diagnosis

▶ Typically diagnosed based on clinical features. In patients with atypical features or when the diagnosis is in question, biopsy may be warranted.

▶ If diagnosis is in question, refer to a dermatologist.

Treatment

- Mild to moderate disease often responds to emollients, low- to mid-potency topical corticosteroids, or topical retinoids.
- Keratolytics may help thin the hyperkeratosis on palms and soles.
- Topical calcineurin inhibitors (eg, pimecrolimus, tacrolimus) may be helpful for facial involvement.
- Severe disease is typically treated with systemic retinoids and, occasionally, immunosuppressants, such as methotrexate, cyclosporine, or azathioprine. Phototherapy has occasionally been helpful, and biologic therapies (namely, ustekinumab) have been reported to be useful in patients with *CARD14* pathogenetic variants.

Prognosis

- Prognosis is variable and difficult to predict and may be related to disease subtype. Remission is noted in a subset of children within a few months of onset, whereas others may have disease that persists for years.
- Patients presenting with 1 form of PRP may occasionally have the PRP evolve into a different subtype.

When to Worry or Refer

- If diagnosis is uncertain.
- If patients have extensive disease or topical therapies fail.

Resource for Families

- Genetic and Rare Diseases Information Center: Pityriasis rubra pilaris. **https://rarediseases.info.nih.gov/diseases/7401/pityriasis-rubra-pilaris**

CHAPTER 54

Seborrheic Dermatitis

Introduction/Etiology/Epidemiology

- Chronic dermatitis of unknown cause. May be related to an inflammatory response to the yeasts of the genus *Malassezia* (formerly *Pityrosporum*).
- Seborrheic dermatitis may be divided into 2 main variants.
  - Infantile: presents from soon after birth to about 1 year of age.
  - Adolescent and adult: occurs primarily in older children (who have experienced adrenarche) or postpubertal individuals.
- In addition to these variants, seborrheic dermatitis may also occasionally occur in toddlers and elementary school-aged children.

Signs and Symptoms

- Infantile
  - Characterized by yellowish greasy scale on the scalp (ie, cradle cap) (Figure 54.1) and erythematous patches with greasy scale that have a predilection for the face and flexural areas (eg, postauricular region, axillae, groin) (Figures 54.2 and 54.3).
  - Occasionally may have near total skin involvement.
  - Shares considerable clinical overlap with atopic dermatitis and infantile psoriasis.
- Adolescent and adult
  - Most common presentation is scaling of the scalp (ie, dandruff).
  - Patients may exhibit erythematous poorly defined scaling patches on scalp (Figure 54.4), ears, eyebrows, nasolabial folds (Figure 54.5), central chest, and beard area in male patients.
  - Pruritus is variable.

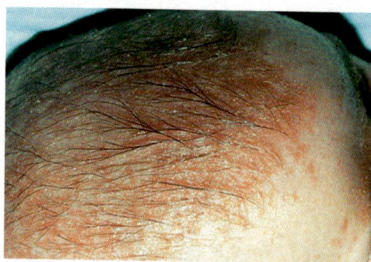

Figure 54.1. Greasy scale on the scalp of an infant (ie, cradle cap).

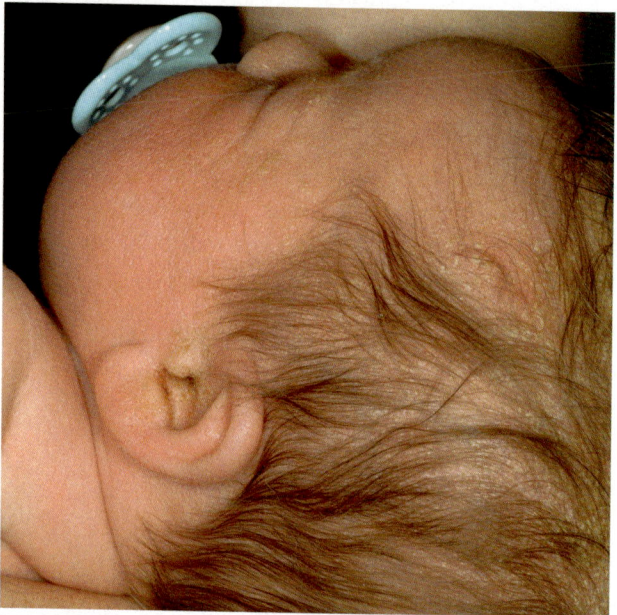

Figure 54.2. Erythematous patches with greasy scale on the face of an infant who has seborrheic dermatitis.

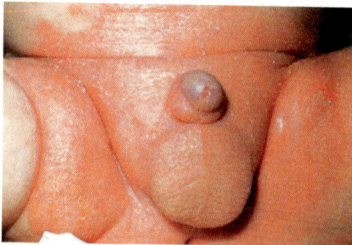

Figure 54.3. In the diaper area, seborrheic dermatitis produces salmon-colored patches with greasy scale that involves the creases and convexities.

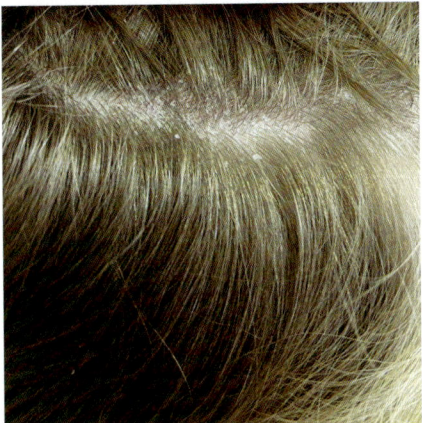

Figure 54.4. This adolescent had scattered adherent scales throughout the scalp that improved with antiseborrheic shampoo and a mid-potency topical steroid solution.

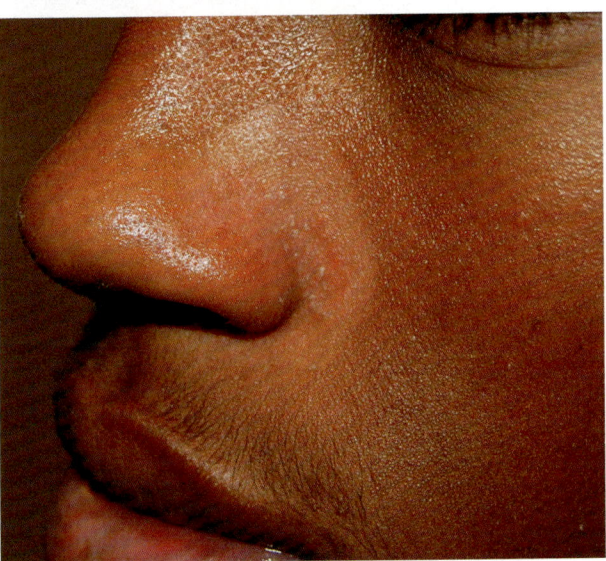

Figure 54.5. Seborrheic dermatitis involving the nasolabial folds has resulted in postinflammatory hypopigmentation.

Look-alikes

Disorder	Differentiating Features
Infantile	
Atopic dermatitis	• Often difficult to distinguish from seborrheic dermatitis. • In infancy, lesions tend to spare flexural areas, particularly diaper area and axillae. • Family history of atopic disorders supports diagnosis.
Scabies	• Papules, pustules, burrows, and vesicles. • Presence of lesions on palms, soles, and genitals. • Marked pruritus usually present. • Diagnosis confirmed by mineral oil preparation performed on scrapings from lesions or by dermoscopy.
Langerhans cell histiocytosis	• Erythematous, yellow or brown scaling papules, with predilection for the scalp, axillae, inguinal creases, palms, and soles. • Petechiae often present. • Lymphadenopathy often present. • Biopsy of lesion will confirm the diagnosis.
Psoriasis	• Tend to be well-defined plaques with thick, adherent, dry scale.
Neonatal lupus erythematosus	• Annular erythematous plaques on sun-exposed regions, especially forehead and periorbital areas. • Minimal scaling; atrophy may be present. • Positive for anti–SS-A (anti-Ro), anti–SS-B (anti-La), or anti-U1RNP antibodies. • Congenital heart block may be present.
Adolescent and Adult	
Psoriasis	• May be difficult to differentiate from seborrheic dermatitis when involvement limited to the scalp or face. • Well-defined papules or plaques with thick, adherent, dry scale. • Pitting of nails may be present.
Periorificial dermatitis	• Erythematous papules and pustules located around mouth, nose, or eyes. • History of corticosteroid use on affected areas may be present.

How to Make the Diagnosis

- The diagnosis is made clinically based on the appearance and location of lesions.

Treatment

- Infantile
  - Scalp
    - May be controlled by gentle brushing to remove scale during daily shampooing. (Baby oil or mineral oil may be applied to loosen scale before shampooing.)
    - If these measures fail, an antiseborrheic shampoo (eg, containing pyrithione zinc or selenium sulfide) may be used as needed.
    - Low-potency topical steroid oil or solution (eg, fluocinolone 0.01%) is occasionally necessary when significant inflammation is present.
  - Skin
    - Lesions may be treated with a low-potency topical corticosteroid (eg, hydrocortisone 1% or 2.5%, alclometasone 0.05% ointment, desonide 0.05% ointment) twice daily as needed.
- Adolescent and adult
  - Scalp
    - More frequent shampooing of the scalp can be helpful.
    - To control scaling: Use an antiseborrheic shampoo (eg, containing pyrithione zinc, selenium sulfide, ketoconazole, tar, or salicylic acid) as needed.
    - To control areas of erythema: Apply a low- or mid-potency topical corticosteroid (eg, fluocinolone, triamcinolone) at bedtime as needed; solution, foam, or lotion vehicle may be preferable to cream or ointment.
  - Skin
    - Lesions may be treated with hydrocortisone 1% or 2.5% and/or ketoconazole cream applied twice daily as needed; topical calcineurin inhibitors (pimecrolimus or tacrolimus) may also be helpful.

Prognosis

- Infantile seborrheic dermatitis has a good prognosis, usually clearing rapidly with appropriate topical therapy.
- Adolescent/adult seborrheic dermatitis often is a chronic condition requiring ongoing therapy.

When to Worry or Refer

- When the diagnosis is uncertain or appropriate therapy fails.
- When petechiae, purpura, or erosions (especially in skinfolds) are present, suggesting possible Langerhans cell histiocytosis.

Resources for Families

- American Academy of Dermatology: Seborrheic dermatitis: overview.
  https://www.aad.org/public/diseases/scaly-skin/seborrheic-dermatitis
- American Academy of Pediatrics: HealthyChildren.org.
  https://www.healthychildren.org/English/ages-stages/baby/bathing-skin-care/Pages/Cradle-Cap.aspx
- MedlinePlus: Information for patients and families (in English and Spanish) sponsored by the US National Library of Medicine and National Institutes of Health.
  https://www.nlm.nih.gov/medlineplus/ency/article/000963.htm
- Society for Pediatric Dermatology: Patient handout on seborrheic dermatitis.
  https://pedsderm.net/for-patients-families/patient-handouts/#Seborrheic%20Dermatitis

Vascular Lesions

CHAPTER 55 — **Cutis Marmorata** 385

CHAPTER 56 — **Cutis Marmorata Telangiectatica Congenita (CMTC)** 387

CHAPTER 57 — **Infantile Hemangioma** 393

CHAPTER 58 — **Kasabach-Merritt Phenomenon** 407

CHAPTER 59 — **Pernio/Chilblains** 411

CHAPTER 60 — **Pyogenic Granuloma** 417

CHAPTER 61 — **Telangiectasias** 421

CHAPTER 62 — **Vascular Malformations** 427

CHAPTER 55

Cutis Marmorata

Introduction/Etiology/Epidemiology

- Cutis marmorata
  - May be present at birth as a benign transient mottling of skin color responsive to cutaneous temperature changes.
  - Caused by vasomotor instability.
  - Most infants exhibit cutis marmorata for a few months.
- Cutis marmorata telangiectatica congenita (congenital phlebectasia) (see Chapter 56)
  - Uncommon congenital vascular process that persists for life.
  - May have associated soft-tissue hypoplasia underlying vascular changes or other developmental anomalies.

Signs and Symptoms

- Cutis marmorata presents as a symmetric, lacy, reticulated, blanching erythematous or violaceous mottled or marbled appearance of the trunk and extremities that becomes more apparent in cooler temperatures (Figure 55.1).
- Usually disappears with rewarming.

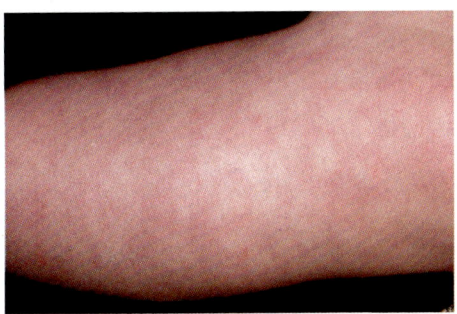

Figure 55.1. Cutis marmorata presents as a lacy, reticulated, or mottled erythema or violaceous appearance.

Look-alikes

Disorder	Differentiating Features
Erythema infectiosum	• Acquired, not congenital. • Erythematous, lacy, reticulated erythema. • After resolution, rash may reappear after activity or sun exposure.
Livedo reticularis	• Appearance may be identical to cutis marmorata. • Acquired form may be associated with many systemic disorders.
Port-wine stain	• Telangiectatic appearance may be present, but primary lesion is an erythematous (vascular) patch. • Reticulated variant may be difficult to distinguish from cutis marmorata telangiectatica congenita early on; with time, features of port-wine stain may become more apparent.

Cutis marmorata telangiectatica congenita	• Reticular vascular pattern present at birth but shows no tendency to resolve with rewarming.
	  – Usually is localized, involving 1 extremity (less likely to be generalized).
	  – Less responsive to environmental temperature changes.
	  – Affected areas may occasionally be slightly atrophic (depressed) or ulcerated.

How to Make the Diagnosis

▶ The diagnosis is made clinically.

Treatment

▶ Cutis marmorata requires no treatment.

Treating Associated Conditions

▶ Cutis marmorata is harmless and self-limited, so no treatment is needed.

▶ Persistent cutis marmorata may be seen in association with hypothyroidism, trisomy 18 syndrome, Down syndrome, and Cornelia de Lange syndrome.

Prognosis

▶ Cutis marmorata resolves spontaneously.

When to Worry or Refer

▶ Consider referral if cutis marmorata persists.

CHAPTER 56

Cutis Marmorata Telangiectatica Congenita (CMTC)

Introduction/Etiology/Epidemiology

- Also known as congenital generalized phlebectasia.
- Distinguished from cutis marmorata by failure of lesions to resolve with rewarming.
- Etiology unknown.
- Presents at or shortly after birth.

Signs and Symptoms

- Reticulated mottling involving one or several limbs (Figures 56.1 and 56.2).
- Occasional truncal or facial involvement.
- May have associated skin atrophy (Figure 56.3), occasional deep purple color, or ulceration.
- Rewarming fails to lead to resolution.
- Ipsilateral limb hypoplasia common (Figure 56.4), usually of no functional significance; limb length discrepancy or limb hyperplasia far less common.
- Less common associations include port-wine stain and ophthalmologic or neurologic manifestations.
- Rare association of macrocephaly, craniofacial and skeletal anomalies, and developmental delay termed *macrocephaly-capillary malformations;* lesions may appear similar to those of cutis marmorata telangiectatica congenita (CMTC) but actually represent reticulate port-wine stains.
- Adams-Oliver syndrome characterized by CMTC in association with transverse limb anomalies and scalp aplasia cutis.

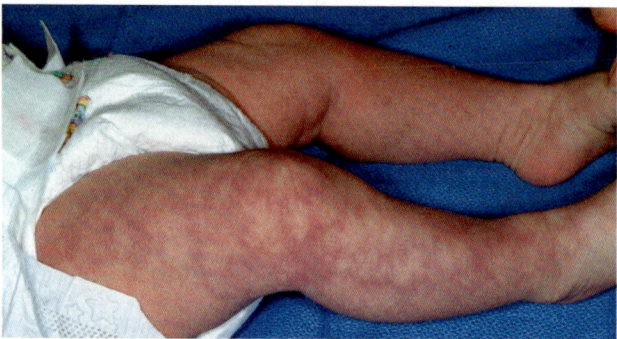

Figure 56.1. Cutis marmorata telangiectatica congenita. Reticulated mottling of the lower extremity.

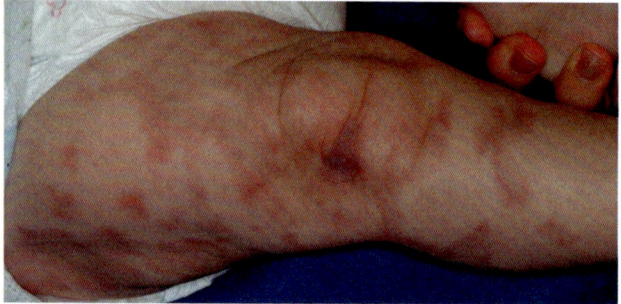

Figure 56.2. Cutis marmorata telangiectatica congenita. Mottling of the lower extremity was present in this infant, with some areas showing more accentuation.

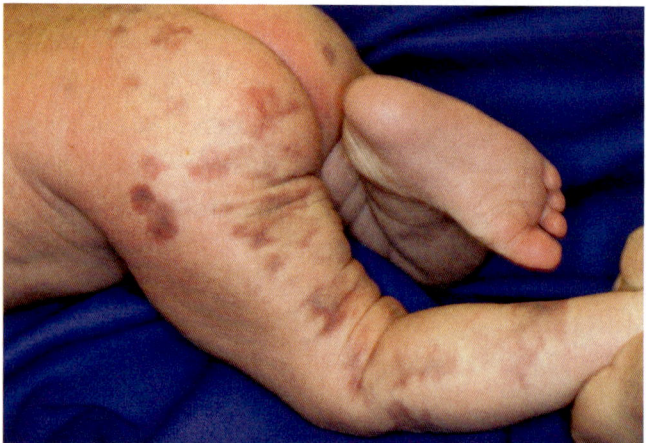

Figure 56.3. Extensive involvement of the buttock and lower extremity with cutis marmorata telangiectatica congenita, with some subtle skin atrophy noted in several of the involved areas.

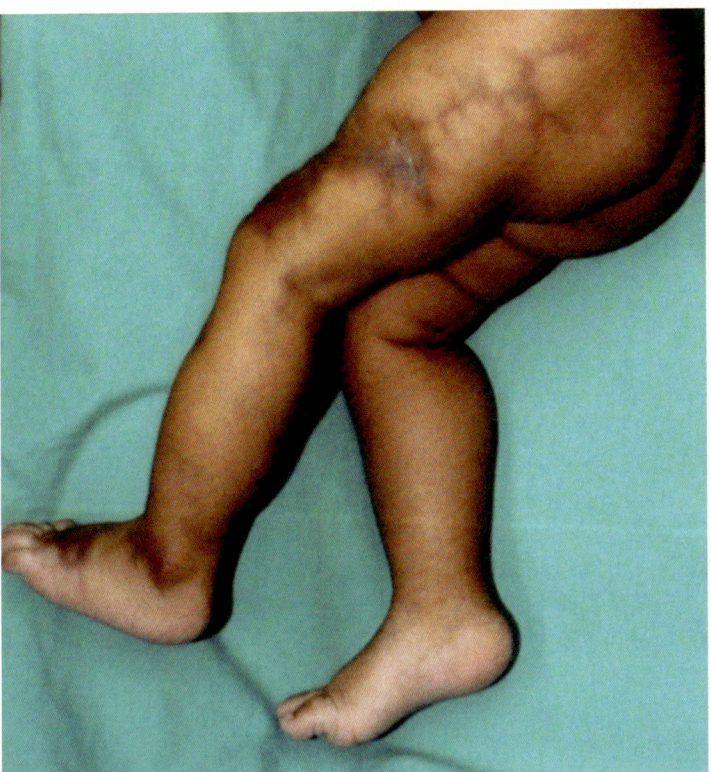

Figure 56.4. Cutis marmorata telangiectatica congenita affecting the left lower extremity. In addition to deep purple mottling, there is hemiatrophy. Reproduced with permission. Leung AKC, Lam JM, Leong KF. Cutis marmorata telangiectatica congenita associated with hemiatrophy. *Case Rep Pediatr.* 2020:88138909.

Look-alikes

Disorder	Differentiating Features
Cutis marmorata	• Disappears with rewarming. • Symmetrically distributed (not limited to one extremity). • Resolves rapidly over first months to 1 year after birth.
Reticulated port-wine stain	• Persists indefinitely. • Less mottled in appearance. • When more extensive, may be associated with macrocephaly and other malformations, overgrowth, or developmental delay.
Klippel-Trénaunay syndrome	• Associated venous varicosities. • Limb overgrowth, instead of hypoplasia. • Port-wine stains present. • Concomitant lymphedema may be present.
Persistent cutis marmorata	• Associated condition usually present (eg, Down syndrome, homocystinuria, Cornelia de Lange syndrome). • Widespread skin involvement.
Livedo reticularis	• Extremely rare in infants. • Associated condition usually present (eg, hematologic disorder, coagulopathy, paraproteinemia, autoimmune disease).

How to Make the Diagnosis

▶ Clinical examination usually sufficient.
▶ Skin biopsy (rarely performed) reveals dilated dermal capillaries and veins.

Treatment

▶ Usually unnecessary.
▶ Lesions fade over several years.

Treating Associated Conditions

▶ Circumferential limb hypoplasia requires no therapy.
▶ Limb length discrepancy extremely rare; if present, refer to orthopedic surgeon or physiatrist.

Prognosis

- The lesions of CMTC generally fade over time with no permanent sequelae.

When to Worry or Refer

- Consider referral to a pediatric dermatologist for patients in whom the diagnosis is in question.
- Consider referral to a pediatric ophthalmologist for patients with extensive or facial involvement; reported rare associations in this setting include glaucoma, retinal detachment, and retinal pigmentation.
- Consider referral to a pediatric neurologist for patients with neurodevelopmental symptoms or concerns.
- Consider referral to a pediatric orthopedist or physiatrist if leg length discrepancy is noted.

Resources for Families

- Cincinnati Children's Hospital Medical Center: Patient information.
  https://www.cincinnatichildrens.org/health/c/cmtc
- National Organization for Rare Disorders: Cutis marmorata telangiectatica congenita.
  https://rarediseases.org/rare-diseases/cutis-marmorata-telangiectatica-congenita
- WebMD: Information for families is contained in Skin Problems and Treatments.
  https://www.webmd.com/skin-problems-and-treatments/cutis-marmorata-telangiectatica-congenita

CHAPTER 57

Infantile Hemangioma

Introduction/Etiology/Epidemiology

- Most common benign tumor of infancy.
- Present in 4% to 5% of infants.
- Composed of benign proliferations of endothelial tissue.
- Most common in white patients, female patients, and preterm neonates and infants.
- Other risk factors include advanced maternal age, placenta previa, multiple gestation pregnancy, and maternal hypertension or preeclampsia.
- Pathogenesis remains speculative; appears to be pathogenic link to placental tissue.
- Typically becomes evident around 1 to 2 weeks after birth, with growth (proliferative) phase for first year, followed by phases of plateau and spontaneous involution.
- May be congenital.
- Most of growth phase occurs during first 5 months after birth.
- Most lesions begin to involute between 6 and 12 months of age, and most involution occurs by age 4 years.
- Involution may not lead to complete resolution of all skin changes.

Signs and Symptoms

- Precursor lesions (sometimes called *pre-hemangiomas*) may present as an area of skin that is pale, ecchymotic, or ulcerated (Figure 57.1) or that has telangiectasias.
- Superficial hemangiomas.
    - Bright red, dome-shaped papules, plaques (Figure 57.2), and tumors. In skin of color, may occasionally appear a darker, ruby red.
    - Rubbery; may compress with palpation.

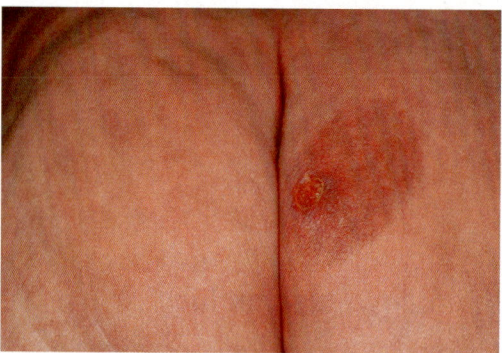

Figure 57.1. Hemangioma precursor. This hemangioma on the medial part of the buttock presented as a vascular patch with focal ulceration before proliferation and thickening.

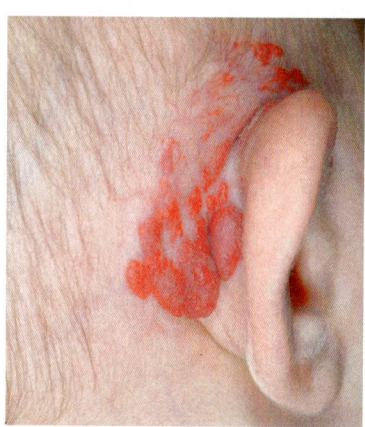

Figure 57.2. Superficial infantile hemangioma.

- Deep hemangiomas
  - Bluish purple subcutaneous nodules and tumors.
  - May have prominent surface telangiectasias (Figure 57.3).
  - May be warm to palpation.
- Combined hemangiomas
  - Superficial and deep components.
  - Bright red (may be a darker, ruby red in skin of color) surface component, deeper blue nodular component (Figures 57.4 and 57.5).

Chapter 57: Infantile Hemangioma

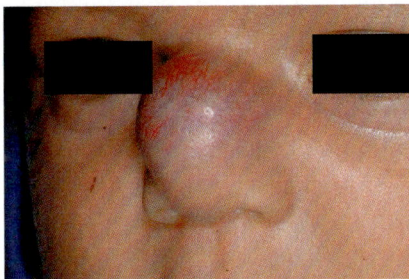

Figure 57.3. Deep infantile hemangioma of the nasal bridge. Note the surface telangiectasias.

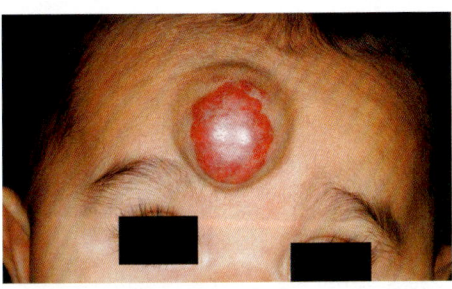

Figure 57.4. Combined infantile hemangioma.

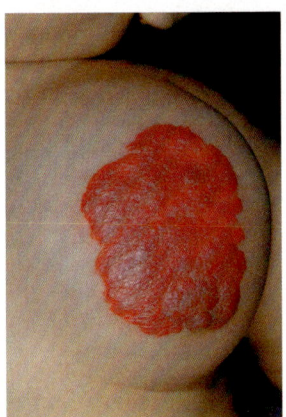

Figure 57.5. Combined infantile hemangioma of the breast.

- ▶ Clinical variants
  - Segmental hemangioma
    - Involve broad anatomic region (Figure 57.6); may be determined by embryonic placodes.
    - Often unilateral, with respect to the midline.
    - Higher incidence of complications (rapid growth, ulceration) and associations (visceral hemangiomatosis; malformations [eg, urogenital anomalies]; PHACES syndrome [see later in this section]).
  - Non-involuting congenital hemangioma (NICH)
    - Well-circumscribed blue nodule with telangiectatic surface and peripheral pallor (Figure 57.7).
    - No spontaneous involution; persists indefinitely.
    - This lesion (and rapidly involuting congenital hemangioma) appears to be an entity distinct from typical infantile hemangioma.

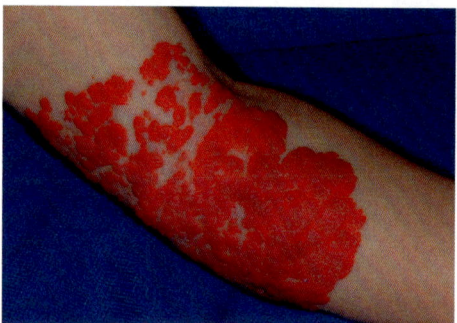

Figure 57.6. Segmental infantile hemangioma. Note the broad anatomic region involved.

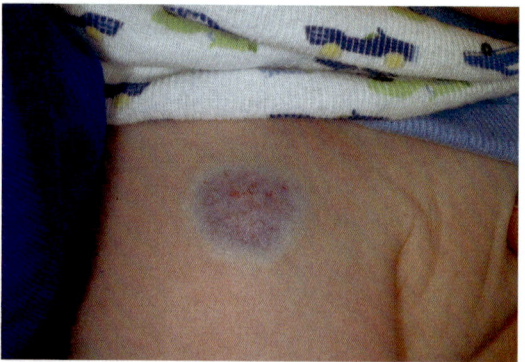

Figure 57.7. Non-involuting congenital hemangioma. A bluish nodule with a peripheral rim of pallor and coarse surface telangiectasias, which presented on the shoulder at birth in this infant.

- Rapidly involuting congenital hemangioma
  - Variety of clinical presentations, including appearances similar to those of NICH (Figure 57.8A) or typical infantile hemangioma and appearance as firm, violaceous tumor.
  - Rapid involution over first year after birth (Figure 57.8B).
- Partially involuting congenital hemangioma
  - Appears similar to rapidly involuting congenital hemangioma early in course.
  - Involutes only partially and assumes appearance more typical of NICH.

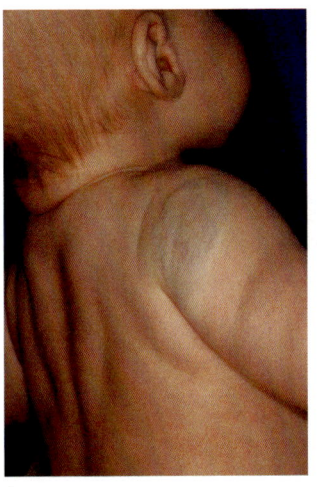 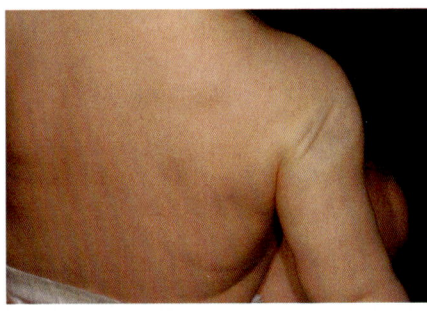

A B

Figure 57.8. Rapidly involuting congenital hemangioma. This blue vascular plaque presented at birth (A), and exhibited rapid involution, leaving behind only some mild atrophy at 10 months of age (B).

- Multiple hemangiomas
  - Multiple cutaneous hemangiomas with (diffuse neonatal hemangiomatosis) or without (benign neonatal hemangiomatosis) extra-cutaneous organ involvement.
  - May range from several (Figure 57.9) to hundreds of lesions.
  - Liver, gastrointestinal tract, and central nervous system most common sites of internal involvement.
  - Greater risk of hepatic involvement with 5 or more skin hemangiomas.
  - Complications include visceral hemorrhage, anemia, and congestive cardiac failure.
  - Infants with liver hemangiomas (especially the diffuse form) may also have associated transient hypothyroidism; evaluation reveals elevated levels of thyroid-stimulating hormone, typical to decreased levels of free thyroxine, decreased levels of free triiodothyronine, and increased levels of reverse triiodothyronine.
  - Abdominal ultrasonography with Doppler study is the most useful screening examination; should be considered in young infants when 5 or more lesions present or in the presence of hepatomegaly or signs and symptoms of congestive heart failure.
- Beard hemangiomas
  - Lesions involve the lower lip, neck, chin, and mandibular regions (Figure 57.10).
  - Increased risk of airway hemangiomatosis.
  - May present with biphasic stridor, hoarseness.
  - If clinically suspected, direct laryngoscopy is indicated.
- PHACES syndrome (posterior fossa anomalies, hemangioma, arterial anomalies, cardiac anomalies, eye anomalies, and sternal clefting or supraumbilical abdominal raphe)
  - Large, segmental facial (or, occasionally, upper trunk or neck) hemangioma in association with other developmental defects; these hemangiomas may be more aggressive in their growth pattern, and ulceration is common.
  - Clinical findings include posterior fossa defects (eg, Dandy-Walker malformation), hemangioma, arterial anomalies (mainly of head and neck vasculature), cardiac anomalies or aortic coarctation, eye anomalies, and sternal clefting or supraumbilical abdominal raphe.
  - Infants are at risk of progressive cerebrovascular disease, including risk of arterial ischemic stroke.

- Lumbosacral hemangiomas
  - May be associated with occult spinal dysraphism and spinal cord defects.
  - Sacral and perineal lesions may also be associated with anorectal or urogenital anomalies.
  - Associated anomalies most likely with extensive lesions or when other lumbosacral findings present (eg, lipoma, gluteal cleft deviation, prominent sacral dimple).
  - PELVIS syndrome has been used to describe infants with *p*erineal hemangioma, *e*xternal genitalia malformations, *l*ipomyelomeningocele, *v*esicorenal anomalies, *i*mperforate anus, and *s*kin tag; this association is also known under the acronym *LUMBAR* syndrome and may also include arterial anomalies and bony deformities.
  - Hemangiomas in this setting may involve not only the perineum but also the lumbosacral region, genitalia, or lower extremities; they are usually of the segmental type.
  - Magnetic resonance (MR) imaging is useful for screening, when indicated.

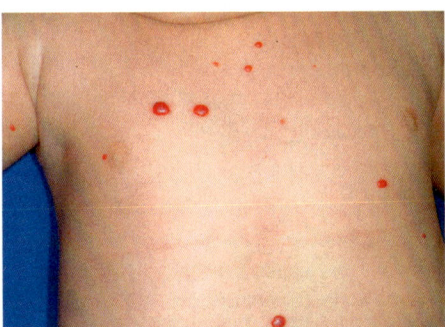

Figure 57.9. Neonatal hemangiomatosis. This infant had multiple small hemangiomas in the liver as well.

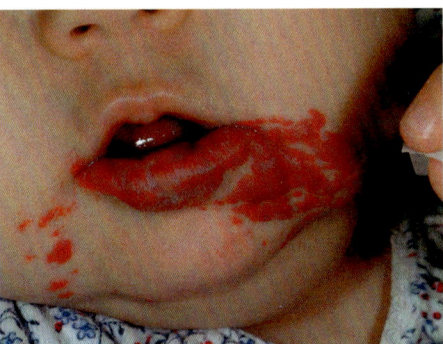

Figure 57.10. Beard distribution infantile hemangioma. This infant also had a subglottic hemangioma.

Look-alikes

Disorder	Differentiating Features
Port-wine stain	• May simulate early superficial hemangioma. • Static lesion, remains flat without proliferation. • Does not involute spontaneously.
Venous malformation	• May simulate deep hemangioma. • Static lesion, lacks natural history of hemangioma. • Does not involute spontaneously. • May develop thromboses, become painful.
Lymphatic malformation	• May simulate deep hemangioma. • Lacks overlying blue hue. • Static lesion, lacks natural history of hemangioma. • Translucent skin-colored to hemorrhagic papules may be present on overlying skin surface (microcystic component).
Arteriovenous malformation	• May simulate superficial or deep hemangioma. • Aggressive growth patterns. • Pulsatile with an audible bruit. • Spontaneous involution does not occur.
Kaposiform hemangioendothelioma	• Reddish purple tumor. • Infiltrative growth nature, may be nodular. • May be associated with Kasabach-Merritt phenomenon (ie, thrombocytopenia, hemolytic anemia).
Pyogenic granuloma	• Small, red papule or nodule. • Moist friable surface, narrow base. • Typically only appears several months after birth (and usually after first year).
Soft-tissue malignancy	• Rhabdomyosarcoma, fibrosarcoma, neuroblastoma. • Growth pattern may be more aggressive. • Usually less homogeneous in appearance. • If diagnosis in question, tissue biopsy indicated.

How to Make the Diagnosis

▶ Clinical examination and history usually suggest the diagnosis.
▶ Ultrasonography, MR imaging occasionally indicated and useful.
  ■ Ultrasonography is most useful in evaluating for liver involvement in patients with multiple skin hemangiomas.
  ■ MR imaging plays a most important role in evaluation for associated visceral or arterial anomalies in patients with more extensive lesions of the face, neck, and upper trunk (PHACES syndrome, in which case both MR imaging and MR angiography of the head and neck are indicated) or anogenital, lumbosacral regions (PELVIS syndrome).

- Tissue biopsy rarely necessary; when in question, diagnosis can be confirmed with immunostaining for glucose transporter 1, FcγRII, merosin, and Lewis-Y antigen; glucose transporter 1 staining is typically negative for NICH and rapidly involuting congenital hemangioma.

Treatment

- Dictated by extent of involvement, lesion location, patient age, and associated complications.
- Goals of therapy are to minimize pain, prevent long-term deformity, prevent life- or function-threatening complications, and minimize psychosocial distress.
- Therapeutic options
  - Active nonintervention
    - Emotional support, guidance, education.
    - Referral to family support groups and educational resources.
  - Local wound care
    - For ulcerated lesions: topical antibiotics (eg, bacitracin, mupirocin, metronidazole), nonstick wound dressings, compresses.
    - Becaplermin (recombinant platelet-derived growth factor) gel; off-label, may be useful for ulcerated lesions.
  - Systemic antibiotic therapy
    - For moderate or severe secondary infection.
  - Pain control
    - For ulcerated lesions.
    - Includes local wound care, oral analgesics, topical anesthetics (sparingly used), pulsed dye laser therapy, oral narcotic analgesics (rarely).
  - Topical corticosteroids
    - Potent formulations may be useful when applied nightly to localized, superficial lesions.
  - Intralesional corticosteroids
    - May be useful for localized lesions; caution with periocular hemangiomas, given risk of ocular arterial embolization.

- Oral corticosteroids
  - Traditional mainstay of therapy.
  - Usually prednisolone or prednisone, 2 to 4 mg/kg/d.
  - Toxicity profile predictable; most infants respond promptly to therapy.
  - Live virus vaccines must be avoided until 1 month after therapy.
  - Transient decrease in linear growth velocity common.
  - Concomitant administration of H_2-receptor antagonist (eg, ranitidine) useful for gastritis prophylaxis.
  - Used relatively rarely in the era of β-blocker therapy.
- Oral propranolol
  - Criterion standard therapy for infantile hemangiomas requiring therapy.
  - Nonselective β-blocker used traditionally for cardiac indications; US Food and Drug Administration approved for treatment of hemangiomas in infants 5 weeks to 5 months of age.
  - Useful for slowing growth and accelerating involution of hemangiomas.
  - Mechanisms of action unclear; may include vasoconstriction, apoptosis, inhibition of angiogenic growth factors.
  - Typically started at dose of 1 to 1.5 mg/kg/d and titrated up to 2 to 3 mg/kg/d, divided 2 to 3 times daily; always administer concomitant with (or after) feeding. Note: The US Food and Drug Administration approval of propranolol hydrochloride suggests a target dose of 3.4 mg/kg/d divided into 2 daily doses; many experts use lower target doses if efficacy is noted.
  - Risks include hypoglycemia, hypotension, bradycardia, bronchospasm, hypothermia, and sleep disruption or night terrors; increased risk of cognitive and motor delay has been suggested by some, although most studies have been reassuring.
  - Contraindicated with sinus bradycardia, hypotension, heart block, and asthma; patients at risk of PHACES syndrome should complete head and neck imaging first and, if arterial anomalies present, therapy started only in consultation with a pediatric neurologist.
  - Baseline heart rate, blood pressure, and (mainly in infants at high risk) electrocardiogram recommended; heart rate typically repeated at 1 hour after initial dose.
  - Propranolol therapy is most effective when started during the proliferative phase (ie, first 6 months after birth) and is typically continued until 9 to 15 months of age in an effort to prevent rebound hemangioma growth.

- Topical timolol
  - Used off-label by many clinicians for superficial, small, uncomplicated, and functionally insignificant hemangiomas.
  - Typically, the gel-forming ophthalmic solution, in a 0.25% to 0.5% concentration; applied as 1 drop rubbed in well 2 to 3 times daily.
  - Adverse events are rare and mainly reported with overapplication of timolol, in larger or deeper hemangiomas, and in preterm newborns and infants.
- Pulsed dye laser therapy
  - Mainly useful for ulcerated lesions or early superficial hemangiomas; may also play a role in treating persistent telangiectasias after involution.
- Recombinant interferon-alfa
  - Reserved for life- and function-threatening hemangiomas that are refractory to other medical therapies.
  - Administered via daily subcutaneous injection, 1 to 3 million $U/m^2/d$.
  - Risk of spastic diplegia; serial neurologic examinations indicated.
- Vincristine
  - Chemotherapeutic agent shown to be beneficial for life-threatening lesions.
  - Administered via central venous catheter.
  - Risks include peripheral neuropathy.
- Surgical excision
  - Useful in selected situations, including involuted lesions, residual scars, or fibrofatty redundant tissue.
  - Use during proliferative phase controversial; usually reserved for function-threatening, medication-resistant lesions and those that are amenable to early surgery (eg, pedunculated, smaller, or localized hemangiomas).

Treating Associated Conditions

- Ulceration
  - See previous discussion.
  - Most common in lesions located on lips, genitals, and perineum and perianal region.
  - Topical antibiotics (eg, bacitracin, mupirocin, metronidazole) are useful.
  - Systemic antibiotics may be necessary.
  - Nonstick wound dressings (eg, petrolatum impregnated gauze) may be useful.
  - Consider bacterial culture, pulsed dye laser therapy, or becaplermin gel when resistant to previously described measures.
  - Pain control is an important aspect of management.
  - Systemic hemangioma therapies (eg, propranolol, prednisolone) may occasionally be necessary.

- Residual skin changes
  - Residual telangiectasias after involution may require pulsed dye laser therapy.
  - Fibrofatty residua or scars remaining after involution may require surgical removal.

- Kasabach-Merritt phenomenon
  - Not associated with infantile hemangioma but, rather, kaposiform hemangioendothelioma or tufted angioma.
  - See Chapter 58.

Prognosis

- Uncomplicated infantile hemangiomas that are not function- or life-endangering have an excellent prognosis, with spontaneous involution over 4 to 5 years.
- In patients with function- or life-endangering lesions, prognosis depends on multiple variables, including location, complications, associated findings, timeliness of therapy, and response to therapy.

When to Worry or Refer

- Referral to a pediatric dermatologist (or other appropriate hemangioma specialist) should be considered for hemangiomas in the following settings:
  - Highest-risk lesions
    - Large (>5 cm) or segmental facial or scalp.
    - Large or segmental lumbosacral or perineal.
    - Multifocal hemangiomas (≥5) and abdominal ultrasonography reveals liver hemangiomas.
    - Periocular hemangiomas causing eyelid asymmetry, lid closure or ptosis, proptosis, or other findings with potential effect on the visual axis.
  - High-risk lesions
    - Large segmental hemangioma on the trunk or extremities.
    - Any facial hemangioma 2 cm or longer (>1 cm if 3 months or younger).
    - Nasal tip or lip hemangioma of any size.
    - Oral hemangioma.
    - Neck or scalp hemangioma longer than 2 cm during growth phase.
    - Breast hemangioma.
    - Ulcerated hemangioma (any site).
- Referral may or may not be indicated for intermediate-risk lesions.
    - Perineal hemangioma.
    - Trunk or extremity hemangioma longer than 2 cm especially in growth phase or if abrupt transition from typical to affected skin (ie, the *ledge effect*) (Figure 57.12).
- Low-risk lesions typically do not require referral to a hemangioma specialist.
    - Hemangioma less than 2 cm on trunk or extremities in areas easily covered by clothing.
    - Hemangioma on trunk or extremities longer than 2 cm if gradual transition from typical to affected skin.

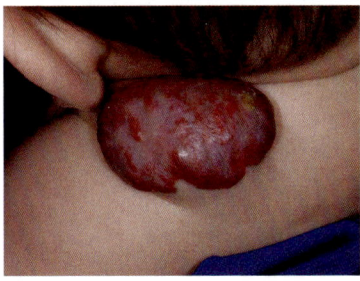

Figure 57.11. Infantile hemangioma with ledge effect in a 3-month-old. Note the abrupt transition from typical to affected skin (ie, steep borders). Although the distribution of this lesion (upper back) does not raise concern for a medical complication, its size and steep borders might justify systemic therapy, given the risk of permanent deformity.

Resources for Families

- American Academy of Pediatrics: HealthyChildren.org.
  https://www.healthychildren.org/English/ages-stages/baby/bathing-skin-care/Pages/Infantile-Hemangiomas-Baby-Birthmarks.aspx
- Hemangioma Investigator Group: Multicenter clinical research consortium and source of patient education and support.
  www.hemangiomaeducation.org
- National Organization for Rare Disorders: Hemangioma Support System: Provides support for parents.
  https://rarediseases.org/organizations/hemangioma-support-system/
  c/o Cynthia Schumerth
  De Pere, WI
  920/336-9399 (after 8:00 pm CT)
- National Organization of Vascular Anomalies: Patient information, resources, and support.
  www.novanews.org
- Society for Pediatric Dermatology: Patient handout (in English and Spanish) on hemangiomas.
  https://pedsderm.net/for-patients-families/patient-handouts/#Anchor-Hemangiomas
- Vascular Birthmarks Foundation: Provides referrals; financial assistance; newsletter; conferences; resource list for advocacy, support, and counseling.
  https://birthmark.org

CHAPTER 58

Kasabach-Merritt Phenomenon

Introduction/Etiology/Epidemiology

- Kasabach-Merritt phenomenon (KMP) refers to the association of a vascular tumor with thrombocytopenia, hemolytic anemia, and coagulopathy.
- Not associated with infantile hemangioma, as traditionally believed.
- Vascular tumor usually kaposiform hemangioendothelioma or tufted angioma.
- May be life-threatening.

Signs and Symptoms

- Usually presents within the first few weeks or months after birth, with sudden enlargement of preexisting vascular lesion (Figure 58.1) and occasional petechiae or purpura.
- Laboratory evaluation reveals thrombocytopenia, anemia, hypofibrinogenemia, elevated D-dimer levels, and prolongation of coagulation studies.
- Ecchymoses, epistaxis, hematuria, and hematochezia may also be present.
- Appearance of preexisting lesions.
  - Kaposiform hemangioendothelioma
    - Firm, violaceous plaque or tumor (Figure 58.2); name derived from histologic resemblance to Kaposi sarcoma.
    - May expand rapidly and tends to be locally aggressive; occasionally involves deep soft tissues and bone.
    - Tends to persist indefinitely.
  - Tufted angioma
    - Brightly erythematous plaque with induration, may be annular.
    - May spontaneously involute or persist indefinitely.

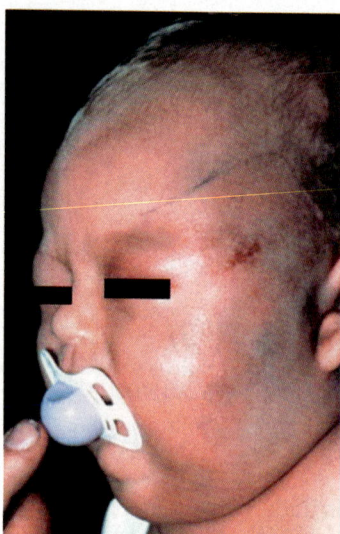

Figure 58.1. Kasabach-Merritt phenomenon. This congenital lesion of the lateral aspect of the face and scalp enlarged in association with thrombocytopenia and coagulopathy.

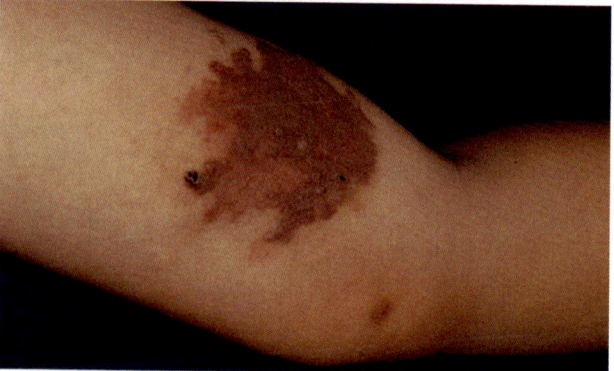

Figure 58.2. Kaposiform hemangioendothelioma. This violaceous, firm plaque presented during early infancy on the medial thigh of this young child and was not complicated by Kasabach-Merritt phenomenon.

Look-alikes

Disorder	Differentiating Features
Infantile hemangioma	• Follows course more typical of hemangioma. • Not associated with thrombocytopenia or coagulopathy. • Sudden enlargement (versus gradual) rare.
Soft-tissue malignancy (ie, rhabdomyosarcoma, fibrosarcoma)	• Usually not associated with coagulopathy. • Histologic features diagnostic.

How to Make the Diagnosis

- Diagnosis is suggested by sudden enlargement of a vascular-appearing tumor.
- Laboratory findings of thrombocytopenia, microangiopathic hemolytic anemia, and coagulopathy are supportive.
- Tissue biopsy with histologic evaluation is confirmatory.

Treatment

- Challenging.
- Small lesions may be amenable to early surgical resection.
- Medical therapy usually is necessary; options include high-dose corticosteroids, vincristine, cyclophosphamide, sirolimus, and antifibrinolytic therapy; everolimus (another mTOR inhibitor, same class as sirolimus) has also been reported effective.
- Vincristine in combination with corticosteroids is considered first-line treatment by many experts.
- Interferon-alfa has lost favor given the associated risk of spastic diplegia in young children.
- Reported response rates to propranolol have been variable.
- Red blood cell transfusions, fresh frozen plasma, or cryoprecipitate may be necessary.
- Platelet transfusions may lead to worsening and should be minimized; antiplatelet therapy (ie, ticlopidine, aspirin) has been used.
- Transcatheter arterial embolization, compression, and radiation therapy occasionally are used.

Treating Associated Conditions

- Kaposiform hemangioendothelioma
  - Wide local excision, if localized and superficial.
  - Treatment otherwise is extremely difficult; oral prednisolone with or without aspirin has been recommended for those requiring treatment but without KMP.
- Tufted angioma
  - Surgical excision, if lesions are small and localized.
  - Laser therapy shows inconsistent results.
  - Low-dose aspirin has been advocated for symptomatic lesions without KMP.

Prognosis

- Mortality rate of 10% to 30%.
- Prognosis poorer for patients with retroperitoneal involvement.

When to Worry or Refer

- Consider referral in any patient with a
  - Rapidly expanding, vascular-appearing tumor.
  - Vascular tumor in conjunction with cutaneous petechiae or purpura, thrombocytopenia, or coagulopathy.

Resources for Families

- Ann & Robert H. Lurie Children's Hospital of Chicago: Kasabach-Merritt phenomenon (KMP).
  https://www.luriechildrens.org/en/specialties-conditions/kasabach-merritt-phenomenon-kmp
- National Organization for Rare Disorders: Kasabach-Merritt phenomenon.
  https://rarediseases.org/rare-diseases/kasabach-merritt-phenomenon

CHAPTER 59

Pernio/Chilblains

Introduction/Etiology/Epidemiology

- Pernio (also known as chilblains) is a disorder marked by an atypical (and often robust) vascular response to cold (nonfreezing) and humid climates.
- May occur after exposure to moistened linings of footwear or gloves.
- Can be seen in younger children, adolescents, and adults.
- Pernio has been reported in patients with impaired thermoregulatory ability such as anorexia nervosa, low body mass index, and palmoplantar hyperhidrosis (excessive hand/foot sweating).
- Minor trauma may predispose acral areas to developing this exaggerated response to cold or wet exposures, although this association has not been verified.
- Although typically idiopathic, can rarely be associated with systemic disorders including systemic lupus erythematosus, hematologic diseases, and malignancy.

Signs and Symptoms

- Patients may experience a variety of symptoms ranging from mild to severe.
- Lesions typically occur after 12 to 24 hours of exposure to the cold or triggering environment.
- Lesions are typically symmetric and can involve fingers, toes, heels, lower extremities, ears, and the nose.
- Lesions may include blanching, pink/red to purple macules and patches (Figures 59.1–59.4), edema, and blistering (which may lead to erosions and crusting).
- Symptoms may include pain, tingling, itching, dysesthesia, or burning.
- Secondary infection may occur.

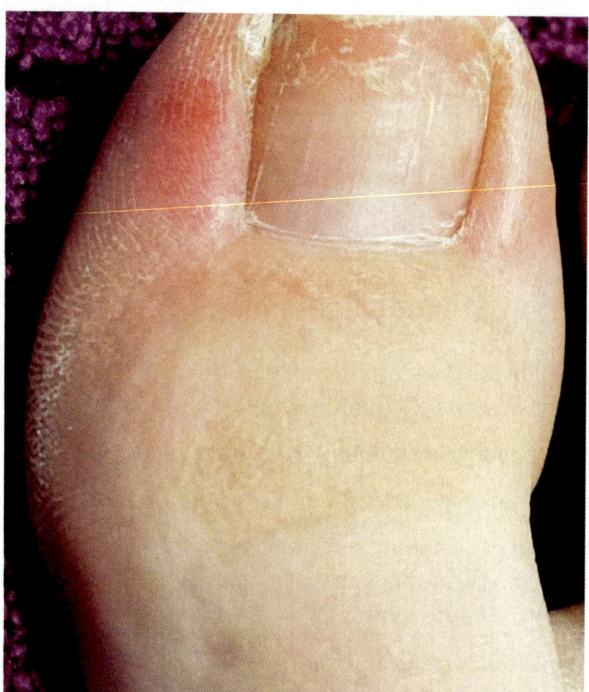

Figure 59.1. Pernio. Focal erythematous macule on toe of a teen after exposure to cold temperatures.

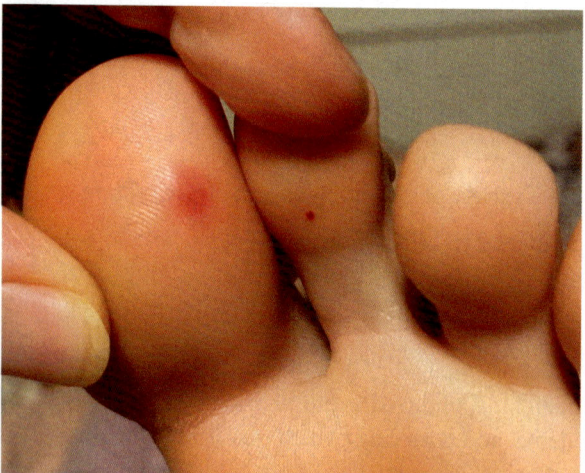

Figure 59.2. Pernio. Erythematous, slightly tender macule on toe of a patient in winter.

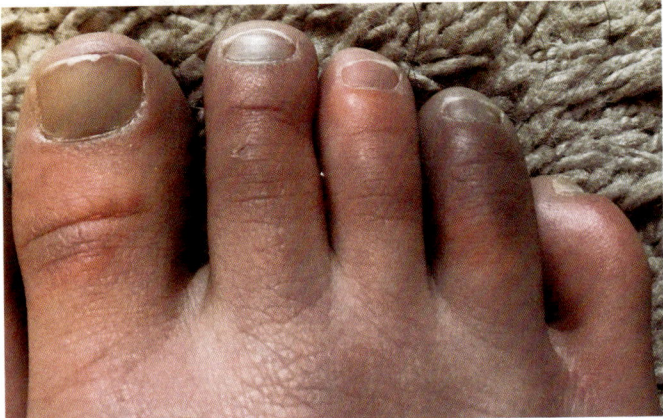

Figure 59.3. Multiple erythematous and purple tender toes in an adolescent with pernio.

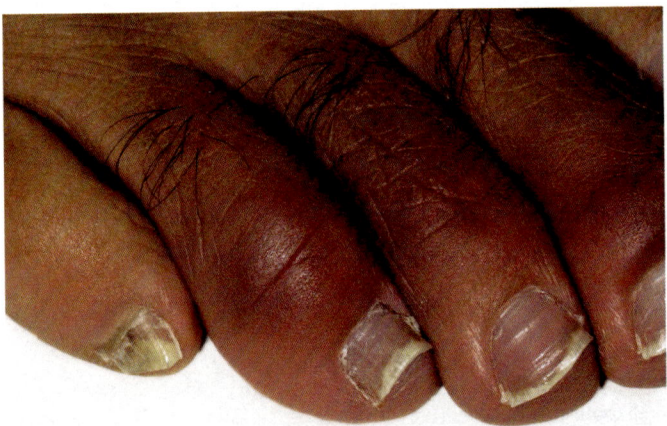

Figure 59.4. Pernio: swelling and erythematous to purple discoloration. In persons with darker skin tones the discoloration may be more difficult to appreciate. Source: NHS. Chilblains. Reviewed July 29, 2022. **https://www.nhs.uk/conditions/chilblains**

Look-alikes

Disorder	Differentiating Features
Frostbite	• Requires actual *freezing* of skin tissue due to extreme freezing/subzero temperatures. • Results in direct cold injury, vasoconstriction, and subsequent inflammatory damage. • Marked erythema and blistering within 1 to 2 days after exposure. • Severe cases can lead to full-thickness tissue loss or, rarely, amputation. • Rapid rewarming of tissue is necessary to reduce cold damage and restore blood flow (warm water with temperature >40 °C [>104 °F]).
Dysproteinemias (cold sensitive)	• Rare collection of disorders in which proteins (ie, cryoglobulins, cryofibrinogens, and cold agglutinins) become insoluble in the blood after they are exposed to cold temperatures. • Wide range of symptoms including palpable purpura, urticaria, bullae, ulcerations, arthralgias, bruising, weakness, pain, and glomerulonephritis.
Acrocyanosis	• Common physiologic phenomenon in newborns and infants in which the feet, hands, and lips develop a purple-bluish hue that is transient. • Occurs when infants hold their breath, during crying spells, or if cold (ie, after a bath). • Mechanism related to vasospasm of cutaneous vessels resulting in venous pooling; transient, mild, and resolves spontaneously.
Raynaud phenomenon	• Transient vasospasm of peripheral arterioles/arteries (in response to cold temperatures or stress) that may have triphasic color changes (white pallor, blue cyanosis, followed by reactive hyperemia from reperfusion). • Fingers most common location. • Many cases are primary (idiopathic). • Recurrent or severe cases may be associated with an underlying connective tissue disease.
Leukocytoclastic (hypersensitivity) vasculitis	• May be triggered by a variety of preceding infections such as an upper respiratory tract infection or group A streptococcal infection. • Not triggered by cold temperatures. • Palpable purpuric lesions, common on buttocks and lower extremities, distal upper extremities. • May have associated arthritis, abdominal pain, renal involvement, gastrointestinal involvement.
Hand, foot, and mouth disease (enterovirus)	• Acute viral illness with fever. • Not triggered by cold temperatures. • Associated with oral erosions (tongue, buccal mucosa, and palate). • Erythematous to gray macules and blisters on hands, feet, and buttocks.
COVID-19 toes	• Occurs in association with SARS-CoV-2 infection (COVID-19), although association is controversial. • Not triggered by cold temperatures. • Often asymptomatic.

How to Make the Diagnosis

- History of preceding exposure to a cold, nonfreezing or wet/humid environment 12 to 24 hours prior to development of characteristic skin lesions usually is sufficient to suggest the clinical diagnosis.
- Biopsy may rarely be necessary to confirm the diagnosis.
- In some patients, additional evaluations may be indicated (and may include antinuclear antibody testing, antiphospholipid antibodies, inflammatory markers, cell counts with peripheral smear, cryoglobulins, and cold agglutinins, among others).

Treatment

- Therapy is usually supportive and includes emollients, oral antihistamines for itching, and keeping affected areas properly covered, warm, and dry.
- Proper drying of hand wear (ie, gloves, mittens) and footwear between uses can minimize acral exposure to wet/humid conditions.
- If hyperhidrosis is present, appropriate treatment is recommended.
- Oral nifedipine, pentoxifylline, or hydroxychloroquine has been used in severe cases.
- In patients whose lesions were triggered by an associated condition, that condition should be appropriately treated.

Prognosis

- The prognosis is generally very good.
- Lesions typically resolve within 1 to 3 weeks.
- Recurrence is common if reexposure occurs or if associated with an underlying untreated causative condition.

When to Worry or Refer

▶ Persistent or atypical presentations may require further consultation and evaluation to assess for an underlying causative condition.

▶ Evaluation by a pediatric dermatologist may be necessary to help verify diagnosis or suggest other diagnostic evaluations.

▶ When severe or chronic/recurrent, referral to a pediatric rheumatologist, geneticist, or oncologist should be considered, depending on clinical features and laboratory findings.

Resources for Families

▶ Cleveland Clinic: Chilblains (pernio).
https://my.clevelandclinic.org/health/diseases/21817-chilblains-pernio

▶ National Organization for Rare Disorders: Perniosis.
https://rarediseases.org/rare-diseases/perniosis

CHAPTER
60

Pyogenic Granuloma

Introduction/Etiology/Epidemiology

- Also known as lobular capillary hemangioma.
- Common in children and young adults.
- Acquired vascular lesion of skin or mucous membranes.
- Cause unknown but appears to represent reactive neovascularization.

Signs and Symptoms

- Solitary red papule or papulonodule, rarely larger than 1 cm.
- May be pedunculated or exophytic (Figure 60.1).
- Surface commonly bleeds or becomes erosive or crusted (Figure 60.2).
- Base of lesion may be surrounded by collarette of scale.
- May develop on surface of port-wine stain (Figure 60.3).
- Occasionally multiple.
- Common locations include hand, finger, face, and oral mucosa.

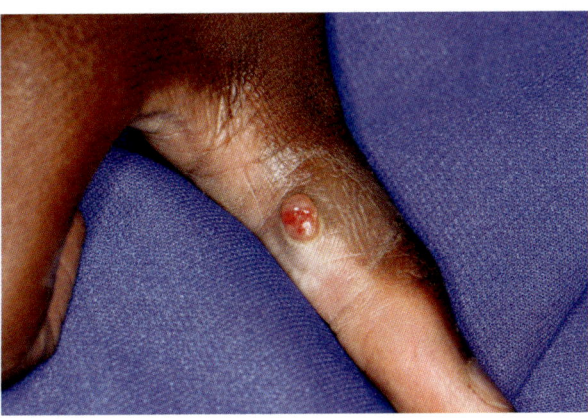

Figure 60.1. Pyogenic granuloma. An eroded, exophytic vascular papule with peripheral collarette of scale, on the finger of a 14-year-old.

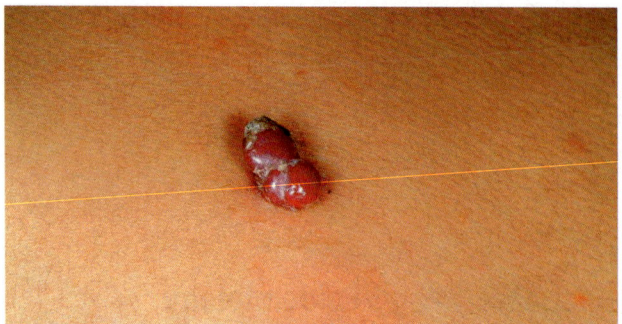

Figure 60.2. Pyogenic granuloma. This multi-lobulated, vascular papule was prone to recurrent bleeding and crusting (as noted at superior portion).

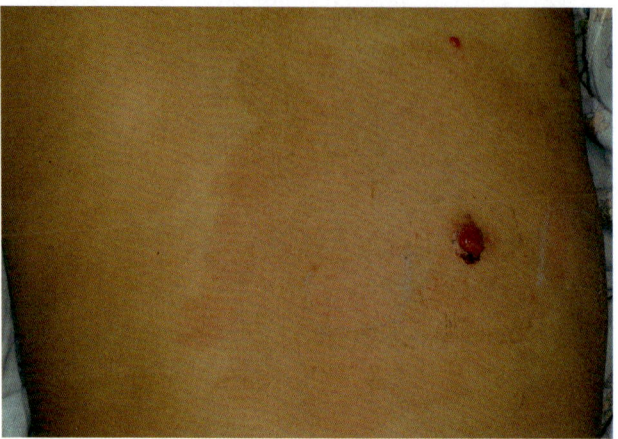

Figure 60.3. Pyogenic granuloma overlying port-wine stain. Note 2 vascular papules, one at the superior pole and the other (eroded) more centrally located.

Look-alikes

Disorder	Differentiating Features
Infantile hemangioma	• Presents in early infancy. • Rarely pedunculated. • Often grows to > 1 cm. • History of proliferation followed by spontaneous involution.
Juvenile xanthogranuloma	• Early lesion may appear vascular, but eventually yellow-orange hue becomes apparent. • Usually sessile (broad-based) rather than pedunculated. • Rarely becomes erosive or crusted on surface.
Spitz nevus	• Slowly growing papule. • Sessile (broad-based) rather than pedunculated. • Rarely becomes erosive or crusted on surface. • Diascopy (pressure with glass slide) may reveal brown pigment. • Dermoscopy (examination with a dermatoscope) may reveal characteristic pigment patterns.
Spider angioma	• May simulate early (small) pyogenic granuloma. • Central papule remains < 3 mm. • Does not become erosive on surface. • Peripheral telangiectatic vessels present.

How to Make the Diagnosis

▶ Pyogenic granuloma is usually diagnosed based on the classic clinical features.

▶ Histologic evaluation is confirmatory after excision.

Treatment

▶ Shave excision followed by electrocautery of the base.

▶ Small lesions may be amenable to pulsed dye laser therapy, topical timolol gel.

▶ Very small lesions with eroded surface may respond to chemical cauterization with silver nitrate.

▶ Full-thickness excision occasionally indicated for larger lesions.

Prognosis

- The prognosis for an uncomplicated pyogenic granuloma is excellent.
- Recurrence is rare but may occur after excision.
- Patients with multiple, clustered (agminated) lesions are more prone to recurrence.

When to Worry or Refer

- Consider referral when the
  - Diagnosis is in question.
  - Patient or parent desires removal.
  - Lesion is erosive or bleeding.

Resources for Families

- American Osteopathic College of Dermatology: Pyogenic granuloma.
  www.aocd.org/?page=PyogenicGranuloma
- MedlinePlus: Information for patients and families (in English and Spanish) sponsored by the US National Library of Medicine and National Institutes of Health.
  https://www.nlm.nih.gov/medlineplus/ency/article/001464.htm
- Society for Pediatric Dermatology: Patient handout on pyogenic granuloma.
  https://pedsderm.net/for-patients-families/patient-handouts/#PyogenicGranuloma
- Verywell Health: An overview of pyogenic granuloma
  https://www.verywellhealth.com/pyogenic-granuloma-1069207

CHAPTER 61

Telangiectasias

Introduction/Etiology/Epidemiology

- Telangiectasias represent dilatations of superficial capillaries.
- May be a manifestation of physical trauma, medications, hormonal differences, autoimmune disease, or genetic disorders.
- Often idiopathic in origin.
- Lesions disappear with diascopy (gentle downward pressure with a microscope slide).
- This discussion includes spider angioma, angioma serpiginosum, hereditary hemorrhagic telangiectasia (HHT), unilateral nevoid telangiectasia, generalized essential telangiectasia, and ataxia-telangiectasia.

Signs and Symptoms

- Spider angioma
  - Also known as nevus araneus.
  - Central red papule with peripheral, radiating telangiectatic vessels.
  - Occasionally, pulsation may be noted.
  - Most common on face (Figure 61.1), upper trunk, arms, and hands; multiple lesions are not unusual in children.
  - Occasionally associated with liver disease, estrogen therapy, pregnancy.

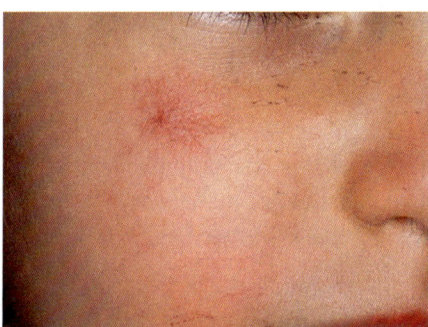

Figure 61.1. Spider angioma. Central vascular papule with numerous radiating telangiectasias on the cheek of a 5-year-old.

- Angioma serpiginosum
  - Rare; usually occurs in first 2 decades after birth, mainly in female patients.
  - Punctate red to violaceous macules, usually in a linear or serpiginous pattern.
  - Most common on the extremities.
- HHT
  - Also known as Osler-Weber-Rendu disease.
  - Autosomal-dominant disorder characterized by mucocutaneous telangiectasias and bleeding diathesis.
  - Caused by variations in endoglin gene *(HHT1)* or activin receptor-like kinase 1 (ALK-1) gene *(HHT2)*.
  - Mutations in *Smad4* result in HHT in association with juvenile polyposis.
  - Patients usually present with epistaxis and anemia secondary to gastrointestinal blood loss; nighttime epistaxis particularly suggestive of HHT.
  - Papular or "mat-like" telangiectasias occur on mucous membranes (ie, lips, tongue, palate, nasal mucosa) and skin (especially ears, palms, fingers, soles); usually first appearing during adolescence or later.
  - May develop arteriovenous malformations, especially in lungs, brain, gastrointestinal tract, liver, and spine.
- Unilateral nevoid telangiectasia
  - Segmental, unilateral distribution of skin telangiectasias (Figure 61.2).
  - May be dermatomal.
  - May be congenital or acquired.
  - May be associated with liver disease, puberty, pregnancy, or hormonal therapy.
- Generalized essential telangiectasia
  - Widespread cutaneous telangiectasias with no bleeding diathesis.
  - More common in adult women, rare in children.
  - Most common site of involvement is the lower extremities.
- Ataxia-telangiectasia.
  - Also known as Louis-Bar syndrome
  - Autosomal-recessive disorder consisting of oculocutaneous telangiectasias, immunodeficiency, cerebellar ataxia, pulmonary infections, and predisposition toward hematologic malignancy.
  - Caused by variation in the ataxia-telangiectasia mutated *(ATM)* gene.

- Presents with truncal ataxia, other neurologic symptoms soon after birth.
- Telangiectasias begin to appear at 3 to 5 years, characteristically involving the bulbar conjunctivae and sun-exposed skin; most common sites of skin involvement are the sun-exposed areas on the face, ears, arms, and upper chest.
- May also have premature aging, pigmentary skin change, noninfectious skin granulomas (most common on the extremities), chronic sinopulmonary infections, bronchiectasis, immunodeficiency, and growth failure.
- Increased risk of Hodgkin disease, non-Hodgkin lymphoma, leukemia, and skin malignancy.

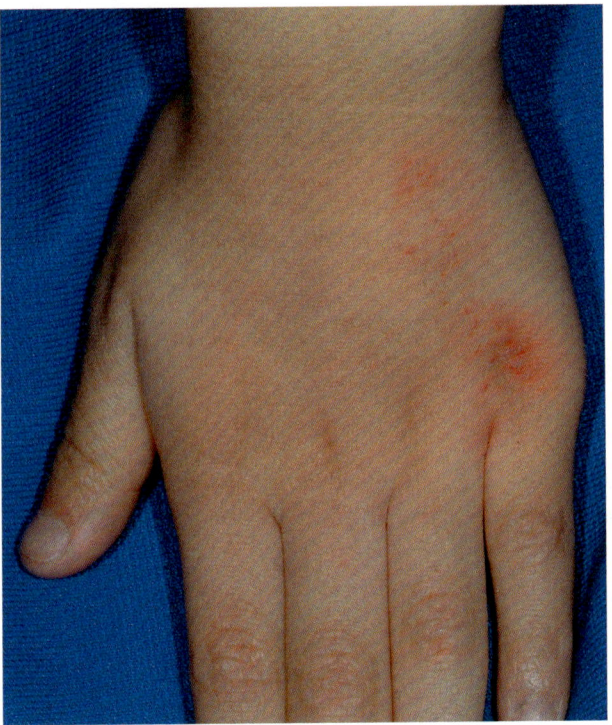

Figure 61.2. Unilateral nevoid telangiectasia. This patient had telangiectatic patches involving the dorsal aspect of the hand and forearm, without any identified predisposing conditions.

Look-alikes

Disorder	Differentiating Features
Pyogenic granuloma, Spitz nevus	• Small lesions may simulate spider angioma. • Lack peripheral telangiectatic network. • With continued growth, both become larger than typical for spider angioma.
Cherry angioma	• Less common in children, typically seen in adults. • Lacks peripheral telangiectatic network.
Pigmented purpura	• May simulate angioma serpiginosum. • More likely bilateral, with extravasated red blood cells noted on biopsy. • Pink to tan or golden-brown patches with petechiae present at diascopic examination.

How to Make the Diagnosis

▶ Spider angioma, angioma serpiginosum, unilateral nevoid telangiectasia, and generalized essential telangiectasia usually are diagnosed based on clinical features.

▶ Skin biopsy may be useful for distinguishing angioma serpiginosum from pigmented purpura.

▶ HHT suspected based on epistaxis history, family history, and examination findings; molecular-based diagnosis available.

▶ Ataxia-telangiectasia usually suspected based on history and clinical examination findings. Elevated α-fetoprotein and carcinoembryonic antigen and spontaneous chromosomal abnormalities support the diagnosis. Molecular-based diagnosis is available if familial variant is known.

Treatment

- Spider angioma: electrocoagulation or pulsed dye laser if desired by the patient.
- Angioma serpiginosum, unilateral nevoid telangiectasia, generalized essential telangiectasia: usually not treated. If desired, pulsed dye laser therapy may be useful.
- HHT: Treatment is dictated by extent of organ involvement; may include embolization, septal dermatoplasty, desmopressin, antifibrinolytic agents, hormonal therapy (estrogen receptor modulators), surgery, laser therapy, and transfusions; gastrointestinal bleeding treated with a variety of medical or surgical therapies.
- Ataxia-telangiectasia: Treatment is mainly supportive; antibiotic therapy if infection present, treatment for bronchiectasis; aggressive surveillance for malignancy is vital, as is vigorous photoprotection (given increased risk of skin malignancy).

Prognosis

- Patients with spider angioma, angioma serpiginosum, unilateral nevoid telangiectasia, or generalized essential telangiectasia, in the absence of associated systemic conditions, have an excellent prognosis with no long-term sequelae related to the skin lesions.
- The prognosis for patients with HHT depends on the extent of organ involvement and associated complications.
- Patients with ataxia-telangiectasia often die from chronic sinopulmonary disease/bronchiectasis, pneumonia, or malignancy.

When to Worry or Refer

- Multiple spider angiomas may be associated with liver disease, pregnancy, or estrogen therapy.
- Consider referral for patients in whom the diagnosis is in question or when laser therapy is requested.
- In the child with a history of recurrent (especially nocturnal) epistaxis and mucocutaneous telangiectasias, consider referral to genetics, otolaryngology, and pediatric dermatology for possible HHT.
- In the child with ataxia, recurrent infections, and oculocutaneous telangiectasias, consider referral to pediatric neurology, genetics, and pediatric dermatology for possible ataxia-telangiectasia.

Resources for Families

- A-T Children's Project: Its mission is to encourage and support excellent laboratory research that will accelerate the discovery of a cure or possible therapies for ataxia-telangiectasia.
  www.atcp.org
- AT Society: Works to improve quality of life and care for people living with ataxia-telangiectasia while promoting research to lengthen lives and find a cure.
  www.atsociety.org.uk
- Cure HHT (HHT Foundation International): Provides support and information for individuals, families, and health care professionals.
  http://curehht.org

CHAPTER 62

Vascular Malformations

Introduction/Etiology/Epidemiology

- ▶ Anomalous blood vessels without endothelial proliferation.
- ▶ Usually present at birth.
- ▶ Persist indefinitely.
- ▶ Although nonproliferative, may gradually increase in size with growth of the individual.
- ▶ Classified by the primary components.
    - Capillary malformation
        - Salmon patch
        - Port-wine stain (PWS)
    - Venous malformation
    - Lymphatic malformation
        - Lymphedema
        - Microcystic lymphatic malformation
        - Macrocystic lymphatic malformation
    - Arteriovenous malformation
    - Combined malformations

Signs and Symptoms

- ▶ Capillary malformation
    - Salmon patch
        - Also known as nevus simplex, stork bite, angel kiss; present in 30% to 40% of newborns.
        - Dull pink macules and patches (Figure 62.1).
        - Posterior neck/scalp (stork bite), glabella (angel kiss), forehead, superior eyelids.
        - Occasional involvement of nose, nasolabial regions, philtrum.
        - No syndrome associations; usually fade by 2 years but may become more prominent with crying, straining, physical exertion.
        - Salmon patches on the posterior neck/scalp may occasionally develop overlying dermatitis, which responds to topical steroids or laser therapy.

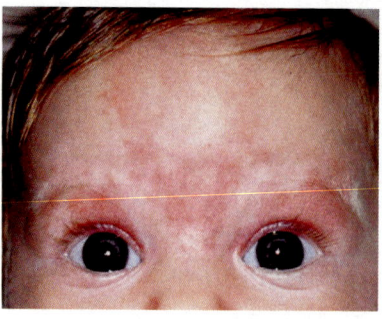

Figure 62.1. Salmon patch. Erythematous patches involving the glabella and upper eyelids.

- PWS
  - Also known as nevus flammeus.
  - May be isolated or associated with syndromes.
  - Caused by variation in *GNAQ* in some patients (same variation involved in Sturge-Weber syndrome).
  - Usually darker red, larger than salmon patch (Figures 62.2 and 62.3).
  - Early lesion may be indistinguishable from infantile hemangioma.
  - May darken and thicken with aging; occasionally develops pyogenic granulomas on surface.
  - Persists indefinitely; may pose psychosocial issue.
  - Syndrome associations outlined in Treating Associated Conditions section.
▶ Venous malformation
  - Although present at birth, may not become obvious until later in life.
  - Blue or blue-purple in color.
  - Subcutaneous, compressible masses (Figures 62.4 and 62.5).
  - May be confused with deep infantile hemangioma in infants.
  - May occur on any part of the body.
  - May be associated with significant distortion, functional compromise.
  - Occasional thromboses, phleboliths may occur.
  - Rare associated syndromes include Maffucci syndrome and blue rubber bleb nevus syndrome.
▶ Lymphatic malformation
  - Lymphedema: may be congenital or acquired; lymph fluid collection in subcutaneous tissues, often extremities; may occur in setting of Turner and Noonan syndromes.
  - Microcystic lymphatic malformation
    - Aggregates of microscopic lymphatic channels.
    - Present as plaques of clear or flesh-colored blebs; may be hemorrhagic (Figure 62.6).
    - Swelling and occasional bruising may occur.

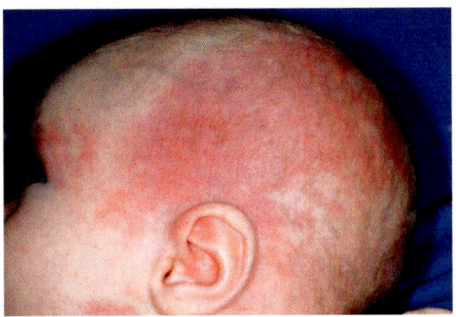

Figure 62.2. Port-wine stain. Dark red, vascular stain involving the scalp, with minimal extension onto the face.

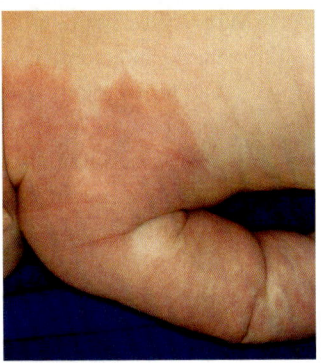

Figure 62.3. Port-wine stain. This lesion involved the upper lateral back, chest, shoulder, and upper extremity of this patient.

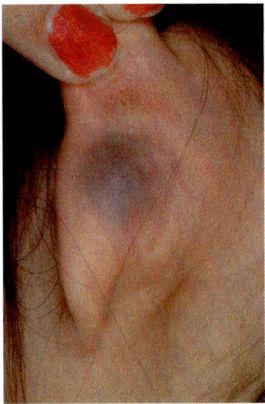

Figure 62.4. Venous malformation. This non-tender, compressible nodule on the posterior helix was present at birth.

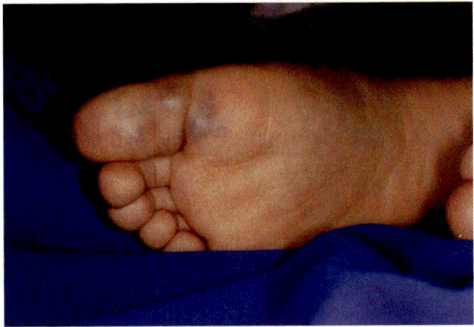

Figure 62.5. Venous malformation. Blue compressible nodules on the plantar surface of the foot and great toe of a 6-year-old.

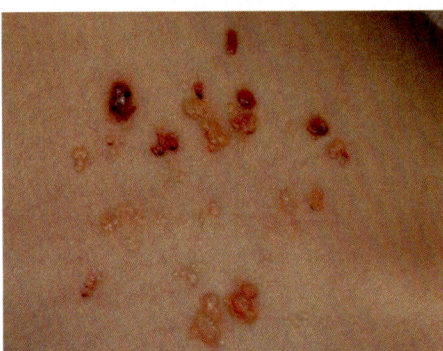

Figure 62.6. Microcystic lymphatic malformation. Translucent, grouped papules, some of which reveal a hemorrhagic component.

- Macrocystic lymphatic malformation
  - Large, interconnected lymphatic channels and cysts.
  - Old terminology: *cystic hygroma, cavernous lymphangioma.*
  - May be associated with Turner syndrome, Down syndrome, trisomy 18 or 13, Noonan syndrome.
  - Any location but favor head, neck, and chest.
  - Present as large, translucent masses (Figure 62.7).
  - Hemorrhage may present with swelling, tenderness, purple appearance.
▶ Arteriovenous malformation
  - Rare vascular malformation with arterial and venous components and arteriovenous shunting.
  - May present as red patch simulating PWS, as pulsating mass with thrills (Figure 62.8), or, occasionally, with necrosis and ulceration.
  - May be classified from stage 1 (pink macules, which may mimic capillary malformation) to stage 4 (larger lesions associated with cardiac compromise).
▶ Combined malformations
  - Combination of 2 or more components (Figure 62.9).
  - Commonly capillary-lymphatic-venous or capillary-venous.

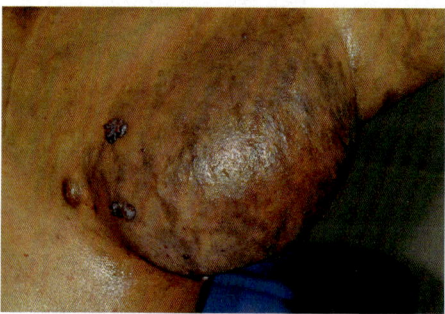

Figure 62.7. Macrocystic lymphatic malformation. A large mass of the lateral chest/anterior axillary region in a young patient. Note hemorrhagic lymphatic blebs on the medial surface.

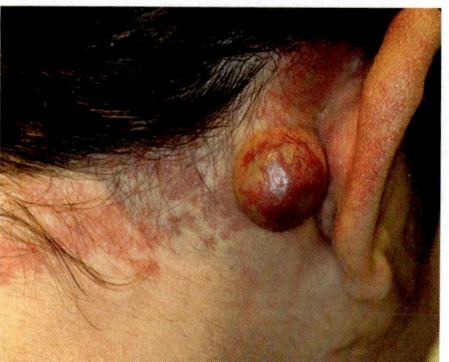

Figure 62.8. Arteriovenous malformation. This 14-year-old had a lifelong history of a red vascular stain involving the right helix and posterior auricular scalp; over time, this superimposed pulsating mass developed.

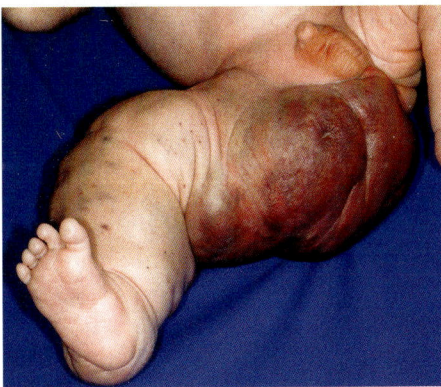

Figure 62.9. Combined vascular malformation. This extensive lesion of the buttock and lower extremity had capillary (red), venous (blue), and lymphatic (deeper aspect of the mass) components.

Look-alikes

Disorder	Differentiating Features
Infantile hemangioma	• Early (superficial) lesion may simulate salmon patch or port-wine stain (PWS). • Proliferates, thickens with time. • May ulcerate, bleed. • Deep lesion may simulate venous malformation. • Natural history of growth during first year helps to distinguish hemangioma from vascular malformations. • Non-involuting congenital hemangioma distinguished by rim of pallor and telangiectatic surface network.
Bruising from birth trauma	• May simulate PWS. • Resolves over first 1 to 2 weeks with color changes typical for ecchymoses.
Warts, molluscum	• May simulate microcystic lymphatic malformation. • Hemorrhage, intermittent swelling, and localization help to distinguish lymphatic malformation.
Herpes simplex virus infection	• May simulate microcystic lymphatic malformation. • Pain, erosions, and rapid healing help to distinguish herpes simplex virus infection.

How to Make the Diagnosis

▶ Clinical examination usually is sufficient for diagnosis.

▶ Venous malformation/macrocystic lymphatic malformation may be confirmed with computed tomography, magnetic resonance imaging, or Doppler ultrasonography.

- Macrocystic lymphatic malformation may be noted on prenatal ultrasonography.
- Arteriovenous malformation confirmed with ultrasonography; may require magnetic resonance imaging or angiography, computed tomography, or arteriography.

Treatment

- Capillary malformation
  - Salmon patch
    - Education and reassurance.
    - Pulsed dye laser may be considered for persistent facial lesions.
  - PWS
    - Pulsed dye laser.
    - Cover-up cosmetics may need to be considered in older children.
- Venous malformation
  - Compression garments may minimize discomfort when lesions are painful.
  - Percutaneous sclerosing therapy for select lesions.
  - Surgical excision, occasionally.
  - Low-dose aspirin (or other antiplatelet/anticoagulant medications) may be useful in patients with recurrent thromboses.
  - Care should be multidisciplinary, when possible; physical therapy may be necessary for patients with more extensive lesions.
- Lymphatic malformation
  - Lymphedema
    - Massage, elevation.
    - Compression garments.
    - Intermittent pneumatic compression.
    - Surgery reserved for severe deformity.
  - Microcystic lymphatic malformation
    - Surgery, if necessary.
  - Macrocystic lymphatic malformation
    - Percutaneous sclerosing therapy.
    - Surgery for select lesions.
    - Systemic sirolimus and sildenafil have been beneficial in some patients.
    - Care should be multidisciplinary, when possible; physical therapy may be necessary for patients with more extensive lesions.

- ▶ Arteriovenous malformation
  - Surgical excision, embolization; amputation occasionally necessary.
  - Multidisciplinary management is optimal.

Treating Associated Conditions

Associated Condition/Syndrome	Comments/Treatment
Pyogenic granuloma located on a port-wine stain (PWS)	• Pulsed dye laser or topical timolol (if small) or excision with electrocautery.
Sturge-Weber syndrome	• Caused by variation in *GNAQ*. • PWS located in a similar distribution as that innervated by the first branch of the trigeminal nerve (now thought to be more associated with patterns of embryonal vascular development) may be associated with glaucoma and leptomeningeal angiomatosis (presents as seizures); multi-dermatomal–type distribution pattern, hemifacial, and extensive forehead (medial or lateral) stains also considered high risk for association with Sturge-Weber syndrome. • Multidisciplinary approach to evaluation/therapy; generally includes referral to neurology, ophthalmology, dermatology. • Pulsed dye laser for PWS.
Phakomatosis pigmentovascularis (PPV)	• PWS in association with pigmented nevus (epidermal nevus, Mongolian spot, nevus spilus) or nevus anemicus. • Mongolian spot and cutis marmorata telangiectatica congenita more recently described as another PPV subtype. • Mosaic activating variations in *GNA11* and *GNAQ* have been found in PPV (as well as extensive dermal melanocytosis). • Occasional systemic differences (including ophthalmologic, neurologic involvement). • Treatment of skin lesions usually unnecessary; pulsed dye laser may be used for PWS.
Klippel-Trénaunay syndrome	• PWS with venous varicosity and tissue (bone and soft tissue) hyperplasia (Figure 62.10). • Most often involves an extremity. • Lymphedema is also often present. • Shown to be associated with *PIK3CA* variations. • Treatment may include compression, laser therapy, sclerosing therapy, pain control, vascular/orthopedic surgical procedures.

(continued)

(continued)

Associated Condition/Syndrome	Comments/Treatment
Proteus syndrome	- May be caused by variation in *AKT1* or *PTEN* in some patients. - PWS in conjunction with tissue overgrowth. - May include cerebriform hyperplasia of palms/soles, lipomas, epidermal nevi, lymphatic/venous malformations, disproportionate overgrowth, macrodactyly, macrocephaly. - Multidisciplinary approach to evaluation/therapy; may include orthopedics, neurology, dermatology. - CLOVES syndrome: similar to Proteus syndrome but consists of congenital lipomatous overgrowth, vascular malformations, epidermal nevi, scoliosis, other skeletal and spinal anomalies (including arteriovenous malformations, tethered spinal cord); lacks cerebriform palmoplantar hyperplasia characteristic of Proteus syndrome; increased risk of Wilms tumor; caused by variations in *PIK3CA*.
Macrocephaly-capillary malformation syndrome	- Also known as megalencephaly-capillary malformation syndrome and megalencephaly-capillary malformation-polymicrogyria syndrome. - Macrocephaly and reticulate PWS; centrofacial PWS common in these patients. - Other features may include atypical growth, craniofacial and skeletal anomalies, developmental delay, anatomic brain defects, connective tissue differences. - Originally designated "macrocephaly-cutis marmorata telangiectatica congenita"; subsequently reclassified when stains noted to be more consistent with reticulate PWS. - Multidisciplinary approach to evaluation/therapy; may include neurology, neurosurgery, dermatology, orthopedics. - Recently shown to be caused by *PIK3CA* variation.
Capillary malformation-arteriovenous malformation (CM-AVM) syndrome	- Caused by variations in *RASA1* and *EPHB4*. - Capillary malformations tend to be multiple and both congenital and acquired, with haphazard distribution; occasionally brown or gray in appearance; some may have a peripheral halo of vasoconstriction (Figure 62.11); may also affect the mucosae (tongue, lips, conjunctivae). - Arteriovenous malformations may be cutaneous, subcutaneous, intramuscular, intraosseous, or cerebral; spinal arteriovenous malformations may also be present. - Multidisciplinary approach to evaluation/therapy; may include neurology, neurosurgery, dermatology, orthopedics. - Divided into CM-AVM1 and CM-AVM2 syndromes, the latter characterized by association with *EPHB4* variation and more frequent findings of Bier spots (vasospastic macules [Figure 62.12]) and telangiectasias (on the lips, perioral regions, and upper trunk).

Associated Condition/ Syndrome	Comments/Treatment
Maffucci syndrome	- Venous malformations and enchondromas. - Risk of hemangioendothelioma, chondrosarcoma. - Caused by variations in *IDH1* and *IDH2*. - Treatment includes orthopedic monitoring/care and malignancy surveillance.
Blue rubber bleb nevus syndrome	- Multiple venous malformations of skin and gastrointestinal tract. - Hemorrhage, iron deficiency anemia possible. - Occasional central nervous system involvement. - Caused by variations in *TEK*. - Treatment supportive; may include sclerosing therapy or band ligation of gastrointestinal tract lesions, bowel resection; oral sirolimus has been reported as helpful, and corticosteroids, interferon-α, and vincristine have also been used; subcutaneous octreotide has been used to decrease gastrointestinal bleeding.

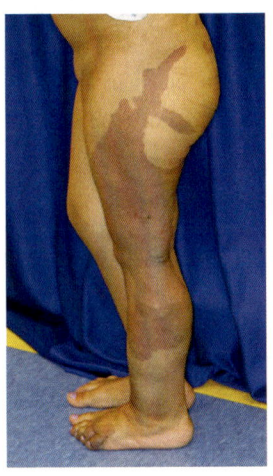

Figure 62.10. Klippel-Trénaunay syndrome. This young patient had extensive port-wine stains, overgrowth, and venous varicosities with lymphedema involving the lower extremity.

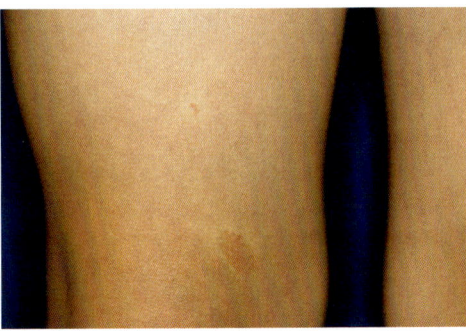

Figure 62.11. Several vascular pink-brown macules on the thigh of a young patient with capillary malformation-arteriovenous malformation syndrome. Note the peripheral halo of vasoconstriction.

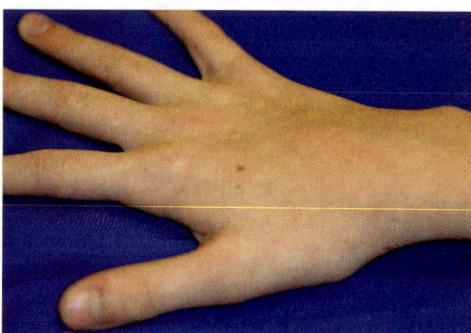

Figure 62.12. Multiple vasospastic macules (Bier spots) on the dorsal aspect of the hand of a young patient with capillary malformation-arteriovenous malformation syndrome.

Prognosis

- Variable.
- Prognosis for salmon patch, nonsyndromic PWS, microcystic lymphatic malformation excellent.
- Prognosis otherwise depends on multiple features, including size of lesion(s), location, complications, and any syndrome associations.

When to Worry or Refer

- Referral should be considered for
  - Any facial PWS.
  - PWS in association with other syndromic findings.
  - Venous malformations that are larger, multiple, or associated with pain, bleeding, function impairment, or overgrowth.
  - Lymphedema or macrocystic lymphatic malformation.
  - Suspected arteriovenous malformation or vascular malformation syndrome.

Resources for Families

- American Academy of Pediatrics: HealthyChildren.org.
  https://www.healthychildren.org/English/ages-stages/baby/bathing-skin-care/Pages/Your-Newborns-Skin-Birthmarks-and-Rashes.aspx
- K-T Support Group: Provides support and resources for patients and families who have Klippel-Trénaunay syndrome and related conditions.
  www.k-t.org
- National Odd Shoe Exchange: A source of footwear for those requiring single shoes or pairs of differing sizes.
  www.oddshoe.org
- National Organization of Vascular Anomalies: Patient information, resources, and support.
  www.novanews.org
- Proteus Syndrome Foundation: Provides support and education for families living with and professionals caring for individuals who have Proteus syndrome.
  www.proteus-syndrome.org
- Society for Pediatric Dermatology: Patient handout on port-wine stains.
  https://pedsderm.net/for-patients-families/patient-handouts/#PWS
- Sturge-Weber Foundation: Provides information and support for patients who have PWSs, Sturge-Weber syndrome, or Klippel-Trénaunay syndrome and their families.
  https://sturge-weber.org/new-to-swf
- Vascular Birthmarks Foundation: Provides referrals, financial assistance, newsletter, biannual conference, resource list for clinics and doctors, advocacy, support, and counseling.
  www.birthmark.org

Disorders of Pigmentation

Hypopigmentation

CHAPTER 63 — **Albinism** 441

CHAPTER 64 — **Pigmentary Mosaicism, Hypopigmented** 445

CHAPTER 65 — **Pityriasis Alba** 451

CHAPTER 66 — **Postinflammatory Hypopigmentation** 455

CHAPTER 67 — **Vitiligo** 459

CHAPTER 63

Albinism

Introduction/Etiology/Epidemiology

▶ Albinism results from a generalized lack of production and distribution of melanin; several phenotypic variants exist.
  - It may be separated into forms that involve the skin, hair, and eyes (oculocutaneous albinism [OCA]) or only the eye (ocular albinism).
  - Nearly all forms of OCA are inherited in an autosomal recessive manner.
▶ The most important biochemical distinction between the more common subtypes is the presence or absence of tyrosinase activity, although this has little clinical relevance. The genetic basis of most variants is now known and can be found in Online Mendelian Inheritance in Man (www.ncbi.nlm.nih.gov/omim).

Signs and Symptoms

There are 7 types of OCA; the 2 most common are discussed here.

▶ OCA type 1: separated into 3 forms depending on whether tyrosinase activity is absent (type A) or reduced (type B) or is temperature sensitive (type TS). In type 1A (ie, tyrosinase-negative OCA), patients are unable to produce melanin and exhibit the following:
  - White hair and white skin (Figure 63.1).
  - Decreased visual acuity, photophobia, nystagmus, and strabismus.
  - Inability to tan or freckle and predisposition to skin cancer.
  - Pale (often gray or blue) irides (Figure 63.1).
  - Foveal hypoplasia.
▶ OCA type 2 (ie, tyrosinase-positive OCA): most common form of OCA, particularly among individuals of African descent. In OCA type 2, patients exhibit the following:
  - Yellow to red or light brown hair; some have metallic-appearing hair.
  - White skin with minimal tanning ability.
  - A tendency to develop freckles and nevi (often red) over time.
  - Ocular findings that are less severe than in OCA type 1.

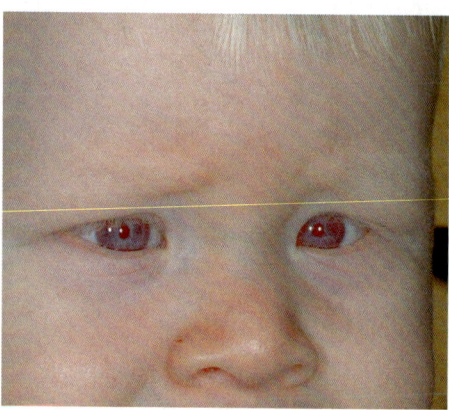

Figure 63.1. Oculocutaneous albinism. Absence of pigment in the skin, hair, and irides.

- ▶ Rare forms of albinism associated with systemic disease are as follows:
  - Hermansky-Pudlak syndrome: autosomal-recessive disorder characterized by OCA and bleeding diathesis related to a platelet storage pool defect; presents with albinism features and multiple ecchymoses (Figure 63.2).
  - Chédiak-Higashi syndrome: autosomal recessive disorder in which patients exhibit partial albinism, silvery hair, immune variations, and eventual neurologic deterioration.

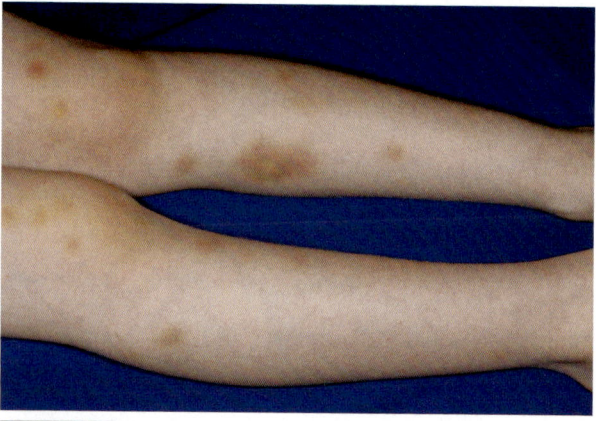

Figure 63.2. Multiple ecchymoses in a young child with oculocutaneous albinism in the setting of Hermansky-Pudlak syndrome.

Look-alikes

Disorder	Differentiating Features
Vitiligo	• Acquired (not congenital) localized pigment loss. • May be widespread but rarely affects total skin surface. • Ocular variations are absent.
Piebaldism	• Congenital localized absence of pigment, often affecting the face or scalp. • Most of the skin surface typical. • May involve small adjacent area of depigmented hair (poliosis or white forelock).
Waardenburg syndrome	• Pigmentary dilution of skin in conjunction with other characteristic features. • Sensorineural deafness common. • White forelock may be present. • Other variations may include synophrys, heterochromia iridis, pseudo-hypertelorism (related to dystopia canthorum, a lateral displacement of the medial canthi).

How to Make the Diagnosis

▶ Patients have very pale skin from birth with no ability to tan in early childhood.

▶ Distinguishing features include white or yellow hair, white skin, pale irides, photophobia, nystagmus, and poor visual acuity.

▶ Molecular genetic testing is available for diagnostic confirmation; variations in the *TYR* gene cause type 1 OCA and in the *OCA2* gene result in type 2 OCA.

Treatment

▶ Strict photoprotection of skin and eyes is imperative from birth.
  ■ Use broad-spectrum sunscreens with a sun protection factor of 30 or higher.
  ■ Use product that provides UV-A and UV-B protection, including eyewear (ie, sunglasses).

▶ Annual skin examination is recommended to observe for photodamage and premalignant or malignant lesions.

▶ Ophthalmologic consultation, with regular follow-up, is indicated.

Treating Associated Conditions

- Bleeding tendency, neurologic symptoms, frequent infections, or other clinical features should prompt a search for associated syndromes.

Prognosis

- As a rule, most children do well. They require lifelong sun protection and surveillance for skin cancer.

When to Worry or Refer

- Changes in existing nevi or the sudden onset of a new lesion (eg, a red nodule) should be cause for concern. In patients who have albinism, melanoma is often amelanotic (ie, may appear red, pink, or white). However, even benign melanocytic nevi in children with OCA are often less brown and more pink.
- Sudden changes in vision require immediate ophthalmologic consultation.

Resources for Families

- Hermansky-Pudlak Syndrome Network: Patient information.
  www.hpsnetwork.org
- National Organization for Albinism and Hypopigmentation: Provides information and support for individuals who have albinism or hypopigmentation.
  www.albinism.org
- Vision for Tomorrow Foundation: Provides support and information on albinism and aniridia.
  www.visionfortomorrow.org

CHAPTER
64

Pigmentary Mosaicism, Hypopigmented

Introduction/Etiology/Epidemiology

- *Pigmentary mosaicism* is the term used to describe a group of disorders in which the skin has a patterned hypopigmentation or hyperpigmentation. In the hypopigmented form discussed in this chapter, affected skin is lighter than the background skin color but not completely depigmented (as would be the case in vitiligo).

- Pigmentary mosaicism is believed to be the result of genetic variations that create a population of cells with more or less pigment potential than the surrounding unremarkable skin. *Mosaicism* refers to the coexistence of 2 genetically distinct populations of cells within the same individual.

- Pigmentary mosaicism may be localized or generalized.

- Terminology used to describe hypopigmented pigmentary mosaicism is inconsistent. Terms such as *nevus depigmentosus, segmental pigmentation disorder, nevoid hypomelanosis,* and *patterned pigmentation* exist in the literature.

- In most cases, localized hypopigmented pigmentary mosaicism is a benign and isolated finding. When more generalized, it can be associated with skeletal, ocular, or neurologic (eg, seizures, developmental delay, macrocephaly) differences, a condition also known as *hypomelanosis of Ito.*

Signs and Symptoms

- Hypopigmentation is present at birth but may be difficult to recognize in neonates with fair skin until background skin color develops and contrast between the 2 areas is appreciated. The hypopigmentation is more noticeable with prolonged sun exposure, as the affected skin does not tan as readily as the unaffected skin.

- Common patterns of mosaic hypopigmentation include a large region or segment of the body (Figure 64.1) and whorled or linear bands (thin or broad) that follow the Blaschko skin developmental lines (Figure 64.2).
- Affected areas are typically sharply demarcated and usually respect the midline.

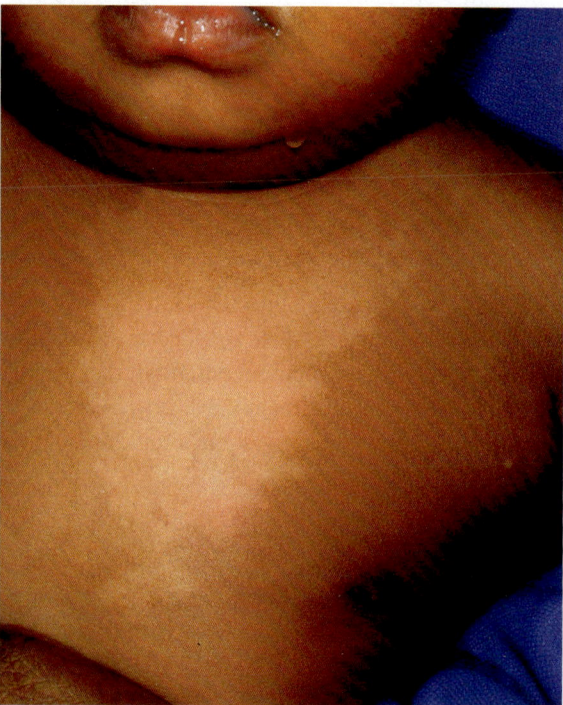

Figure 64.1. Pigmentary mosaicism, hypopigmented type. A large, shaggy-bordered, hypopigmented patch on the chest that respects the midline. This lesion often is called a *nevus depigmentosus,* which is a misnomer, as the lesion is not depigmented.

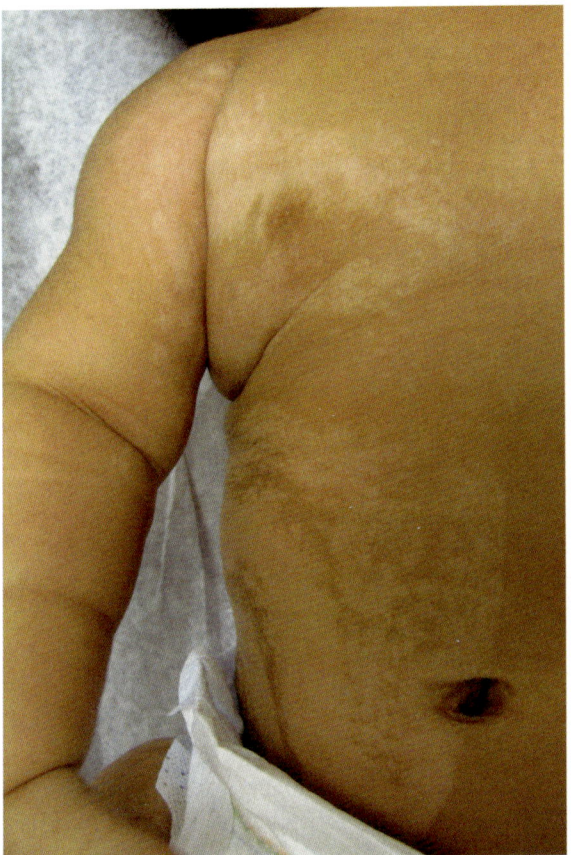

Figure 64.2. Pigmentary mosaicism, hypopigmented type. Whorled and curvilinear streaks of hypopigmentation that represent the Blaschko lines and respect the midline.

Look-alikes

Disorder	Differentiating Features
Lichen striatus (hypopigmented phase)	• Usually begins in childhood; not present at birth. • Begins as skin-colored to pink papules (sometimes scaly). • Typically lesions appear proximally on an extremity and extend distally. • Over time, papules resolve and linear hypopigmentation or hyperpigmentation remain. • Eventual spontaneous resolution (unlike pigmentary mosaicism, which persists indefinitely).
Goltz syndrome (focal dermal hypoplasia)	• X-linked dominant inheritance. • Telangiectatic and atrophic streaks (along the Blaschko lines) and soft papules due to fat herniation. • Associations may include dental, ophthalmologic, and skeletal anomalies.
Incontinentia pigmenti (fourth stage)	• X-linked dominant inheritance. • Inflammatory papules and pustules are usually the initial presentation in newborn (first stage), distributed along the Blaschko lines. • Warty lesions (second stage) give rise to hyperpigmentation (third stage) in a similar distribution pattern, followed by eventual hypopigmentation (fourth stage). • Hypopigmentation may be accompanied by atrophy and loss of hair. • Associations may include dental, ophthalmologic, neurologic, and skeletal anomalies.
Piebaldism	• Congenital depigmentation (as opposed to hypopigmentation) affecting the midline of the head or torso with focal and symmetric involvement of the extremities. • Associated poliosis (white forelock) may be present. • May be an isolated cutaneous finding or associated with Waardenburg syndrome.
Vitiligo (segmental form)	• Usually begins in childhood or adolescence, not infancy. • Affected area is depigmented, not hypopigmented. • Borders tend to be more sharply demarcated, less shaggy.

How to Make the Diagnosis

▶ The diagnosis of hypopigmented pigmentary mosaicism is usually made based on the history and physical examination findings. A Wood lamp can help differentiate hypopigmented skin from depigmented skin.

▶ Consider ophthalmologic examination to evaluate for ocular anomalies in children with the generalized type.

- If other malformations or neurodevelopmental differences are absent, further workup is not indicated. If they are present, consultation with the appropriate specialist(s) is warranted.
- Rarely, karyotype analysis is performed (on blood or skin biopsy tissue) searching for chromosomal mosaicism.

Treatment

- There are no specific treatments for hypopigmented pigmentary mosaicism. Daily sunscreen and photoprotection can help reduce contrasting pigment accentuation.

Prognosis

- In most cases, hypopigmented pigmentary mosaicism is a benign, isolated skin finding not associated with other medical concerns.
- In the rare patient who has generalized involvement, prognosis depends on the nature of any other organ differences.

When to Worry or Refer

- Referral to dermatology is warranted when the diagnosis is uncertain.
- Referral to other specialists (eg, ophthalmology, neurology, genetics, orthopedics) is warranted when applicable.

Resources for Families

- American Academy of Pediatrics: HealthyChildren.org.
  https://www.healthychildren.org/English/ages-stages/baby/bathing-skin-care/Pages/Your-Newborns-Skin-Birthmarks-and-Rashes.aspx
- NORD—National Organization for Rare Disorders: Hypomelanosis of Ito.
  https://rarediseases.org/rare-diseases/hypomelanosis-of-ito
- Society for Pediatric Dermatology: Patient handout on pigmentary mosaicism.
  https://pedsderm.net/for-patients-families/patient-handouts/#pigmentary%20mosaicism

CHAPTER
65

Pityriasis Alba

Introduction/Etiology/Epidemiology

- Pityriasis alba is thought to represent postinflammatory hypopigmentation.
- It is most often observed in children who have atopic dermatitis.

Signs and Symptoms

- Pityriasis alba appears as poorly defined macular areas of hypopigmentation (Figure 65.1), perhaps with very fine scale.
- Lesions are transient and may be located on face (most common by far) (Figure 65.2), trunk, or extremities.
- Lesions may become more apparent after sun exposure, as unaffected skin tans but affected areas do not.

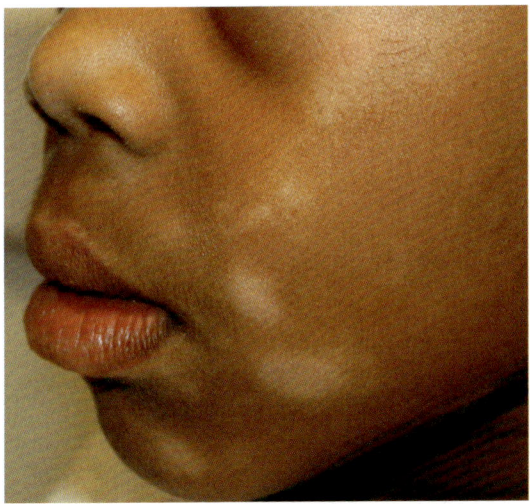

Figure 65.1. Pityriasis alba. Hypopigmented macules with indistinct borders.

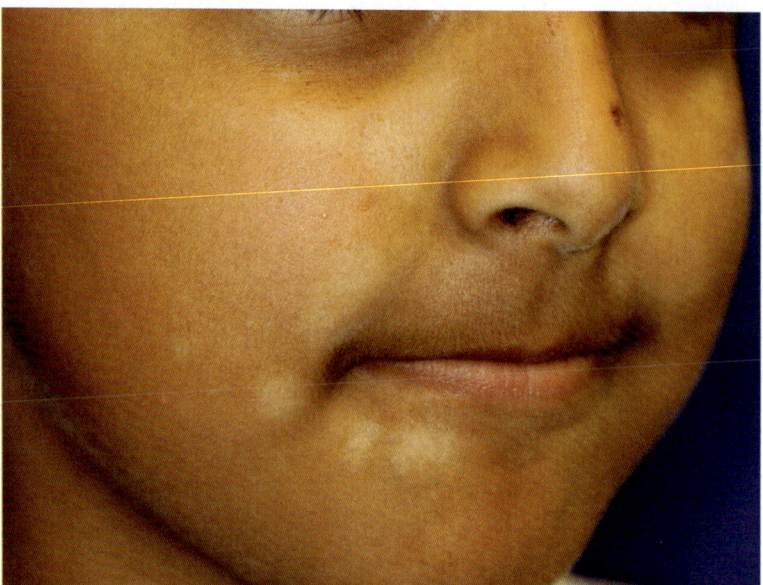

Figure 65.2. Pityriasis alba. Hypopigmented macules on the face in a young patient with atopic dermatitis.

Look-alikes

Disorder	Differentiating Features
Vitiligo	• Lesions are depigmented (not hypopigmented) and well defined. • Hairs within affected areas depigmented. • Accentuation with Wood lamp examination. • Tends to occur over joints, around orifices, and in areas prone to trauma.
Tinea versicolor	• Lesions well defined and typically concentrated on the trunk; individual lesions may coalesce into large patches. • Facial involvement less common. • Generally *not* seen in prepubertal patients. • Performance of a potassium hydroxide preparation on scale from lesions may reveal short hyphae and spores (ie, "spaghetti and meatballs").

How to Make the Diagnosis

▶ The diagnosis is made clinically based on the observation of poorly defined macules or patches of hypopigmentation that have fine scale.

▶ Atopic history (ie, presence of atopic dermatitis, asthma, or allergic rhinoconjunctivitis) common and supports the diagnosis.

Treatment

- Application of an emollient is adequate for treatment in most cases.
- Some advise application of a topical corticosteroid, topical calcineurin inhibitor, or topical phosphodiesterase 4 inhibitor, particularly if the lesions are erythematous or pruritic. This will treat underlying inflammation and may help to accelerate repigmentation.
- Counsel the patient and family that months will be required for return of typical pigmentation.
- Sun protection will help minimize tanning of surrounding skin, thereby reducing the contrast between unaffected and affected skin.

Treating Associated Conditions

- Treat associated atopic dermatitis and xerosis if present.

Prognosis

- Lesions of pityriasis alba typically improve over time, but new lesions may intermittently recur.
- The condition tends to resolve by mid-adolescence.

When to Worry or Refer

- Diagnostic uncertainty exists or lesions do not respond to therapy.

Resource for Families

- MedlinePlus: Information for patients and families (in English and Spanish) sponsored by the US National Library of Medicine and National Institutes of Health.
  https://www.nlm.nih.gov/medlineplus/ency/article/001463.htm

CHAPTER
66

Postinflammatory Hypopigmentation

Introduction/Etiology/Epidemiology

- Hypopigmented macules and patches that result from inflammatory damage to melanocytes.
- Often a history of preceding inflammation, such as dermatitis, arthropod bite, or abrasion.

Signs and Symptoms

- Hypopigmentation with indistinct margins and no surface change (Figure 66.1).
- No associated symptoms.
- May have associated scar.

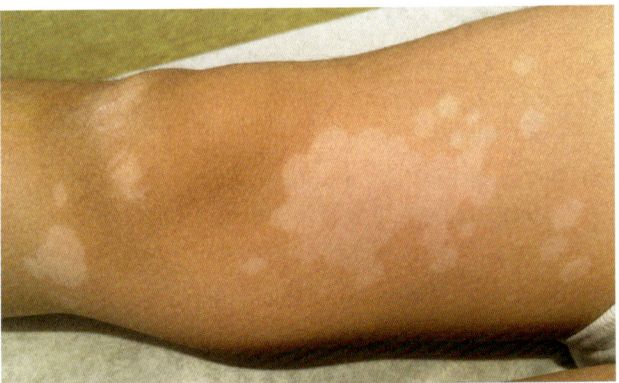

Figure 66.1. Postinflammatory hypopigmentation. Hypopigmented macules located at sites of prior bullous impetigo lesions.

Look-alikes

Disorder	Differentiating Features
Pityriasis alba	• Likely represents a form of postinflammatory hypopigmentation. • Macules with indistinct borders and, occasionally, scale. • Usually seen in the setting of atopic dermatitis. • Most often occurs on the face.
Vitiligo	• Well-defined depigmented (not hypopigmented) macules or patches. • Accentuation with Wood lamp examination. • Tends to occur over joints, around orifices, and in areas prone to trauma.
Tinea versicolor	• Well-defined hypopigmented macules and patches located on the trunk, proximal surfaces of the arms, and sides of neck. • Potassium hydroxide preparation of scale from lesions reveals short hyphae and spores (ie, "spaghetti and meatballs").
Piebaldism	• Congenital absence of pigment usually limited to one area. • Well-defined depigmented (versus hypopigmented) macules or patches. • May involve small adjacent area of depigmented hair (poliosis or white forelock).

How to Make the Diagnosis

▶ History of preceding inflammation is most useful clue.

▶ Lesions are hypopigmented (not depigmented).

Treatment

▶ No treatment necessary or available.

▶ It is important to educate caregivers that postinflammatory hypopigmentation is the result of preceding skin inflammation, and not a side effect of topical therapies (eg, topical corticosteroids).

▶ Counsel the patient and family that months may be required for pigmentation to return to as expected.

▶ Sun protection is vital (tanning of surrounding skin will make lesions more visible).

Treating Associated Conditions

- If preceding inflammatory condition is treatable and flares can be minimized (ie, atopic dermatitis), this will diminish the risk of additional postinflammatory changes.

Prognosis

- If no associated scarring, repigmentation is typical, although months to years may be required for this to occur.

When to Worry or Refer

- Refer if uncertainty exists regarding the diagnosis.

Resource for Families

- National Organization for Albinism and Hypopigmentation: Provides information and support for individuals who have albinism or hypopigmentation.
  www.albinism.org

CHAPTER 67

Vitiligo

Introduction/Etiology/Epidemiology

- Vitiligo represents an acquired complete depigmentation of skin due to melanocyte destruction that is thought to be autoimmune in nature.
- Two main forms have been described: generalized and segmental (ie, involves one area of the body and typically does not cross the midline).
- Vitiligo develops in childhood or adolescence in about half of patients.

Signs and Symptoms

- Vitiligo presents as well-defined macules or patches of complete depigmentation (ie, the skin is completely white) with typical texture (Figure 67.1).
  - It may begin with speckled areas of hypopigmentation that continue to lose pigment and coalesce over time.
  - Lesions may be faintly erythematous (especially the periphery) early in the course.
  - Areas prone to trauma or pressure (eg, knees, elbows, small joints such as metacarpophalangeal joints, hips) are most frequently involved (Figure 67.2); this distribution may represent the Koebner phenomenon (ie, appearance of lesions at sites of injury).
  - Other common locations include eyelids, perioral regions (Figure 67.3), axillae, and the groin.
- Generalized vitiligo often starts symmetrically on the arms, legs, or periorbital areas and may progress to involve large areas.
- Localized segmental vitiligo often follows a dermatomal distribution.
- Trichrome vitiligo is a variant seen in children; unaffected, hypopigmented, and depigmented patches are present simultaneously in an involved area.
- Halo nevi (Figure 67.4) are more common in children with vitiligo and may precede the diagnosis by months to years.

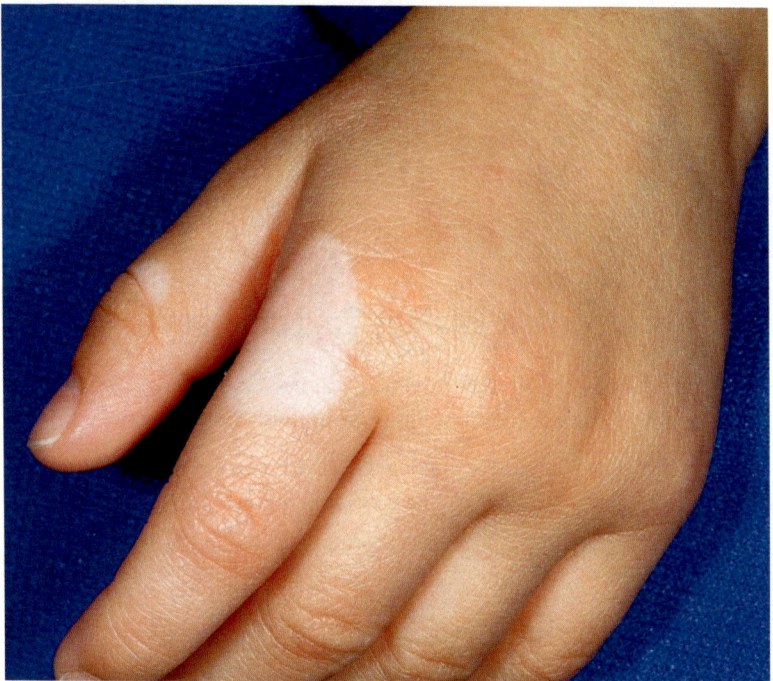

Figure 67.1. Vitiligo appears as well-defined areas of complete loss of pigmentation (ie, depigmentation).

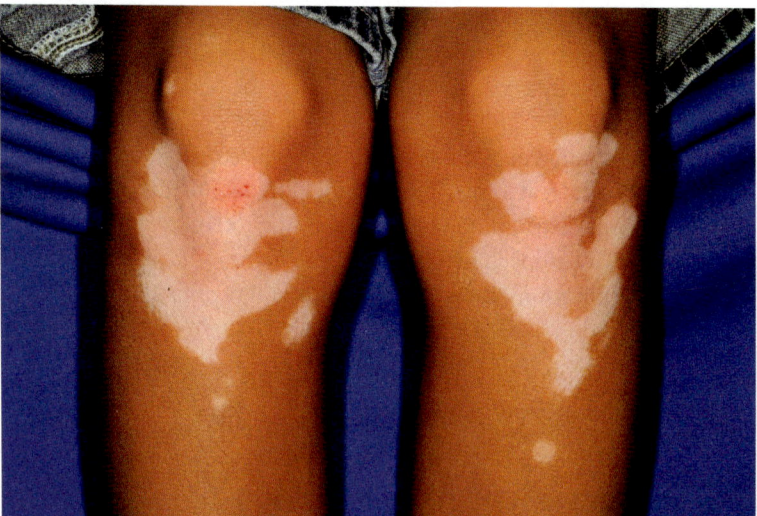

Figure 67.2. Vitiligo. This young patient had depigmented macules and patches on bilateral knees, elbows, and hips.

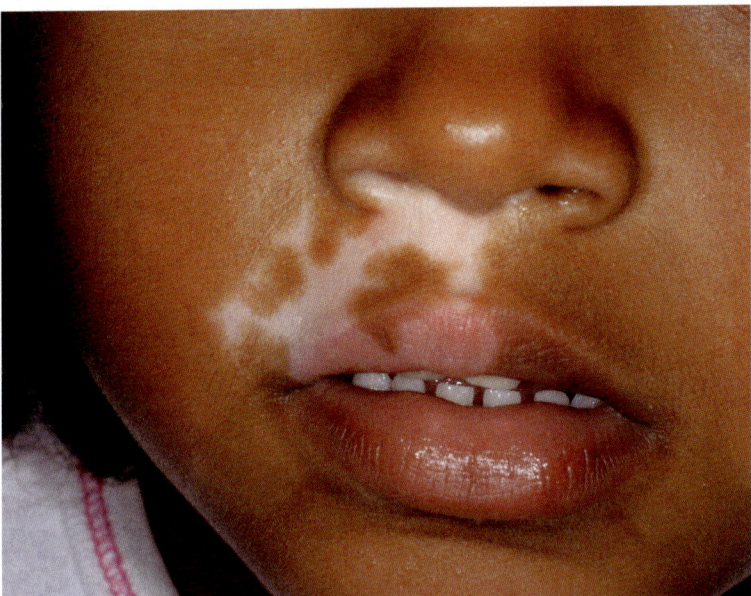

Figure 67.3. Segmental vitiligo. This young patient had right-sided depigmented patches around the mouth and on the upper lip. Notice the sharp midline demarcation as well as the islands of repigmentation (associated with the patient's response to topical therapy).

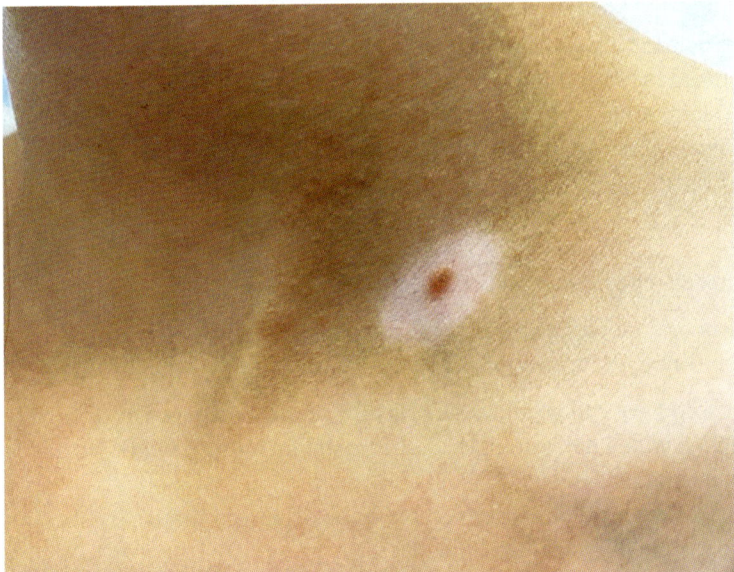

Figure 67.4. Halo nevus is a melanocytic nevus that develops a surrounding rim of hypopigmentation or depigmentation. They are more common in children with vitiligo.

Look-alikes

Disorder	Differentiating Features
Pityriasis alba	• Poorly defined areas of macular hypopigmentation (not depigmentation), often with associated scale. • Atopic history common.
Tinea versicolor	• Well-defined hypopigmented (not depigmented) macules and patches located on the trunk, upper arms, or neck. • Lesions often have associated fine scale and may be pruritic.
Piebaldism	• Congenital absence of pigmentation localized to one area. • May involve small adjacent area of depigmented hair (poliosis or white forelock).
Waardenburg syndrome	• Pigmentary dilution of skin in conjunction with other characteristic features. • Sensorineural deafness common. • White forelock may be present. • Other differences may include synophrys, heterochromia iridis, pseudo-hypertelorism (related to dystopia canthorum, lateral displacement of the medial canthi).

How to Make the Diagnosis

▶ The diagnosis of vitiligo is made clinically based on typical features (well-defined macules or patches of depigmentation).

▶ The distinction between hypopigmentation and depigmentation may be enhanced by examining the patient with a Wood lamp in a darkened room. Depigmented areas are well defined and strikingly prominent, while hypopigmented areas are less well defined.

Treatment

▶ Spontaneous repigmentation occurs in a few patients.

▶ Treatment options to date are variably effective, with numerous anecdotal topical and systemic agents having limited value.

▶ Patients who have vitiligo and desire therapy are best managed by or in consultation with a dermatologist. Some treatment options might include
  ▪ Topical corticosteroids.
  ▪ Topical calcineurin inhibitors (eg, tacrolimus, pimecrolimus): most useful for facial lesions.

- Topical ruxolitinib cream (Janus kinase inhibitor now US Food and Drug Administration approved for treatment of nonsegmental vitiligo in patients 12 years and older).
- Photochemotherapy using psoralens plus UV-A: often used in adolescents older than 12 years (rarely used in younger children).
- Narrowband UV-B phototherapy.
- Excimer laser therapy.

▶ For patients who do not desire specific medical therapy, options include application of a camouflage cream matched to the child's skin color and application of sunscreen (to protect depigmented skin and reduce tanning of unaffected skin).

▶ Treatment options generally limited to adult patients with vitiligo include autologous skin grafting, mini-grafting with UV light exposure, and treatment of remaining pigmented areas with 20% monobenzyl ether of hydroquinone (which results in permanent skin depigmentation).

Treating Associated Conditions

▶ Generalized (nonsegmental) vitiligo is associated with an increased risk of autoimmune disease in the affected individual and first-degree relatives. While most children who have vitiligo have no other associated conditions, it is important to gather a family history and be observant for the development of symptoms suggestive of inflammatory eye disease (light sensitivity, change in vision) or other autoimmune disease (eg, type 1 diabetes, pernicious anemia, hypothyroidism, hypoparathyroidism, celiac disease, Addison disease, autoimmune hepatitis).

▶ Most experts recommend thyroid function screening and antithyroid antibody levels for patients with vitiligo, with other testing performed only if indicated based on clinical signs or symptoms.

Prognosis

▶ Variable and unpredictable.
▶ Repigmentation, whether spontaneous or therapeutic, appears as perifollicular macules that coalesce to gradually fill in the area of depigmentation or as radial repigmentation in a centripetal pattern (ie, from outside toward the center).

When to Worry or Refer

- Vitiligo is widespread or rapidly progressive, and phototherapy is being considered.
- Vitiligo develops along with inflammatory eye disease or another autoimmune disorder (in which case consultation with the appropriate pediatric subspecialist is warranted). Consultation also may be of value if the patient has a first-degree relative with 2 autoimmune disorders. Rarely, vitiligo may be associated with autoimmune polyglandular syndromes, most notably type 1.

Resources for Families

- American Vitiligo Research Foundation: Provides education and support for persons who have vitiligo.
  www.avrf.org
- Society for Pediatric Dermatology: Patient handout on vitiligo.
  https://pedsderm.net/for-patients-families/patient-handouts/#Vitiligo
- Vitiligo Research Foundation: Provides information and links to physicians for patients who have vitiligo.
  https://vrfoundation.org
- Vitiligo Support International: Provides education and support for persons who have vitiligo.
  https://vitiligosupport.org

Disorders of Pigmentation

Hyperpigmentation

CHAPTER 68 — **Acanthosis Nigricans** 467

CHAPTER 69 — **Acquired Melanocytic Nevi** 471

CHAPTER 70 — **Café au Lait Macules** 477

CHAPTER 71 — **Congenital Melanocytic Nevi (CMN)** 481

CHAPTER 72 — **Ephelides** 487

CHAPTER 73 — **Lentigines** 489

CHAPTER 74 — **Congenital Dermal Melanocytosis** 493

CHAPTER 75 — **Melanonychia Striata** 497

CHAPTER 76 — **Pigmentary Mosaicism, Hyperpigmented** 501

CHAPTER 68

Acanthosis Nigricans

Introduction/Etiology/Epidemiology

- Represents epidermal proliferation process with minimal increase in melanin.
- Believed to be due to insulin resistance and its effect on the skin.
- May be seen in the following settings:
  - Obesity
  - Insulin resistance syndromes
  - Endocrinologic disorders (eg, type 2 diabetes mellitus, Addison disease, Cushing disease, hypothyroidism, hyperandrogenism, hypogonadism, polycystic ovary syndrome)
  - Medications (oral contraceptives, nicotinic acid)
- Malignancy: In adults, sudden onset of acanthosis nigricans may herald a malignant tumor, but no such association is recognized in childhood.

Signs and Symptoms

- Velvety thickening of the skin creates a brown to gray-black color that may be mistaken by patients as dirt (Figure 68.1).
- Most commonly observed on the nape or sides of the neck, axillae, and groin (crural creases); some patients may exhibit lesions over the knuckles (Figure 68.2) and around the mouth.

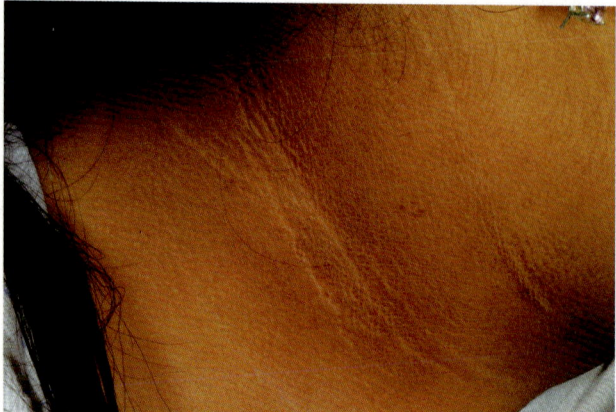

Figure 68.1. Velvety, hyperpigmented thickening of the skin characterizes acanthosis nigricans, seen here over the lateral aspect of the neck.

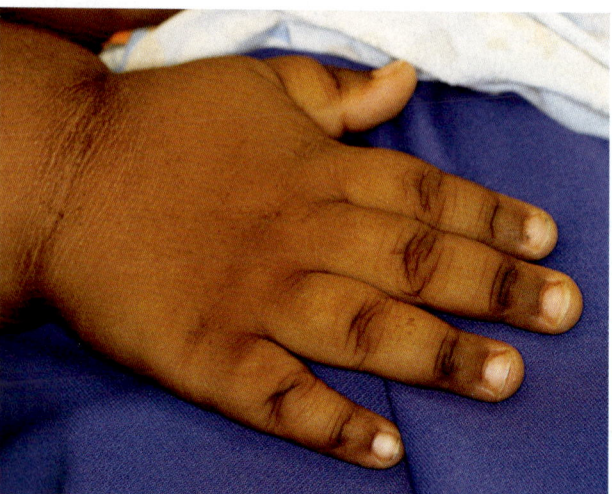

Figure 68.2. In this 4-year-old who had morbid obesity, changes of acanthosis nigricans were present in a diffuse pattern, including classic locations, as well as overlying the knuckles and in the wrist folds, as demonstrated here.

Look-alikes

Disorder	Differentiating Features
Postinflammatory hyperpigmentation	• Lacks the velvety texture of acanthosis nigricans.
Lichenification (ie, thickening of the skin) associated with chronic atopic or contact dermatitis	• Lacks the velvety texture of acanthosis nigricans. • Other features of atopic dermatitis often present. • Pruritus common (acanthosis nigricans not pruritic).

How to Make the Diagnosis

▶ The diagnosis is made clinically based on the clinical appearance (ie, velvety thickening of skin) in typical locations.

Treatment

▶ Evaluate patient for underlying cause based on history and physical examination.
  - Evaluate the patient for the possibility of type 2 diabetes and hyperlipidemia.
  - Consider obtaining an insulin level or other endocrinologic testing if the patient does not have obesity.

▶ Treatment of acanthosis nigricans is difficult and often unsatisfactory.
  - Consider application of keratolytic preparation (ie, one containing lactic or salicylic acid) or a retinoid.
  - Extensive acanthosis nigricans may benefit from carbon dioxide laser resurfacing.
  - If otherwise indicated, metformin may improve acanthosis due to reduced insulin resistance.
  - Changes often (but not always) improve with weight loss (and resultant improved insulin sensitivity).

Treating Associated Conditions

▶ If an underlying disorder is identified in a patient who has acanthosis nigricans, it should be managed appropriately.

▶ Acanthosis nigricans is an important marker for insulin resistance, hyperlipidemia, and metabolic syndrome.

Prognosis

- Familial acanthosis nigricans has an excellent prognosis.
- If associated with other disorders, the prognosis depends on the other conditions and is variable.

When to Worry or Refer

- Consider referral to a nutritionist or consultation for management of associated conditions.

Resources for Families

- MedlinePlus: Information for patients and families (in English and Spanish) sponsored by the US National Library of Medicine and National Institutes of Health.
  https://www.nlm.nih.gov/medlineplus/ency/article/000852.htm
- Society for Pediatric Dermatology: Patient handout on acanthosis nigricans.
  https://pedsderm.net/for-patients-families/patient-handouts/#Acanthosis%20Nigricans
- WebMD: Information for families is contained in Skin Problems and Treatments.
  www.webmd.com/skin-problems-and-treatments/acanthosis-nigricans-overview

CHAPTER 69

Acquired Melanocytic Nevi

Introduction/Etiology/Epidemiology

- Acquired melanocytic nevi are common.
- Begin to appear after 2 to 3 years of age.
- Increase in number and reach a peak during the third decade.
- Often disappear with advancing age.

Signs and Symptoms

- Pigmented macules, papules, and plaques with variable surface changes.
- Sometimes classified based on appearance.
  - Junctional nevus: uniformly hyperpigmented (often brown) macule (Figure 69.1).
  - Compound nevus: uniformly hyperpigmented (often brown) slightly elevated papule (Figure 69.2).
  - Intradermal nevus: often light brown to flesh-colored and elevated (Figure 69.3).
- Variants of acquired nevi
  - Halo nevi
    - Acquired nevi that develop a surrounding ring of hypopigmentation or depigmentation (Figure 69.4).
    - Likely represents an immunologic response to melanocytes; often coexists with vitiligo (and may precede or follow this diagnosis).
    - Nearly always benign in children; refer for evaluation if the ring of hypopigmentation is incomplete or the nevus is atypical using ABCDE criteria (see When to Worry or Refer section).
    - Nevus and hypopigmentation ultimately resolve.

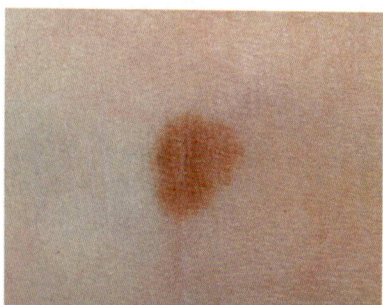

Figure 69.1. Junctional nevus.

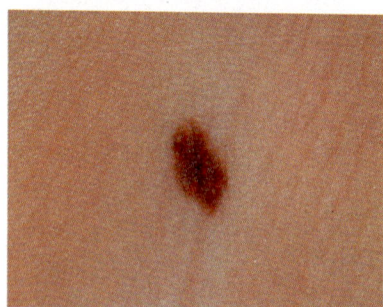

Figure 69.2. Compound nevus.

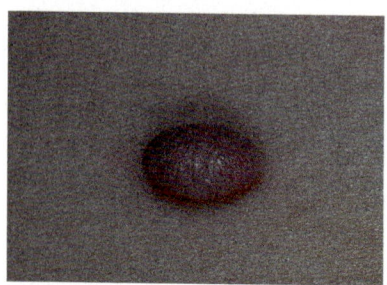

Figure 69.3. Intradermal nevus.

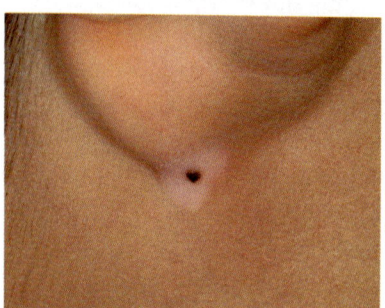

Figure 69.4. A halo nevus is an acquired nevus with a ring of surrounding hypopigmentation or depigmentation.

- Atypical nevi
  - Often larger (5–12 mm) than common acquired nevi; have irregular and ill-defined borders (Figure 69.5).
  - Color often is variegated with shades of brown, tan, or pink (Figure 69.6).
  - Individuals who have large numbers of atypical nevi or those who have a family history of melanoma in first-degree relatives have an increased risk of developing melanoma.
- "Eclipse" nevi
  - Nevus with central elevation simulating the appearance of a sunny-side up fried egg (see Figure 69.6).
  - Periphery often darker compared with the lighter central portions.
  - This phenotype is common on the scalps of older children and teenagers, and these nevi tend to behave in benign fashion.

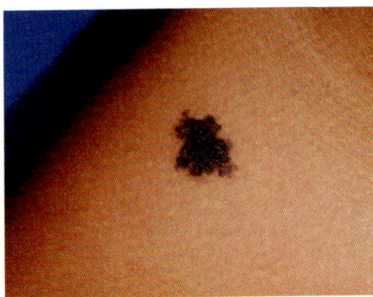

Figure 69.5. Atypical nevi are often larger (often 5–12 mm in diameter) and have irregular borders.

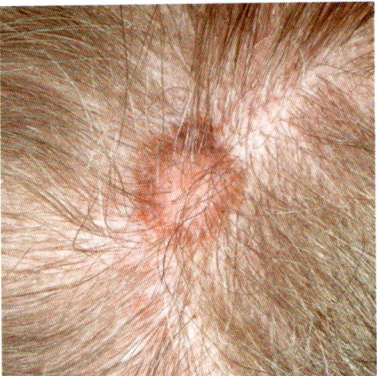

Figure 69.6. This benign "eclipse" nevus reveals pink and brown color; the lighter center is elevated, causing the lesion to have the appearance of a sunny-side up fried egg.

Look-alikes

Disorder	Differentiating Features
Ephelides	• Small, hyperpigmented macules located in sun-exposed areas such as the face, upper chest, shoulders, and back. • Become darker following sun exposure. • Often fade when sun exposure is minimal. • Unlike melanocytic nevi, have no change in surface texture. • No malignancy potential.
Lentigines	• Small, hyperpigmented macules not limited to sun-exposed areas. • Unlike melanocytic nevi, have no change in surface texture. • No malignancy potential.
Café au lait macules	• Hyperpigmented macules that are not elevated and have no change in surface texture; most often tan in color. • Typically larger than acquired melanocytic nevi. • No malignancy potential.

How to Make the Diagnosis

▶ The diagnosis is made clinically based on the typical appearance of acquired nevi.

Treatment

▶ Benign-appearing nevi that are asymptomatic do not require removal.

▶ Rapidly changing, symptomatic, or significantly atypical nevi must be assessed for possible malignant transformation.

Treating Associated Conditions

▶ Familial atypical mole/melanoma syndrome should be considered in a patient who has atypical (ie, dysplastic) moles and several family members with atypical (ie, dysplastic) nevi and at least one relative with melanoma. These patients require close surveillance to assess for the development of melanoma.

Prognosis

- Ordinary acquired nevi are typically inconsequential (unless in a cosmetically compromising region); however, all nevi should be monitored using ABCDE criteria (see When to Worry or Refer section).
- Atypical nevi may imply an increased risk for the development of melanoma.

When to Worry or Refer

- Melanoma is the malignant neoplasm of melanocytes that may arise de novo or from preexisting nevus. Consider the possibility of melanoma when a nevus exhibits any of the following ABCDE criteria:
  - *A*symmetry
  - *B*order irregularity
  - *C*olor variation (especially red, blue, black)
  - *D*iameter larger than about 6 mm
  - *E*volving lesion that is changing quickly
- Recently, it has been suggested that applying these traditional ABCDE criteria in addition to modified ABCD criteria may facilitate earlier detection of melanoma in children. The modified ABCD criteria (and explanation) are as follows:
  - *A*melanotic (as pediatric melanoma may be nonpigmented).
  - *B*leeding, bump (bleeding lesions; lumps or bumps [ie, papulonodules or papules]).
  - *C*olor uniformity (as the color may be consistent and uniform throughout the lesion).
  - *D*e novo, any diameter (new papular lesions; lesions may be <6 mm).
- Refer patients who have atypical nevi and a family history of atypical nevi or melanoma to a dermatologist.
- Refer patients who have atypical-appearing halo nevi (eg, those with an incomplete ring of hypopigmentation or depigmentation or an atypical appearance according to ABCDE criteria) to a dermatologist.

Resources for Families

- American Academy of Dermatology: Diseases and conditions (search options include "moles" and "melanoma").
  https://www.aad.org/public/diseases
- Society for Pediatric Dermatology: Patient handout on moles and melanoma.
  https://pedsderm.net/for-patients-families/patient-handouts/#Anchor-Moles

CHAPTER 70

Café au Lait Macules

Introduction/Etiology/Epidemiology

- Isolated café au lait macules (also known as café au lait spots) occurs in up to 2% of all infants and 10% of Black infants.
- The frequency of café au lait macules in older children is estimated at 13% for white and 27% for Black children.
- Small, solitary lesions are inconsequential, whereas multiple or large lesions may signal a syndromic association.

Signs and Symptoms

- Tan, homogeneous macules with well-defined borders (Figures 70.1, 70.2, and 70.3).

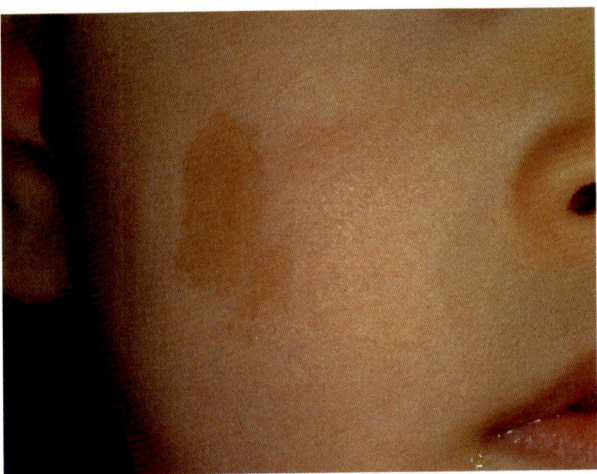

Figure 70.1. Café au lait macule on the face.

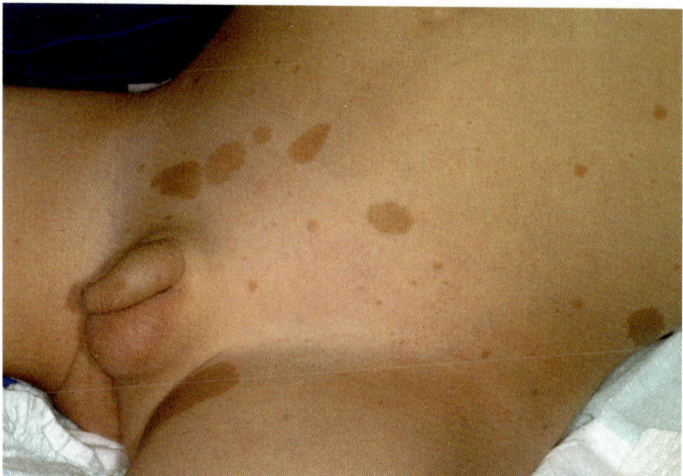

Figure 70.2. Multiple café au lait macules in a child who has neurofibromatosis type 1.

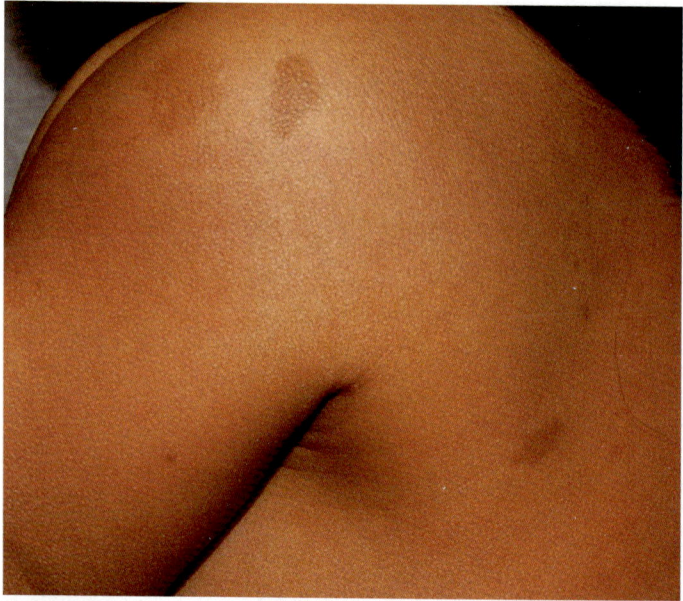

Figure 70.3. Multiple café au lait macules in a child with skin of color. The lesions are somewhat darker than in individuals with a lighter skin tone.

Look-alikes

Disorder	Differentiating Features
Ephelides (freckles)	• Small (typically smaller than café au lait macules), hyperpigmented macules in sun-exposed areas.
Lentigines	• Small (typically smaller than café au lait macules), hyperpigmented macules that are not related to sun exposure.
Congenital melanocytic nevus	• Typically more deeply pigmented than café au lait macules. • Often slightly elevated and have a surface textural change. • Hypertrichosis within lesion is common.
Postinflammatory hyperpigmentation	• History of preceding inflammatory process. • Borders of lesions not well-defined.

How to Make the Diagnosis

▶ Diagnosis is made clinically based on the appearance of the macules or patches.

Treatment

▶ No treatment is needed for café au lait macules.

▶ Multiple or very large lesions suggest the need to investigate for possible associated conditions.

Treating Associated Conditions

Numerous disorders may be associated with multiple café au lait macules. Some of the more common are summarized here.

▶ Neurofibromatosis type 1 (see Chapter 89).
▶ McCune-Albright syndrome.
  ■ Large segmental café au lait macule or patch with very irregular (ie, "coast of Maine") borders; may be present at birth or develop later.
  ■ Bony variations.
    – Polyostotic fibrous dysplasia: replacement of bone with fibrous tissue resulting in asymmetry and pathologic fractures.
    – Bony lesions often are ipsilateral to café au lait macule.
  ■ Endocrine variations: precocious puberty (mainly in girls), hyperthyroidism, Cushing syndrome.

- Silver syndrome: triangular face, short stature, skeletal asymmetry, and atypical pubertal development.
- Bloom syndrome: short stature, facial telangiectasias and erythema, and characteristic facies (ie, narrow face, prominent nose and ears).
- Watson syndrome: café au lait macules, intellectual disability, axillary freckling, and pulmonic stenosis.

Prognosis

- Isolated café au lait macules persist and are harmless (and have no malignant potential).

When to Worry or Refer

- Refer or obtain consultation for patients who have multiple or large lesions or when clinical features suggest a possible associated syndrome.

CHAPTER 71

Congenital Melanocytic Nevi (CMN)

Introduction/Etiology/Epidemiology

- Congenital melanocytic nevi (CMN) are found at birth in about 1% of newborns.
- CMN have an increased risk of malignant transformation.
  - The risk of malignant transformation in small (<1.5 cm) congenital nevi is quite low and considered by most experts to be no greater than the baseline risk of malignant melanoma in the general population.
  - The risk of malignant transformation in medium (1.5–20 cm), large (>20–40 cm), or "giant" (>40 cm) congenital nevi is higher than the baseline risk in the general population but difficult to quantify; some studies of giant congenital nevi have estimated this risk to be as high as 10% to 15%.
  - Importantly, a substantial number of the melanomas arising within a large or giant congenital melanocytic nevus may occur in the central nervous system, rather than the skin.

Signs and Symptoms

- CMN usually are present at birth but may appear during the first 6 months after birth.
- Most lesions are small (<1.5 cm in diameter). Large CMN occur in about 1 in 20,000 newborns and giant CMN in around 1 in 500,000 newborns.
  - Congenital nevi are typically larger than acquired nevi and have significant hair growth within them (Figure 71.1).
  - They are usually slightly elevated and have surface texture changes (Figure 71.2).
- Occasionally, lesions are larger, measuring 20 cm or more (Figure 71.3).
- Large and giant CMN are often accompanied by satellite lesions (Figure 71.4).

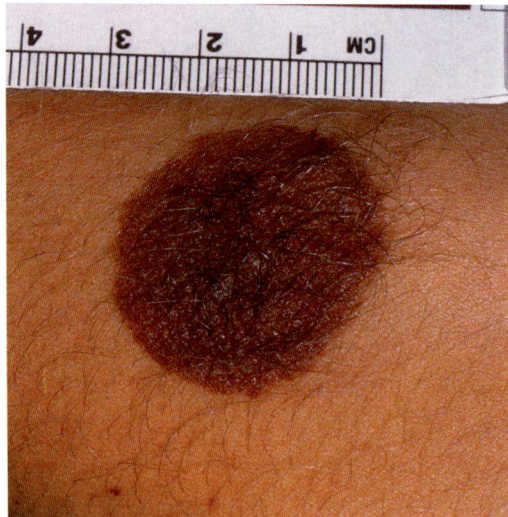

Figure 71.1. Congenital melanocytic nevus with superimposed hypertrichosis.

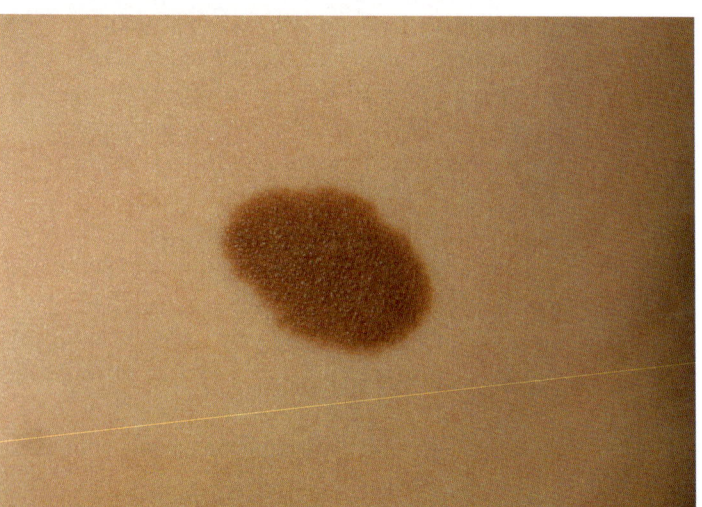

Figure 71.2. Congenital melanocytic nevus demonstrating surface textural change.

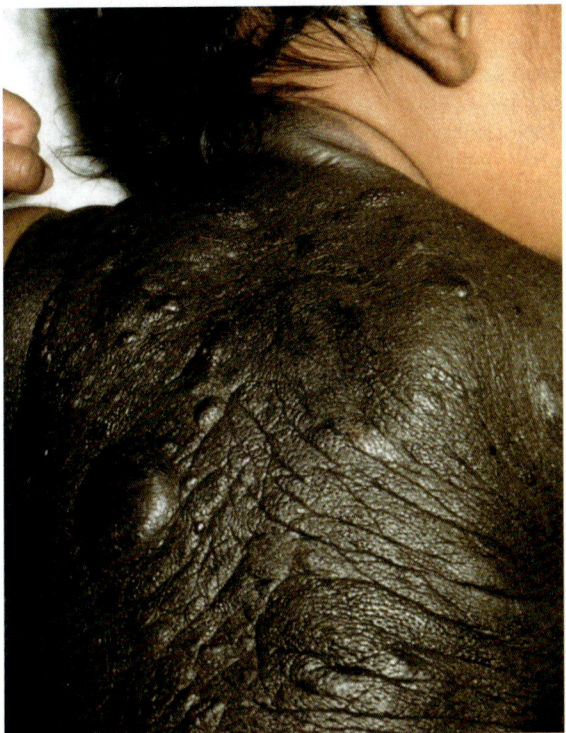

Figure 71.3. A giant congenital melanocytic nevus involving the entire posterior trunk.

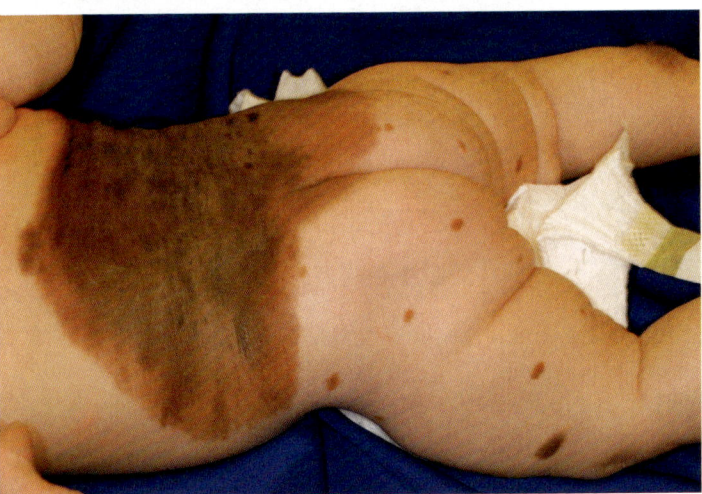

Figure 71.4. A large congenital melanocytic nevus involving the posterior trunk. There are multiple satellite nevi present as well.

Look-alikes

Disorder	Differentiating Features
Ephelides	• Small, hyperpigmented macules located in sun-exposed areas such as the face, upper chest, and back. • Ephelides become darker after sun exposure and may lighten during times of less sun exposure. • Unlike congenital melanocytic nevi (CMN), have no change in surface texture, hypertrichosis, or malignancy potential.
Lentigines	• Small, hyperpigmented macules not limited to sun-exposed areas. • Unlike CMN, have no change in surface texture, hypertrichosis, or malignancy potential.
Café au lait macules	• Hyperpigmented macules that are not elevated and have no change in surface texture, hypertrichosis, or malignancy potential.
Becker melanosis (Becker nevus)	• Hyperpigmented patch usually distributed on the upper trunk of adolescents. • No increased malignancy potential.
Plexiform neurofibroma	• May present with "bag of worms" consistency on palpation (representing enlarged nerve roots). • May be associated with pain, atrophy, muscle loss. • Risk of malignant degeneration into malignant peripheral nerve sheath tumor. • Associated with neurofibromatosis type 1 (considered one of the diagnostic criteria) (see also Chapter 89).

How to Make the Diagnosis

▶ The diagnosis is made clinically based on the history and typical appearance of the lesion.

Treatment

▶ Small CMN that are asymptomatic and not changing may be observed or excised at puberty (malignant change before puberty is extraordinarily rare).

▶ Infants who have larger lesions should be referred to a plastic surgeon for discussion of possible excision and to a dermatologist for clinical surveillance (if not excised).

Treating Associated Conditions

▶ Infants with extensive CMN on the head or overlying the midline of the back, and especially in those with large numbers of satellite nevi, are at risk of central nervous system involvement (ie, neurocutaneous melanosis). Magnetic resonance imaging of the brain and spinal cord should be performed.

Prognosis

▶ Medium, large, and giant CMN are at increased risk of melanoma development and should be considered for excision, when feasible.
▶ Close clinical follow-up for atypical progression (eg, ulceration, new nodular components, bleeding, color change) with biopsy of suspicious areas is vital for patients who have not had such larger congenital nevi excised.

When to Worry or Refer

▶ Melanoma is the malignant neoplasm of melanocytes that may arise de novo or from preexisting nevi. Consider the possibility of melanoma when a CMN exhibits any of the following ABCDE criteria:
  - *A*symmetry.
  - *B*order irregularity.
  - *C*olor variation (especially red, blue, black).
  - *D*iameter larger than about 6 mm (but this criterion is less useful for CMN, as they are often larger than this very early after birth).
  - *E*volving lesion that is changing quickly.
▶ Recently, it has been suggested that applying these traditional ABCDE criteria *in addition to* modified ABCD criteria may facilitate earlier detection of melanoma in children. The modified ABCD criteria (and explanation) are as follows:
  - *A*melanotic (as pediatric melanoma may be nonpigmented).
  - *B*leeding, *b*ump (bleeding lesions; lumps or bumps [ie, papulonodules or papules]).
  - *C*olor uniformity (as the color may be consistent and uniform throughout the lesion).
  - *D*e novo, any *d*iameter (*new* papular lesions; lesions may be <6 mm).
▶ Patients with CMN that are medium, large, or giant in size or which show atypical features or any symptoms (eg, rapid evolution, nonhealing sores or bleeding) should be referred for prompt dermatologic evaluation.

Resources for Families

- American Academy of Pediatrics: HealthyChildren.org.
  https://www.healthychildren.org/English/ages-stages/baby/bathing-skin-care/Pages/Your-Newborns-Skin-Birthmarks-and-Rashes.aspx
- Nevus Network: Provides support and information for patients who have congenital nevi.
  www.nevusnetwork.org
- Nevus Outreach: Provides support and information for patients who have large nevi or neurocutaneous melanosis.
  www.nevus.org
- Society for Pediatric Dermatology: Patient handout on CMN.
  https://pedsderm.net/for-patients-families/patient-handouts/#CongenitalNevus

CHAPTER
72

Ephelides

Introduction/Etiology/Epidemiology

- Ephelides (freckles) most often occur in white children and adults with fair skin and red hair.

Signs and Symptoms

- Small, red to tan (≤5 mm) macules without change in skin surface markings (Figure 72.1).
- Located on sun-exposed areas such as the face, upper chest, and back; do not occur on mucous membranes.
- Darken in summer and lighten during winter.

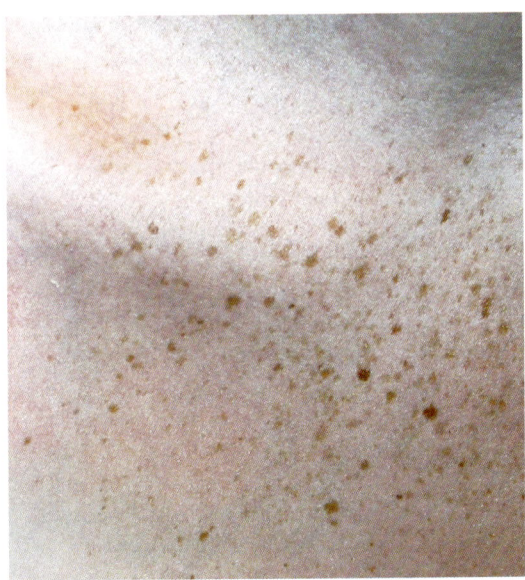

Figure 72.1. Ephelides (freckles) are small tan or red macules that appear in sun-exposed areas.

Look-alikes

Disorder	Differentiating Features
Café au lait macules	• Hyperpigmented macules typically larger than ephelides and not limited to sun-exposed areas.
Lentigines	• Small, hyperpigmented macules not limited to sun-exposed areas.
Melanocytic nevi	• Typically more deeply pigmented than ephelides. • Often slightly elevated and have surface textural change.

How to Make the Diagnosis

▶ The diagnosis is made clinically based on the appearance of the lesions.

Treatment

▶ Photoprotection, including the use of sunscreen.
▶ If desired for cosmetic reasons, laser therapy may be considered.

Prognosis

▶ Lesions persist and darken with sun exposure.

When to Worry or Refer

▶ An ephelis that suddenly grows or turns black in color (may represent transforming junctional nevus rather than an ephelis).
▶ Numerous ephelides early after birth after sun exposure, especially if history of severe sunburn reactions (could represent xeroderma pigmentosum or other photosensitivity disorder).

CHAPTER
73

Lentigines

Introduction/Etiology/Epidemiology

- Lentigines are persistent macular areas of hyperpigmentation that can occur on any skin or mucosal surface, regardless of sun exposure.
- The incidence is unknown, but isolated lentigines appear to be very common.

Signs and Symptoms

- Lentigines are usually small (≤5 mm), hyperpigmented macules that mimic ephelides (ie, freckles).
  - Lentigines may be brown to black, are well-defined, and may be widely distributed (ie, not limited to sun-exposed areas).
  - Lesions do not become more apparent after sun exposure.
  - Isolated lentigines have no clinical significance.
- Multiple lentigines may be associated with systemic disorders; the most common of these are as follows:
  - LEOPARD syndrome: *LEOPARD* is an acronym for the major defects in this autosomal dominantly inherited disorder: *l*entigines, *e*lectrocardiographic abnormalities, *o*cular hypertelorism, *p*ulmonic stenosis, *a*bnormal genitalia, *r*etarded (delayed) growth, and sensorineural *d*eafness (Figure 73.1).
  - Peutz-Jeghers syndrome: autosomal dominant disorder consisting of face, lip, and oral mucosa lentigines associated with benign intestinal polyposis (Figure 73.2). These patients may also have lentigines on the fingers, toes, palms, and soles.
  - Lentiginosis with cardiocutaneous myxomas consists of multiple lentigines associated with cardiac and subcutaneous myxomas. Disorders considered within this disease category include the following:
    - Carney complex: lentigines, cardiac and other myxomas, and endocrine tumors.

- LAMB syndrome: *l*entigines, *a*trial myxomas, *m*ucocutaneous myxomas, and *b*lue nevi.
- NAME syndrome: *n*evi, *a*trial myxomas, *m*yxoid neurofibromas, ephelides, and *e*ndocrine neoplasia.

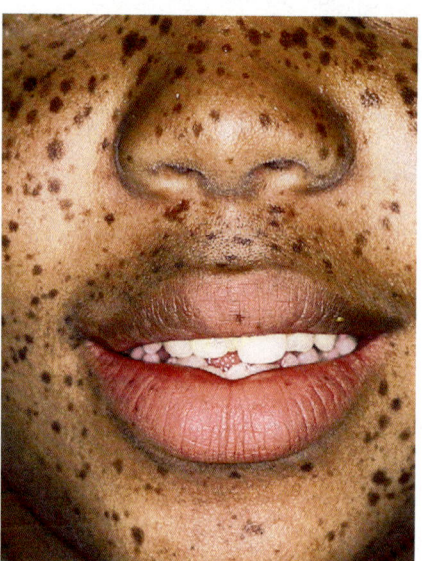

Figure 73.1. Patient with LEOPARD syndrome. Multiple lentigines with relative sparing of the mucous membranes. Reproduced with permission from Cohen BA. *Pediatric Dermatology.* 3rd ed. Mosby; 2005:144.

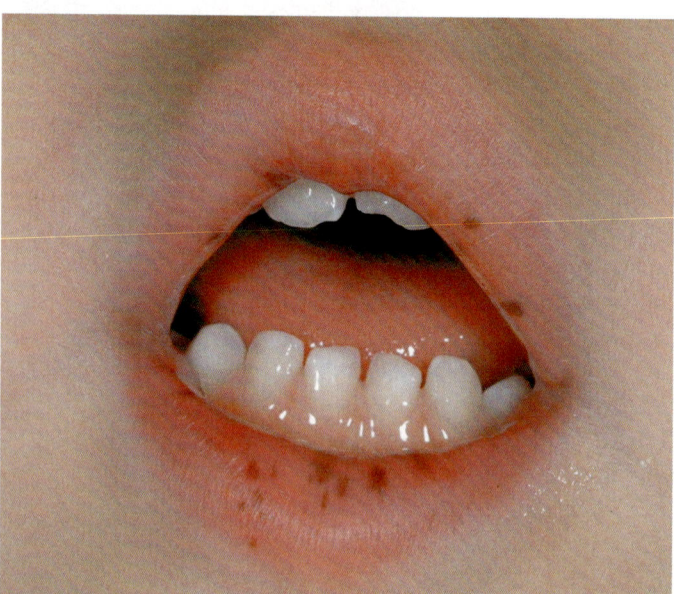

Figure 73.2. In Peutz-Jeghers syndrome, lentigines appear on the face, lips, and oral mucosa. They are associated with gastrointestinal polyposis.

Look-alikes

Disorder	Differentiating Features
Ephelides	• Small, hyperpigmented macules located in sun-exposed areas such as face, upper chest, and back. • Unlike lentigines, ephelides become darker after sun exposure and often fade in absence of sun (ie, winter months).
Café au lait macules	• Hyperpigmented macules typically larger than lentigines.
Labial melanotic macule	• Small (1–8 mm), brown to dark brown or black macule. • Most often on the lower lip; typically solitary (Figure 73.3).
Melanocytic nevi	• Typically more deeply pigmented than lentigines. • Often slightly elevated and have surface textural change. • May develop hypertrichosis.

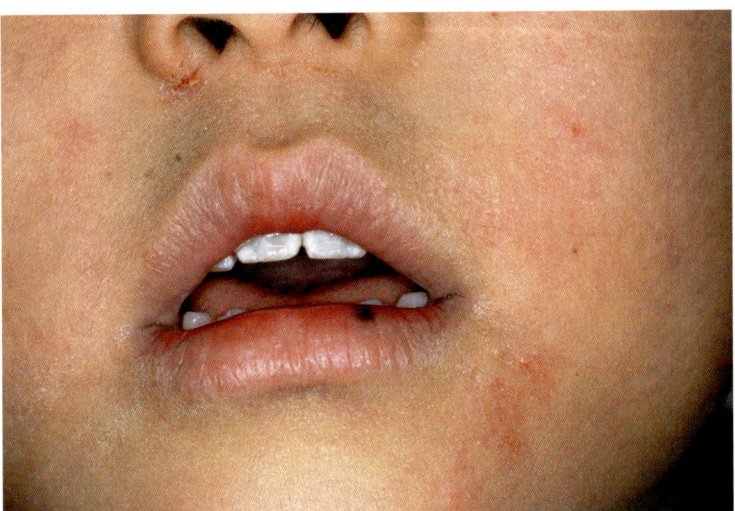

Figure 73.3. Labial melanotic macule. Small, dark brown, solitary macule on the left side of the lower lip of a young child with eczema.

How to Make the Diagnosis

▶ The diagnosis is made clinically on the basis of the appearance and distribution (ie, not limited to sun-exposed areas) of lesions.

Treatment

- Lentigines do not require treatment unless desired for cosmetic reasons.
- Identification of multiple lentiginosis syndromes is of paramount importance.

Treating Associated Conditions

- If multiple lentigines are present, assess for clinical features of an associated syndrome (eg, LEOPARD, Peutz-Jeghers, lentiginosis with cardiocutaneous myxomas) and consider dermatology and genetics referral.
- If multiple lentigines without mucosal lentigines, consider electrocardiography, echocardiography, hearing test, endocrine evaluation.
- If multiple lentigines including mucosal lentigines, consider referral to gastroenterology.

Prognosis

- Excellent if isolated lentigines. Lesions that appear early in life may fade or spontaneously resolve.
- Presence of an associated syndrome alters prognosis.

When to Worry or Refer

- Multiple or mucosal lentigines are observed (may indicate the presence of an associated disorder).

CHAPTER 74

Congenital Dermal Melanocytosis

Introduction/Etiology/Epidemiology

- The most common form of cutaneous hyperpigmentation seen in neonates.
- Common in newborns of color; occurs in approximately 90% of Black and Native American, 80% of Asian, 70% of Hispanic, and 10% of white neonates.
- Underlying disease is dermal melanocytosis (spindle-shaped melanocytes located in the dermis, likely as the result of arrested migration from the neural crest during embryogenesis).
- Formerly known as Mongolian spots.

Signs and Symptoms

- Slate gray macular pigment present at birth (Figure 74.1). Lesions may be single or multiple and vary in size.
- Common locations are the buttocks and mid-sacral area, but larger surfaces of the back, shoulders, and extremities may be involved (Figure 74.2).

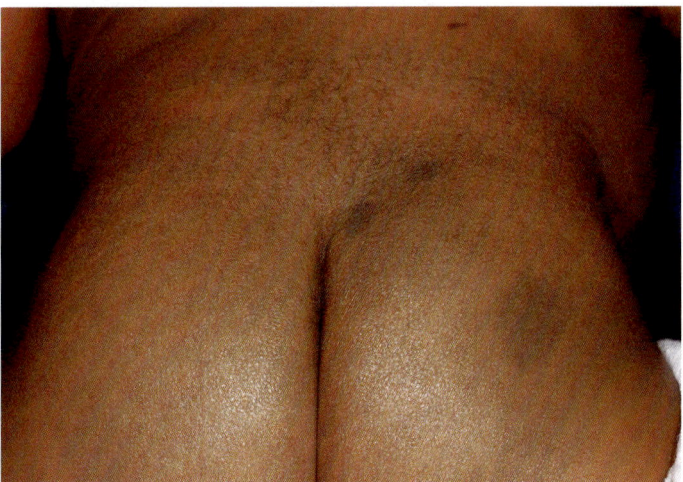

Figure 74.1. Congenital dermal melanocytosis. Blue-gray macules over the buttocks.

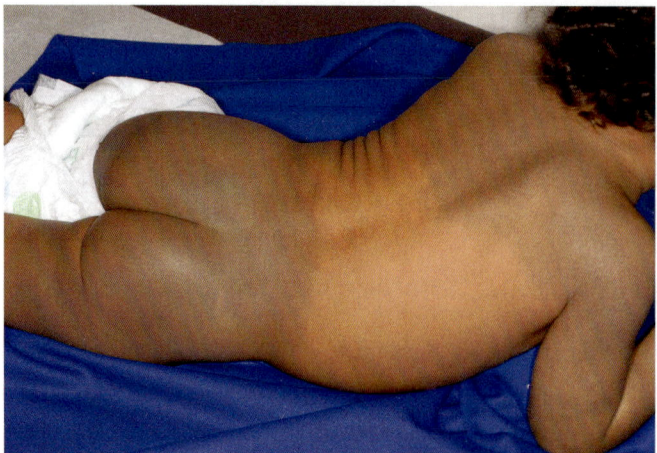

Figure 74.2. Congenital dermal melanocytosis. Blue-gray patches over the buttocks and upper back and extremity.

Look-alikes

Disorder	Differentiating Features
Nevus of Ota	• Blue-gray hyperpigmentation (also due to dermal melanocytosis) of skin surrounding the eye; usually present at birth. • Does not lighten or resolve with time. • Scleral hyperpigmentation may be present. • Distinction from congenital dermal melanocytosis based primarily on location and scleral involvement; histologic findings in these 2 conditions may have overlapping features.
Nevus of Ito	• Blue-gray hyperpigmentation (also due to dermal melanocytosis) that appears on shoulder. • Does not lighten or resolve with time. • Distinction from congenital dermal melanocytosis based primarily on location; histologic findings in these 2 conditions may have overlapping features.
Blue nevus	• Usually smaller than congenital dermal melanocytosis, with better-defined borders. • Usually solitary. • Does not resolve spontaneously with time.
Bruise	• History of trauma may be present. • Lesion typically tender to palpation. • Lesion evolves with typical color changes as erythrocytes degrade and eventually resolves.
Minocycline hyperpigmentation	• History of minocycline use. • Slate gray diffuse or focal hyperpigmentation. • Often involves the pretibial regions, sclerae/conjunctivae, and/or gingivae.

How to Make the Diagnosis

- The diagnosis is made clinically. The presence of congenital dermal melanocytosis should be documented in the medical record in the event concern is later raised that the lesions represent bruises.

Treatment

- No treatment is needed.

Prognosis

- Congenital dermal melanocytosis is a harmless condition, and the lesions often fade before adulthood.

When to Worry or Refer

- Extensive congenital dermal melanocytosis occasionally has been observed with GM_1 gangliosidosis or Hurler syndrome. Widespread lesions of congenital dermal melanocytosis associated with cutaneous vascular lesions may suggest a rare syndrome called *phakomatosis pigmentovascularis*.

Resources for Families

- American Academy of Pediatrics: HealthyChildren.org.
  https://www.healthychildren.org/birthmarks
- MedlinePlus: Information for patients and families (in English and Spanish) sponsored by the US National Library of Medicine and National Institutes of Health.
  https://www.nlm.nih.gov/medlineplus/ency/article/001472.htm
- Society for Pediatric Dermatology: Patient handout on dermal melanocytosis.
  https://pedsderm.net/for-patients-families/patient-handouts/#DermalMelanocytosis

CHAPTER 75

Melanonychia Striata

Introduction/Etiology/Epidemiology

- Pigmented band of the nail unit; also known as longitudinal melanonychia.
- May present at any age, including in children.
- Common in individuals with skin of color, especially Black individuals (present in up to 77%, with nearly 100% developing the finding by 50 years of age; often involves multiple digits); seen in up to 20% of Japanese individuals and approximately 1% of white individuals.
- Underlying disease may represent melanocytic activation or melanocytic hyperplasia.
- May represent either a benign (ie, lentigo or benign nevus) or malignant (ie, melanoma) process, despite similar clinical presentations in both settings.
- Approximately 5% to 10% of cases in adults result from a subungual melanoma; subungual melanoma as a cause for melanonychia is rare in children.

Signs and Symptoms

- Longitudinal, pigmented (tan, brown, dark brown, or black) streak of the nail plate (Figures 75.1 and 75.2).
- May or may not have associated nail deformity.
- Hutchinson sign (melanin pigmentation extends to skin and soft tissue proximal to the nail plate) is traditionally considered pathognomonic for subungual melanoma. However, noting some periungual pigmentation is not necessarily a positive Hutchinson sign; pseudo-Hutchinson sign (reflection of pigmentation through the cuticle/nail fold) is reported more frequently in pediatric patients.

▶ Other concerning features for malignancy include sudden or rapid change in the width of the pigmented band and irregular or blurred borders (see When to Worry or Refer section).

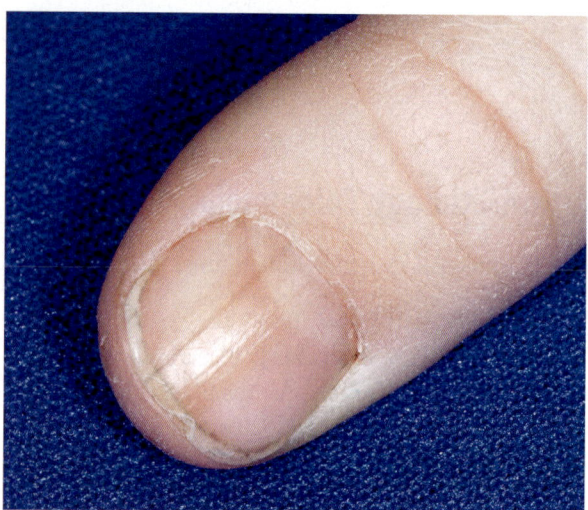

Figure 75.1. Solitary, well-demarcated, light tan longitudinal band of the thumb in an 8-year-old.

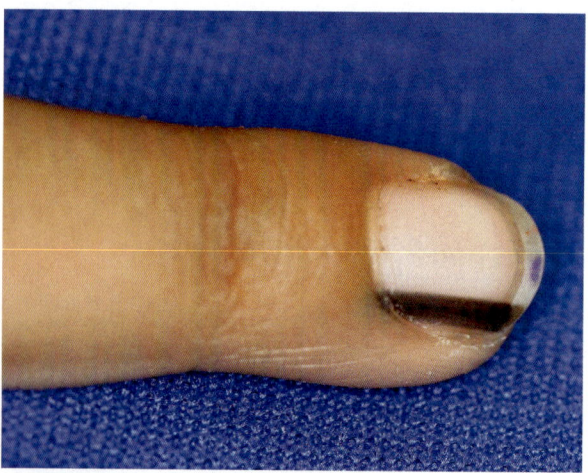

Figure 75.2. Very dark-brown linear streak on the index finger of a 5-year-old. This lesion continued to change and was eventually biopsied, revealing a benign nevus in the nail matrix area.

Look-alikes

Disorder	Differentiating Features
Physiologic melanonychia	• Commonly caused by chronic local nail trauma (ie, nail biting and cuticle trauma during a pedicure). • Other causes include pregnancy, certain drugs, some systemic diseases. • May affect multiple nails, especially in individuals with skin of color.
Onychomycosis	• Dermatophyte fungal infection of the nail plate. • May rarely be associated with partial or complete melanonychia of one or more nails. • Typically associated with a thickened nail plate that may separate from the nail bed, as well as yellow or white discoloration of nail plate. • Treatment for fungal infection results in reversal of nail discoloration.
Addison disease	• Adrenal insufficiency may darken skin, mucosae, and nails. • Longitudinal melanonychia can be the first (and occasionally only) sign of Addison disease. • Nail pigmentation disappears after treatment of the primary disease.
Laugier-Hunziker syndrome	• Idiopathic macular hyperpigmentation on mucosal lips (<5-mm macules typically), oral cavity, and nails. • Benign disease with no systemic involvement.
Peutz-Jeghers syndrome	• Combination of pigmentary macules (lips, around and inside mouth, perianal, hands, and feet) with predisposition toward intestinal hamartomatous polyposis. • Variation of the *SKT11* gene. • Melanonychia of one or multiple nails can rarely be seen. • Must evaluate for associated gastrointestinal polyps and other potential malignancies (with long-term surveillance).

How to Make the Diagnosis

▶ The diagnosis is typically made clinically based on the typical appearance of a pigmented longitudinal streak of the nail plate.

▶ The presence of multiple bands, as occasionally noted in patients with skin of color, is reassuring and typically lessens the likelihood of a malignant cause.

Treatment

▶ No treatment is necessary for benign melanonychia striata.

▶ Avoid trauma, as feasible.

▶ Rapid changes or sudden darkening in color must be assessed for possible malignant transformation.

- When there is a clinical concern for possible malignancy, biopsy of the nail matrix for histologic evaluation is indicated.
- Higher-grade atypical melanocytic lesions and melanoma are treated with complete surgical excision.

Prognosis

- Melanonychia striata has an excellent prognosis when caused by a benign nail matrix lesion such as lentigo or benign nevus.
- When subungual melanoma is present, the prognosis depends on a variety of histologic features as well as depth of the primary lesion.

When to Worry or Refer

- Refer patients who have melanonychia striata with atypical features or a family history of melanoma to a dermatologist for evaluation and follow-up; additional evaluations may include dermoscopy and/or nail matrix biopsy.
- Atypical features in melanonychia striata may include older age (older adults are at far greater risk for subungual melanoma than children are), rapid evolution, greater (>3 mm) width of the band, blurred borders, irregular pigmentation, extension of pigment onto adjacent skin (Hutchinson sign), having a mass under the nail plate (with lifting of the plate), bleeding or ulceration, and pain (if there is extension to bone).

Resources for Families

- Verywell Health: Brown line on nails: vitamin deficiencies and other medical causes.
  www.verywellhealth.com/what-is-longitudinal-melanonychia-1069479
- WebMD: Information for families is contained in Skin Problems and Treatments.
  https://www.webmd.com/skin-problems-and-treatments/what-to-know-melanonychia

CHAPTER 76

Pigmentary Mosaicism, Hyperpigmented

Introduction/Etiology/Epidemiology

- *Pigmentary mosaicism* is the term used to describe a group of disorders in which the skin has a patterned hypopigmentation or hyperpigmentation. In the hyperpigmented form discussed in this chapter, affected skin is darker than the background skin color.

- Pigmentary mosaicism is believed to be the result of genetic variations that create a population of cells with more or less pigment potential than the surrounding typical skin. *Mosaicism* refers to the coexistence of 2 genetically distinct populations of cells within the same individual.

- Pigmentary mosaicism may be localized or generalized.

- The terminology used to describe hyperpigmented pigmentary mosaicism is inconsistent. Terms such as *giant* or *segmental café au lait patch* or *spot*, *segmental pigmentation disorder*, *linear* and *whorled nevoid hypermelanosis*, and *patterned pigmentation* are present in the literature.

- In most cases, localized hyperpigmented pigmentary mosaicism is a benign and isolated finding. When more generalized, it may be associated with skeletal, ocular, or neurologic variations.

Signs and Symptoms

- Hyperpigmentation is noticed at birth or early in infancy, although its appreciation may be difficult to recognize in some young infants (who may initially present later, at 1–2 years of age). Affected areas are darker than the background skin color and may be more noticeable after sun exposure.

- One pattern of mosaic hyperpigmentation affects 1 or several large regions or segments of the body and has been termed, in some cases, *segmental pigmentation disorder* (Figure 76.1). Another typical pattern is whorled or linear bands (thin or broad) that follow the Blaschko lines (Figures 76.2 and 76.3). In some cases, patients may have a mixture of hypopigmentation and hyperpigmentation, making it difficult to determine the typical background skin type (Figure 76.4).

- Affected areas are typically sharply demarcated and often stop at the midline.

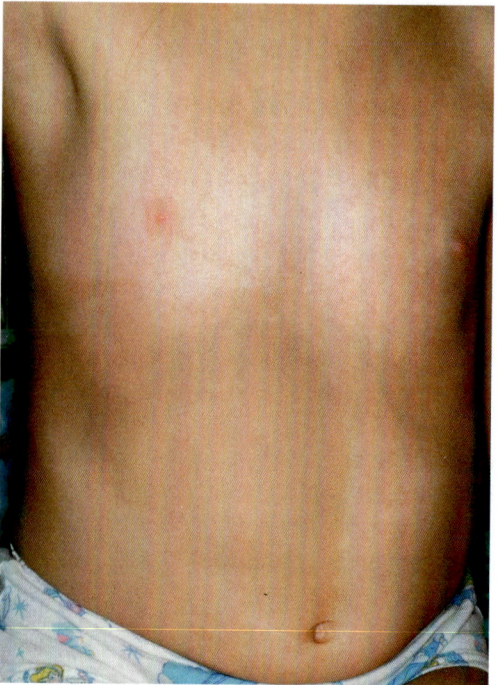

Figure 76.1. Pigmentary mosaicism, hyperpigmented type. This young child has a large hyperpigmented patch involving a large region of the right side of the abdomen (segmental pigmentation type).

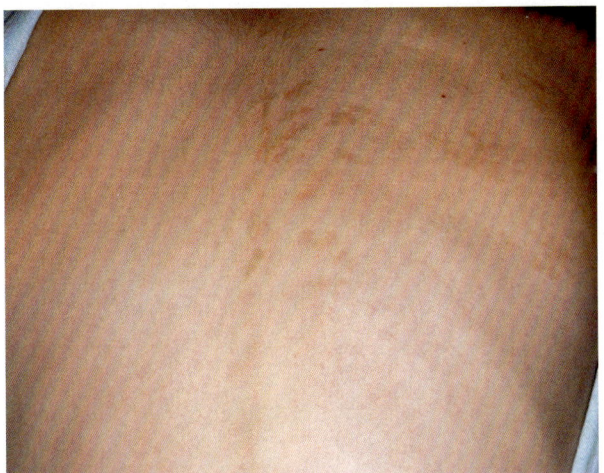

Figure 76.2. Pigmentary mosaicism, hyperpigmented type. This child has linear and curvilinear hyperpigmented patches that follow the Blaschko lines, limited to the right side of the upper back.

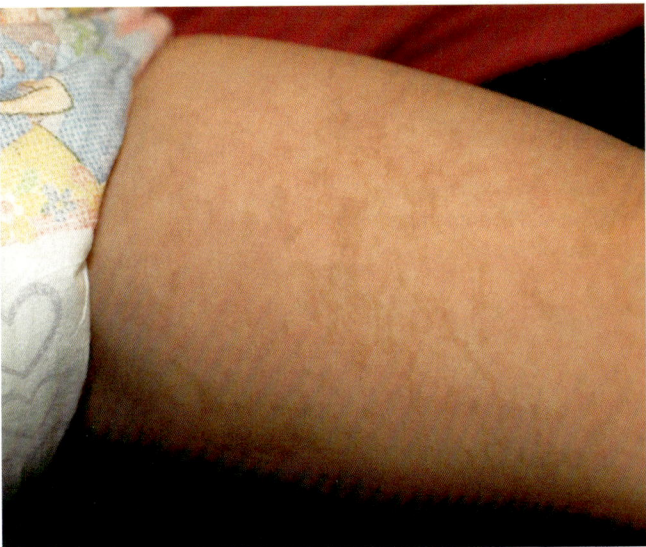

Figure 76.3. Pigmentary mosaicism, hyperpigmented type. There is an area of hyperpigmentation composed of coalescent shaggy-bordered macules and patches.

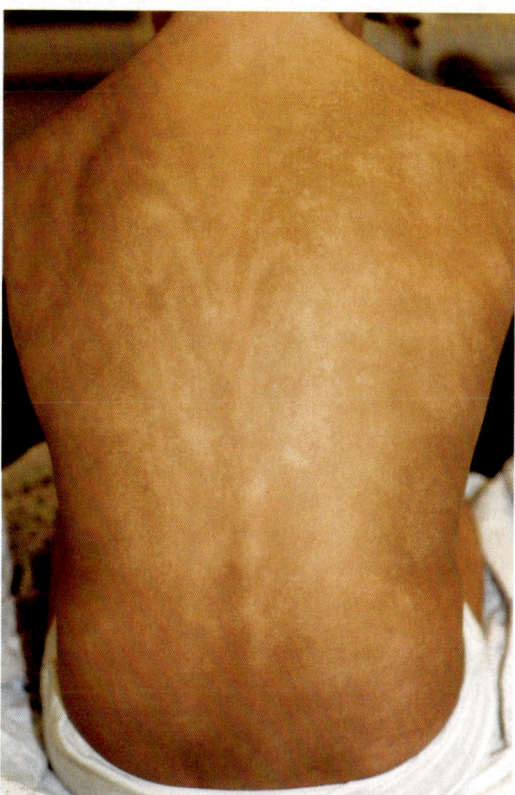

Figure 76.4. Pigmentary mosaicism with mixed pattern of hyperpigmentation and hypopigmentation that follows the Blaschko lines on the back.

Look-alikes

Disorder	Differentiating Features
McCune-Albright syndrome	• In addition to large café au lait patches with a "coast of Maine" (rough or shaggy-bordered) appearance (which may appear similar to segmental pigmentation type of pigmentary mosaicism), polyostotic fibrous dysplasia (often presenting as fractures) and endocrine hyperfunction (which may present as precocious puberty) are seen. • Skin and bone changes are typically unilateral (although this is also the case with localized pigmentary mosaicism).
Incontinentia pigmenti (third stage)	• X-linked dominant inheritance. • Vesicles are usually the initial presentation in newborn (first stage), distributed along the Blaschko lines. • Warty lesions (second stage) give rise to eventual hyperpigmentation (third stage) in a similar distribution pattern. • Associations may include dental, ophthalmologic, neurologic, and skeletal anomalies; irregular patches of scalp alopecia may also be present.
Becker nevus (pilar and smooth muscle hamartoma)	• An irregular hyperpigmented patch, plaque, or band occurring on the torso, often over the shoulder region. • Often presents or enlarges around the time of puberty. • Associated hypertrichosis and a pseudo-Darier sign (contraction of prominent arrector pili muscles) may be visible after stroking.
Plexiform neurofibroma (in neurofibromatosis type 1)	• In addition to hyperpigmentation, may have a "bag of worms" consistency at palpation. • May have overlying hypertrichosis. • Other signs of neurofibromatosis type 1 are present.

How to Make the Diagnosis

▶ The diagnosis of hyperpigmented pigmentary mosaicism is usually made based on history and physical examination.

▶ Consider a formal ophthalmologic examination to evaluate for ocular anomalies in children with the generalized type.

▶ If other malformations or neurodevelopmental variations are absent, further workup is not indicated. If they are present, consultation with the appropriate specialists is warranted.

▶ Rarely, karyotype analysis is performed (on blood or skin biopsy tissue) to search for chromosomal mosaicism.

Treatment

▶ There are no specific treatments for hyperpigmented pigmentary mosaicism.

Prognosis

▶ In most cases, hyperpigmented pigmentary mosaicism is a benign, isolated skin finding not associated with other medical concerns.

▶ In the rare patient who has generalized involvement, prognosis depends on the nature of any other organ variations.

When to Worry or Refer

▶ Referral to dermatologic examination is warranted when diagnosis is unclear.

▶ Referral to other specialists (eg, ophthalmology, neurology, genetics, orthopedics) is warranted when applicable.

Resources for Families

▶ American Academy of Pediatrics: HealthyChildren.org.
https://www.healthychildren.org/English/ages-stages/baby/bathing-skin-care/Pages/Your-Newborns-Skin-Birthmarks-and-Rashes.aspx

▶ Society for Pediatric Dermatology: Patient handout on pigmentary mosaicism.
https://pedsderm.net/for-patients-families/patient-handouts/#pigmentary%20mosaicism

Lumps and Bumps

CHAPTER 77 — **Cutaneous Mastocytosis** 509

CHAPTER 78 — **Dermoid Cysts** 517

CHAPTER 79 — **Epidermal Nevi** 521

CHAPTER 80 — **Granuloma Annulare** 525

CHAPTER 81 — **Juvenile Xanthogranuloma** 529

CHAPTER 82 — **Pilomatricoma** 533

CHAPTER 83 — **Spitz Nevus** 539

CHAPTER 77

Cutaneous Mastocytosis

Introduction/Etiology/Epidemiology

- Three types of disease
  - Solitary mastocytoma
  - Urticaria pigmentosa (also known as maculopapular cutaneous mastocytosis)
  - Diffuse cutaneous mastocytosis
- Increased number of mast cells present in the dermis in all forms.
- Most often occurs sporadically, although some reports of familial cases.
- In pediatric disease, most lesions appear prior to 2 years of age.

Signs and Symptoms

- Solitary mastocytoma (single lesion, Figures 77.1 and 77.2) and urticaria pigmentosa (multiple lesions, Figure 77.3) present as skin-colored, red to brown macules and papules.
- Some have a peau d'orange (orange peel–like) surface (see Figure 77.1).
- Children with diffuse cutaneous mastocytosis may have only a cobblestone or diffuse peau d'orange pattern noted of the skin.
- Lesions can occur on any part of the body.
- Infants may develop numerous blisters (bullous mastocytosis) (Figure 77.4).
- Darier sign is positive (the lesion urticates [becomes red and swollen] or blisters after stroking) (see Figure 77.2).
- As the lesions age, around teenage years to young adulthood, many mastocytomas will become just hyperpigmented macules.
- Macules can further resolve and leave typical-appearing skin.
- Systemic manifestations may include itching, flushing, headache, abdominal cramping, diarrhea, nausea, bone pain, and pulmonary symptoms (less common in pediatric disease). Anaphylaxis is rare.

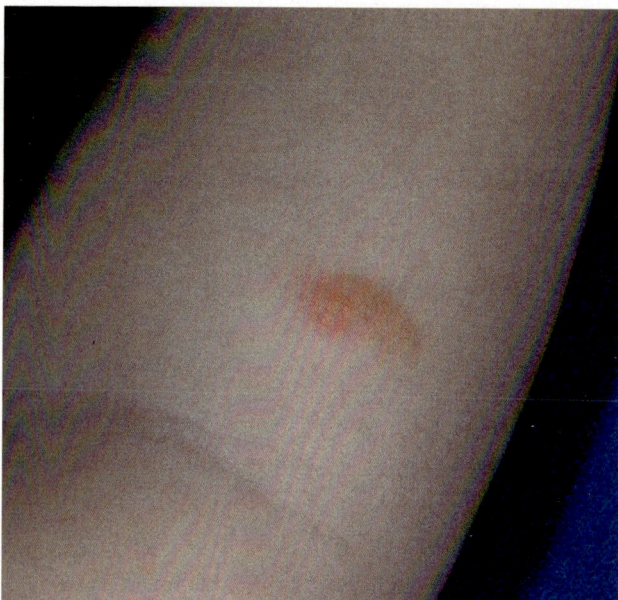

Figure 77.1. Solitary mastocytoma. A pink-orange plaque with a peau d'orange surface on the forearm of an infant.

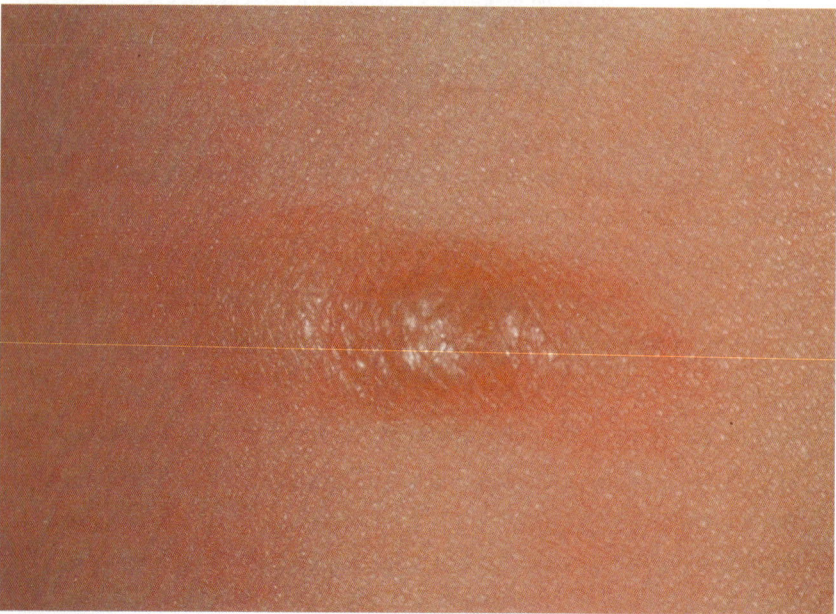

Figure 77.2. Mastocytoma with a positive Darier sign after stroking; the lesion has become red and more elevated.

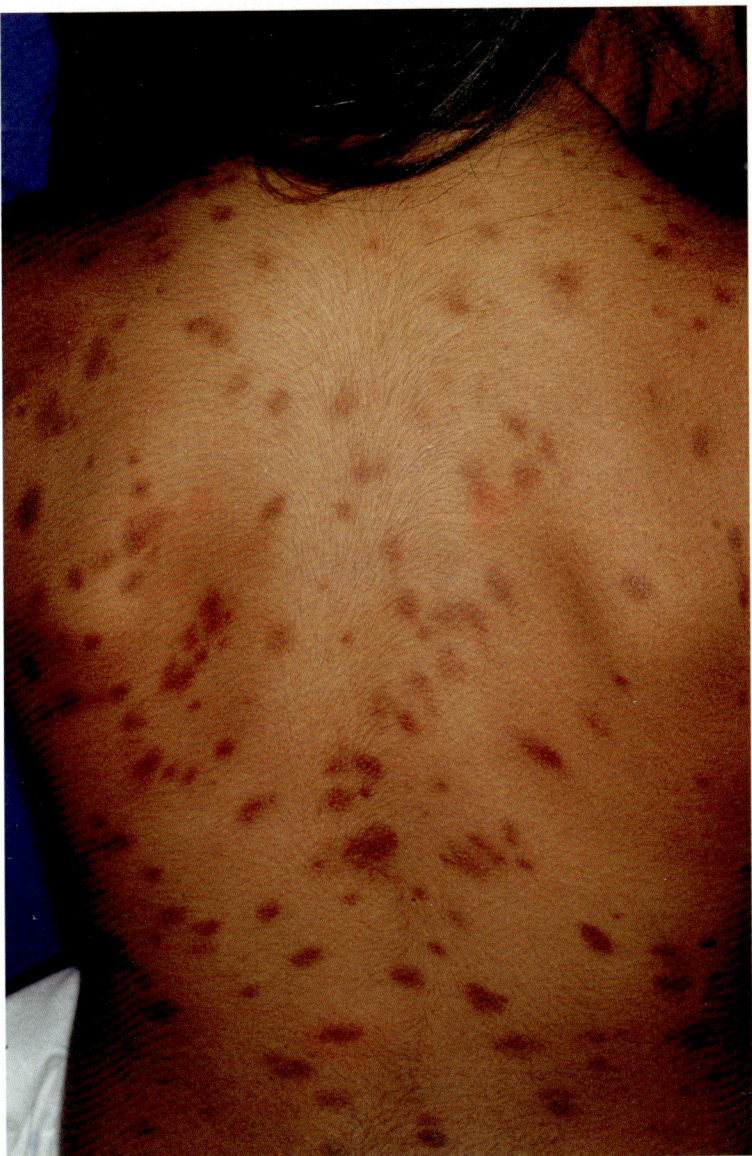

Figure 77.3. In urticaria pigmentosa, multiple hyperpigmented macules and papules are present. On close inspection, lesions have an orange peel–like (peau d'orange) appearance.

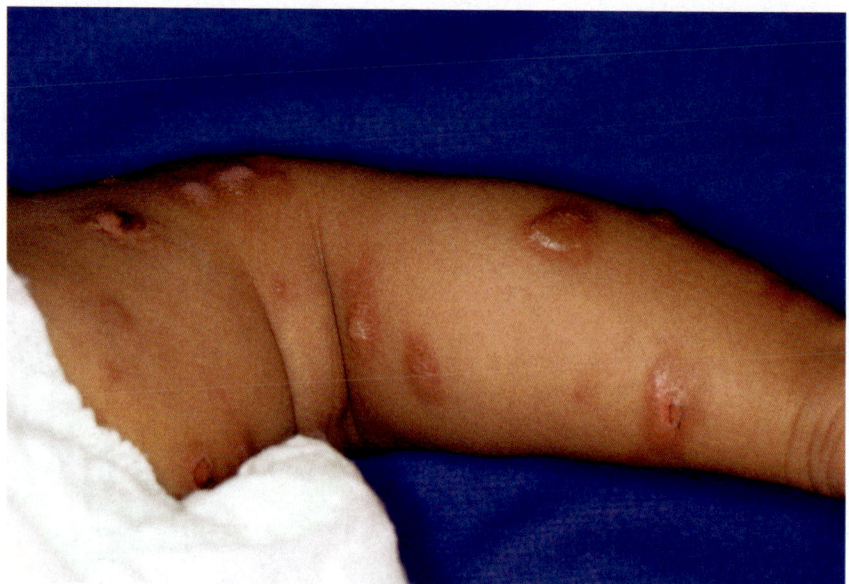

Figure 77.4. Bullous mastocytosis. This young infant with diffuse urticaria pigmentosa developed multiple vesicles and bullae, which eventually ceased to occur by around 3 years of age.

Look-alikes

Disorder	Differentiating Features
Solitary Mastocytoma	
Melanocytic nevus	• Negative Darier sign. • No peau d'orange surface appearance. • May have hypertrichosis. • May have dark-brown pigmentation.
Nevus sebaceus	• Most often located on the scalp. • Negative Darier sign. • May have a linear patterning. • Most prominent color of appearance is yellow.
Juvenile xanthogranuloma	• Negative Darier sign. • Most prominent color of appearance is yellow, although early lesions may be erythematous. • Dome-shaped papule or nodule.
Bullous impetigo	• Recurrent blistering in same location unusual. • Once resolved, no residual papule visible. • Bacterial culture result positive for *Staphylococcus aureus*.
Cutaneous herpes simplex virus infection	• Recurrent blistering may occur in same location but appears as clustered vesicles on background of erythema. • Tingling or pain commonly present before blisters appear. • May leave residual scarring, but no papular lesion. • Viral culture or polymerase chain reaction result positive for herpes simplex virus.
Urticaria Pigmentosa	
Urticaria	• Duration of each lesion is hours, with frequent waxing and waning. • After resolution the skin looks unremarkable, without residual hyperpigmentation or papules. • Blister formation does not typically occur.
Arthropod bites	• Often a central punctum is present on close inspection. • Pruritus common, often severe. • Lesions may be clustered in linear groupings. • Usually located on exposed areas of the body, with the exception of bedbug bites.
Nodular scabies	• Papules and nodules that persist after scabies infestation. • Darier sign only occasionally positive. • Lesions most common in flexures, on the penis and scrotum, or on the areolae. • Other family members may have a history of scabies infestation.
Café au lait macules/ neurofibromatosis	• Negative Darier sign. • Lesions are flat and non-palpable (and peau d'orange appearance is absent). • Axillary/inguinal freckling; neurofibromas may be present in those who have neurofibromatosis type 1.

How to Make the Diagnosis

- The diagnosis is usually based on clinical findings.
- Positive Darier sign (in appropriate clinical setting) is confirmatory.
- Skin biopsy reveals increased mast cells in the dermis (confirmed by special stains).

Treatment

- Below are possible triggers to potentially avoid, which may cause mast cell degranulation (avoidance usually not necessary with solitary lesions). It is important to note that items on this list will not necessarily cause a reaction in all affected individuals.
  - Heat (eg, hot baths) or overly cold exposures
  - Pressure or other physical stimuli
  - Aspirin
  - Alcohol
  - Ibuprofen
  - Codeine and morphine
  - Certain anesthetic agents
  - Radiocontrast dye
- Topical corticosteroids may occasionally be useful for solitary mastocytoma to decrease inflammation and bulla formation.
- Antihistamines may decrease urtication, minimize blister formation, and improve systemic symptoms.
  - A nonsedating H_1 antagonist-type antihistamine (eg, loratadine, cetirizine, levocetirizine, fexofenadine) is helpful as a first-line agent.
  - For those whose symptoms do not improve or are severe, consider adding one of the following:
    - Sedating H_1 antihistamine (eg, hydroxyzine, cyproheptadine): these may be administered at bedtime to avoid daytime sedation.
    - In severe disease, an H_2 receptor antagonist may also be useful in conjunction with H_1 blockers.
- Oral cromolyn sodium may be useful for associated gastrointestinal symptoms.
- Surgery can be considered for solitary lesions in an accessible location, when clinically indicated or requested.
- Pimecrolimus cream and biologic agents have also been reported as useful.

Prognosis

- The prognosis for solitary mastocytoma and pediatric urticaria pigmentosa is excellent, with resolution occurring in most (but not all) patients over several years.
- The resolution of diffuse cutaneous mastocytosis or familial mastocytosis is not as predictable.

When to Worry or Refer

- Consider referral to a dermatologist for patients who have severe or extensive disease, in whom the diagnosis is in question, or in whom standard treatment is not effective.

Resources for Families

- The Mast Cell Disease Society: Provides information for patients, families, and medical professionals.
  https://tmsforacure.org
- Mastokids: Provides information and support for patients who have pediatric mastocytosis and their families.
  www.mastokids.org
- Society for Pediatric Dermatology: Patient handout on mastocytosis.
  https://pedsderm.net/for-patients-families/patient-handouts/#Mastocytosis

CHAPTER 78

Dermoid Cysts

Introduction/Etiology/Epidemiology

- Developmental epithelium-lined cysts that result from entrapment along the lines of embryonic closure.
- In contrast with epithelial cysts, dermoid cysts may have appendageal elements, including hair follicles, in addition to keratin.
- They are present at birth, although they may not become clinically apparent until later.
- These developmental remnants are distinct from dermoids of the ovary (ovarian teratomas) and do not contain multiple tissues such as teeth, bone, or thyroid.

Signs and Symptoms

- Dermoid cysts most commonly occur on the head or face; the most common location is on the orbital ridge, often the outer third of the eyebrow (Figures 78.1 and 78.2).
- They may also occur in the nasal midline (glabella, dorsal aspect of the nose) and on the scalp.
- Midline lesions may be associated with deep extension and, occasionally, central nervous system communication.
- Some lesions reveal an overlying central punctum or sinus, and protruding hairs may be present; with midline lesions, the presence of an overlying pit may suggest a higher risk for intracranial extension.
- Dermoid cysts are most often solitary, non-tender, and mobile; the overlying epidermis is usually unremarkable in appearance.

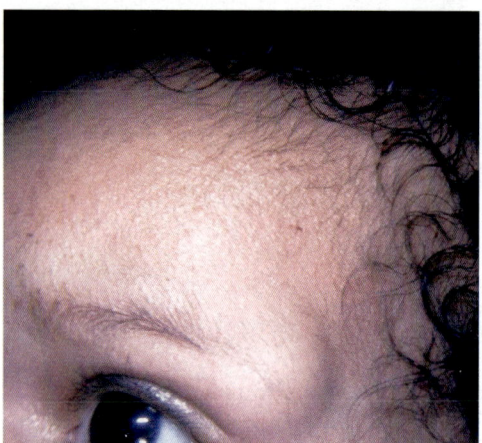

Figure 78.1. Dermoid cyst of the lateral eyebrow in a 3-week-old.

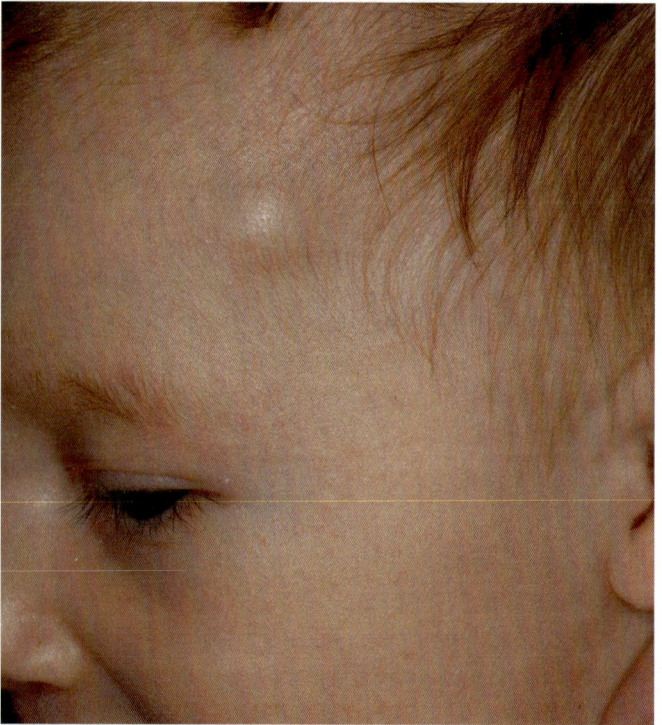

Figure 78.2. Dermoid cyst on the mid-lateral forehead in a 2-month-old.

Look-alikes

Disorder	Differentiating Features
Other epithelial cysts	• More common in adolescents and adults. • Usually acquired, rather than congenital. • Common locations include the scalp, face, neck, and upper trunk.
Milia	• Small (usually 1–2 mm) and more superficial. • Often multiple. • Whitish in color.
Cutaneous bronchogenic cyst	• Typically located on the midline of the chest, near the sternal notch. • May be firmer. • May have connection to underlying structures or a draining sinus.
Infantile hemangioma (deep type)	• Most often become clinically evident between 2 and 4 weeks of age. • Gradual enlargement over 6 to 10 months of age. • Blue hue, sometimes with surface telangiectasias.
Pilomatricoma	• Usually acquired, rather than congenital. • Often blue in appearance. • Very firm to palpation.

How to Make the Diagnosis

▶ The diagnosis is usually made clinically based on the characteristic presentation and location.

▶ Can be confirmed through imaging with ultrasonography when the diagnosis is in question; however, with midline lesions, magnetic resonance imaging or computed tomography is preferable to evaluate for underlying tract or central nervous system connection.

Treatment

▶ Clinical observation may be appropriate if small and uncomplicated and of no psychosocial concern.

▶ Surgical excision is the modality of choice for problematic or cosmetically displeasing lesions. Excision can help prevent episodes of inflammation or infection as well as tissue deformity (when relevant based on size/location).

▶ Midline lesions should be imaged prior to any surgical procedure.

Prognosis

- The prognosis is excellent for uncomplicated dermoid cysts.

When to Worry or Refer

- Lesions that are inflamed, draining, rapidly growing, or symptomatic should be referred for surgical excision.
- Midline cysts or sinuses should undergo magnetic resonance imaging or computed tomography to assess for a tract and intracranial connection prior to excision or other surgical manipulation.

Resource for Families

- Medscape: Provides a discussion of cutaneous dermoid cysts. http://emedicine.medscape.com/article/1112963-overview

CHAPTER
79

Epidermal Nevi

Introduction/Etiology/Epidemiology

- Epidermal nevi are benign congenital hamartomas derived from the ectoderm and associated with mosaicism.
- They typically present at birth or during infancy; they often continue to expand during childhood and become more prominent (ie, thicker, more verrucous) at puberty.
- Several subtypes have been identified, including keratinocytic epidermal nevi (focus of this chapter), nevus comedonicus, and nevus sebaceus (of Jadassohn) (see Chapter 107).
- Somatic variations in fibroblast growth factor receptor 3 (*FGFR3*), *PIK3CA*, *HRAS*, *KRAS*, and *NRAS* have been identified in some patients.

Signs and Symptoms

- Usually asymptomatic.
- Epidermal nevi present as skin-colored to tan or brown verrucous plaques (Figure 79.1).
- They are often linear or curvilinear; larger lesions reveal distribution pattern along Blaschko lines.
- With time, they may become thicker and more verrucous and/or develop papules that look like acrochordons.
- When more extensive lesions occur in a unilateral fashion (Figure 79.2), the term *nevus unius lateris* has been used.
- When diffuse, widespread lesions present, they may be part of epidermal nevus syndrome, which may include congenital anomalies, including variations in the central nervous system, eyes, and skeleton.

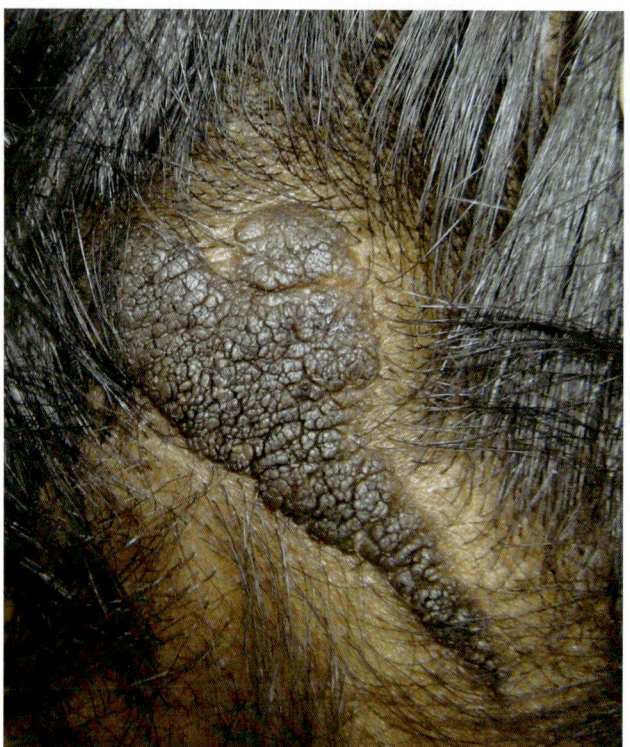

Figure 79.1. Epidermal nevus on the scalp. A verrucous, brown linear plaque.

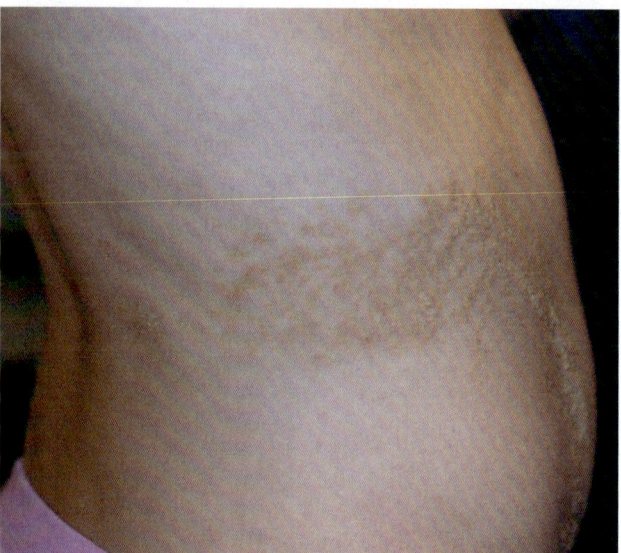

Figure 79.2. Large epidermal nevus on the right side of the trunk. This more diffuse presentation has been termed *nevus unius lateris*.

Look-alikes

Disorder	Differentiating Features
Lichen striatus	• Also presents in a linear fashion but usually composed of erythematous scaly papules. • Acquired, not congenital. • Spontaneously resolves over months to years with residual dyspigmentation.
Incontinentia pigmenti	• Similar pattern of lesions (distributed in a linear or whorled pattern along Blaschko lines) may be present. • In the neonate, usually presents with red papules and vesicles (stage 1). • Several subsequent phases of lesions may evolve with time, including verrucous (stage 2), hyperpigmented (stage 3), and hypopigmented (stage 4). • Most often diagnosed in girls because of X-linked dominant inheritance. • Other variations may be present, including dental, ophthalmologic, neurologic, musculoskeletal.
Verruca vulgaris (wart)	• May be confused with smaller or more patchy epidermal nevi. • Although multiple warts may be linear (from koebnerization), they do not follow the distribution of Blaschko lines. • May resolve spontaneously.
Inflammatory linear verrucous epidermal nevus	• Linear distribution of erythematous, scaly papules coalescing into plaques; not typically as brown. • Pruritus often severe. • May mimic other inflammatory conditions such as psoriasis, lichen striatus, lichen planus.

How to Make the Diagnosis

▶ The diagnosis of epidermal nevus is usually made clinically.

▶ If the diagnosis is in question, skin biopsy for histologic analysis can be performed and reveals acanthosis and papillomatosis.

▶ Some lesions may reveal histologic changes of epidermolytic hyperkeratosis.

Treatment

- Treatment is challenging and is necessary only if requested by the patient or parents.
- Destructive therapies (ie, curettage or cryotherapy) may result in scarring. Additionally, some lesions may recur after treatment.
- Laser ablation may be effective, but response is unpredictable.
- Surgical excision is the most definitive treatment but may be limited by the resultant scarring.
- Topical therapies (eg, retinoids, topical chemotherapy) have been used with variable success; photodynamic therapy has been reported to be beneficial.

Prognosis

- The prognosis for epidermal nevi is excellent; most lesions are uncomplicated, the most significant concern being the potential for psychosocial ramifications.
- The prognosis for epidermal nevus syndrome is variable, depending on the extent of extracutaneous involvement.

When to Worry or Refer

- Referral to a dermatologist is appropriate for assistance with the diagnosis (if in question) and recommendations for further evaluation or therapy.
- Referral to other specialists, as appropriate, is indicated for patients with epidermal nevus syndrome.

Resources for Families

- MedlinePlus: Information for patients and families sponsored by the US National Library of Medicine and National Institutes of Health.
  http://ghr.nlm.nih.gov/condition/epidermal-nevus
- Society for Pediatric Dermatology: Patient handout on epidermal nevus (also available in Spanish).
  https://pedsderm.net/for-patients-families/patient-handouts/#EpidermalNevus

CHAPTER 80

Granuloma Annulare

Introduction/Etiology/Epidemiology

- Granuloma annulare is a common skin disorder in children.
- Most commonly occurs in school-aged children.
- Although a potential association with diabetes has been suggested in adults, this association has not been confirmed in children.

Signs and Symptoms

- Presents as annular (ringlike), skin-colored, erythematous or violaceous, non-scaling papules and plaques (Figures 80.1 and 80.2).
- Outer border often composed of numerous smaller papules.
- Common locations are areas of trauma (eg, dorsal surfaces of feet and hands, ankles and wrists).
- Subcutaneous lesions (most common in children) present as firm nodules with typical overlying skin (Figure 80.3); most often seen on anterior tibiae, fingers, feet, and scalp.
- Lesions can be solitary or multiple and are painless.

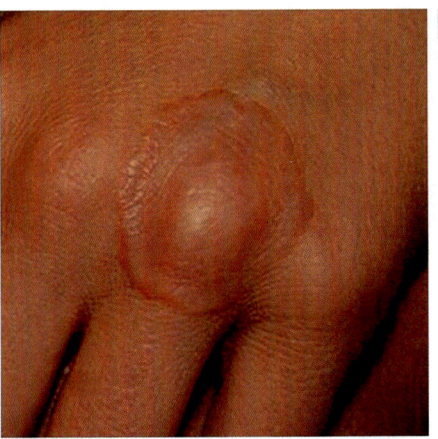

Figure 80.1. Annular plaque of granuloma annulare.

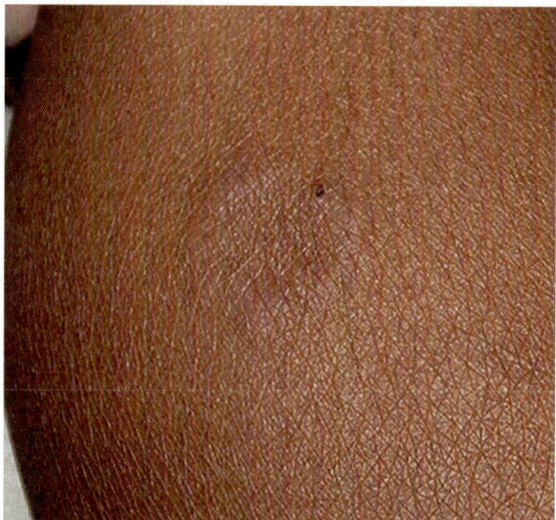

Figure 80.2. Granuloma annulare: an annular erythematous plaque in a patient with skin of color. (There is a small crust at approximately 1:30, the result of mild trauma unrelated to granuloma annulare.)

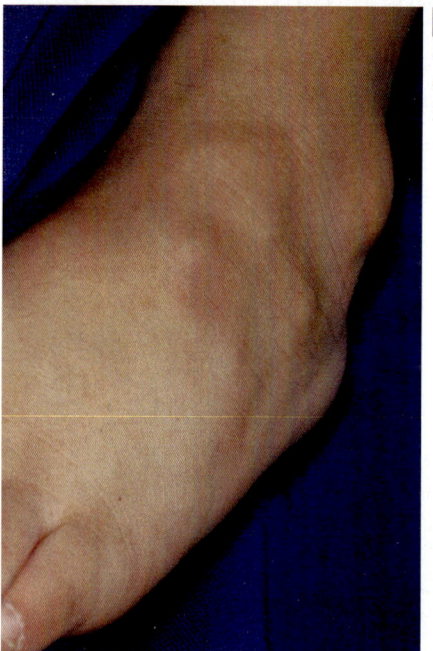

Figure 80.3. Subcutaneous granuloma annulare. Several firm nodules on the dorsolateral surface of the foot of a 5-year-old.

Look-alikes

Disorder	Differentiating Features
Tinea corporis	• Erythematous plaques, also annular but with scale. • May spread in a pattern of autoinoculation. • Potassium hydroxide preparation of skin scrapings reveals hyphae. • Pruritus common.
Nummular eczema	• Scaly, often crusted red papules and plaques. • Central clearing less common. • Pruritus very common.
Soft-tissue malignancy	• May be confused with subcutaneous granuloma annulare. • Other classic lesions of cutaneous granuloma annulare absent. • Biopsy may be necessary to rule out malignancy.
Rheumatoid nodules	• May be confused with subcutaneous granuloma annulare. • Usually overlying affected joints in patients with history of rheumatoid arthritis or another autoimmune condition.
Sarcoidosis	• Cutaneous lesions may present as annular plaques. • Color tends to be more violaceous. • Face and nose most common locations. • Scarring possible. • May be associated with pulmonary symptoms, uveitis, or hilar adenopathy.

How to Make the Diagnosis

▶ The diagnosis is usually made from clinical findings.
▶ A biopsy shows focal collagen degeneration with reactive inflammation.

Treatment

▶ Reassurance and anticipatory guidance.
▶ Steroids used topically or intralesionally can sometimes decrease inflammation but must be used cautiously to prevent atrophy; most often, no treatment recommended.

Treating Associated Conditions

- Not typically applicable.
- An association between granuloma annulare and other disorders (eg, diabetes mellitus, hyperlipidemia, thyroid disease) has been suggested by some authors but remains controversial.

Prognosis

- The lesions of granuloma annulare tend to resolve over months to several years, leaving behind no permanent sequelae.
- Recurrence common.

When to Worry or Refer

- Consider referral to a dermatologist for patients in whom the diagnosis is in question.

Resource for Families

- MedlinePlus: Information for patients and families (in English and Spanish) sponsored by the US National Library of Medicine at the National Institutes of Health.
  https://medlineplus.gov/ency/article/000833.htm

CHAPTER 81

Juvenile Xanthogranuloma

Introduction/Etiology/Epidemiology

- Juvenile xanthogranulomas (JXGs) are benign nodular lesions occurring particularly in infants and young children.
- They are collections of xanthomatous cells, but no association with systemic hyperlipidemia exists.
- Lesions may be present at birth.
- JXG is a common form of non-Langerhans cell histiocytosis; the course is self-limited, with resolution of lesions over several years.
- Iris lesions can mimic retinoblastomas and may result in hyphema and/or glaucoma.

Signs and Symptoms

- Characterized by orange or yellow-brown firm papules or papulonodular lesions (Figures 81.1 and 81.2). In patients with darker skin tones, they may be skin-colored or dark red or brown (Figure 81.3).
- Early lesions erythematous; eventually become lipidized, with yellow color predominating clinically.
- Often located in the head and neck area, although can be on any area of the body.
- May be solitary or multiple.
- Extra-cutaneous sites of involvement include eye (most common); less commonly, soft tissues, muscle, lung, liver, spleen, central nervous system, kidneys, and adrenal glands.

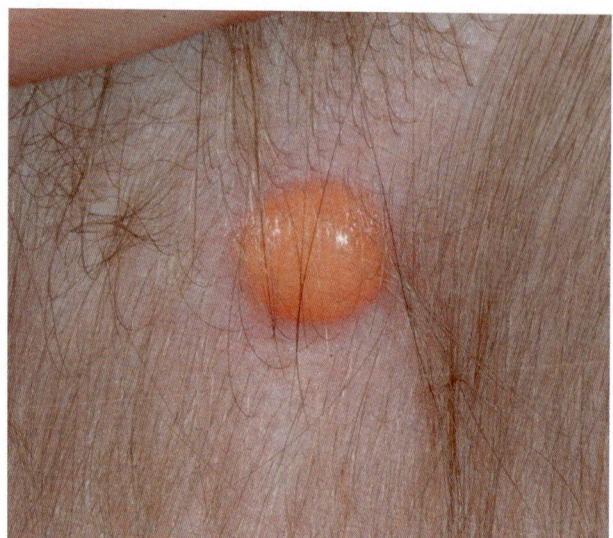

Figure 81.1. Juvenile xanthogranuloma of the scalp.

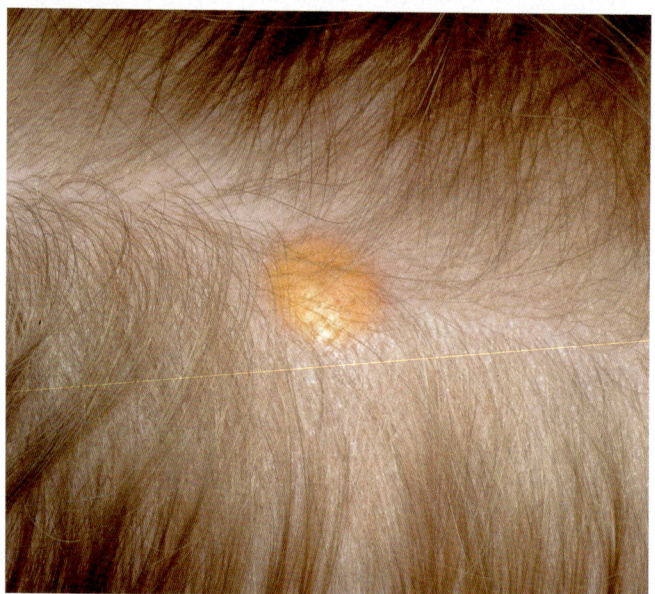

Figure 81.2. Juvenile xanthogranuloma of the scalp. A small yellow-orange papule.

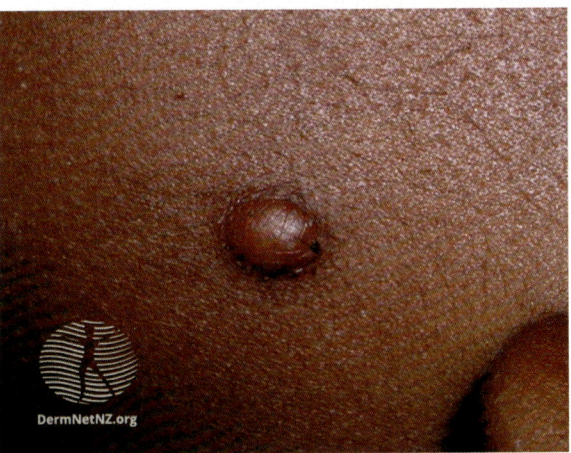

Figure 81.3. In persons with darker skin tones, a juvenile xanthogranuloma may be skin colored or, as in this patient, red-brown. Reproduced with permission from DermNet NZ.

Look-alikes

Disorder	Differentiating Features
Spitz nevus	• Most often an erythematous papule. • Does not undergo lipidization, so does not become yellow. • May see brown pigment with dermoscopy or diascopy (compressing lesion and viewing through a glass slide).
Solitary mastocytoma	• Red-brown papule with a peau d'orange surface. • Urticates (becomes red and more elevated) with stroking (Darier sign).
Melanocytic nevus	• Usually tan to brown. • May have associated hypertrichosis, especially if congenital.

How to Make the Diagnosis

▶ The diagnosis is usually made based on clinical findings.

▶ Biopsy of the lesion will show foamy, multinucleated histiocytic giant cells with scattered eosinophils.

Treatment

- Observation and reassurance.
- Most lesions resolve spontaneously over several years.
- Surgical excision, when requested or clinically indicated (ie, for rapid growth, ulceration, or concern for cosmetic deformity).

Treating Associated Conditions

- Children with multiple or facial lesions should be referred to ophthalmology for eye examination.
- Patients with neurofibromatosis type 1 and JXGs may have an increased risk of juvenile chronic myelogenous leukemia and should be monitored appropriately.

Prognosis

- The prognosis for children with isolated cutaneous JXGs is excellent.

When to Worry or Refer

- See the Treating Associated Conditions section.
- Consider referral to a dermatologist when the diagnosis is in question.
- Neonates or infants with multiple lesions merit an evaluation for systemic involvement.

Resources for Families

- Medscape: Dermatologic manifestations of juvenile xanthogranuloma.
  http://emedicine.medscape.com/article/1111629-overview
- Society for Pediatric Dermatology: Patient handout on juvenile xanthogranuloma (JXG).
  https://pedsderm.net/for-patients-families/patient-handouts/#JXG

CHAPTER 82

Pilomatricoma

Introduction/Etiology/Epidemiology

- Benign tumor of the hair matrix.
- Usually presents in the first 2 decades after birth.
- Also known as a pilomatrixoma or calcifying epithelioma of Malherbe.

Signs and Symptoms

- Most often presents as a solitary, asymptomatic, slowly growing, firm nodule located on the head, neck, or upper extremities.
- Lesions often have an overlying blue or pink color (Figures 82.1 and 82.2).
- The lesions are very firm to palpation because of calcification.
- Two maneuvers may assist in diagnosis.
  - "Teeter-totter" sign: Downward pressure on one edge of the lesion will cause the opposite edge to become elevated (Figure 82.3).
  - "Tent" sign: The multifaceted shape of the lesion (like the sides of a tent) is observed when the overlying skin is compressed (Figure 82.4).

PEDIATRIC DERMATOLOGY

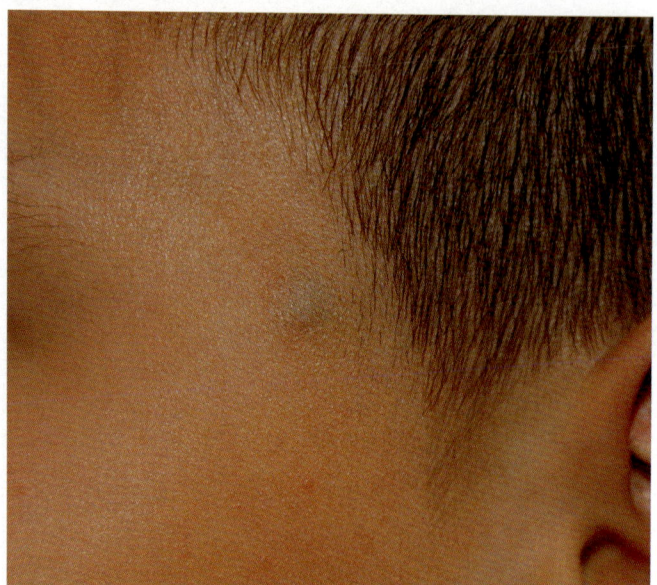

Figure 82.1. A pilomatricoma in the temporal fossa has an overlying blue color.

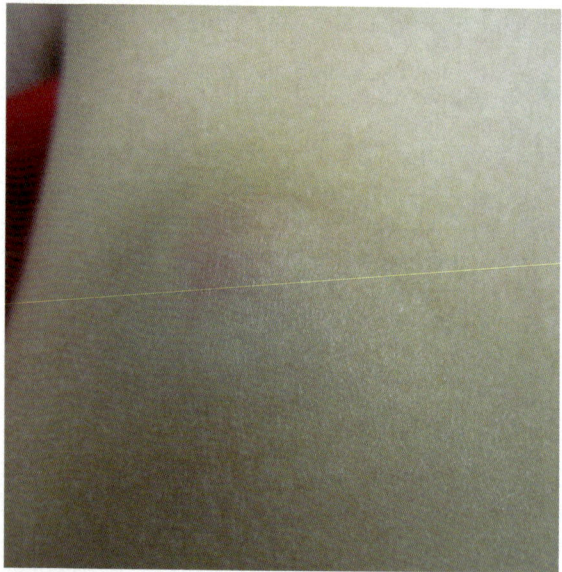

Figure 82.2. A pilomatricoma with an overlying pink color.

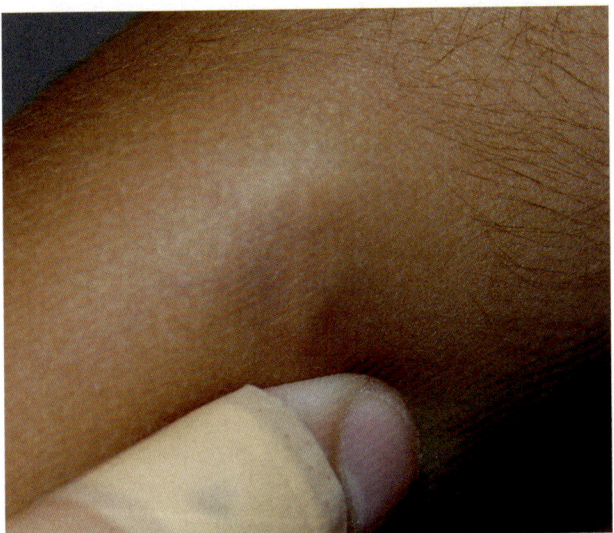

Figure 82.3. The "teeter-totter" sign in pilomatricoma. Depressing the inferior margin of the lesion causes the upper margin to elevate.

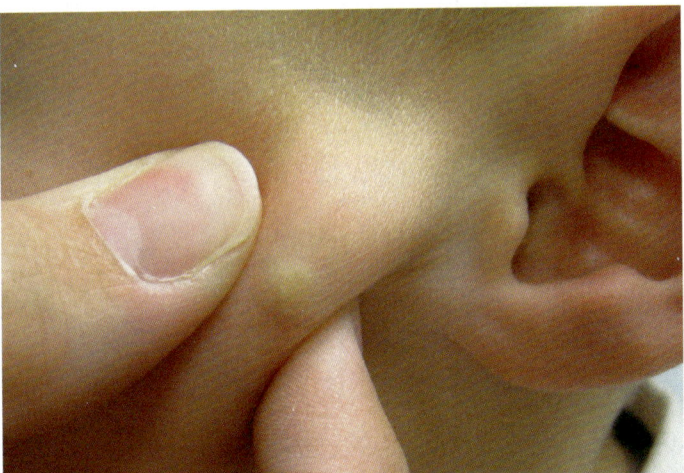

Figure 82.4. The "tent" sign in pilomatricoma. Compressing the skin overlying the lesion reveals its multifaceted shape.

Look-alikes

The firm nature of pilomatricomas and their overlying blue or pink color usually distinguish them from many other papules or nodules.

Disorder	Differentiating Features
Dermoid cyst	• Usually congenital. • Skin-colored nodule; blue color typically lacking. • Usually located along the orbital ridge, often the outer third of the eyebrow.
Other epithelial cysts	• Skin-colored papule or nodule; blue color typically lacking. • May have central punctum.
Milia	• White in color. • Small (usually 1–2 mm) and more superficial. • Often multiple.
Venous malformation	• Blue in color but soft and compressible.
Branchial cleft cyst	• Usually located on the lateral aspect of the neck along the anterior border of the sternocleidomastoid muscle. • Typically a skin-colored compressible cyst.
Cutaneous bronchogenic cyst	• Typically located on the midline chest near the sternal notch. • May have connection to underlying structures or a draining sinus.
Thyroglossal duct cyst	• Located on the midline of the neck. • Moves with swallowing. • Typically a skin-colored compressible cyst.
Metastatic neuroblastoma	• Typically multiple papules or nodules. • Lesions may blanch on palpation. • Primary tumor mass detected with computed tomography or magnetic resonance imaging.

How to Make the Diagnosis

▶ The diagnosis is suspected clinically and confirmed with pathologic examination of the excised lesion.

Treatment

▶ Because pilomatricomas do not resolve spontaneously, surgical excision often is recommended, especially for lesions that are painful or become inflamed.

Prognosis

- The prognosis is excellent for solitary uncomplicated pilomatricomas.
- Patients who have multiple pilomatricomas may have associated disorders, especially myotonic dystrophy and Gardner syndrome, and should be evaluated/referred accordingly.

When to Worry or Refer

- Referral to a dermatologist is appropriate for assistance with diagnosis and recommendations for management.
- Referral to other specialists, as appropriate, is indicated for patients with multiple pilomatricomas in whom concern exists for associated disorders.

Resource for Families

- Society for Pediatric Dermatology: Patient handout on pilomatricoma. https://pedsderm.net/for-patients-families/patient-handouts/#Pilomatricoma

CHAPTER 83

Spitz Nevus

Introduction/Etiology/Epidemiology

- Spitz nevus (also called *spindle cell nevus*) is considered a benign, acquired form of a melanocytic nevus that usually presents in childhood or adolescence. It rarely presents in adults.
- It was previously called a "benign juvenile melanoma" because it shares some histologic features with melanoma but does not have the same aggressive behavior.
- The etiology and pathogenesis are unknown.

Signs and Symptoms

- Spitz nevi tend to be solitary and appear on the head, neck, or extremities. Uncommonly, they can be clustered (agminated) or, rarely, disseminated.
- Spitz nevus usually presents as a smaller than 1 cm, dome-shaped, round, pink (Figure 83.1), red (Figure 83.2), brown, or brown-black papule. It grows rapidly in the first few months and then plateaus with the possibility of regressing over time.
- Pink or hypopigmented Spitz nevi usually have a dotted or polymorphous vascular pattern at dermoscopy (an illuminated magnification tool often used by dermatologists). Pigmented Spitz nevi typically have a very dark-brown to black color and, at dermoscopy, have a globular, negative network or starburst pattern.

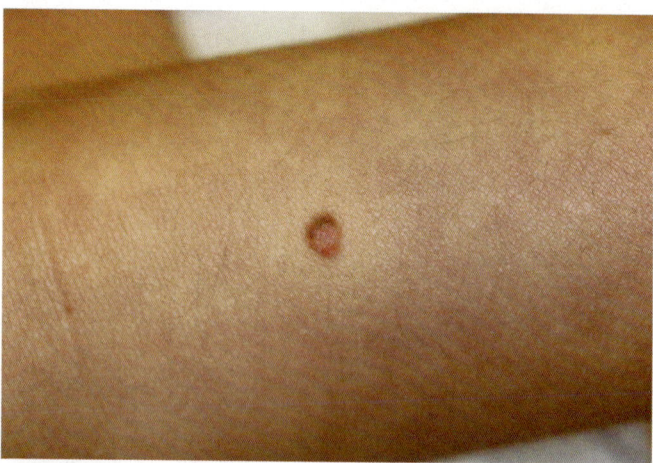

Figure 83.1. Spitz nevus. This patient had a rapidly growing pink papule with a crescent of brown pigmentation on the upper extremity. The lesion was excised, and histologic examination revealed a Spitz nevus without atypia.

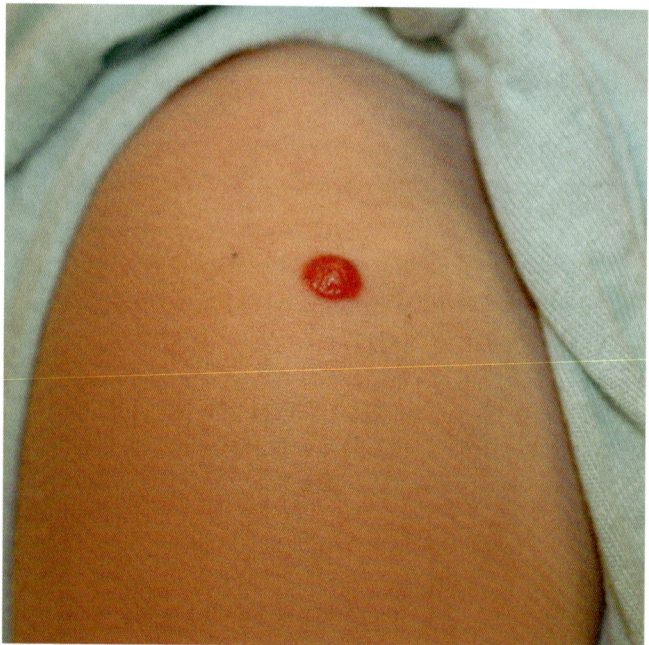

Figure 83.2. Spitz nevus of shoulder presenting as a bright red, well-circumscribed papule.

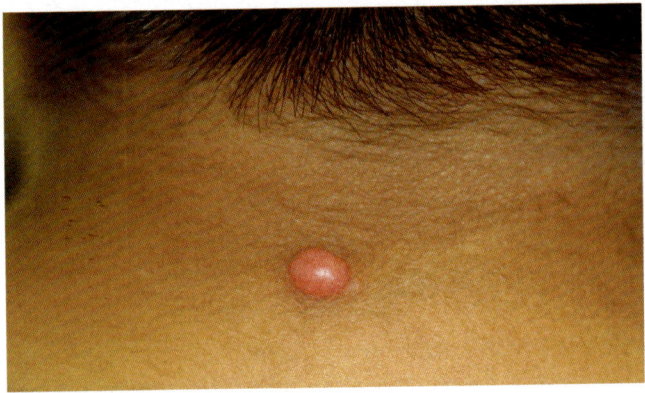

Figure 83.3. This patient had a rapidly enlarging pink papule on the posterior aspect of the neck. The lesion was excised, and histologic examination revealed a Spitz nevus with atypical features. As a result, re-excision was performed with adequate margins and without recurrence to date.

Look-alikes

Disorder	Differentiating Features
Pyogenic granuloma	• Typically of acute onset. • Bright red, friable papule, which may be pedunculated. • Peripheral collarette typically present around base. • Bleeds easily; surface may be eroded. • Vascular lacunae are noted at dermoscopy with no melanocytic features.
Intradermal melanocytic nevus	• Pink, skin-colored, brown, or dark-brown papule. • Typically slow growing. • May see brown pigment with diascopy (compressing lesion and viewing through a glass slide).
Juvenile xanthogranuloma	• Orange to yellow-brown papule; early lesions may be more pink to red in appearance, sometimes mimicking a Spitz nevus. • Slowly grows and then involutes over time. • No melanocytic features at dermoscopy.
Verruca vulgaris	• Surface of the papule is rough (ie, verrucous). • Thrombosed capillaries (ie, purple or black specks) may be seen within the lesion. • No melanocytic features at dermoscopy.

How to Make the Diagnosis

- The history, physical examination, and, when used, appearance at dermoscopy can help in making a diagnosis.
- Definitive diagnosis often depends on excisional biopsy with histologic confirmation.

Treatment

- Typical Spitz nevi are benign, but uniform management recommendations are lacking; many advocate for excision of all lesions, while some follow the lesions clinically and excise only if atypical clinical features develop.
- Importantly, pediatric melanoma often presents in an amelanotic fashion, which clinically translates into a red papule that may mimic Spitz nevus.
- When lesions are excised, most experts recommend complete excision to prevent recurrence that can be misinterpreted as a melanoma and to allow for accurate dermatopathic interpretation.

Prognosis

- Classic Spitz nevi are considered benign, and excision is curative.
- "Atypical spitzoid tumors" occasionally present in children, and the prognosis for these lesions is variable (Figure 83.3).

When to Worry or Refer

- Patients who have a suspected Spitz nevus should be referred for pediatric dermatologic evaluation.
- For any such lesion that is rapidly growing, ulcerating, or bleeding, urgent referral should be requested because prompt surgical excision is indicated.

Resource for Families

- Society for Pediatric Dermatology: Patient handout on Spitz nevus. https://pedsderm.net/for-patients-families/patient-handouts/#spitznevus

Bullous Diseases

CHAPTER 84 — **Childhood Dermatitis Herpetiformis** 545

CHAPTER 85 — **Epidermolysis Bullosa (EB)** 551

CHAPTER 86 — **Linear IgA Dermatosis** 561

CHAPTER 84

Childhood Dermatitis Herpetiformis

Introduction/Etiology/Epidemiology

- A rare immunobullous disorder in children.
- Associated with celiac disease (ie, gluten-sensitive enteropathy) in 75% to 95% of patients who are affected.
- Typically seen in children between 2 and 7 years of age.
- Children with celiac disease diagnosed have circulating immunoglobulin A antibodies to tissue transglutaminase and endomysium.

Signs and Symptoms

- Characterized by intensely pruritic papulovesicular lesions (Figure 84.1) with a bilateral, symmetric distribution.
- Most often located on the extensor aspects of knees and elbows, sacrum, buttocks, posterior aspect of the neck, scalp, and shoulders (Figures 84.2 and 84.3).
- Mucous membrane involvement usually absent.

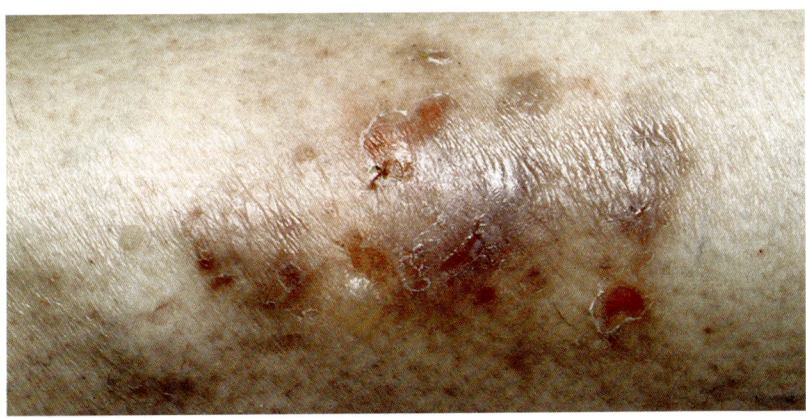

Figure 84.1. Dermatitis herpetiformis. Vesicles and erosions are present.

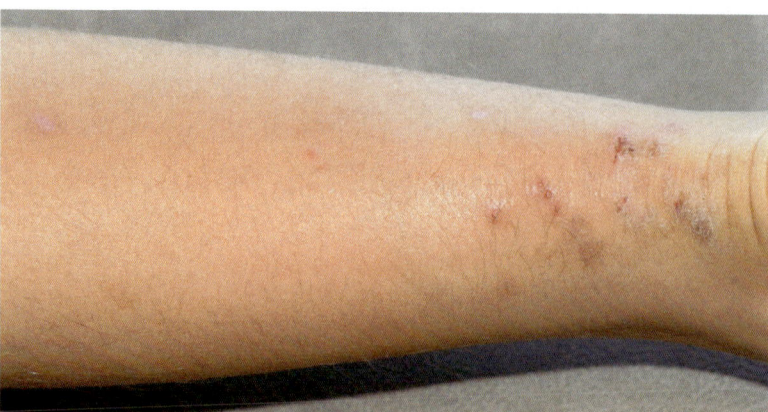

Figure 84.2. Intensely pruritic lesions of dermatitis herpetiformis on the leg of a patient with celiac disease.

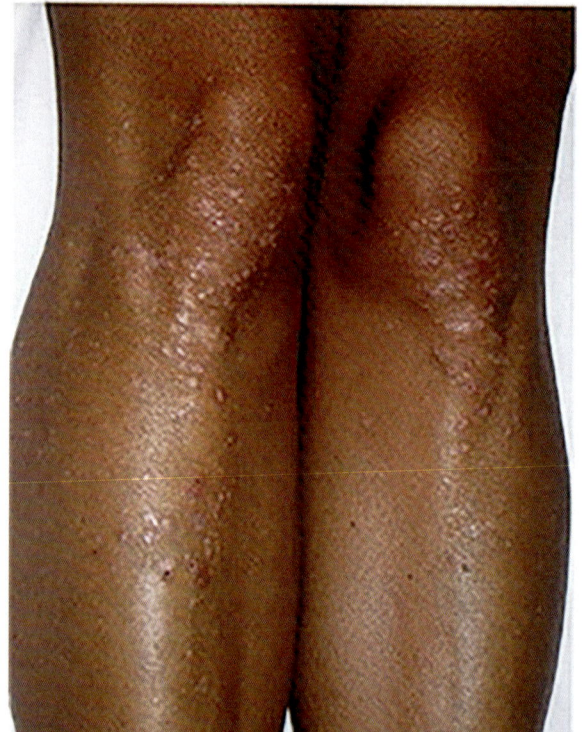

Figure 84.3. Grouped papules, vesicles, and erosions on the knees and legs of a patient with skin of color with dermatitis herpetiformis. Reproduced with permission from Antiga E, et al. Dermatitis herpetiformis: novel perspectives. *Front Immunol.* 2019;10.

Look-alikes

Disorder	Differentiating Features
Linear immunoglobulin A dermatosis	• Bullae tend to be larger. • "Cluster (or string) of jewels" pattern (annular grouping of bullae) often noted. • Not as symmetric in distribution, less often pruritic. • Direct immunofluorescence and immunoblotting studies help confirm diagnosis.
Bullous lupus erythematosus	• Other features of systemic lupus erythematosus usually present. • Concentrated in sun-exposed areas. • Bullae tend to be larger, not typically pruritic. • Antinuclear antibody (and other serological studies) will confirm diagnosis of systemic lupus erythematosus. • Direct immunofluorescence and immunoblotting studies help confirm the diagnosis.
Bullous pemphigoid	• Urticarial plaques present in addition to tense blisters. • Bullae tend to be larger. • Pruritus common with early lesions. • Direct immunofluorescence and immunoblotting studies help confirm the diagnosis.
Herpes simplex virus infection	• Most often clustered vesicles and erosions on an erythematous base. • Often occur inside or around the mouth. • Tend to be painful, less often pruritic. • More often focal.
Arthropod bites and papular urticaria	• Papules may have a central punctum at close inspection. • Usually concentrated on exposed areas of skin. • Linear groupings of papules may be observed owing to exposure to crawling (and feeding) insects.
Scabies	• Mixture of papules, linear burrows, crusted papules or (especially in infants) nodules. • Palm and sole lesions very common, as is involvement of the areolae and penis. • Other family members often report lesions and/or pruritus. • Microscopic examination of skin scrapings with mineral oil confirms the diagnosis (visualization of scabies mites, eggs, or fecal pellets). • Pruritus worse in the evening.
Pityriasis lichenoides et varioliformis acuta	• Scaly, red papules with necrotic surface changes. • Usually not pruritic. • Associated fever may be present. • Usually responds to treatment with oral erythromycin or tetracycline.

(continued)

Look-alikes (continued)

Disorder	Differentiating Features
Epidermolysis bullosa	• Inherited (not acquired) mechanobullous disease. • Usually begins in neonatal period or during early infancy. • Vesicles and bullae induced by friction, pressure, or trauma. • Blisters usually larger than those seen in dermatitis herpetiformis (with exception of some simplex forms of epidermolysis bullosa). • Certain subtypes may reveal nail dystrophy, milia, extensive scarring, mitten deformities. • Molecular genetic testing confirms the diagnosis; immunofluorescence antigen mapping and electron microscopy of skin biopsy specimens used less often in current era.
Acquired epidermolysis bullosa	• Acquired autoimmune blistering disease. • Blisters induced by trauma. • Scarring common. • Direct fluorescence and immunoblotting studies will help confirm diagnosis. • Blisters and erosions usually larger than those seen in dermatitis herpetiformis.

How to Make the Diagnosis

▶ The diagnosis is suggested clinically and confirmed by means of skin biopsy with immunofluorescence study, which reveals immunoglobulin A at dermal papillary tips in a granular pattern.

▶ Circulating serum antibodies to tissue transglutaminase or endomysium may be present (in patients sensitive to gluten).

Treatment

▶ Dapsone at 1 to 2 mg/kg/d is usually very effective (must first confirm appropriate glucose-6-phosphate dehydrogenase level and follow complete blood cell counts and liver function tests).

▶ Sulfapyridine may be an effective alternative for therapy.

▶ Gluten-free diet may be effective in certain patients, although challenging for children and parents.

Treating Associated Conditions

▶ Patients with gluten sensitivity should be referred to an experienced gastroenterologist for baseline and follow-up care.

Prognosis

▶ The prognosis for children with dermatitis herpetiformis is unpredictable.
▶ Many recommend indefinite continuation of the gluten-free diet in individuals sensitive to gluten, as even small amounts of gluten exposure can lead to disease relapse.

When to Worry or Refer

▶ Consider referral to a dermatologist for confirmation of diagnosis and comanagement.

Resources for Families

▶ Gluten Intolerance Group: Provides information about dermatitis herpetiformis.
  https://gluten.org
▶ National Institute of Diabetes and Digestive and Kidney Diseases: Celiac disease.
  www.niddk.nih.gov/health-information/health-topics/digestive-diseases/celiac-disease/Pages/facts.aspx

CHAPTER 85

Epidermolysis Bullosa (EB)

Introduction/Etiology/Epidemiology

- Epidermolysis bullosa (EB) is a group of rare genetic skin disorders characterized by fragile skin and the formation of vesicles or bullae in response to mild frictional trauma.
- Occurs in approximately 1 per 50,000 births.
- Sexes affected equally.
- Classified into 3 general categories according to the level of the cleavage plane within the dermal–epidermal junction.
  - EB simplex (EBS)
    - Autosomal dominant
    - Caused by defects in keratin genes *K5* or *K14*.
    - Three major forms: localized, generalized intermediate, and generalized severe.
    - Also, EBS with muscular dystrophy (autosomal recessive; caused by variation in plectin) and some rarer forms caused by variations in transglutaminase 5, plakophilin-1, desmoplakin, and plakoglobin.
  - Junctional EB (JEB)
    - Autosomal recessive
    - Caused by defects in the following:
      - Laminin 332 (formerly laminin 5) (Herlitz type; JEB, generalized severe).
      - Integrin $\alpha_6\beta_4$ (JEB with pyloric atresia).
      - Collagen XVII (non-Herlitz type; JEB, generalized intermediate).
  - Dystrophic EB (DEB)
    - Autosomal dominant and recessive forms.
    - Caused by defects in collagen VII.

Signs and Symptoms

- EBS
  - EBS, localized (Weber-Cockayne type).
    - Blisters primarily on the hands and feet (Figure 85.1).
    - May not present until adolescence or early adulthood in some patients.
    - Hyperhidrosis common.
  - EBS, generalized intermediate (Koebner type)
    - Generalized blisters from birth or during infancy, especially on the arms and legs.
    - Mild mucosal involvement.
    - Occasional nail dystrophy.
  - EBS, generalized severe (Dowling-Meara type)
    - Vesicles arranged in a herpetiform pattern.
    - Blisters may be large during infancy, with significant oral mucosal involvement.
    - Blistering tends to become milder with age.
  - EBS with muscular dystrophy
    - Resembles mild EBS.
  - Muscular dystrophy may develop anytime between infancy and third decade.

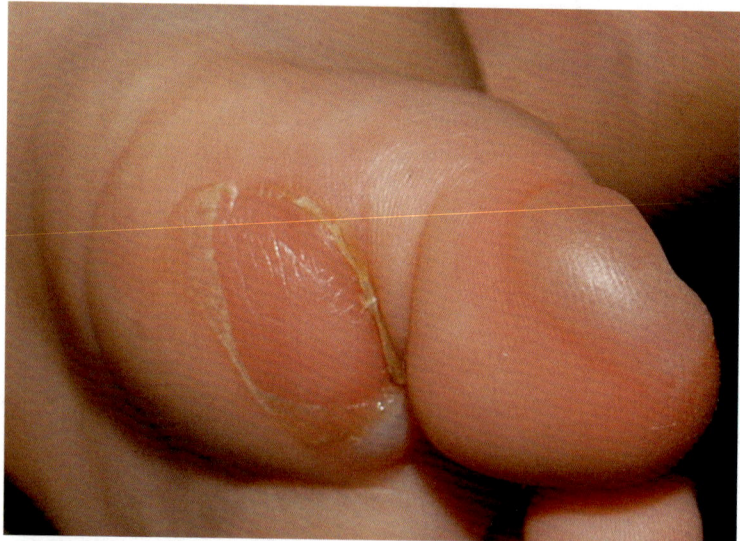

Figure 85.1. Epidermolysis bullosa simplex (localized or Weber-Cockayne type). This patient has a bulla involving the great toe and a healing bulla on the ball of the foot.

- JEB
  - JEB, generalized severe (Herlitz type)
    - Among children who are affected, 50% die in infancy, usually from sepsis, dehydration, or respiratory complications.
    - Lesions are typically seen at birth or soon after (Figure 85.2).
    - Blisters occur anywhere on the body, including mucous membranes.
    - Granulation tissue in perioral area is common.
    - Laryngeal involvement may be present, with hoarseness.
    - Growth retardation and anemia are common.
    - Nail dystrophy or anonychia often are present.
  - JEB with pyloric atresia (Figure 85.3)
    - Pyloric atresia and genitourinary anomalies are possible.
    - Prognosis is poor.
  - JEB, generalized intermediate (non-Herlitz type)
    - Similar to Herlitz type but milder.
    - Mucosal involvement is less severe.

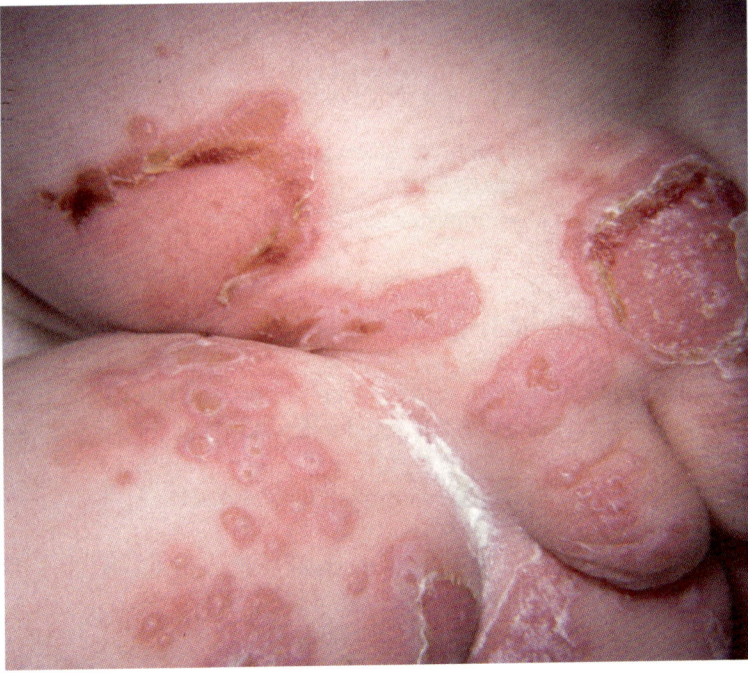

Figure 85.2. Numerous bullae and erosions in a patient with junctional epidermolysis bullosa, generalized severe (Herlitz type).

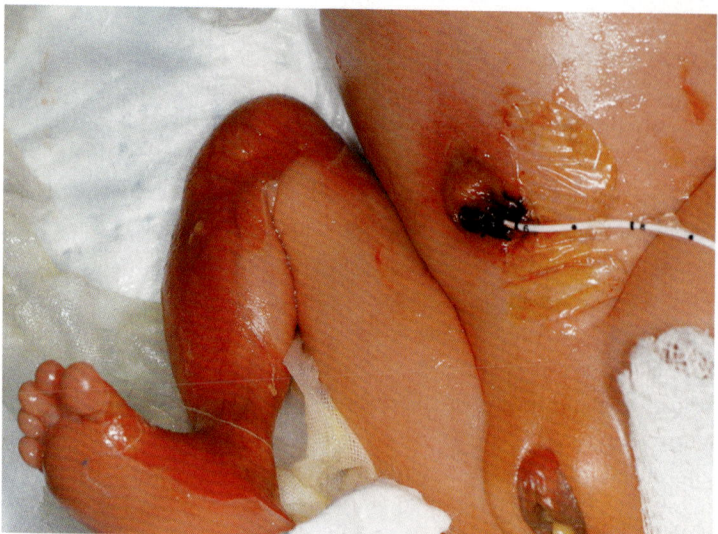

Figure 85.3. Denudation of the lower leg and foot in a newborn with junctional epidermolysis bullosa with pyloric atresia. She died from overwhelming infection shortly after birth.

- ▶ DEB
  - Dominant DEB
    - Blistering most prominent on distal extremities, elbows, and knees.
    - Milia are common (Figure 85.4).
    - Scarring is present at prior blister sites.
    - Nail dystrophy is common.
  - Recessive DEB
    - Blisters are noted at birth and involve the skin and mucous membranes.
    - Widespread blistering with scarring is present (Figure 85.5).
    - Mitten deformities of hands and feet develop with digital fusion (Figure 85.6).
    - Teeth often are carious; delayed eruption may be noted.
    - Microstomia develops from scarring.
    - Other complications include difficulty swallowing (esophageal scarring), chronic anemia, growth failure, conjunctival scarring, and predisposition to squamous cell carcinoma.

Chapter 85: Epidermolysis Bullosa (EB)

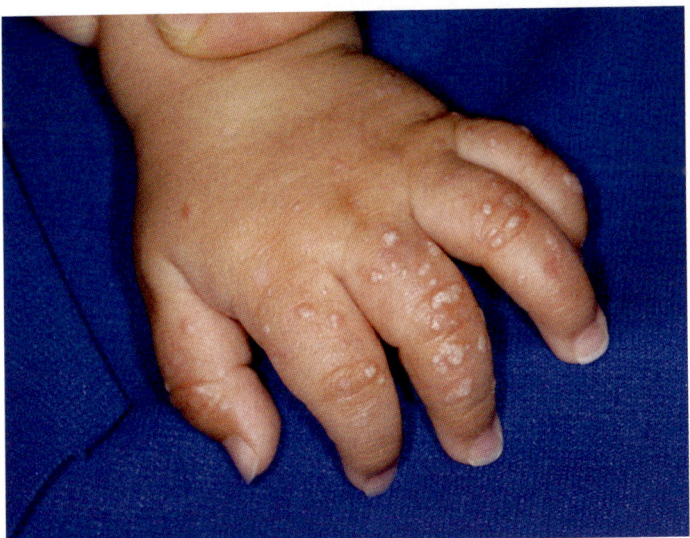

Figure 85.4. Multiple milia with scarring over the dorsal aspect of the hand and fingers of a 1-year-old with dominant dystrophic epidermolysis bullosa.

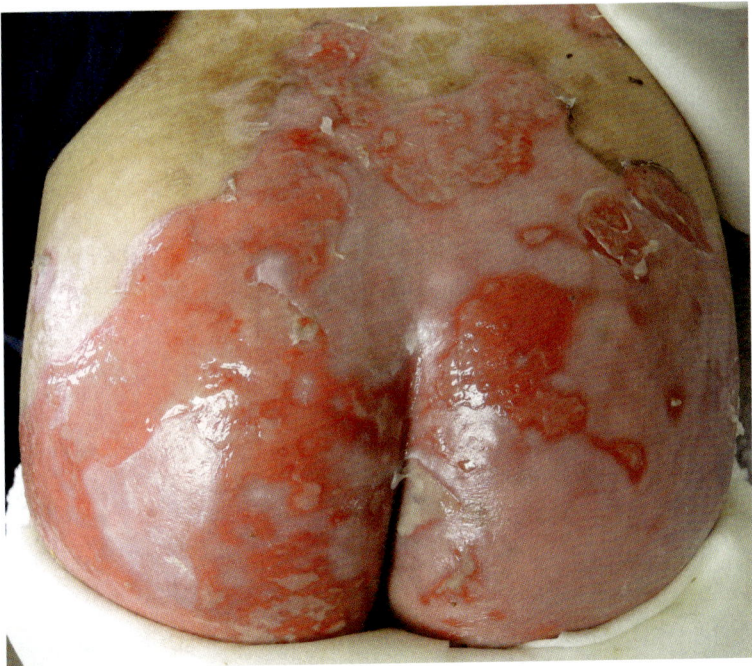

Figure 85.5. This young adult with recessive dystrophic epidermolysis bullosa has widespread bullae and erosions that heal with scarring.

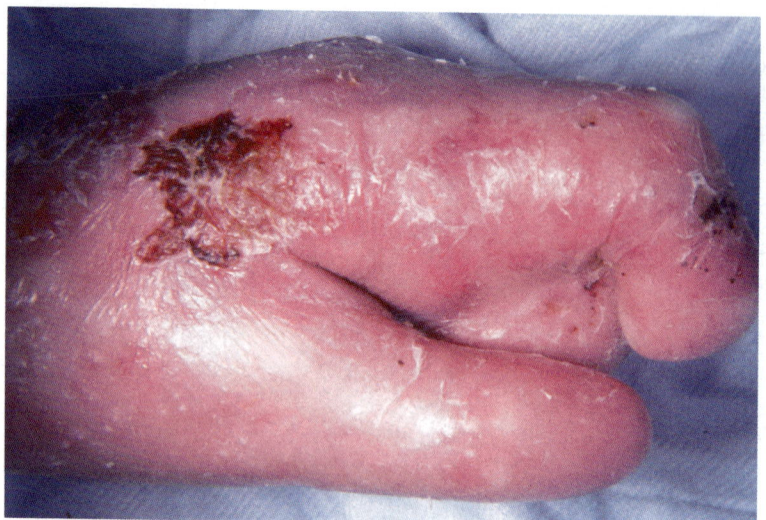

Figure 85.6. Mitten deformity of the hand of a patient with recessive dystrophic epidermolysis bullosa.

Look-alikes

Disorder	Differentiating Features
Bullous congenital ichthyosiform erythroderma	• Blisters may be present soon after birth, similar to epidermolysis bullosa. • Thickened areas of skin with ridging often present during infancy or develop with time. • Eventuates into an ichthyosis disorder (epidermolytic hyperkeratosis), with less propensity toward blistering.
Incontinentia pigmenti	• Small vesicles occur in clusters. • Blisters are arranged in a linear or whorled pattern, along Blaschko lines. • Subsequent to blister stage, skin lesions appear verrucous or hyperpigmented. • Most patients are female (X-linked dominant). • Blisters not trauma induced.
Bullous impetigo	• Does not usually present as a recurrent or chronic condition. • Involvement more focal. • Mucous membranes not involved. • Blisters rupture easily, leaving superficial erosions with peripheral collarettes of scale. • Blisters not trauma induced.
Herpes simplex virus infection	• Most often clustered vesicles and erosions with an erythematous surround. • Usually more focal. • Blisters not trauma induced.

Look-alikes

Disorder	Differentiating Features
Bullous pemphigoid	• Urticarial plaques present in addition to tense blisters. • Blisters not trauma induced. • Pruritus common with early lesions. • Direct fluorescence and immunoblotting studies will help confirm diagnosis.
Dermatitis herpetiformis	• Usually presents as tiny vesicles and erosions. • Most often clustered on elbows, knees, shoulders, sacrum, and buttocks. • Blisters not trauma induced. • Pruritus is intense. • May be associated with gluten sensitivity.
Erythema multiforme major	• Typical target lesions may be present. • Only occasionally bullous, and bullae are not trauma induced. • Oral mucous membrane erosions common. • Palms and soles usually involved. • History of herpes simplex virus infection or drug ingestion may be present.
Acquired epidermolysis bullosa	• Acquired autoimmune blistering disease, not genetic. • Direct fluorescence and immunoblotting studies will help confirm diagnosis.
Linear IgA dermatosis	• Acquired autoimmune blistering disorder, not genetic. • "Cluster of jewels" pattern (annular grouping of bullae) often noted. • Blisters not trauma induced. • Mucosal involvement not as extensive as in epidermolysis bullosa.

How to Make the Diagnosis

▶ Molecular genetic testing is recommended to confirm the diagnosis and aid in prognosis and decision-making.

▶ Skin biopsy for immunomapping, when available, may provide for more prompt diagnosis.

▶ Electron microscopy may be helpful when genetic testing or immunomapping is not available or does not provide conclusive results, but this is rarely used in the current era.

▶ Prenatal genetic testing is possible and should be considered when applicable.

Treatment

- Treatment is palliative and supportive.
- Avoidance of trauma, treatment of infections, pain control, and nutritional counseling are all vital.
- Bullae may be drained with sterile needle and syringe for pain control.
- Antibiotic ointment and protective dressings can be applied to areas of open or blistered skin to promote healing and prevent secondary infection.
- Patient and family education, psychologic support, and referral to support group organizations are important.

Treating Associated Conditions

- Multidisciplinary treatment teams are important to decrease morbidities associated with EB.
- Care teams may include representation from primary care and pediatrics, dermatology, nursing, plastic surgery, ophthalmology, gastroenterology, general surgery, hematology, dentistry, genetics, and nutrition.
- Growth failure is treated with aggressive nutritional rehabilitation; gastrostomy tube placement may be required for infants with severe forms of EB.
- Esophageal involvement with dysphagia may require dietary modifications or dilatation procedures.
- Mitten deformities of the hand require physical therapy and surgical intervention (degloving procedures).

Prognosis

- Prognosis depends on the subtype of EB.
- Children with most forms of EBS, non-Herlitz JEB, and dominant DEB tend to have a fairly good prognosis.
- EBS, generalized severe (Dowling-Meara) subtype, may be severe during infancy and is occasionally fatal.
- Children with Herlitz JEB and JEB with pyloric atresia have a poor prognosis.

- Patients with recessive DEB have a chronic course marked by complications and diminished quality of life. Squamous cell carcinoma, if it occurs, is usually rapidly progressive and invasive, leading to death in most of these patients.

When to Worry or Refer

- Patients with possible EB should be referred to an experienced dermatologist for confirmation of the diagnosis and coordination of multidisciplinary care.
- Because of the increased risk of cutaneous squamous cell carcinoma, biopsy should be performed in any suspicious lesion in patients with recessive DEB.

Resources for Families

- American Academy of Dermatology: Epidermolysis bullosa: overview. **https://www.aad.org/public/diseases/a-z/epidermolysis-bullosa-overview**
- Dystrophic Epidermolysis Bullosa Research Association (debra) of America: Provides information, support, and resources for patients who have epidermolysis bullosa and their families. **www.debra.org**
- Dystrophic Epidermolysis Bullosa Research Association (debra) UK: Located in the United Kingdom, this organization provides information for patients who have epidermolysis bullosa and their families. **www.debra.org.uk**
- Epidermolysis Bullosa Medical Research Foundation: Dedicated to supporting research in EB: Provides information for patients and families. **https://www.ebmrf.org**

CHAPTER 86

Linear IgA Dermatosis

Introduction/Etiology/Epidemiology

- Also known as chronic bullous disease of childhood.
- A rare, acquired autoimmune blistering disorder.
- Most often occurs in children younger than 5 years.
- Occasionally preceded by an upper respiratory illness.
- Usually idiopathic but can be drug induced. There are also reports of occurrence after vaccinations, although causality is not proven.

Signs and Symptoms

- Vesiculobullous lesions occur on the extremities (Figure 86.1), face, and trunk.
- Bullae may form a ring around margins of an older crusted lesion, forming the "cluster of jewels" configuration (Figure 86.2).
- Pruritus tends to be mild, but pain may be significant.
- Mucous membranes may be involved.
  - Oral erosions most common type of mucous membrane involvement.
  - Eye involvement occurs less commonly.

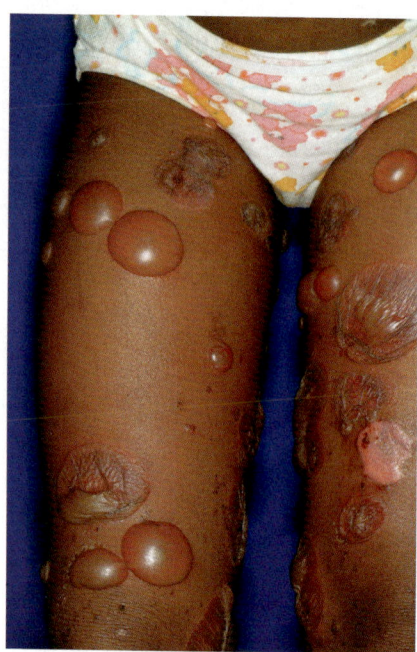

Figure 86.1. Multiple tense bullae in a young patient who has linear IgA dermatosis.

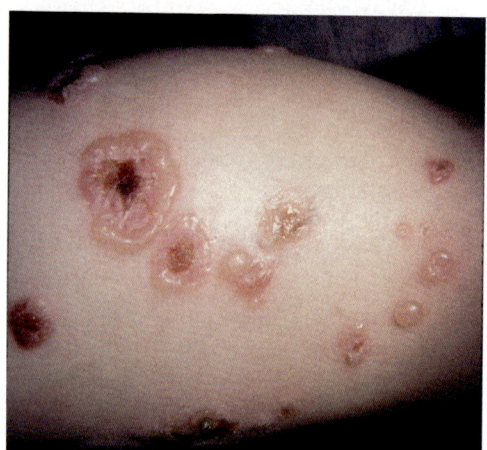

Figure 86.2. Linear IgA dermatosis lesions showing bullae surrounding a crust—the "cluster of jewels" configuration.

Look-alikes

Disorder	Differentiating Features
Bullous impetigo	• Does not usually present as a recurrent or chronic condition. • Involvement more focal. • Mucous membranes not involved. • Blisters rupture easily, leaving superficial erosions with peripheral collarettes of scale.
Herpes simplex virus infection	• Most often clustered vesicles and erosions on an erythematous base. • Usually more focal.
Bullous pemphigoid	• Urticarial plaques present in addition to tense blisters. • Pruritus common with early lesions. • Direct fluorescence and immunoblotting studies will help confirm diagnosis.
Dermatitis herpetiformis	• Usually presents as tiny vesicles and erosions. • Most often clustered on elbows, knees, shoulders, sacrum, and buttocks. • Pruritus is intense. • May be associated with gluten sensitivity.
Stevens-Johnson syndrome (SJS) or *Mycoplasma pneumoniae*–induced rash and mucositis (MIRM) or reactive infectious mucocutaneous eruption (RIME)	• Typical target lesions may be present (with SJS, which more commonly has significant skin component compared with MIRM and RIME). • Bullae in setting of these disorders do not typically present in "cluster of jewels" pattern. • Erosions of 2 or more mucous membranes typically present. • Palms and soles often involved in SJS, occasionally in MIRM or RIME. • History of *Mycoplasma,* herpes simplex virus, or other viral infection or drug ingestion may be present.
Epidermolysis bullosa	• Inherited (not acquired) mechanobullous disease. • Usually begins in neonatal period or during early infancy. • Blisters induced by trauma. • Certain subtypes may reveal nail dystrophy, milia, extensive scarring, mitten deformities of the hand. • Mutation analysis or immunomapping of skin biopsy specimens confirms diagnosis.
Bullous lupus erythematosus	• Other features of systemic lupus erythematosus usually present. • Concentrated in sun-exposed areas. • Antinuclear antibody (and other serological studies) will confirm diagnosis of systemic lupus erythematosus. • Direct immunofluorescence and immunoblotting studies help confirm the diagnosis.

(continued)

Look-alikes (continued)

Disorder	Differentiating Features
Acquired epidermolysis bullosa	• Blisters induced by trauma. • Scarring common. • Direct fluorescence and immunoblotting studies will help confirm diagnosis.
Bullous insect bites	• Typically occur in the summer months. • Pruritus present. • Linear groupings of lesions may be present. • Central punctum may be visualized. • Other, more typical urticarial papules may be present.

How to Make the Diagnosis

▶ The diagnosis is suggested clinically and confirmed with skin biopsy.
  ▪ Histopathologic analysis reveals a subepidermal blister.
  ▪ Direct immunofluorescence examination shows a linear band of IgA along the dermal-epidermal junction.

Treatment

▶ Dapsone has historically been the drug of choice for this condition. After confirming reference glucose-6-phosphate dehydrogenase levels, dapsone is used initially at a dose of 0.5 to 1 mg/kg/d.

▶ Patients receiving dapsone require monitoring for decreased hemoglobin and leukopenia, as well as hepatotoxicity (rare).

▶ Systemic steroids may be useful during acute stage of therapy (often in conjunction with dapsone) but should not be used chronically.

▶ Other treatments that have been used with success include topical steroids, rituximab, omalizumab, etanercept, sulfapyridine, erythromycin, dicloxacillin, azathioprine, colchicine, mycophenolate mofetil, and intravenous immunoglobulin.

Treating Associated Conditions

▶ If conjunctival involvement is present, regular ophthalmologic evaluations are indicated.

Prognosis

- Most children with linear IgA dermatosis experience spontaneous remission within 5 years of onset, but treatment of the disorder can be challenging.

When to Worry or Refer

- Dermatology referral should be made early for diagnostic confirmation and initiation of therapy.

Resource for Families

- DermNet NZ: Linear IgA bullous disease.
  http://dermnetnz.org/immune/linear-iga.html

Genodermatoses

CHAPTER 87 — **Ichthyosis** 569

CHAPTER 88 — **Incontinentia Pigmenti** 577

CHAPTER 89 — **Neurofibromatosis (NF)** 583

CHAPTER 90 — **Tuberous Sclerosis Complex (TSC)** 591

CHAPTER 91 — **Ectodermal Dysplasia** 599

CHAPTER 87

Ichthyosis

Introduction/Etiology/Epidemiology

- Ichthyosis refers to a large group of heterogeneous skin disorders having the common clinical feature of thick fishlike scales.
- The most common form of nonsyndromic ichthyosis is ichthyosis vulgaris, with an occurrence of 1:250.
- The nonsyndromic forms most likely to be encountered are discussed herein.

Signs and Symptoms

- Ichthyosis vulgaris: occurrence 1:250, autosomal semidominant inheritance (disease is milder in those with a pathogenic variant in one allele but more pronounced in those with pathogenic variants in both alleles).
  - Usually not present at birth.
  - Fine brown-gray scales most prominent on distal extremities (Figure 87.1); flexural areas are typically spared.
  - Striking accentuation of palmar and plantar skin creases.
  - Often accompanies atopic dermatitis and other atopic disorders (eg, asthma, allergic rhinoconjunctivitis).
  - Diagnosis: clinical.
  - Caused by pathogenic variants in the filaggrin gene (*FLG*).
- Recessive X-linked ichthyosis: occurrence 1:1,500 male patients.
  - The defect is a pathogenic variant or complete deletion of the *ARSC1* gene that encodes steroid sulfatase.
  - Female carriers have deficient placental steroid sulfatase and associated perinatal problems, including delayed onset of labor and failure to progress.
  - Usually presents in the first 3 months with scaling; may present at birth with a thin collodion membrane.
  - "Dirty" brown fine scale that involves the flexures, preauricular areas, lateral neck, and flanks; palms and soles are spared (Figure 87.2).
  - 50% of patients and 30% of carriers have corneal opacities.

- Patients with recessive X-linked ichthyosis have an increased incidence of cryptorchidism and may have increased risk of testicular cancer.
- Diagnosis: clinical, enzyme assay (reduced steroid sulfatase activity), fluorescent in situ hybridization.

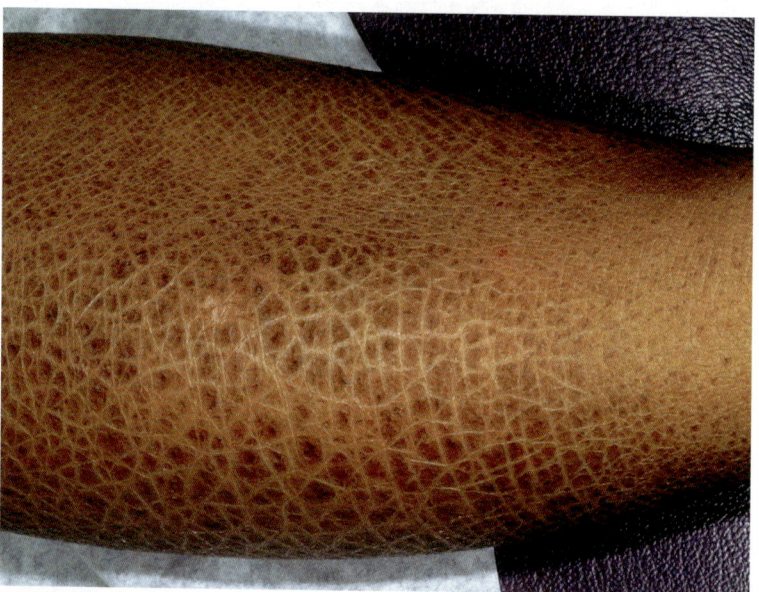

Figure 87.1. In ichthyosis vulgaris, fine scales with a "pasted on" appearance are observed on the distal extremities.

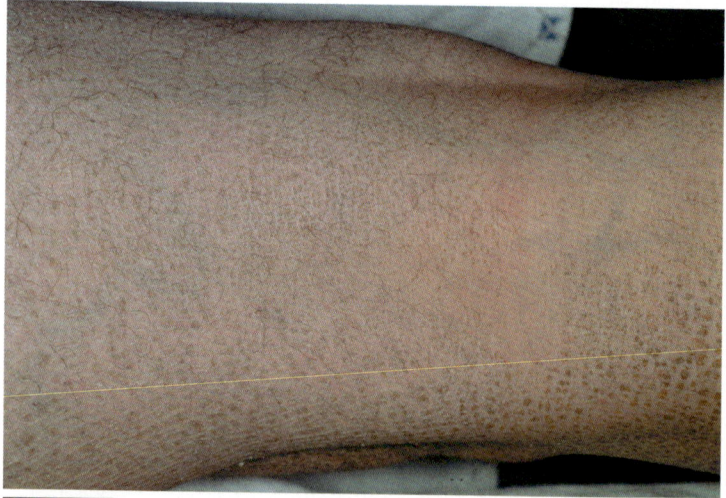

Figure 87.2. Recessive X-linked ichthyosis. There is "dirty" brown fine scale.

- Lamellar ichthyosis
  - One of the more severe ichthyoses; categorized as one of the autosomal recessive congenital ichthyoses (ARCIs), which have an occurrence of 1:300,000 to 1:100,000.
  - Usually present at birth.
    - Often, the neonate is covered with a collodion membrane (Figure 87.3) and exhibits ectropion and eclabium.
    - Neonates may have increased transepidermal water loss and resulting hypernatremic dehydration.
  - Characterized by thick, dark, platelike scale over the entire body (Figure 87.4); ectropion; eclabium; entrapment of hair; entrapment of sweat ducts (leading to risk of hyperthermia from reduced sweating); and atypical nails.
  - Once the lamellar scales have matured and dried, water retention (ie, sweat retention) becomes more problematic.
  - Diagnosis: clinical, histopathology, electron microscopy, molecular genetic testing.
  - Often related to pathogenic variant in transglutaminase 1 (*TGM1*); however, ARCIs have been related to pathogenic variants in 13 known genes (most related to congenital ichthyosiform erythroderma [CIE]).

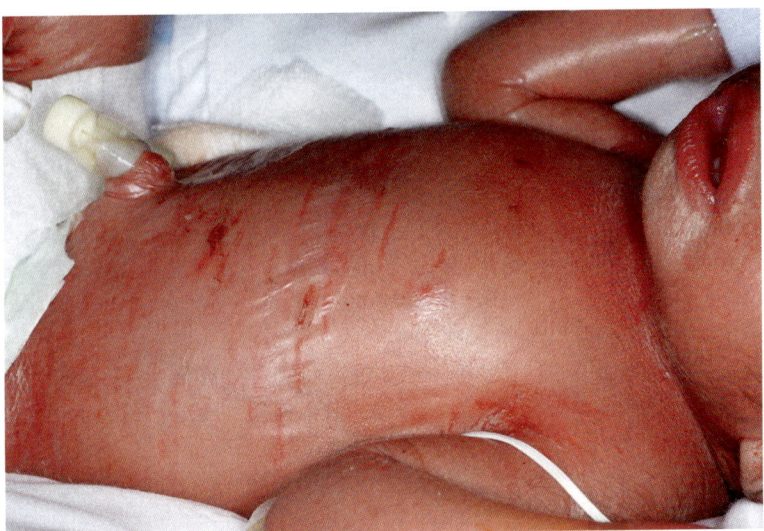

Figure 87.3. This neonate is covered with a thick collodion membrane and there is mild eclabium.

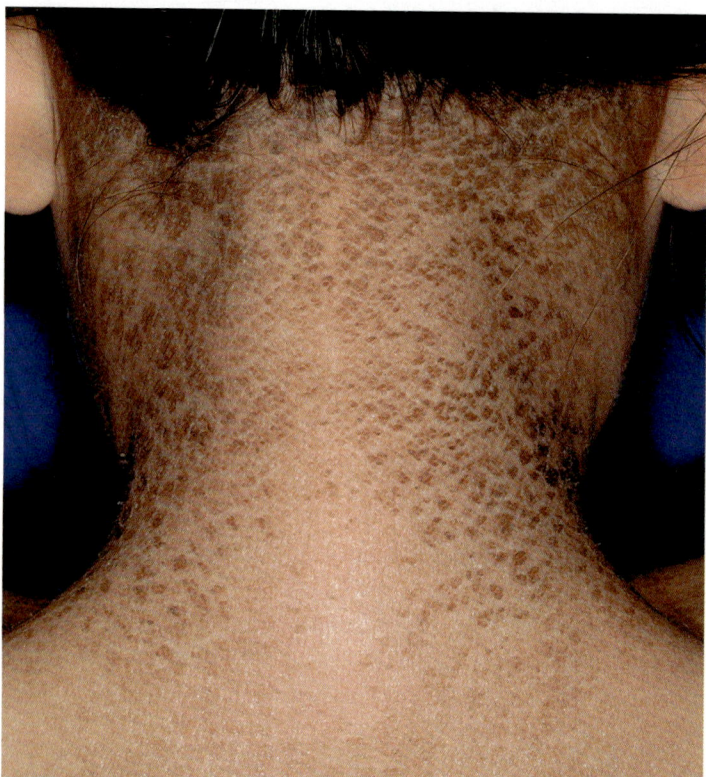

Figure 87.4. Lamellar ichthyosis is characterized by thick, platelike scales.

- CIE
  - Also categorized as a subtype of ARCI.
  - Clinically similar to lamellar ichthyosis in onset (often born with collodion membrane), chronicity, and proclivity to encased scalp, eyelids (causing ectropion), and lips (causing eclabium).
  - Unique features of CIE are the presence of erythroderma and fine whitish scales on the trunk (Figure 87.5).
  - Distal extremities, as in lamellar ichthyosis, may exhibit thick, dark, large, platelike scales.
  - Some patients may improve after puberty.
  - Diagnosis: clinical, histopathology, electron microscopy, molecular genetic testing.
  - May be related to pathogenic variants in *TGM1, ALOXE3, ALOX12B, LIPN,* or several others.

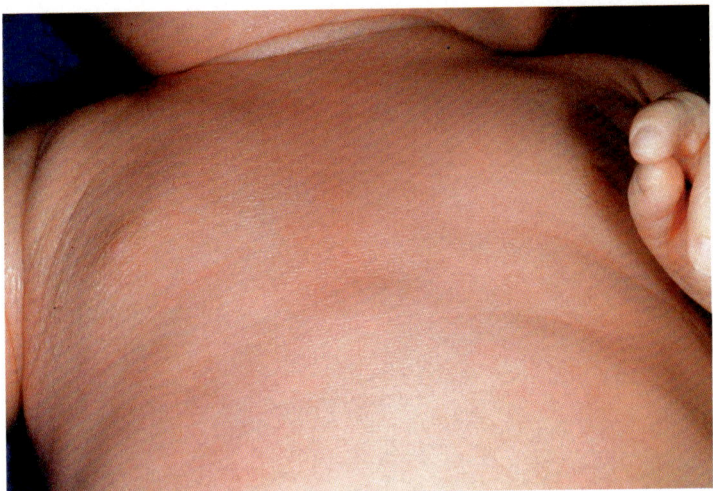

Figure 87.5. Patients who have non-bullous congenital ichthyosiform erythroderma exhibit diffuse erythema and fine scaling.

- ▶ Epidermolytic ichthyosis (formerly *bullous CIE* and *epidermolytic hyperkeratosis*): occurrence 1:300,000, autosomal-dominant inheritance.
  - Considered one of the keratinopathic ichthyoses, which also include the rare disorder superficial epidermolytic ichthyosis (formerly *ichthyosis bullosa of Siemens*).
  - Presents as a severe blistering disease in the newborn. Sheets of epidermis are shed, leaving a widespread glistening redness of the skin (ie, erythroderma). The differential diagnosis may include staphylococcal scalded skin syndrome or epidermolysis bullosa during the neonatal phase.
  - Patches of thick, dark scales eventually develop over the first few weeks to months after birth, especially around flexures.
    - Scales become dark, thickened, and quill-like (Figure 87.6).
    - Blistering diminishes by age 1 year, but skin remains fragile and may blister with trauma in older children.
    - Skin changes typically associated with malodor and colonization by bacteria and *Candida* organisms.
  - Diagnosis: clinical, histopathology, molecular genetic testing.
  - Caused by pathogenic variants in keratin 1 (*KRT1*) or keratin 10 (*KRT10*) genes; superficial epidermolytic ichthyosis is caused by pathogenic variants in keratin 2 (*KRT2*).

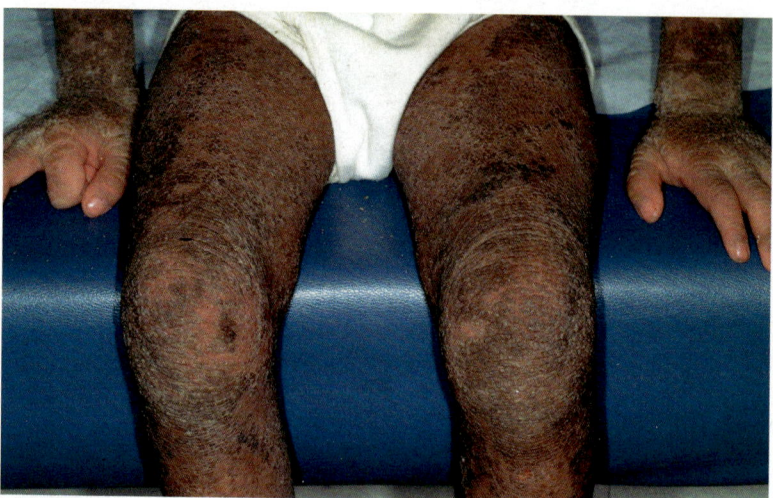

Figure 87.6. Epidermolytic ichthyosis. The skin takes on a cobblestone appearance on the extremities.

Look-alikes

The features described previously assist in differential diagnosis.

How to Make the Diagnosis

- Diagnosis is based on clinical features and testing for individual disorders (as discussed previously).
- Molecular genetic testing is available for diagnostic confirmation and prenatal testing.

Treatment

- Newborns: careful attention to the fluid and electrolyte balance, temperature, protein intake, and infection risk.
- Older children: The specific type of ichthyosis will dictate therapy. Children with types other than ichthyosis vulgaris are best managed in consultation with a pediatric dermatologist. Elements of treatment may include
  - Application of an emollient.
  - Application of a keratolytic (used with caution if the skin surface is compromised due to concerns about systemic absorption); this includes α-hydroxy acid products such as lactic or glycolic acid and urea-containing lotions.

- Topical vitamin D preparations are helpful in some patients.
- Preservation of range of motion when thick scale surrounds joints.
- Use of topical and systemic retinoids for severe cases.

Treating Associated Conditions

▶ Ichthyosis may be the cutaneous manifestation of a variety of other disorders. Consider this possibility if the patient exhibits differences of the central nervous, cardiovascular, or skeletal systems or if the patient has hepatomegaly or experiences metabolic disturbances.

Prognosis

▶ Prognosis depends on the type of ichthyosis. The prognosis is excellent for ichthyosis vulgaris; those with more severe forms will experience lifelong difficulties with dry skin, fissuring, infections, overheating, and thick scales.

When to Worry or Refer

▶ Severe platelike scale, skin fragility, ectropion, infection, metabolic disturbance, hyperthermia, and other anomalies.

Resource for Families

▶ Foundation for Ichthyosis & Related Skin Types: Provides information and support for patients and families, as well as links to health care professionals.
www.firstskinfoundation.org

CHAPTER 88

Incontinentia Pigmenti

Introduction/Etiology/Epidemiology

- X-linked dominant disorder that is usually lethal in male embryos (although rare cases may result from mosaicism or XXY genotype).
- Due to a pathogenic variant in the inhibitor of nuclear factor kappa B kinase regulatory subunit gamma (*IKBKG*) gene.

Signs and Symptoms

- Four stages are recognized and constitute the major diagnostic criteria (the presence of 1 major criterion is sufficient to establish the diagnosis).
  - Stage 1 (vesicular)
    - Often presents at birth with vesicles on erythematous bases distributed in a linear arrangement on limbs or in a whorled pattern on the trunk (conforming to Blaschko lines) (Figure 88.1).
    - Vesicles occur in crops for weeks to months.
  - Stage 2 (verrucous)
    - Begins at about 1 month of age and consists of warty, red-brown papules with scale (Figure 88.2).
    - Typically resolves by 4 to 6 months of age.
  - Stage 3 (hyperpigmented)
    - Linear and swirled hyperpigmentation (along Blaschko lines) (Figure 88.3).
    - May persist for years.
  - Stage 4 (hypopigmented)
    - Hypopigmented atrophic streaks (Figure 88.4).
    - Follicular atrophoderma.
    - Observed in some patients.
- Important to recognize that although the stages typically proceed in order, not all stages may present clinically, they may occur nonsequentially, and there may be overlap between stages.

- Other clinical features (minor criteria) support the diagnosis. These include differences of the teeth (eg, partial or complete absence of teeth, pegged teeth [common]), hair (eg, alopecia, woolly hair), nails (eg, ridging, pitting), and retina (ie, peripheral neovascularization). Affected individuals may also have other ocular differences (eg, optic atrophy, microphthalmos, cataracts, myopia, strabismus) and central nervous system anomalies (eg, seizures, developmental delay).

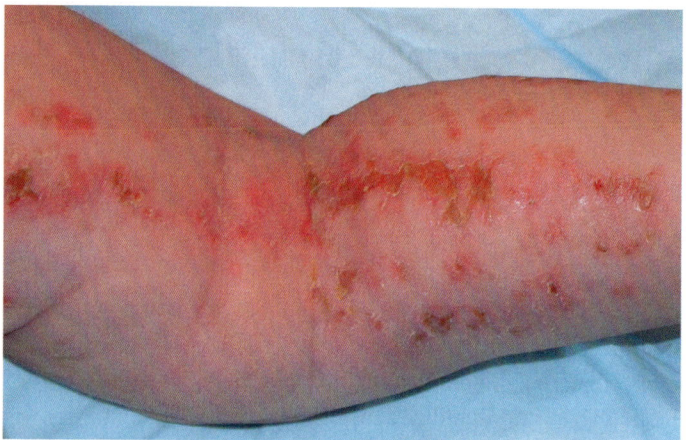

Figure 88.1. In the first stage of incontinentia pigmenti, vesicles and crusting appear in a linear arrangement on the limbs or in a whorled distribution on the trunk.

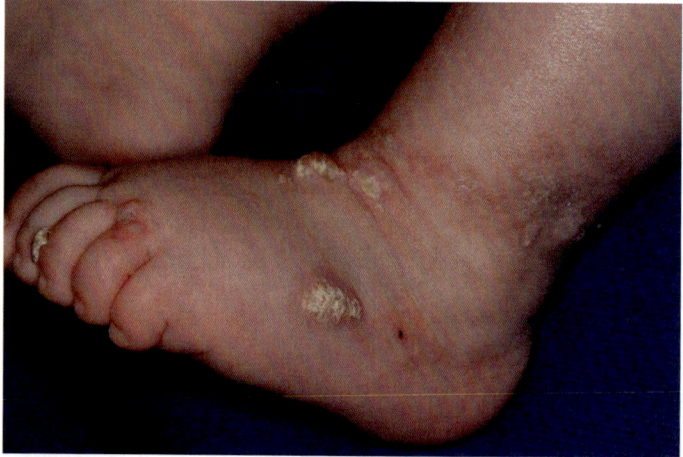

Figure 88.2. Warty papules in an infant, who has the second stage of incontinentia pigmenti.

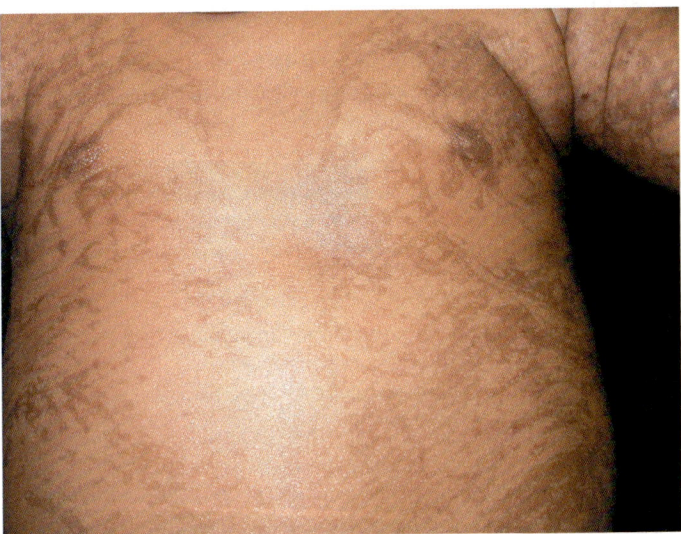

Figure 88.3. Whorled and linear hyperpigmentation, arranged along the Blaschko lines, are observed in the third stage of incontinentia pigmenti.

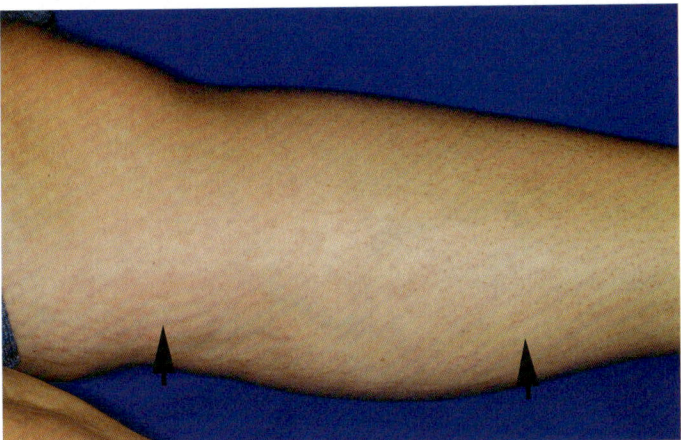

Figure 88.4. Hypopigmented atrophic streaks (arrows) are observed in the fourth stage of incontinentia pigmenti.

Look-alikes

The differential diagnosis of vesicles appearing in the neonatal period is presented here. In none of these disorders are vesicles distributed in a linear or whorled pattern as they are in incontinentia pigmenti.

Disorder	Differentiating Features
Erythema toxicum	• Individual vesicles or pustules on erythematous bases. • Blotchy erythematous patches that wax and wane quickly.
Miliaria crystallina	• Fragile vesicles without surrounding erythema.
Bullous impetigo	• Flaccid bullae or ruptured bullae forming round or oval crusted erosions; vesicles occasionally are present. • Gram stain or bacterial culture will reveal *Staphylococcus aureus*.
Scabies	• Occurs rarely during the first month after birth. • Generalized eruption; may have vesicles but usually will be accompanied by erythematous papules or nodules and burrows. • Palm and sole involvement common.
Neonatal herpes simplex virus infection	• Typically, clustered vesicles on an erythematous base (although solitary vesicles occasionally occur). • Vesicles concentrated on head, particularly at sites of trauma (eg, that caused by a scalp electrode). • Infants may have signs of sepsis (in disseminated disease) or seizures or coma (in central nervous system disease).
Infantile acropustulosis	• Usually begins in first months after birth (not in first days). • Recurrent vesicles or pustules that are limited to the hands and feet, including palms, soles, wrists, and ankles.
Eosinophilic pustular folliculitis	• Papules and pustules typically located on scalp. • Marked pruritus present. • Exhibits chronic, intermittent course.

How to Make the Diagnosis

▶ Diagnosis is typically made clinically based on the appearance and distribution (ie, linear and whorled; in Blaschko's lines) of lesions and confirmed with skin biopsy.
▶ Exclude other diagnoses of importance (eg, herpes simplex virus infection, impetigo).
▶ Skin biopsy can be used to confirm the diagnosis when necessary.
▶ Molecular genetic testing is available for diagnostic confirmation.
▶ Examination of affected mothers may reveal scarring alopecia, nail dystrophy, and atrophic linear hairless streaks (Figure 88.5).

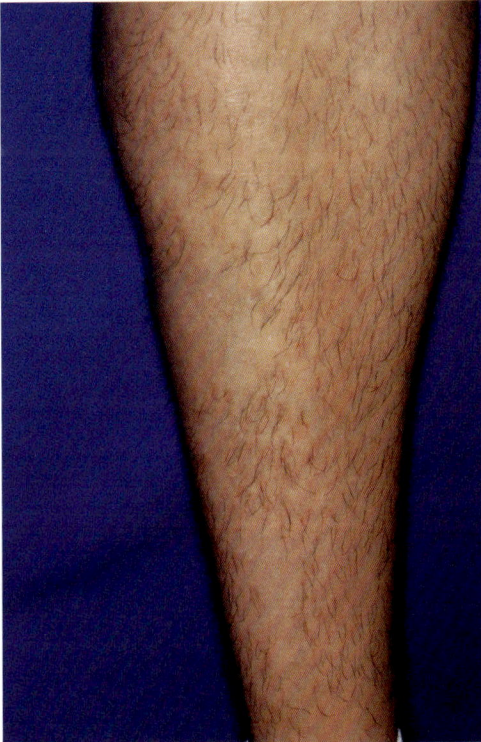

Figure 88.5. Hairless, atrophic streaks on the leg of the affected mother of an infant with incontinentia pigmenti.

Treatment

- Infants in the vesicular stage should be treated with a topical antibiotic ointment applied to open areas to prevent secondary bacterial infection; lesions spontaneously resolve over weeks to months.
- Warty stage lesions may improve temporarily with application of keratolytic agents containing urea or salicylic acid.
  - Beware of the increased percutaneous absorption of these agents, which might lead to systemic toxicity.
  - Application of an emollient to the warty lesions may suffice, as they eventually resolve spontaneously.
- Pediatric ophthalmologic consultation should be obtained as soon after birth as possible, with close follow-up during the first 3 years.
- Male patients should have a karyotype performed, and genetics consultation should be considered.

- Early dental evaluation is recommended with appropriate follow-up.
- Additional evaluation should be based on observation of other features, such as seizures, developmental delay, or skeletal anomalies.

Treating Associated Conditions

- Neurodevelopmental, ocular, skeletal, and dental problems should be addressed as they develop.

Prognosis

- Prognosis is generally excellent but is influenced by involvement of other areas, particularly the central nervous system.

When to Worry or Refer

- Refer all patients for dental and ophthalmologic evaluation; consider genetics referral for diagnostic confirmation and genetic counseling.
- Refer to dermatology, neurology, or orthopedic surgery as clinically indicated.

Resources for Families

- National Foundation for Ectodermal Dysplasias: Provides information and support on incontinentia pigmenti.
  https://www.nfed.org/blog/welcome-incontinentia-pigmenti-families
- National Institute of Neurological Disorders and Stroke: Provides information about incontinentia pigmenti and links to relevant organizations.
  https://www.ninds.nih.gov/Disorders/All-Disorders/Incontinentia-pigmenti-Information-Page

CHAPTER 89

Neurofibromatosis (NF)

Introduction/Etiology/Epidemiology

- Neurofibromatosis (NF) is a cluster of syndromes sharing common features.
  - NF type 1 (NF1) is transmitted as an autosomal dominant trait (50%) or occurs as a spontaneous pathogenic variant (50%). The gene responsible (*NF1* gene) is located on chromosome 17 and encodes the protein neurofibromin.
  - Inheritance of NF type 2 (NF2) is autosomal dominant, with 50% spontaneous new pathogenic variants. The gene responsible (*NF2* gene) is located on the long arm of chromosome 22 and encodes the protein merlin.

Signs and Symptoms

- NF1
  - Two or more of the following clinical features are necessary for the diagnosis of NF1:
    - Café au lait macules (Figure 89.1).
      - Six or more measuring more than 0.5 cm in infants and children or more than 1.5 cm in postpubertal individuals. (The majority of children who have ≥6 café au lait macules ultimately will have NF1 diagnosed.)
      - Have smooth borders ("coast of California").
      - Nearly all patients who have NF1 meet this criterion.
    - Two or more neurofibromas of any type (Figure 89.2) or 1 or more plexiform neurofibromas (Figure 89.3).
    - Axillary or inguinal freckling (Figure 89.4); occurs in 85% of patients.
    - Optic glioma; present in 15% to 20% of pediatric patients with NF1; most commonly detected in those younger than 6 years.
    - Two or more Lisch nodules (iris hamartomas); these are rarely seen before 3 years of age (Figure 89.5).
    - Characteristic osseous lesion (eg, dysplasia of the sphenoid bone; dysplasia of long bone cortex, which often manifests as anterolateral bowing of long bones [ie, the tibia]; and pseudarthrosis).
    - A parent who meets the diagnostic criteria for NF1.

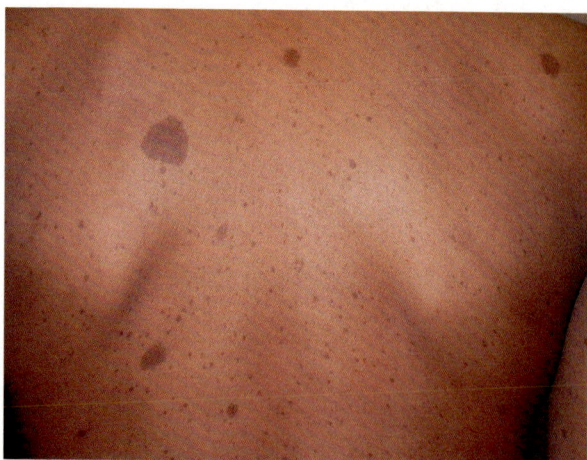

Figure 89.1. Multiple café au lait macules in a patient who has neurofibromatosis type 1.

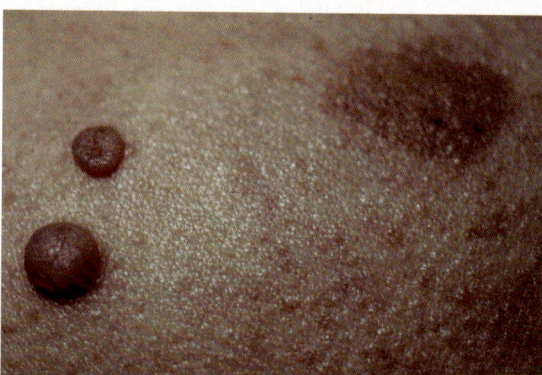

Figure 89.2. Neurofibromas and a café au lait macule in a patient who has neurofibromatosis type 1.

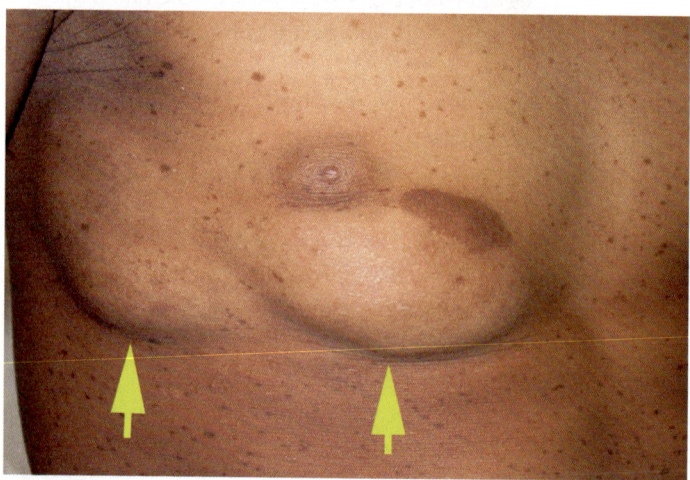

Figure 89.3. Plexiform neurofibromas (ie, large, subcutaneous masses [arrows]) in a patient who has neurofibromatosis type 1.

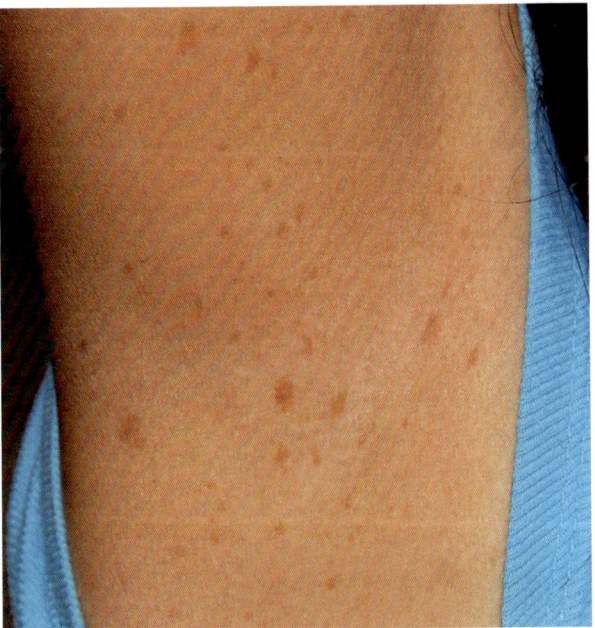

Figure 89.4. Axillary freckling in a patient who has neurofibromatosis type 1.

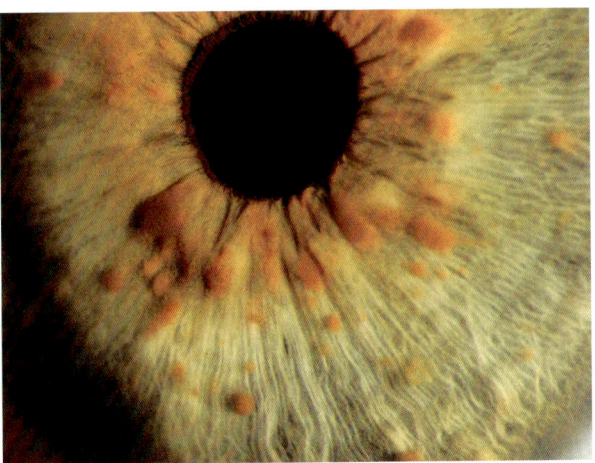

Figure 89.5. Lisch nodules (iris hamartomas) are observed in patients who have neurofibromatosis type 1.

- Other common features observed in patients who have NF1 include the following:
  - Macrocephaly (independent of tumors or severity).
  - Short stature.
  - Precocious puberty.
  - Scoliosis.
  - Hypertension (may be due to renal artery stenosis or pheochromocytoma).
  - Learning disabilities observed in as many as 40% of children; attention-deficit/hyperactivity disorder and autism spectrum disorder also may occur.
  - Intellectual disability seen in approximately 5% of patients.
  - Epilepsy occurs in as many as 7% of individuals.

▶ NF2-related schwannomatosis
- In children, the diagnosis should be suspected when 2 or more of the following are present:
  - A schwannoma at any location, including intradermal.
  - Skin plaques present at birth or in early childhood (often plexiform schwannomas at histologic examination).
  - A meningioma, particularly non-meningothelial (non-arachnoidal) cell in origin.
  - A cortical wedge cataract.
  - A retinal hamartoma.
  - A mononeuropathy, particularly causing a facial nerve palsy, foot or wrist drop, or third nerve palsy.
- Other features include the following:
  - Fewer cutaneous neurofibromas than in patients who have NF1.
  - Small numbers of large, pale café au lait macules.

Look-alikes

The constellation of features observed in patients who have NF1 generally suggests the diagnosis and excludes other disorders. Some other diseases characterized by multiple café au lait macules are presented as follows:

Disorder	Differentiating Features
McCune-Albright syndrome	• Large segmental café au lait macule(s), often with "coast of Maine" (shaggy border) appearance. • Bony variations (eg, polyostotic fibrous dysplasia). • Endocrine variations.
Silver-Russell syndrome	• Triangular face. • Short stature. • Skeletal asymmetry. • Atypical pubertal development.
Bloom syndrome	• Short stature. • Facial telangiectasias and erythema. • Narrow face, prominent nose and ears.
Multiple café au lait macules without neurofibromatosis	• Multiple café au lait macules without other features of neurofibromatosis type 1. • Some of these patients may have Legius syndrome (caused by *SPRED1* pathogenic variant), characterized by multiple café au lait macules and, in some cases, intertriginous freckling, lipomas, macrocephaly, learning disabilities, attention-deficit/hyperactivity disorder, and developmental delay.

How to Make the Diagnosis

▶ The diagnosis of NF1 or NF2 is usually made clinically, satisfying the criteria listed previously.

▶ Molecular genetic testing is available for NF1 and NF2 and may be used to confirm a clinical diagnosis or evaluate a patient in whom diagnostic uncertainty exists. It may also be used in counseling those affected who are planning a pregnancy or in prenatal diagnosis once pregnant.

Treatment

▶ There is no specific therapy for NF1. Management is directed primarily at identifying and treating complications. Those providing health care for patients who have NF1 should consult the American Academy of Pediatrics clinical report, "Health Supervision for Children With Neurofibromatosis Type 1" (*Pediatrics.* 2019;143[5]:e20190660). Elements of surveillance include the following:
- Genetic evaluation.
- At all health maintenance visits monitor growth, head circumference, and blood pressure; perform a complete examination concentrating on cardiac, cutaneous, ophthalmologic, neurologic, and skeletal systems; monitor for precocious puberty; and assess development and behavior, vision, and hearing.
- Ophthalmologic examination annually until puberty, then as needed.
- Head magnetic resonance imaging: The role of this procedure (eg, to determine whether an optic glioma is present) in individuals without symptoms is controversial and should be determined on a case-by-case basis in collaboration with an ophthalmologist.
- Selumetinib (an inhibitor of mitogen-activated protein kinase kinase enzyme, or MEK inhibitor) is approved by the US Food and Drug Administration for treatment of children 2 years or older with symptomatic inoperable plexiform neurofibromas).

▶ There is no specific therapy for NF2. Management should include the following:
- Genetic evaluation.
- Surveillance for vestibular schwannomas by means of magnetic resonance imaging, audiometry, or brainstem auditory evoked response.

Treating Associated Conditions

▶ NF1: Learning disabilities, optic gliomas, plexiform neurofibromas, and other complications should be addressed if they develop.
▶ NF2: Vestibular schwannomas or hearing loss should be addressed if present.

Prognosis

- The prognosis for NF is variable, depending on the severity of involvement and development of malignancy.
- The spectrum of severity ranges from individuals with minimal effect on quality of life to those with profound effect or who require multiple procedures and coordinated multispecialty care.

When to Worry or Refer

- NF1: Development of pain in or sudden growth of a plexiform neurofibroma; sudden changes in visual acuity; development of headache, hypertension, scoliosis, or variations of long bones.
- NF2: Development of hearing loss, tinnitus, difficulties with balance, headache, or other signs of increased intracranial pressure.
- Subspecialties that may be involved in the care of patients with NF include genetics, neurology, ophthalmology, surgery (ie, orthopedic, general, plastic), dermatology, otolaryngology, and oncology.

Resources for Families

- Children's Tumor Foundation: Education and links to support and physicians for patients who have NF and their families.
  www.ctf.org
- Neurofibromatosis Consortium: Information about ongoing clinical trials and links to NF clinical centers.
  www.uab.edu/nfconsortium
- Neurofibromatosis Network: Provides support and information for patients and families.
  www.nfnetwork.org

CHAPTER 90

Tuberous Sclerosis Complex (TSC)

Introduction/Etiology/Epidemiology

- Tuberous sclerosis complex (TSC) is a neurocutaneous syndrome and a multisystem disorder with highly variable features.
- TSC is caused by pathological variants in either *TSC1* on chromosome 9 (encoding hamartin) or *TSC2* on chromosome 16 (encoding tuberin).
- The disorder is transmitted as an autosomal dominant trait with high penetrance but markedly variable expressivity; up to two-thirds of cases are new pathological variants.

Signs and Symptoms

TSC involves variations in the following systems:

- Skin
  - Hypomelanotic macules (traditionally referred to as *ash leaf spots*) present at birth or soon thereafter; occur in 87% to 100% of patients (Figure 90.1).
  - Facial angiofibromas (ie, adenoma sebaceum).
    - Erythematous papules located in the nasolabial folds, nose, cheeks, or chin (Figure 90.2).
    - Appear between 2 and 6 years of age; occur in 47% to 90% of patients.
  - Shagreen patches: plaques with a peau d'orange texture usually observed in the lumbosacral region (Figure 90.3); occur in 20% to 80% of patients.
  - Fibrous cephalic plaques (formerly called *fibrous forehead plaques*): connective tissue nevi that may be present at birth.
  - Periungual fibromas: usually appear after puberty; observed in 17% to 80% of patients (Figure 90.4).

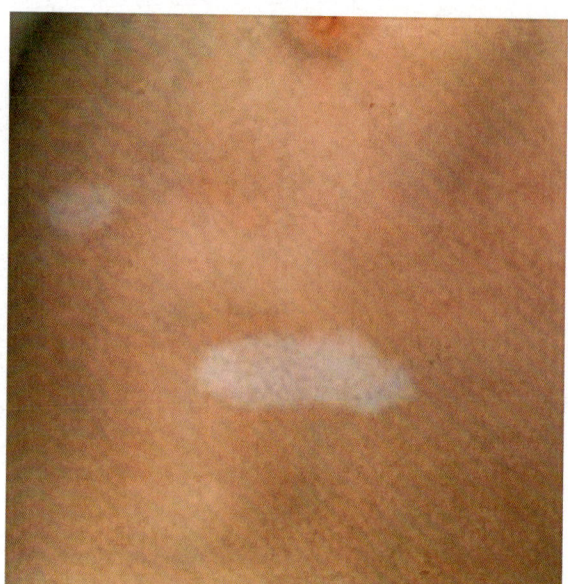

Figure 90.1. Hypopigmented macules on the chest of a child who has tuberous sclerosis complex.

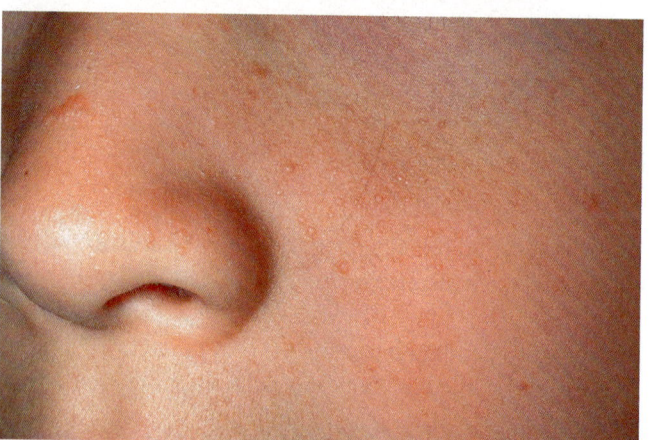

Figure 90.2. Facial angiofibromas are pink to red papules (occasionally may appear more flesh-colored in skin of color) that are most prominently distributed on the nose, cheeks, nasolabial folds, and chin, as seen in this teenager with tuberous sclerosis complex.

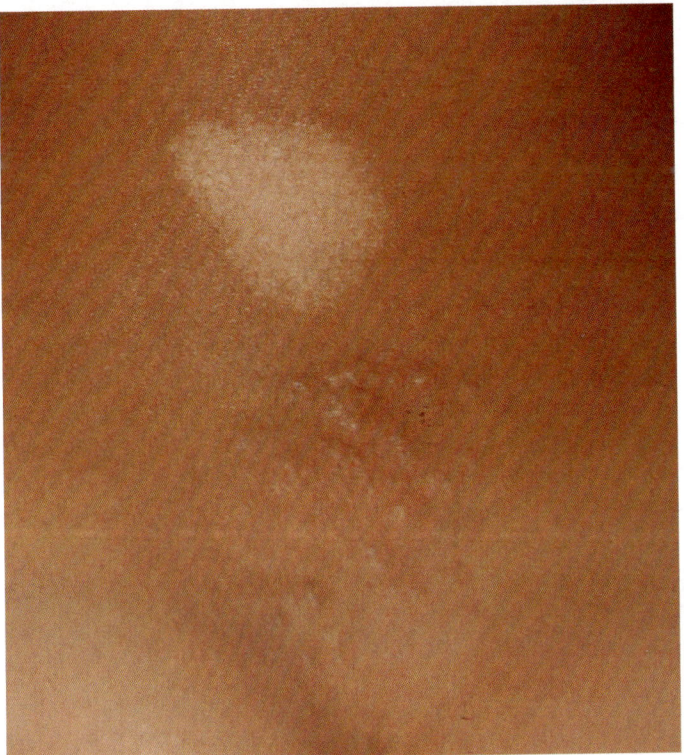

Figure 90.3. Shagreen patches have an orange peel or cobblestone texture and often are located over the lumbosacral spine. This patient with skin of color also has a hypomelanotic patch above the shagreen patch.

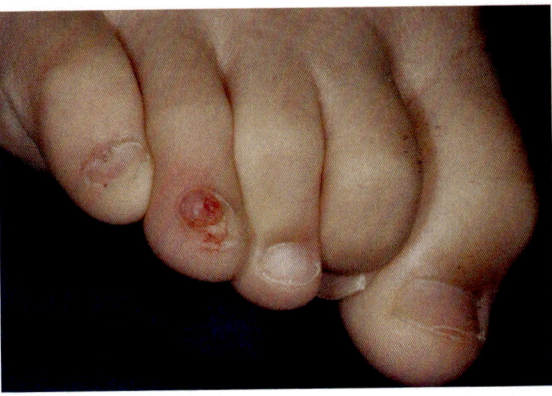

Figure 90.4. Periungual fibromas usually appear after puberty in patients who have tuberous sclerosis complex.

- Brain: subependymal nodules (90%); TSC-associated neuropsychiatric disorder, including autism spectrum disorder, cognitive disorders, and others (90%); seizures, including infantile spasms (80%); cortical tubers (70%); subependymal giant cell astrocytoma (SEGA)
- Kidney: angiomyolipomas (70%), cysts
- Heart: rhabdomyomas (47%–67%), arrhythmia
- Eye: astrocytic hamartoma of the retina, optic disc, or both (up to 50% of patients)
- Lungs: lymphangioleiomyomatosis (LAM) (30% of women)

Look-alikes

The constellation of clinical findings suggests the diagnosis of TSC and excludes other disorders. The differential diagnosis of hypopigmented macules and angiofibromas is presented here; however, in each of the conditions listed, other features of TSC would be absent.

Disorder	Differentiating Features
Hypopigmented Macules	
Vitiligo	• Acquired disorder. • Affected areas exhibit complete pigment loss (ie, depigmentation), not hypopigmentation. • Predilection for elbows, knees, ankles, hips, fingers, and periorificial regions. • Tends to occur in symmetric fashion.
Pityriasis alba	• Acquired disorder. • Poorly defined areas of macular hypopigmentation often with associated scale; most commonly involves the face. • Atopic history common.
Tinea versicolor	• Acquired disorder. • Seen mainly in individuals after puberty. • Well-defined hypopigmented macules and patches located on the trunk, proximal arms, or neck. • Lesions often have associated fine scale and may be pruritic.
Pigmentary mosaicism–nevus depigmentosus type	• Present at birth but may not become noticeable for months to years. • Hypopigmentation with a shaggy border. • Usually occurs unilaterally and respects the midline. • Typically larger than a hypopigmented macule. • Geographic or segmental distribution common.

Look-alikes

Disorder	Differentiating Features
Pigmentary mosaicism—hypomelanosis of Ito type	• Present at birth but may not become noticeable for months to years. • Hypopigmentation that follows the Blaschko lines (ie, lines representing patterns of embryonic cell migration from the neural crest); presents as streaky lines on the extremities and whorls on the trunk.
Piebaldism	• Congenital absence of pigmentation localized to 1 area. • Associated poliosis (depigmentation of hair) may be present when involving face and scalp. • Rare associations with other variations (eg, Waardenburg syndrome).
Nevus anemicus	• Congenital area of pallor (may resemble hypopigmentation) resulting from diminished vascular flow to the affected region. • Diascopy (compressing the lesion with a glass slide) will cause blanching of surrounding typical skin, causing border of the lesion to disappear.
Angiofibromas	
Acne	• Often appears later than angiofibromas. • Comedones (ie, blackheads and whiteheads) and pustules usually present. • Involvement of forehead, chest, shoulders, and back common. • Early acne often limited to T zone (ie, forehead, and the middle face including chin, nose, and occasionally medial portion of cheeks).
Molluscum contagiosum	• Usually translucent papules that may have a central umbilication. • Usually not symmetrically distributed and may be present at other (non-facial) sites.
Periorificial dermatitis	• Typically exhibits small pustules and acneiform papules. • Erythema and scaling may be present, especially in nasolabial folds. • Concentrated in perioral, perinasal, and periorbital regions.
Keratosis pilaris	• Small, rough-feeling (sandpaper-like), skin-colored or erythematous papules. • Keratin plug or hair emerging from follicular orifice may be observed or palpated. • Often located at other non-facial sites as well (eg, upper arms, thighs, buttocks).

How to Make the Diagnosis

- Definite TSC requires the presence of 2 major features or 1 major and 2 or more minor features.
- Possible TSC requires the presence of 1 major feature or 2 or more minor features.
- Molecular genetic testing is available for diagnostic confirmation and prenatal diagnosis.

Major Features

- Hypomelanotic macules (≥3 at least 5 mm in diameter)
- Facial angiofibromas (≥3) or fibrous cephalic plaque
- Ungual fibromas (≥2)
- Shagreen patch (connective tissue nevus)
- Multiple retinal nodular hamartomas
- Multiple cortical tubers and/or radial migration lines
- Subependymal nodules (≥2)
- SEGA
- Cardiac rhabdomyoma
- LAM
- Renal angiomyolipoma (≥2)

Minor Features

- "Confetti" hypopigmented macules
- Dental enamel pits (>3)
- Intraoral fibromas (≥2)
- Retinal achromic patch
- Multiple renal cysts
- Nonrenal hamartoma
- Sclerotic bone lesions

Treatment

- Prompt diagnosis, early identification and treatment of seizures, surveillance for additional features and complications, and genetic counseling form the fundamental approach to management.
- Multidisciplinary care is vital. Neurology and genetics generally are involved in the care of all patients with TSC. Other subspecialties that may be involved include ophthalmology, dermatology, nephrology, cardiology, oncology, pulmonology, orthopedic surgery, psychiatry and psychology, and dentistry.
- Essential studies if considering the diagnosis include brain magnetic resonance imaging (MRI), neurodevelopmental testing, ophthalmologic evaluation, electrocardiography, echocardiography, and abdominal MRI (preferred over renal ultrasonography).
- Sun protection is important, as ultraviolet radiation–induced DNA damage can lead to progression of angiofibromas.
- Several topical or systemic inhibitors of mammalian target of rapamycin are available for various manifestations of TSC.
    - Everolimus has been approved for use in the treatment of SEGA and seizures (and select other complications) associated with TSC.
    - Systemic mammalian target of rapamycin inhibitors are used to treat growing renal angiomyolipoma and severe lung disease caused by LAM.
    - Topical sirolimus (rapamycin) is used to treat facial angiofibromas.

Treating Associated Conditions

- Complete evaluation, as noted previously, should identify most of the associated problems; these should be managed appropriately.
- Brain MRI should be repeated every 1 to 3 years in individuals without symptoms who are younger than 25 years to monitor for SEGA.
- Abdominal MRI (preferred over renal ultrasonography) should be performed every 1 to 3 years to monitor for angiomyolipoma and renal cystic disease.
- High-resolution chest computed tomography should be performed routinely in women older than 18 years (to screen for pulmonary LAM) and in any patient if pulmonary symptoms are present.
- Monitor for associated neuropsychiatric manifestations.

Prognosis

Prognosis depends on the following:

- The extent of neurologic involvement and the development of central nervous system complications. Central nervous system tumors are the leading cause of morbidity and mortality.
- Complications in other organ systems.
  - Renal: Renal disease is the second leading cause of early death in patients who have TSC.
  - Cardiovascular: rhabdomyomas (often regress spontaneously), cardiac arrhythmias.
  - Pulmonary: pulmonary LAM (usually affects adult women).

When to Worry or Refer

- Any infant or young child suspected of having TSC should be referred to a pediatric neurologist as soon as possible (to evaluate for epilepsy). Also refer if brain, cardiac, renal, or pulmonary tumors are suspected or present.
- Consider referral for neurodevelopmental testing.

Resources for Families

- National Institute of Neurological Disorders and Stroke: Provides information about tuberous sclerosis complex and links to organizations providing support.
  https://www.ninds.nih.gov/health-information/disorders/tuberous-sclerosis-complex
- TSC Alliance: Provides support and information (in English and Spanish) for affected patients and their families. The organization also maintains a list of TSC clinics in the United States.
  www.tsalliance.org
- Tuberous Sclerosis Association: A site in the United Kingdom that provides information for patients and medical providers.
  www.tuberous-sclerosis.org

CHAPTER 91

Ectodermal Dysplasia

Introduction/Etiology/Epidemiology

- The ectodermal dysplasias are a large group of genetic disorders characterized by defects in 2 or more ectodermal structures (ie, teeth, hair, nails, and sweat glands).
- There are nearly 200 forms of ectodermal dysplasia.
- Hypohidrotic ectodermal dysplasia (1:100,000 births) is a classic example.

Signs and Symptoms

- Depending on the syndrome, there are combinations of defects in teeth, hair, nails, and sweat glands.
- Many ectodermal dysplasias have additional variations, such as eczema, hearing defects or deafness, cleft lip and palate, vision differences, limb deformities, developmental delay or intellectual disability, and urinary tract anomalies.
- Two forms that are most likely to be encountered are
  - Anhidrotic (hypohidrotic) ectodermal dysplasia (Christ-Siemens-Touraine syndrome).
    - Characterized by reduced sweating, hypotrichosis, and defective dentition.
    - Neonates appear red and scaly at birth.
    - Scalp and body hair are sparse and light colored (Figure 91.1).
    - Decreased sweat glands with decreased sweating (hypohidrosis) and risk of hyperthermia.
    - Delayed tooth eruption; conical or misshapen teeth (Figure 91.2).
    - Characteristic facial features include saddle nose, midface hypoplasia, and periorbital hyperpigmentation (Figure 91.3).
    - Most often occurs in male patients because of X-linked recessive pathogenic variant in ectodysplasin A.

- Hidrotic ectodermal dysplasia (Clouston syndrome).
  - Characterized by sparse scalp and sexual hair, nail variations, and keratoderma (marked thickening) of palms and soles. Sweat glands are intact (thus termed *hidrotic*).
  - Hair loss is usually gradual and more pronounced after puberty.
  - Nails may be typical at birth and gradually become thickened and misshapen.
  - Keratoderma increases with age.
  - Caused by an autosomal-dominant pathogenic variant in *GJB6*.

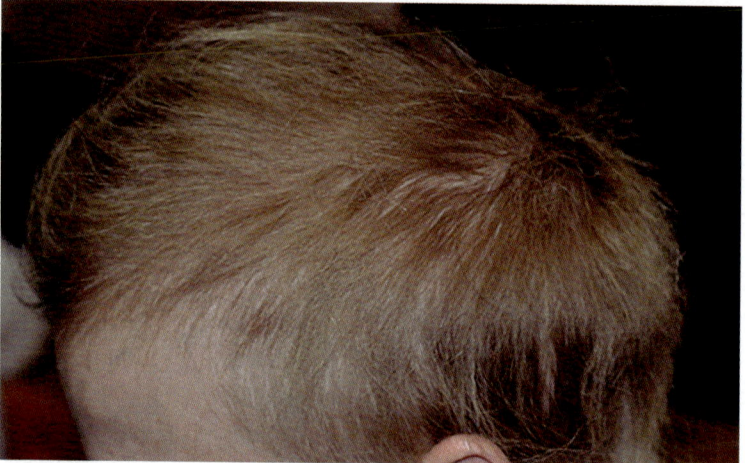

Figure 91.1. Light-colored, short, sparse hair is seen in this young patient with anhidrotic (hypohidrotic) ectodermal dysplasia.

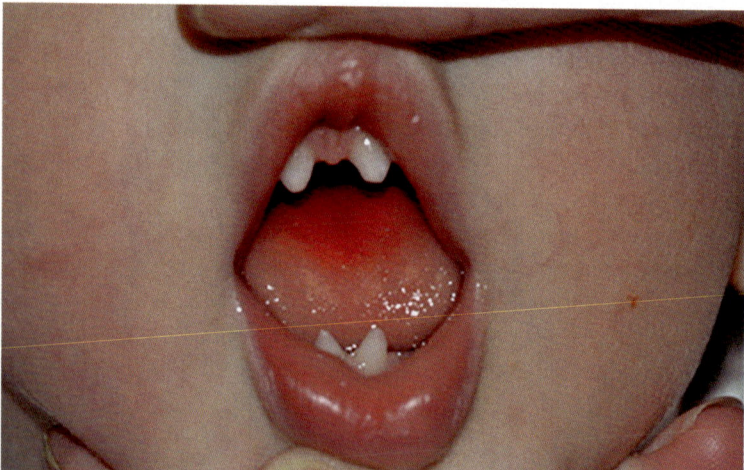

Figure 91.2. This infant with anhidrotic (hypohidrotic) ectodermal dysplasia has conical teeth.

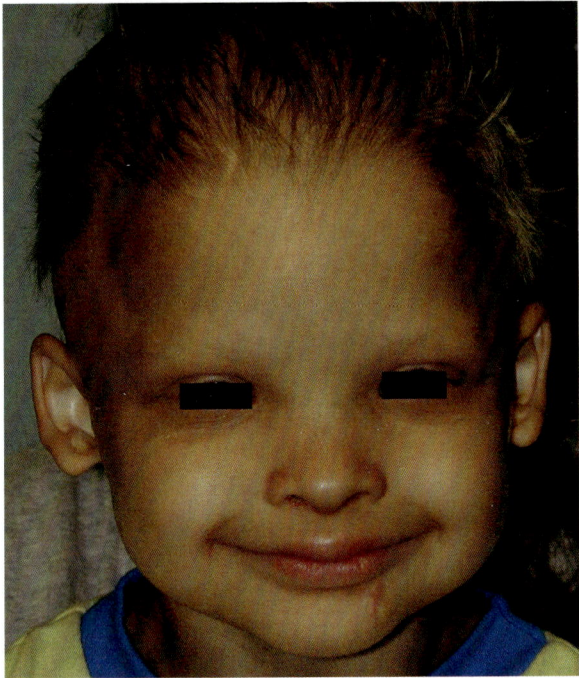

Figure 91.3. This patient with anhidrotic (hypohidrotic) ectodermal dysplasia exhibits the typical facial features, including depressed nasal bridge, midface hypoplasia, periocular hyperpigmentation, and sparse hair.

Look-alikes

For anhidrotic ectodermal dysplasia, the facial features, hypotrichosis, and atypical dentition are unique and, in the absence of other differences (eg, major skeletal anomalies, immunodeficiency), usually are sufficient for diagnosis and to distinguish it from other entities.

Disorder	Differentiating Features
Pachyonychia congenita	• Distinguished by absence of keratoderma and hypotrichosis.
Keratosis-ichthyosis-deafness syndrome	• Distinguished by milder nail dystrophy and presence of sensorineural deafness.

How to Make the Diagnosis

▶ Diagnosis is typically based on the distinct clinical features and family history.

▶ Genetic testing can confirm many types of ectodermal dysplasia.

Treatment

- There is no cure for ectodermal dysplasia.
- Gentle skin care and frequent moisturizing can help with dry or itchy skin.
- Urea cream (20% or 40%) may help improve nail thickening and aid in trimming.
- Dental variations can be corrected with implants or dentures, and early dental evaluation is vital.
- Hair prostheses may be helpful for some patients.
- For patients with hypohidrosis, precautions should be taken to avoid overheating, such as cool baths, cooling suits, use of spray misters, air-conditioning, and light clothing.
- Lubricating eye drops and nasal irrigation may be necessary.
- Genetic counseling is recommended to determine the need for molecular genetic testing, carrier testing, or prenatal testing.

Prognosis

- Most patients with ectodermal dysplasia have a typical life expectancy.
- Some patients have an increased susceptibility toward respiratory infections, which can contribute to morbidity and mortality.

When to Worry or Refer

- Dentists, pediatric dermatologists, and genetic specialists should be involved in the patient's care and can aid in making the diagnosis.
- Refer to other specialists as indicated based on affected systems.

Resources for Families

- National Foundation for Ectodermal Dysplasias.
  https://www.nfed.org
- NORD—National Organization for Rare Disorders: Ectodermal dysplasias.
  https://rarediseases.org/rare-diseases/ectodermal-dysplasias

Hair Disorders

CHAPTER 92 — **Alopecia Areata** 605

CHAPTER 93 — **Androgenetic Alopecia** 615

CHAPTER 94 — **Hypertrichosis and Hirsutism** 619

CHAPTER 95 — **Loose Anagen Syndrome** 623

CHAPTER 96 — **Telogen Effluvium** 629

CHAPTER 97 — **Traction Alopecia** 635

CHAPTER 98 — **Trichotillomania** 639

CHAPTER
92

Alopecia Areata

Introduction/Etiology/Epidemiology

- Alopecia areata is a common cause of non-scarring hair loss (alopecia) in children and adults.
- Prevalence is estimated at approximately 0.2% of the population, and lifetime risk is believed to be between 1% and 2%.
- Genetic and environmental factors may be important; approximately 1 in 5 patients has a family member who is affected. Recent studies have identified nucleotide polymorphisms that appear to be associated with alopecia areata.
- Believed to be an organ-specific autoimmune disease; melanocyte peptides are the suspected antigen.
- Patients may be more frequently affected by atopic diseases such as asthma, allergic rhinitis, and atopic dermatitis. Patients may have a family history positive for alopecia areata.
- May be associated with other autoimmune or systemic disorders, including thyroid disease, vitiligo, diabetes, systemic lupus erythematosus, and inflammatory bowel disease; risk of potential associations remains unclear and controversial.
- Also rarely reported in association with HIV and other immunodeficiency diseases.

Signs and Symptoms

- Most patients have a history of asymptomatic sudden hair loss, which is often rapidly progressive.
- The affected scalp usually has round to oval, smooth, well-circumscribed patches of complete hair loss (Figure 92.1).
- Alopecia may range from a small solitary patch to many patches of variable sizes (Figure 92.2).

PEDIATRIC DERMATOLOGY

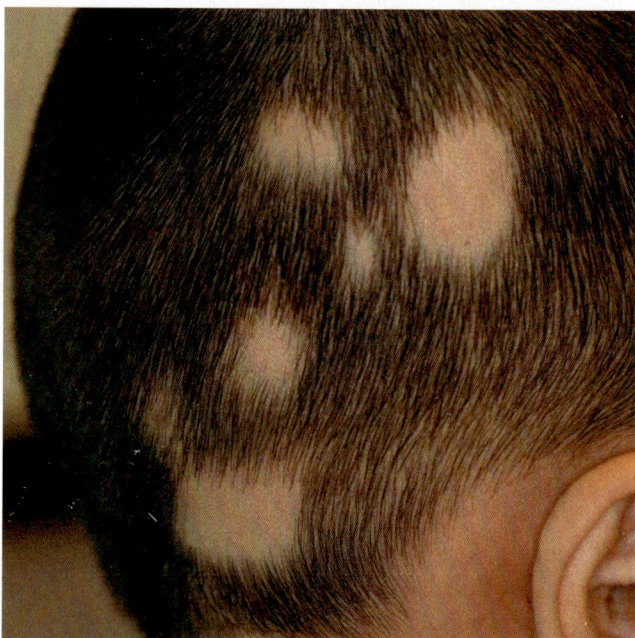

Figure 92.1. Smooth, well-defined patches of complete hair loss in a child with alopecia areata.

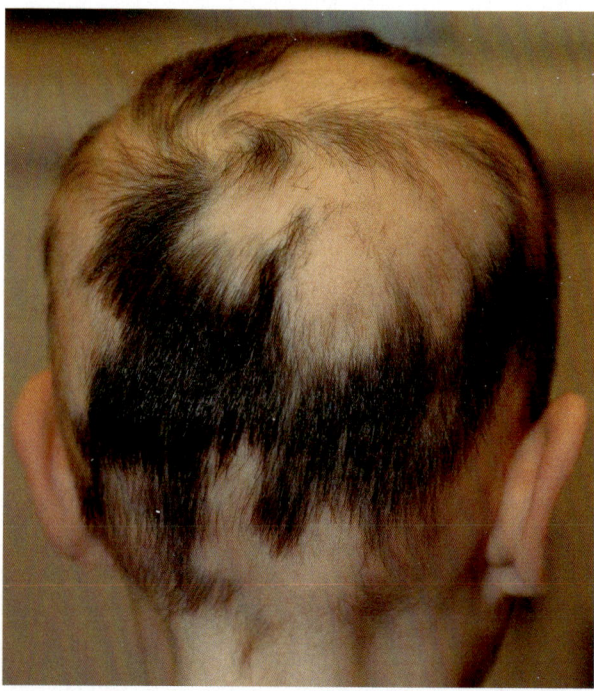

Figure 92.2. Extensive patchy hair loss in a child with alopecia areata.

- Less commonly, a patient may present with an ophiasis distribution in which there is circumferential hair loss extending around the temporal and occipital hairlines; this form has a poorer prognosis and is often recalcitrant to treatment.
- Occasionally, the condition can progress to complete loss of more than 90% of scalp hair (alopecia totalis) (Figure 92.3) or complete alopecia of all hair-bearing surfaces, including eyelashes, eyebrows (Figure 92.4), nose hairs, and body hair (alopecia universalis).
- Rarely, alopecia areata may present with diffuse scalp hair thinning that may resemble telogen effluvium.
- Usually, there are no associated scalp findings of scale or inflammation, although histologically, there is evidence of a perifollicular lymphocytic infiltration. Sometimes the affected skin has a peachy hue.
- In some patients, finding of exclamation point hairs, short hairs that taper proximally and are thicker distally (Figure 92.5), can further support the diagnosis.
- Dermoscopy (magnified light examination) reveals exclamation point hairs and yellow perifollicular dots; dermatologists may use this modality if the diagnosis is in question.
- Nail changes occur in roughly one-half of patients with alopecia areata and (not specific for alopecia areata) include the following:
  - Multiple small pits (often linear) (Figure 92.6).
  - Trachyonychia (thin, longitudinal ridges giving the nail plates a diffuse sandpaper-like texture).
  - Separation of the distal nail plate from the nail bed (onycholysis).

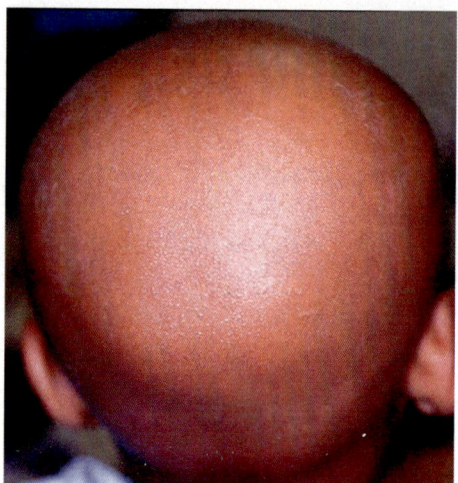

Figure 92.3. Nearly complete hair loss in a child with severe alopecia areata (alopecia totalis).

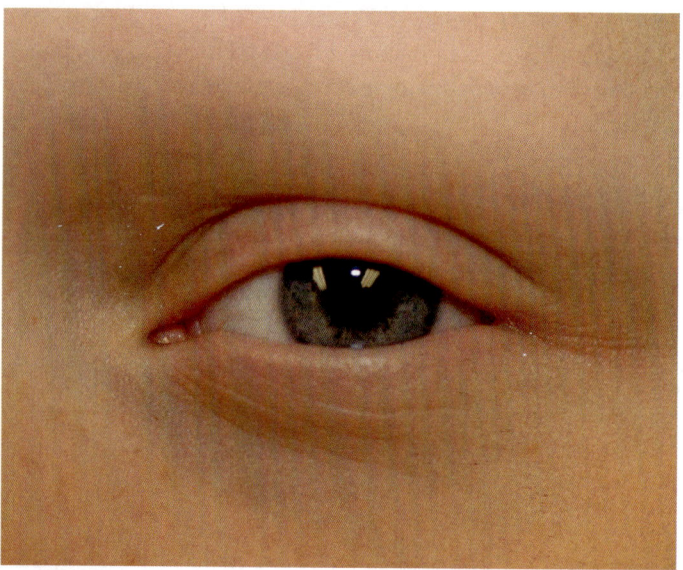

Figure 92.4. Complete loss of eyelashes and eyebrows in a child with alopecia universalis.

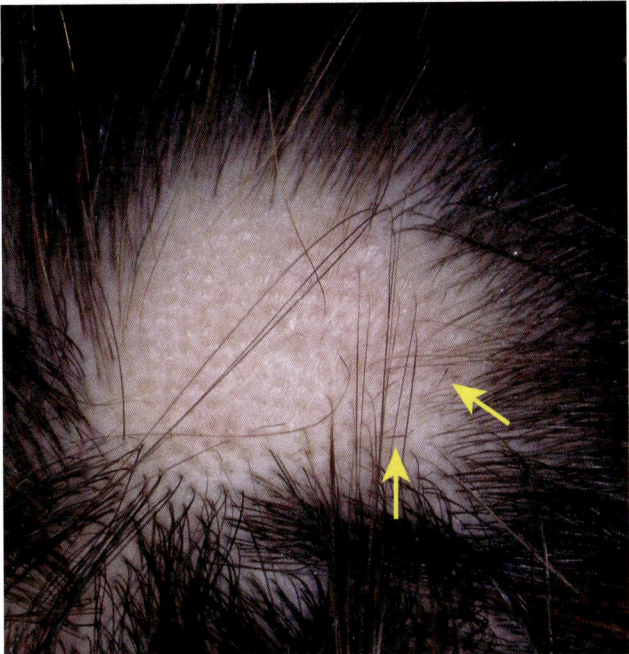

Figure 92.5. Exclamation point hairs (arrows) noted along right edge of a patch of alopecia areata.

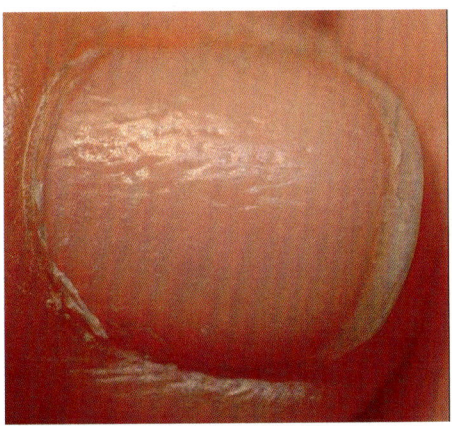

Figure 92.6. Multiple small nail pits may be observed in patients who have alopecia areata.

Look-alikes

Nail changes would not be expected in any of the conditions listed herein, unless otherwise noted.

Disorder	Differentiating Features
Tinea capitis	• Scaling or inflammation (pustules, nodules) of the scalp usually present. • Black dot hairs may be observed. • Regional lymphadenopathy (cervical, suboccipital) may be present. • Fungal (dermatophyte) culture or potassium hydroxide preparation result is positive.
Traction alopecia	• Symmetric bilateral involvement typical. • Thinning or complete hair loss, especially around hairline or in areas where hair is parted. • Most common in Black female patients; hair styling usually suggestive with tight braids or heavy hair adornments.
Trichotillomania	• Irregular, asymmetric areas of incomplete alopecia. • Broken-off hairs are present with hairs of differing lengths in affected regions (because hairs cannot be broken all at the same time). • Secondary findings (excoriations, crusting) or features of nail-biting may be present.
Loose anagen syndrome	• Typical onset during preschool years in blond girls. • No complete hair loss; rather, diffusely thin and lusterless hair. • Hair grows slowly; history of no (or few) haircuts common. • Hair mount of easily extracted hairs confirms diagnosis (reveals ruffled cuticle and dystrophic anagen bulb).
Telogen effluvium	• Usually acute, diffuse thinning without areas of complete hair loss. • Typically associated with preceding physical or emotional trauma or illness, which is believed to trigger conversion from anagen to telogen phase of hair growth. • Self-limited; gradual improvement within months.
Androgenetic alopecia	• Not typically seen in younger children. • Classic distribution: symmetric thinning over vertex and frontal hairline. No smooth, bald areas. Occurs over months to years. • May occur in adolescent male or, less commonly, female patients. • May be associated with signs of hyperandrogenism.

How to Make the Diagnosis

- Diagnosis is usually clinical, based on the typical findings.
- In some patients, there may be associated loss of eyebrows, eyelashes, or nose hairs. Characteristic nail changes occur in approximately one-half of patients.
- Skin biopsy is rarely necessary to confirm the diagnosis; findings include perifollicular lymphocytic infiltration.

Treatment

- The most commonly used first-line therapy for alopecia areata is topical or intralesional corticosteroids.
  - Used primarily in mild to moderate patchy disease; often not practical in patients with extensive hair loss.
  - Patients receiving high-potency (Classes I–II) topical steroids or injected steroids should be monitored for cutaneous atrophy; hypothalamic-pituitary-adrenal axis suppression possible with long-term corticosteroid therapy (mainly with ultra-potent topical preparations or repeated intralesional therapy). Patients are typically treated for weeks at a time, with a short treatment holiday to minimize risk of atrophy.
  - Intralesional steroid injections usually not tolerated well in younger children and, hence, used infrequently before 10 to 12 years of age.
- Other treatments for patchy or localized alopecia areata (all off-label) include the following:
  - Topical minoxidil solution or foam; oral minoxidil may be an option in older, recalcitrant cases.
  - Topical calcineurin inhibitors (tacrolimus ointment or pimecrolimus cream).
  - Topical 1% anthralin (short contact therapy; gradually applied for up to 1 hour nightly and then washed off).
  - Topical immunotherapy (contact sensitization with squaric acid or other agents).
  - Janus kinase (JAK) inhibitors (oral or topical tofacitinib; topical 1% ruxolitinib cream).
  - Excimer laser therapy.

- For alopecia totalis, some clinicians use more aggressive systemic immunosuppressive modalities, but careful analysis of the risk versus benefit ratio must be considered. Systemic corticosteroids may be considered for select patients, and usually only as a bridge to halt severe progression of hair loss, while topical therapies are also started; potential side effects make this a rarely used modality in young children.

- Oral JAK inhibitors may be considered in older patients with more severe or recalcitrant disease; oral ritlecitinib is a JAK inhibitor approved by the US Food and Drug Administration for severe alopecia areata (defined as ≥ 50% scalp hair loss) in patients 12 years or older. Oral baricitinib is another JAK inhibitor approved for severe alopecia areata but currently is indicated only in adults.

- Intermittent recurrence of disease activity is common in patients with alopecia areata.

- Hair loss can be psychosocially devastating for the patient as well as family members; in patients or family members struggling with the effect of chronic or extensive hair loss, referral to a psychologist or local mental health provider may be helpful.

- Education about other supportive resources, including the National Alopecia Areata Foundation, may be very beneficial (see Resources for Families section).

- Hair prosthesis should be considered for children with severe hair loss who express interest in this modality. Students should be allowed to wear hair prostheses, hats, or other scalp coverings in school or public settings if they desire.

- Some patients may simply opt for no therapy or may wish to take treatment holiday periods.

Treating Associated Conditions

- Because alopecia areata can occur more commonly in the setting of other autoimmune disorders, a comprehensive family history and review of systems should be performed for other autoimmune disorders, including thyroid disease, type 1 diabetes, and inflammatory bowel disease.

- Laboratory workup should be based on findings from the history and physical examination.

- Alopecia areata has been reported in the setting of autoimmune polyglandular syndromes.

Prognosis

- Because response to therapy is unpredictable, prognosis is difficult to predict and extremely variable.
- Many children with an isolated episode of localized patchy hair loss will have spontaneous hair regrowth without therapy.
- In children with rapid and extensive hair loss, especially when progressing to complete loss, therapy usually works poorly.
- Prepubertal onset and family history of alopecia areata are associated with a poorer prognosis.

When to Worry or Refer

- Referral to a pediatric dermatologist should be considered in children with more extensive or chronic hair loss or when the diagnosis of alopecia areata is uncertain.
- Referral may also be beneficial if the primary care physician is not experienced in treating the disorder.
- If the patient has a second autoimmune disorder or a first-degree relative who has 2 autoimmune disorders, consultation with a pediatric endocrinologist is warranted.

Resources for Families

- American Academy of Pediatrics: HealthyChildren.org.
  https://www.healthychildren.org/hairloss
- Hair Club for Kids.
  https://hairclub.com/hair-club-kids
- Locks of Love: Public nonprofit organization that provides hairpieces to children in the United States and Canada who are financially disadvantaged.
  https://locksoflove.org/about
- National Alopecia Areata Foundation: Information, support, and resources for patients and families.
  www.naaf.org
- Society for Pediatric Dermatology: Patient handout on alopecia areata.
  https://pedsderm.net/for-patients-families/patient-handouts/#AlopeciaAreata

CHAPTER 93

Androgenetic Alopecia

Introduction/Etiology/Epidemiology

▶ Androgenetic alopecia is hair loss that occurs due to the effects of circulating hormones in individuals who are genetically susceptible.
  - Can occur in male or female patients and is the most common type of hair loss in adults.
  - Early onset disease starts in the teenage years, rarely earlier. Earlier onset disease tends to be more pronounced.
  - This type of hair loss can be inherited from either or both parents. Occurrence in male patients is common and does not require workup. In female patients, consider hormone evaluation.

Signs and Symptoms

▶ Most patients first note diffuse thinning of the hair, sometimes accompanied by mild shedding.

▶ Hair loss occurs in a predictable pattern in male and female patients, and it is therefore sometimes called *pattern* alopecia.
  - The earliest form of male pattern alopecia is triangular recession of the frontal hairline (Figure 93.1). The crown of the scalp is the next to be affected, and eventually hair loss can affect most of the scalp, often sparing a band along the inferior scalp.
  - Female pattern alopecia is typically milder and begins with thinning of hair density on the midline scalp (from frontal to crown), leading to widening of the central hair part (Figure 93.2). Thinning can progress to involve the entire crown of the scalp.

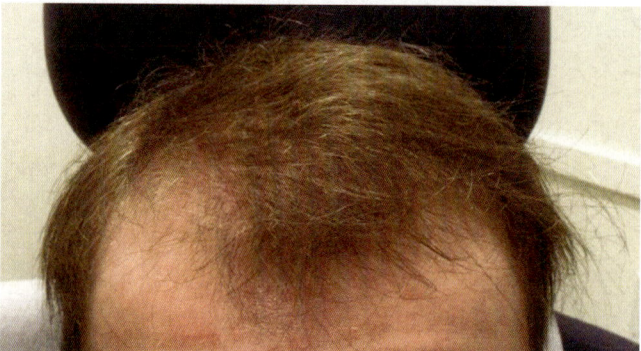

Figure 93.1. This adolescent patient has triangular recession of the frontal hairline.

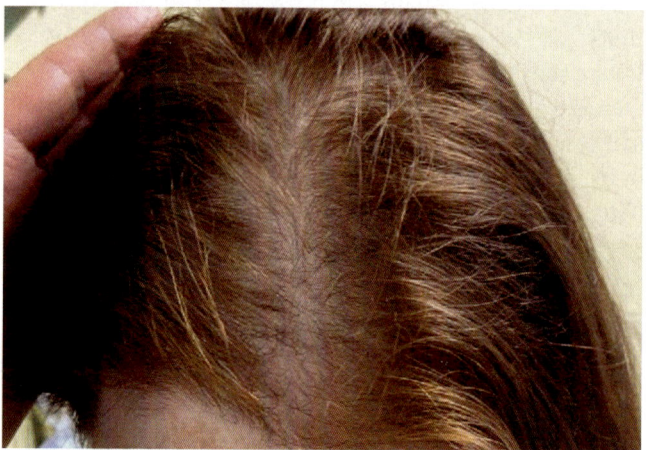

Figure 93.2. This adolescent patient has thinning of the midline scalp hair, leading to a widened part with visible scalp.

Look-alikes

Disorder	Differentiating Features
Telogen effluvium	• Increased shedding of the hair, often noticed with washing or brushing. • Causes diffuse hair loss throughout the entire scalp; no distinct pattern is present. • History of a severe illness or stressor 6 weeks to 4 months before onset of the hair loss.
Alopecia areata	• Usually causes localized hair loss, but occasionally can be widespread. • Round or oval areas of complete hair loss. • May have associated nail pitting.
Scarring alopecia	• The end result of an inflammatory process in and around the hair follicles; multiple causes. The scalp appears smooth and shiny with absence of visible hair follicles. • History or presence of papules, pustules, or plaques preceding the hair loss. • Typically preceded by scalp symptoms, including pain or pruritus.

How to Make the Diagnosis

▶ The diagnosis of androgenetic alopecia is often made clinically on the basis of examination findings and family history.
  ▪ If the diagnosis is in question, scalp biopsy may be helpful (has characteristic features, including a miniaturized follicle).
  ▪ Laboratory testing is not indicated in male patients; consider hormone evaluation in female patients, including free testosterone, dehydroepiandrosterone sulfate, luteinizing hormone, follicle-stimulating hormone, and androstenedione.

Treatment

▶ Without treatment, the condition is progressive.
  ▪ Topical minoxidil 5% (solution or foam) can prevent further loss and promote hair growth in both male and female patients. Apply carefully to avoid unwanted hair on forehead and face.
  ▪ Off-label oral treatment options and those not approved by the US Food and Drug Administration include finasteride (approved by the US Food and Drug Administration for 18 years and older), spironolactone (female patients only; works via inhibiting effects of androgens), and low-dose oral minoxidil.

Prognosis

▶ Topical and oral treatments are generally effective, but recurrent hair loss can be expected if treatment is discontinued.

When to Worry or Refer

▶ Female patients with other features of hormone excess should be referred to specialists in endocrinology or gynecology for evaluation.

Resources for Families

▶ American Academy of Dermatology: Thinning hair and hair loss: could it be female pattern hair loss?
www.aad.org/public/diseases/hair-loss/types/female-pattern

▶ American Academy of Dermatology: What is male pattern hair loss, and can it be treated?
www.aad.org/public/diseases/hair-loss/treatment/male-pattern-hair-loss-treatment

▶ MedlinePlus: Information for patients and families sponsored by the US National Library of Medicine and National Institutes of Health.
https://medlineplus.gov/genetics/condition/androgenetic-alopecia/

CHAPTER 94

Hypertrichosis and Hirsutism

Introduction/Etiology/Epidemiology

- ▶ Hypertrichosis is the presence of excessive hair on the body, either generalized or localized.
- ▶ Localized hypertrichosis can be seen as an isolated patch (nevoid circumscribed hypertrichosis) or as a characteristic of other skin neoplasms such as melanocytic nevi or smooth muscle hamartomas. It can also be seen in association with developmental defects, such as a lumbosacral hair tuft seen overlying a tethered spinal cord.
- ▶ Generalized hypertrichosis can be a feature of:
  - An inherited disorder, such as congenital generalized hypertrichosis terminalis or hypertrichosis lanuginosa.
  - A syndrome such as Cornelia de Lange syndrome.
  - A systemic condition such as certain neurologic disorders, hypothyroidism, or malnutrition.
  - Prolonged exposure to medications such as phenytoin or cyclosporine.
- ▶ Hirsutism is a type of hypertrichosis that refers to excess hair in children or female patients that is present in what would be considered a "male" (androgen-dependent) pattern, including a mustache or beard distribution, sideburns, chest, breasts, and upper inner thighs.
  - Idiopathic hirsutism is excess hair without an underlying endocrine or metabolic disorder.
  - Hirsutism can be the result of an endocrine disorder including late-onset congenital adrenal hyperplasia, virilizing tumors, Cushing syndrome, polycystic ovary syndrome, or other.

Signs and Symptoms

- Localized hypertrichosis presents as a patch of hair seen in apparently typical skin or in association with another skin neoplasm.
- Generalized hypertrichosis presents as excess hair growth throughout the body (Figure 94.1A and Figure 94.1B). There is no definition of the amount that is excessive, so patients should be compared with others in that population.
- Hirsutism presents as excess male-pattern hair such as on the upper lip, sideburns, chin (Figure 94.2), chest, arms, and legs. The presence of menstrual difficulties, severe acne, or other signs of androgen excess should prompt workup for an endocrine disorder.

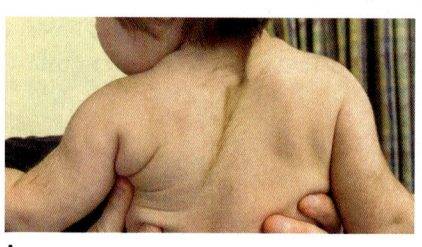
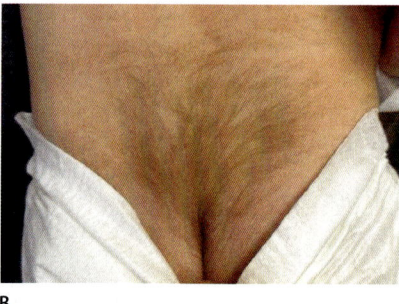

A B

Figure 94.1. This toddler had generalized hypertrichosis after presumed percutaneous absorption of topical minoxidil used daily by his father.

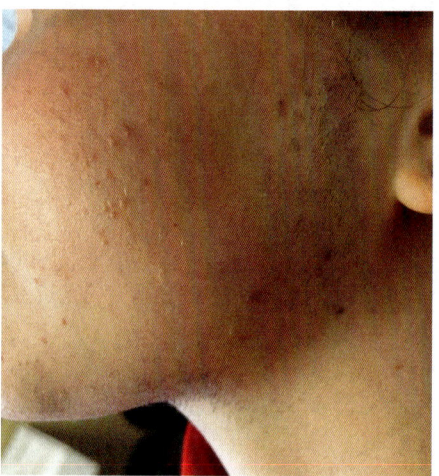

Figure 94.2. This adolescent girl had male-pattern facial hair in the setting of polycystic ovary syndrome.

Look-alikes

Disorder	Differentiating Features
Excess body hair as a biological variant	• Genetic background can influence the amount of hair present on the face or body. • Hair growth that is deemed excessive by 1 population may be considered typical in another.

How to Make the Diagnosis

▶ The diagnosis of hypertrichosis or hirsutism is usually made clinically.

▶ Consider examining other family members to assess quantity of hair in these genetically similar individuals, given that some genetic groups tend to have more hair than others.

▶ Assess for menstrual difficulties or other features of androgen excess (eg, deepened voice, severe acne) that would prompt an endocrinologic workup in patients with hirsutism.

▶ Preliminary laboratory evaluation in this setting may include 17-hydroxyprogesterone, free testosterone, dehydroepiandrosterone sulfate, cortisol, luteinizing hormone, and follicle-stimulating hormone. In the prepubertal child, a bone age test can also be helpful.

Treatment

▶ Treat any underlying disorders that are identified.
  - For patients with medication-induced hypertrichosis, discuss with the prescribing provider whether there is an acceptable alternative medication.

▶ Hair removal techniques can be considered if the excess hair is problematic. These include:
  - Mechanical: cutting, shaving, plucking, waxing (the latter may not be tolerated in young children).
  - Chemical: depilatories (use caution, as these may be irritating, and there is potential for systemic absorption).
  - Electrolysis and laser therapy (painful and typically not covered by insurance).

- Systemic medications can be used to control hirsutism, often in combination. These include:
  - Estrogen-progestin combination oral contraceptive pills.
  - Antiandrogen therapy (spironolactone, flutamide, or finasteride).
  - Insulin sensitizers (metformin).

Prognosis

- Medication-induced hypertrichosis is expected to improve after the medication is withdrawn.
  - Congenital hypertrichosis is lifelong, and hair removal can be considered.
  - The response to medical therapies for hirsutism is variable. Patients often seek hair removal in addition to use of systemic medications.

When to Worry or Refer

- Consult with the appropriate specialists in endocrinology and gynecology if an underlying disorder is suspected and for management with systemic medications.

Resources for Families

Hirsutism:

- Medline Plus: Information for patients and families (in English and Spanish) sponsored by the US National Library of Medicine and National Institutes of Health.
  https://medlineplus.gov/ency/article/007622.htm

Hypertrichosis:

- DermNet NZ: Hypertrichosis.
  https://dermnetnz.org/topics/hypertrichosis

CHAPTER
95

Loose Anagen Syndrome

Introduction/Etiology/Epidemiology

- In loose anagen syndrome, the actively growing anagen hairs (see human hair growth phases in Chapter 96, Telogen Effluvium) are poorly anchored and more easily removed from the scalp than they typically are.
- Characteristically seen in children, typically blond girls between 2 and 5 years of age, although it may occur in boys and in patients with darker hair types.
- Possibly an autosomal-dominant disorder, although many cases appear to be sporadic.

Signs and Symptoms

- Classic presentation is a child presenting with fine, limp hair that does not grow well (Figures 95.1 and 95.2).
- Parent may report that the child "does not need haircuts because the hair grows so slowly."
- Hair loss may be patchy or diffuse, and the hair is often irregular in length (often shorter in the front and longer in the back).
- Hairs are easily removed from the scalp with gentle traction, although shedding is cyclic, so inability to extract hair does not rule out the diagnosis.
- Usually no associated nail or skin alterations or systemic manifestations.

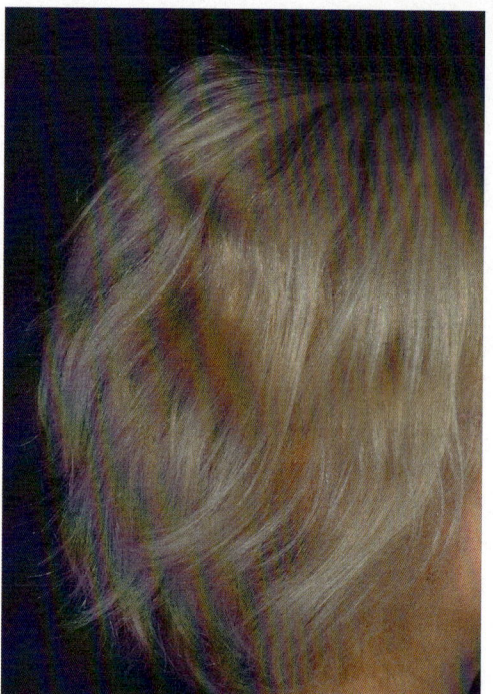

Figure 95.1. Typical appearance of a patient with loose anagen syndrome: short, fine, blond hair that does not grow well.

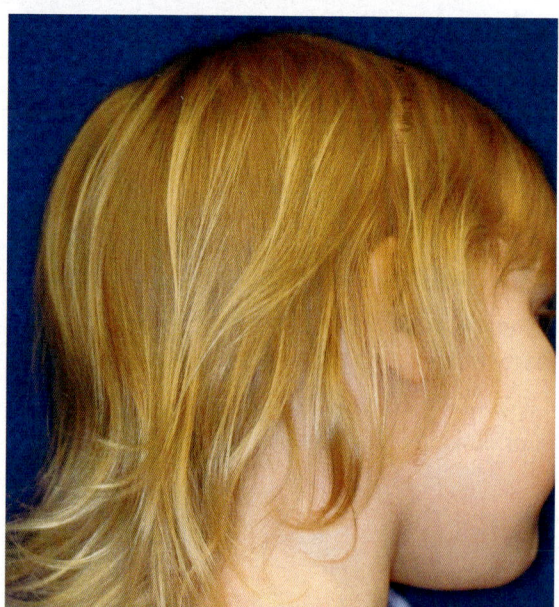

Figure 95.2. Fine, short, lightly pigmented hair that does not grow well in a young patient with loose anagen syndrome.

Look-alikes

Disorder	Differentiating Features
Telogen effluvium	• Acquired condition; affected children usually have history of previously typical hair texture and rate of growth. • History of inciting trigger (eg, febrile illness, surgery, anesthesia) common. • Hairs of typical length, diffusely thin. • Hair pull reveals multiple telogen hairs rather than dystrophic anagen hairs (identified at microscopy). • Improves spontaneously over 3 to 6 months.
Alopecia areata	• Usually causes patches of complete alopecia; may have loss of eyebrows or eyelashes. • Affected areas often have a smooth, bald appearance. • May have associated nail pitting. • May see exclamation point hairs.
Trichotillomania	• Acquired condition; usually localized, not diffuse. • Areas of hair loss often have angulated, irregular borders. • Hairs of differing lengths in affected areas. • Broken-off hairs are present. • Easily extracted anagen hairs not present.
Ectodermal dysplasia	• Distinct facial features (eg, dark circles under eyes, frontal bossing, full lips). • May have associated nail/skin/dental variations (including missing or conical teeth). • Congenital condition; usually does not improve with age. • Large group of inherited disorders that may have additional systemic manifestations, including reduced ability to sweat.
Hair shaft abnormalities (eg, trichorrhexis nodosa, monilethrix)	• Structural variations of the hair shaft often result in hair fragility and breakage, leading to sparse, short hair that appears dry or lusterless, unkempt. • Microscopic examination of hairs often diagnostic, but consultation with a pediatric dermatologist advised if this diagnosis is being considered.

How to Make the Diagnosis

▶ The diagnosis is usually suggested clinically.
▶ Diagnostic confirmation can be made by performing a gentle hair pull and examining the extracted anagen hairs microscopically. The distinctive microscopic findings include a ruffled cuticle and distorted/misshapen anagen hair bulb (Figure 95.3).

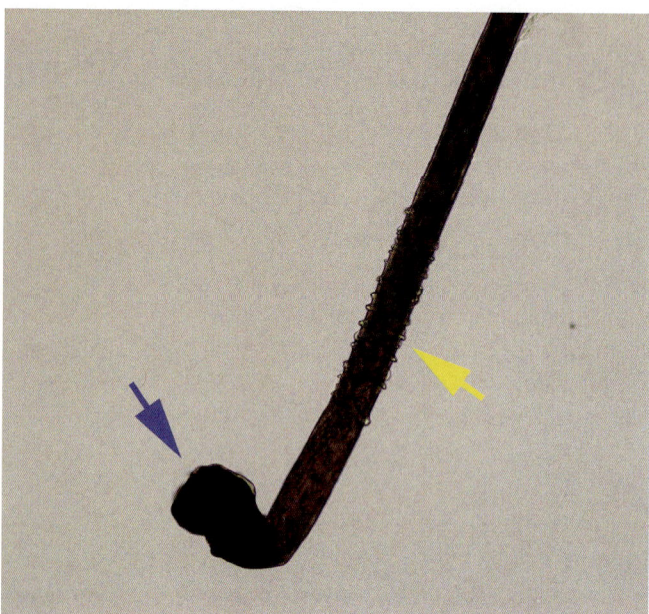

Figure 95.3. Light microscopy of loose anagen syndrome. A dysplastic anagen hair with a "ruffled sock" or "floppy sock" appearance of the cuticle (yellow arrow) and a distorted hair bulb (blue arrow).

Treatment

- There is no treatment available for loose anagen syndrome.
- Volumizing shampoos and conditioners are commonly recommended but do not affect the condition itself.
- Gentle hairstyling should be encouraged to minimize further hair loss (avoiding tight braids or other styles that place tension on the hair shafts).

Prognosis

- The prognosis is good; the condition usually improves over time.
- Although the condition has been reported in the setting of Noonan syndrome, most patients do not have systemic associations.

When to Worry or Refer

- If associated nail, dental, or cutaneous alterations are present, referral to a pediatric dermatologist to evaluate for possible ectodermal dysplasia or other genodermatoses should be considered.
- Also consider referral when the diagnosis is in question, if other variations of the hair shaft are detected at microscopic examination, or in children with potential systemic variations.

CHAPTER 96

Telogen Effluvium

Introduction/Etiology/Epidemiology

- One of the most common forms of non-scarring alopecia in children.
- Human hair follicle has 3 distinct phases.
  - Anagen phase: approximately 80% to 90% of hairs in this growing phase; can last from 2 to 6 years (average 3 years).
  - Catagen phase: brief, approximately 3-week period of involution.
  - Telogen phase: resting phase typically lasting 3 months; approximately 10% of hairs at any time; an average of 50 to 100 telogen hairs shed daily and simultaneously replaced.
- It is unclear what stimuli trigger anagen hairs to enter the catagen phase under typical circumstances, although there are several known events that may interrupt the typical hair cycle and cause large numbers of hairs to prematurely enter the catagen, then telogen phase in concert (resulting in greater than typical hair loss). Telogen effluvium typically occurs when more than 25% of the scalp hairs enter the telogen phase.
  - Most common forms of telogen effluvium include physiologic hair loss of newborns and postpartum women (in which case childbirth is believed to be the trigger).
  - There are also several physical injuries and illnesses that may cause large numbers of anagen hairs to prematurely enter the telogen phase, including
    - High fever
    - Surgery
    - General anesthesia
    - Serious infections
    - Thyroid disease (hypothyroidism or hyperthyroidism)
    - Iron deficiency
    - Malnutrition related to underlying medical problems (eg, celiac disease, anorexia nervosa) or crash diets insufficient in calories or protein

- Essential fatty acid, zinc, or biotin deficiency
- Medications (eg, angiotensin-converting enzyme inhibitors, anticonvulsants [eg, valproic acid, carbamazepine], β-blockers, cimetidine, lithium, oral contraceptives)

▶ Usually, the onset of hair loss occurs 6 weeks to 4 months after the preceding trigger event/condition.

Signs and Symptoms

▶ Patients usually present with a history of increased shedding of the hair or hair falling out at the root (often noticed after washing or brushing hair).

▶ Process is generally diffuse and very subtle, even undetectable, to the clinician.

▶ Condition usually is much more apparent to the affected patient or family members and may be more noticeable when comparing the child's appearance with photographs taken prior to the onset.

▶ Patients lack other symptoms, and the scalp generally appears unremarkable with no evidence of scale, inflammation, or regional lymphadenopathy.

▶ There usually are no completely smooth, bald areas but rather diffuse thinning of the scalp hair (Figures 96.1–96.3).

▶ It may occasionally be associated with Beau lines on the nails (horizontal bands or grooves in same area of several or all nails).

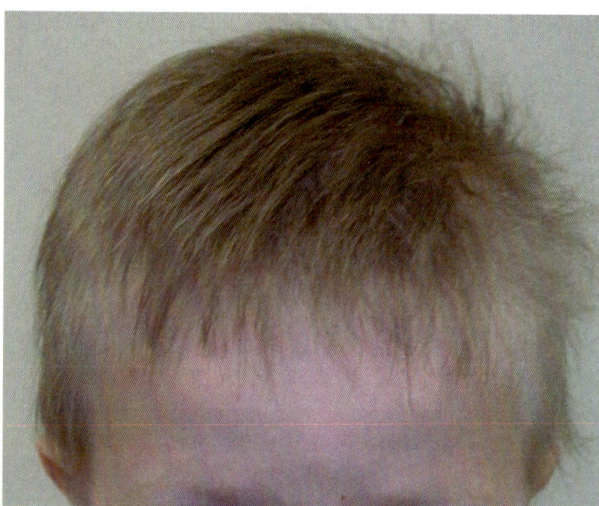

Figure 96.1. Diffuse thinning of scalp hair typical of telogen effluvium. This child experienced complete regrowth of the scalp hair within several months.

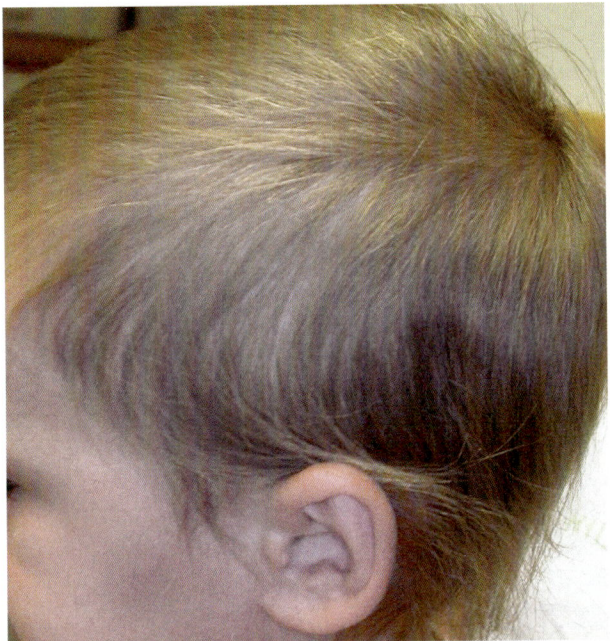

Figure 96.2. Diffuse thinning of the scalp hair in this child with telogen effluvium.

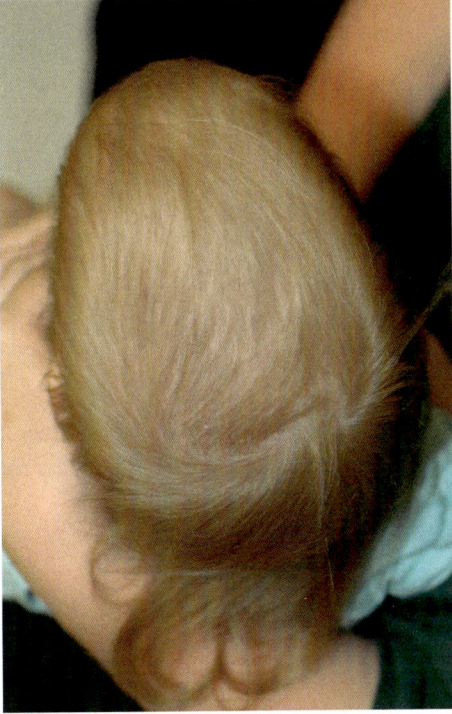

Figure 96.3. Patient with diffuse thinning of telogen effluvium after an illness.

Look-alikes

Disorder	Differentiating Features
Tinea capitis	• Usually causes more localized hair loss. • Scaling or inflammation of the scalp usually present. • Black dot hairs may be observed. • Regional lymphadenopathy (cervical, suboccipital) may be present. • Fungal culture or potassium hydroxide preparation result is positive.
Traction alopecia	• Usually causes localized hair loss with symmetric bilateral involvement. • Thinning or complete hair loss, especially around hairline or in areas where hair is parted/under tension. • Most common in Black girls; hair styling usually suggestive with tight braids or heavy hair adornments.
Trichotillomania	• Usually causes localized hair loss. • Irregularly shaped areas of incomplete alopecia. • Hairs of differing lengths in affected areas. • Broken-off hairs are present.
Alopecia areata	• Usually causes localized hair loss (occasionally may be widespread). • Round or oval areas of complete alopecia. • May have associated nail pitting, trachyonychia (rough nails).
Loose anagen syndrome	• Typically long history of diffusely thin and lusterless hair. • Hair grows slowly; history of no (or few) haircuts common. • Hair mount of easily extracted hairs confirms the diagnosis (reveals ruffled cuticle and dystrophic anagen bulb).

How to Make the Diagnosis

▶ The diagnosis of telogen effluvium is most commonly made based on a clinical history of hair shedding beginning 2 to 4 months after a significant physical illness, injury, or other stressful event.

▶ Examination usually reveals an absence of scalp changes, and hair loss is usually diffuse and subtle.

▶ Hair pull examination can be done by firmly placing a lock of hair between the thumb and forefinger and applying steady traction. If more than 6 hairs are removed, this is suggestive of active hair shedding.

▶ Microscopic examination of extracted hairs can confirm the pulled hairs are in the telogen phase. Typical appearance of telogen hair reveals nonpigmented root with club shape.

- If clinical examination is suggestive of telogen effluvium but there is no supportive history, other hair loss disorders should be considered.
  - Careful diet history and growth evaluation should be obtained to rule out underlying nutritional deficiencies or history of crash dieting.
  - A medication history also should be elicited.
  - Laboratory investigation for iron deficiency anemia or thyroid disease should be considered.
- Cessation of hair loss within 3 to 4 months followed by gradual regrowth is consistent with the diagnosis.

Treatment

- The clinician's main responsibility is to provide reassurance to the patient or parents about the expectation of complete regrowth of hair, usually within 6 months.
- Treatment should be directed toward any underlying medical conditions, such as correction of iron deficiency anemia or thyroid disease, or management of any identified nutritional deficiencies.

Prognosis

- The prognosis for telogen effluvium is excellent.
- Complete hair regrowth usually occurs within 6 months.
- Can occasionally be chronic or relapsing.

When to Worry or Refer

- If an underlying trigger cannot be elicited via comprehensive history, physical examination, or laboratory studies, the clinician should consider referral to a dermatologist.
- If progressive hair loss persists for more than 6 months, dermatology referral is recommended.

Resources for Families

▶ American Hair Loss Association: Provides information about various causes of hair loss.
www.americanhairloss.org

▶ British Association of Dermatologists: Patient information leaflet on telogen effluvium.
https://www.bad.org.uk/pils/telogen-effluvium

CHAPTER 97

Traction Alopecia

Introduction/Etiology/Epidemiology

▶ Traction alopecia is a common cause of hair loss that is most commonly seen in Black children, particularly girls.
▶ The condition is due to styling with tight braids, cornrows, or ponytails, especially when using artificial hair integrations (hair extensions) and/or heavy hair adornments that increase tension further on the already-stressed hair.
▶ African American hair has inherently lower strength, which may predispose to hair loss under conditions of increased tension or weight on the hair.

Signs and Symptoms

▶ Usually characterized by thinning of the hair, particularly around the frontal and parietotemporal hairlines.
  - Alopecia or thinning of the hair may extend circumferentially around the hairline, depending on how the hair is styled; may result in a higher hairline over time.
  - Hair loss also may be observed between the tight braids where the hair has been parted (Figures 97.1 and 97.2).
  - Fine vellus hairs may be observed in affected areas.
▶ There usually are no associated scalp changes, although occasionally, perifollicular inflammation can be observed, including erythema or papules and pustules (most often representing sterile folliculitis related to application of greasy pomades).

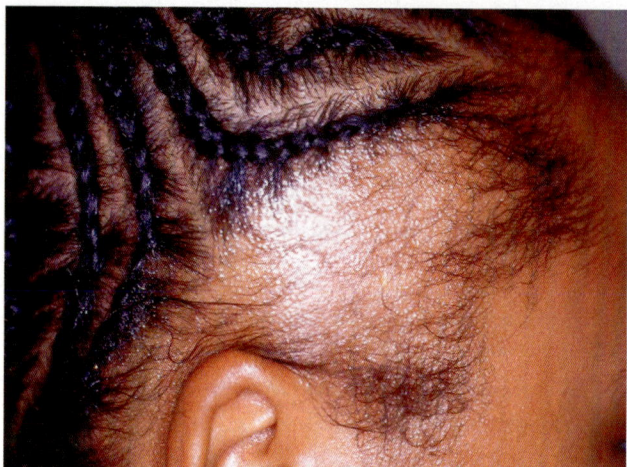

Figure 97.1. Marked thinning of the temporal scalp due to traction alopecia. Note the hairstyle with many small, tight braids typically seen in children with this disorder.

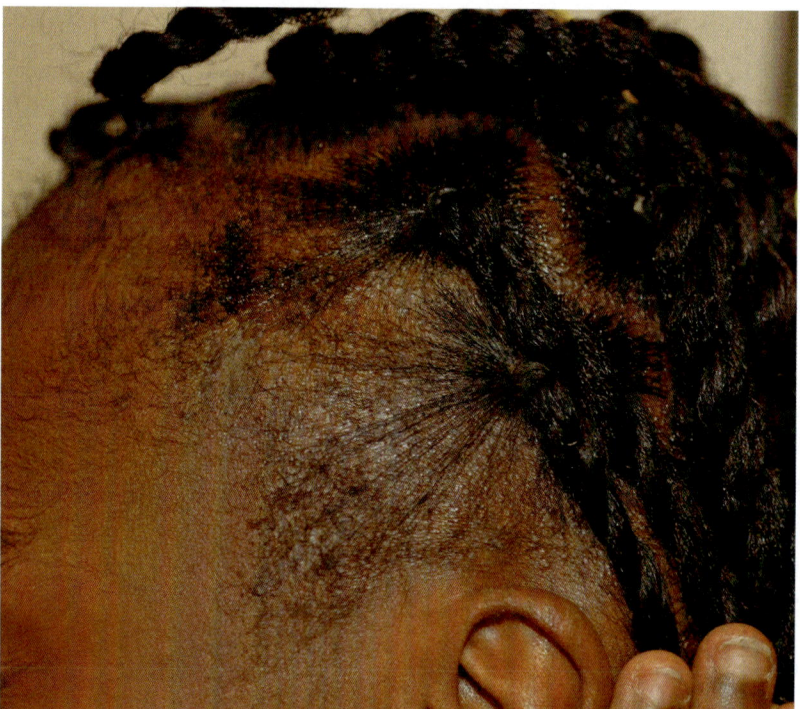

Figure 97.2. Partial alopecia involving the hairline in this child with traction alopecia. Note the tightly pulling braids.

Look-alikes

Presented here are causes of localized hair loss. Hair loss is usually not symmetric in any of these conditions.

Disorder	Differentiating Features
Tinea capitis	• Scaling or inflammation of scalp usually present. • Black dot hairs may be observed. • Regional lymphadenopathy (cervical, suboccipital) may be present. • Fungal (dermatophyte) culture or potassium hydroxide preparation is positive.
Trichotillomania	• Irregularly shaped areas of incomplete alopecia. • Hairs of differing lengths in affected areas. • Broken-off hairs are present.
Alopecia areata	• Round or oval smooth areas of complete alopecia. • Lesions may be scattered throughout scalp, not limited to frontal or parietotemporal hairlines or areas between braids. • Nail pits or trachyonychia (rough nails) may be present.

How to Make the Diagnosis

▶ The diagnosis usually is made clinically based on the pattern of hair loss.

▶ When suspecting traction alopecia, a careful history should be obtained on hairstyling practices, including braids, ponytails, hair adornments, and chemical processing or heat-related procedures.

Treatment

▶ The mainstay of treatment is aimed at changing the hairstyling practices to ones that avoid any undue tension, trauma, or weight on the involved hair.

▶ Loose hairstyles without braids or hair adornments should be encouraged.

▶ Gentle treatment of the hair with avoidance of chemical processing or heat-related procedures also should be emphasized.

Treating Associated Conditions

▶ Sterile folliculitis is treated best by withdrawing the application of greasy pomades to the scalp.

▶ If follicular pustules are present, bacterial and fungal cultures should be performed to rule out bacterial infection and tinea capitis, respectively.

Prognosis

- If the condition is recognized promptly and the appropriate changes made in hairstyling, the prognosis is excellent, with complete regrowth of hair expected.
- In patients with more chronic traction alopecia (years), permanent hair loss may result.

When to Worry or Refer

- Consider referral to a dermatologist if the diagnosis is in doubt or for patients with chronic symptoms because permanent hair loss may result.

Resources for Families

- American Academy of Pediatrics: HealthyChildren.org.
  https://www.healthychildren.org/English/health-issues/conditions/skin/Pages/Hair-Loss-Alopecia.aspx
- British Association of Dermatologists: Traction alopecia printable leaflet.
  https://www.bad.org.uk/pils/traction-alopecia
- Skin of Color Society: Traction alopecia.
  https://skinofcolorsociety.org/discover-patients-public/patient-education/traction-alopecia

CHAPTER 98

Trichotillomania

Introduction/Etiology/Epidemiology

- Trichotillomania (ie, hairpulling disorder), the loss of hair because of hairpulling, plucking, twirling, or twisting, is a common cause of hair loss in children.
- Classified in the past as an impulse control disorder and, more recently, in *Diagnostic and Statistical Manual of Mental Disorders,* 5th Edition, as an obsessive-compulsive disorder.
- Seen more frequently in children and adolescents than in adults and more common in female patients.
- Exact frequency is unknown, but some reports indicate prevalence of up to 1 in 200 persons by 18 years of age.
- May involve pulling or twisting of the hairs of the scalp (most commonly affected site), eyelashes, eyebrows, or other hair-bearing areas.
- Most patients and parents deny pulling or twisting (some may not even be cognizant of the behavior), which can make accurate diagnosis a challenge.
- An often chronic condition that may vary greatly in severity, from a short-lived habit with localized hair loss to a more severe condition with associated psychologic or psychiatric morbidity.
- Patients often have an associated sense of tension before the act of hairpulling or twisting, which is typically followed by a sense of relief or gratification; may occur more often when patients are tired, bored, or falling asleep.

Signs and Symptoms

- Localized, well-circumscribed areas of hair loss, often with angular or irregular borders (Figures 98.1 and 98.2).
- Careful examination reveals hairs of variable length within the affected region (unlike the complete hair loss of alopecia areata) (Figures 98.3 and 98.4).

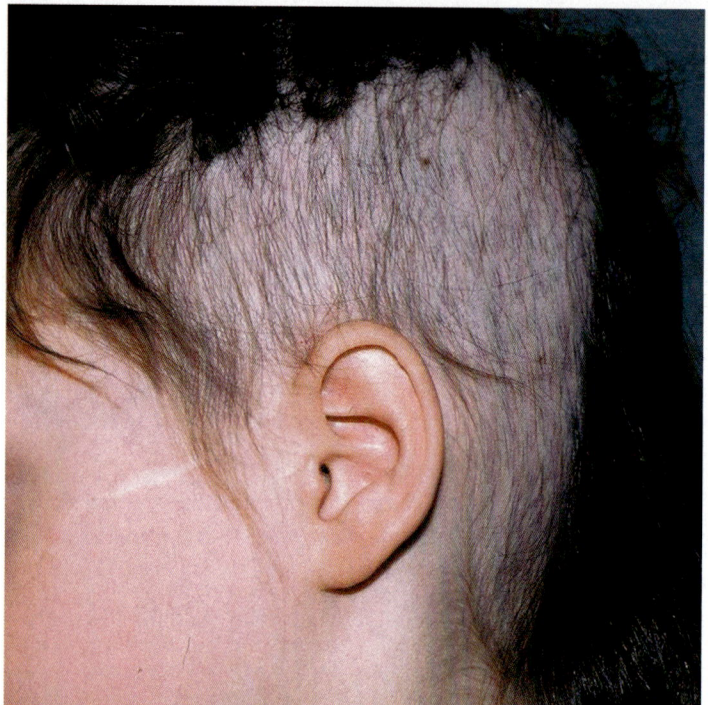

Figure 98.1. Trichotillomania. There is a well-defined patch of relative alopecia within which hairs are of differing lengths. The hair in the affected area has a bristlelike feel.

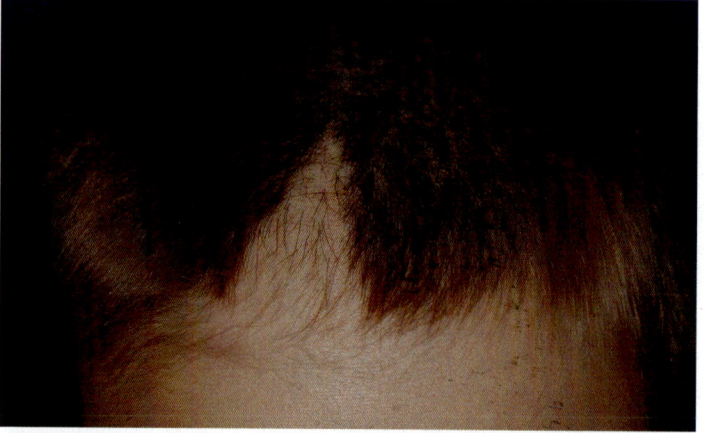

Figure 98.2. Trichotillomania. Irregular patch of alopecia with broken-off hairs in this school-aged child with a history of obsessive-compulsive behavior and anxiety.

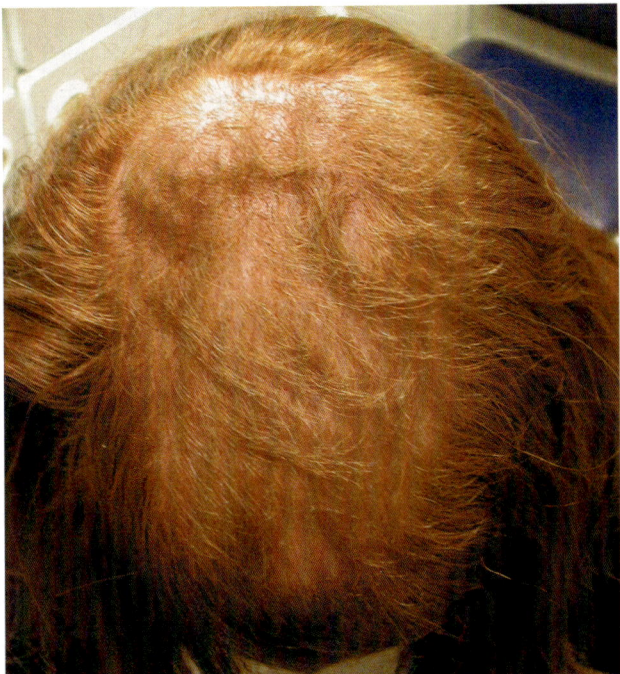

Figure 98.3. Trichotillomania involving the vertex scalp. Note the well-demarcated area of affected scalp and variation in hair length within the affected areas.

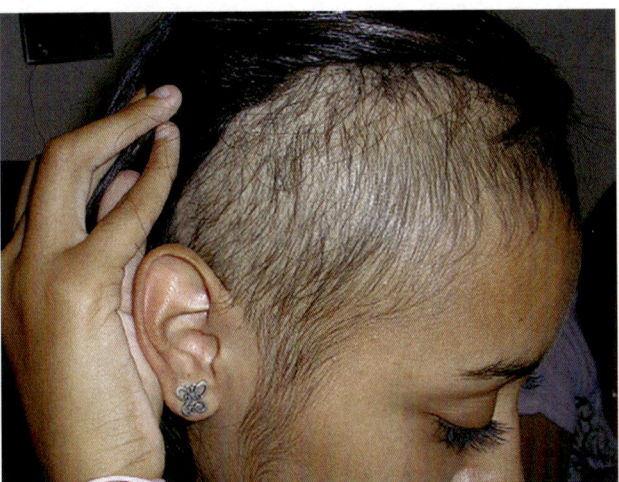

Figure 98.4. Trichotillomania in a patient with skin of color. Note the large patch of alopecia on the right frontal and temporal scalp within which are short hairs of varying lengths. Reproduced with permission from Usatine RP, Smith MA, Chulley HS, et al. *The Color Atlas of Pediatrics.* McGraw-Hill Education.

- Frontal, temporal, and parietal scalp usually affected; eyelashes and eyebrows involved less often (Figures 98.5, 98.6, 98.7, and 98.8).
- Affected area often has a rough, bristlelike texture due to hair stubble (Figure 98.1).
- Usually no associated scalp variations, although some erosions may be present.
- Classically occurs on the contralateral side of the dominant hand.
- Associated findings may include nail-biting (onychophagia), skin or nose picking, and lip biting.

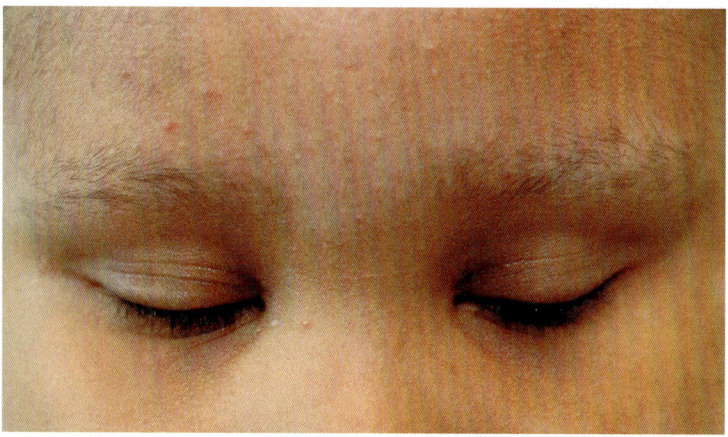

Figure 98.5. Patchy, irregular loss of eyebrows and eyelashes in this patient with trichotillomania.

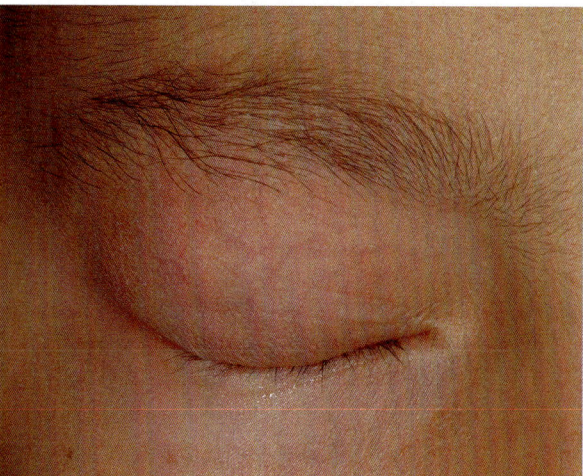

Figure 98.6. Trichotillomania localized to the eyelashes. Note the lashes of differing lengths within the affected upper eyelid margin.

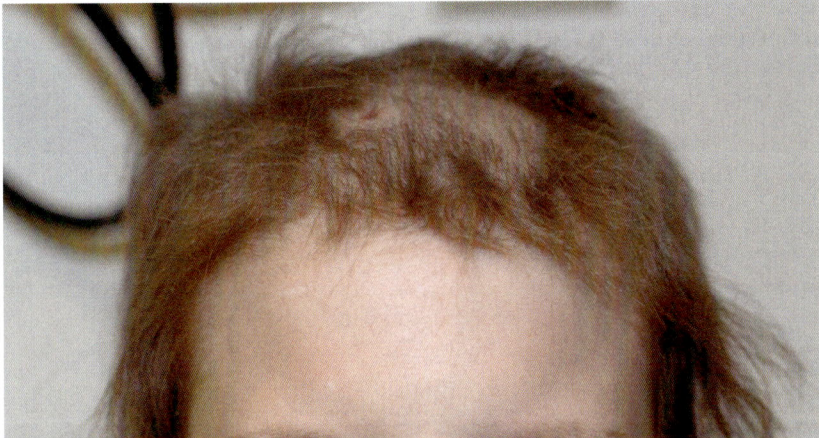

Figure 98.7. Trichotillomania. Patient with hair loss on vertex of scalp from hairpulling.

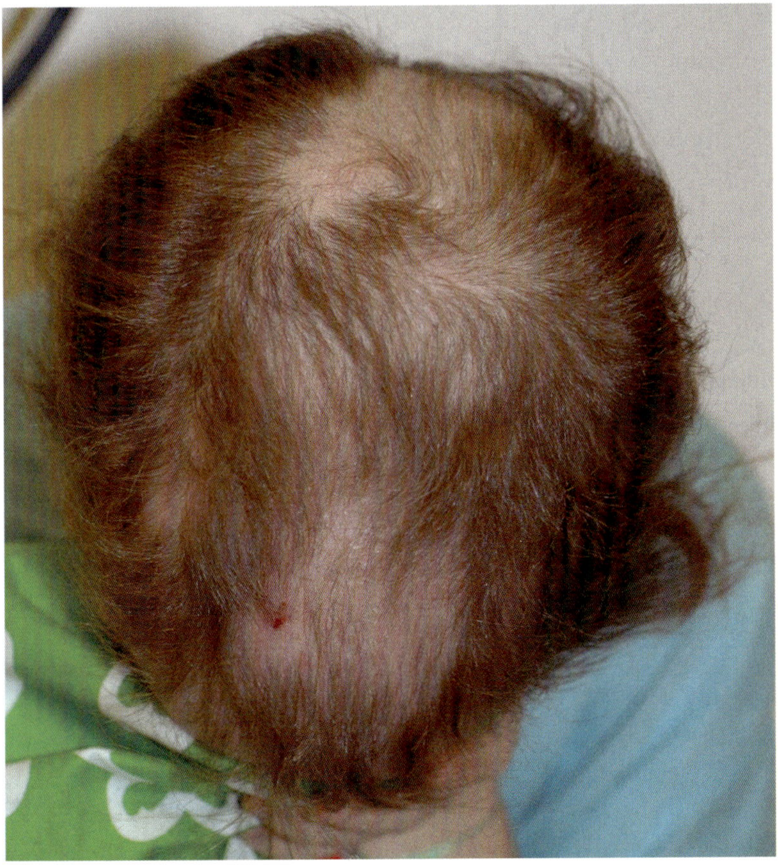

Figure 98.8. Trichotillomania. Same patient as in Figure 98.7; note excoriations on the scalp.

Look-alikes

Disorder	Differentiating Features
Tinea capitis	• Black dot hairs may be observed. • Regional lymphadenopathy (cervical, suboccipital) may be present. • Fungal culture or potassium hydroxide preparation result is positive.
Alopecia areata	• Round or oval areas (angular borders not observed) of complete hair loss. • Exclamation point hairs may be observed. • Nail pitting or trachyonychia (rough nails) may be present. • Hairs have similar length during regrowth phase. • Broken-off hairs are absent.
Traction alopecia	• Symmetric bilateral involvement present. • Thinning or complete hair loss, especially around hairline or in areas where hair is parted. • Broken-off hairs are typically absent.

How to Make the Diagnosis

▶ The diagnosis can be very challenging because many patients and parents deny the behavior of hairpulling or twisting.

▶ In younger children, parents may observe and report the behavior of hairpulling or twisting, whereas in older children and adolescents, the behavior usually occurs in private and family members are not aware of the habit.

▶ The diagnosis is made clinically based on the characteristic pattern of irregular and bizarre patterns of hair loss, presence of broken-off hairs, and exclusion of other potential causes (eg, tinea capitis).

▶ Although generally not necessary, skin biopsy may be helpful in making the diagnosis. Histologic findings include follicular plugging, melanin casts, distorted hair shafts (trichomalacia), hemorrhage, and an increase in hair follicles in the catagen phase.

▶ Special care and sensitivity must be used when the potential diagnosis of trichotillomania is discussed with the patient and family members.

Treatment

- There are no specific therapies for trichotillomania.
- Close collaboration with a child psychologist or psychiatrist is often necessary to reverse the behavior.
  - In some patients, behavior modification strategies alone can be helpful (including positive reinforcement and redirectional therapy).
  - In others, a combination of behavior modification and pharmacological therapy, such as selective serotonin reuptake inhibitors or N-acetylcysteine, may be necessary, but data on these treatments are limited.

Treating Associated Conditions

- Psychiatric comorbidities (eg, obsessive-compulsive disorder, depression, anxiety disorder) should be addressed by a pediatric psychologist or psychiatrist; such comorbidities are unlikely in younger patients.
- Trichophagia and trichobezoar should be considered in patients presenting with symptoms suggestive of gastric obstruction.

Prognosis

- Patients with trichotillomania are a heterogeneous group, so the prognosis varies from excellent in those individuals with an isolated habit to poor in individuals who have associated psychiatric morbidity.
- In general, younger children appear to have a more favorable outcome than do those with a later onset of disease.

When to Worry or Refer

- Referral to a pediatric dermatologist may be helpful when the diagnosis is uncertain.
- Once the diagnosis is suspected, patients may benefit from referral to a behavioral pediatrician, child psychologist, or psychiatrist experienced in the disorder.

Resources for Families

- The TLC Foundation for Body-Focused Repetitive Behaviors: Provides information, resources, and links for patients and families. **https://www.bfrb.org**
- Trichotillomania Support: Website in the United Kingdom that provides information and support for patients who have trichotillomania. **https://trichotillomania.co.uk/**

Skin Disorders in Neonates/Infants

CHAPTER 99 — **Aplasia Cutis Congenita** **649**

CHAPTER 100 — **Collodion Baby** **655**

CHAPTER 101 — **Diaper Dermatitis** **659**

CHAPTER 102 — **Eosinophilic Pustular Folliculitis** **669**

CHAPTER 103 — **Erythema Toxicum** **671**

CHAPTER 104 — **Infantile Acropustulosis** **675**

CHAPTER 105 — **Intertrigo** **677**

CHAPTER 106 — **Miliaria** **681**

CHAPTER 107 — **Nevus Sebaceus (of Jadassohn)** **685**

CHAPTER 108 — **Transient Neonatal Pustular Melanosis** **689**

CHAPTER 109 — **Subcutaneous Fat Necrosis (SFN)** **693**

CHAPTER 99

Aplasia Cutis Congenita

Introduction/Etiology/Epidemiology

- Aplasia cutis congenita (ACC) is a congenital defect of the skin that results in localized absence of the epidermis; dermis; and, occasionally, subcutaneous tissue.

- The cause is unknown, and most cases are sporadic, although autosomal dominant inheritance has been suggested in some reports. A link with maternal antithyroid medication (especially methimazole) use during pregnancy has been suggested.

- ACC is a feature of Adams-Oliver (with transverse limb defects and vascular and cardiac irregularities) and oculocerebrocutaneous (Delleman) syndromes and may occur in those who have trisomy 13 syndrome.

Signs and Symptoms

- Usually presents as a solitary, round, oval, or stellate, 1- to 2-cm ulcer (Figure 99.1) or scar (Figure 99.2) located on the scalp near the origin of the hair whorl (although other body sites occasionally are affected). A minority of patients have multiple lesions (typically 2 or 3).

- In some patients, the defect is covered by a thin membrane and surrounded by long dark hairs (the hair collar sign [Figure 99.3]). This membranous form of ACC is postulated to be a mild form of cranial neural tube closure defect.

- Occasionally may present as bullous ACC, with the appearance of a blister overlying the ACC, and often an associated hair collar sign (Figure 99.4); this form may be a forme fruste of a neural tube defect, and histologic evaluation may reveal changes of cephalocele or meningocele.

- Large lesions (>4 cm) may be associated with underlying skull defects that may predispose to sagittal sinus hemorrhage or thrombosis, local infection, or meningitis.

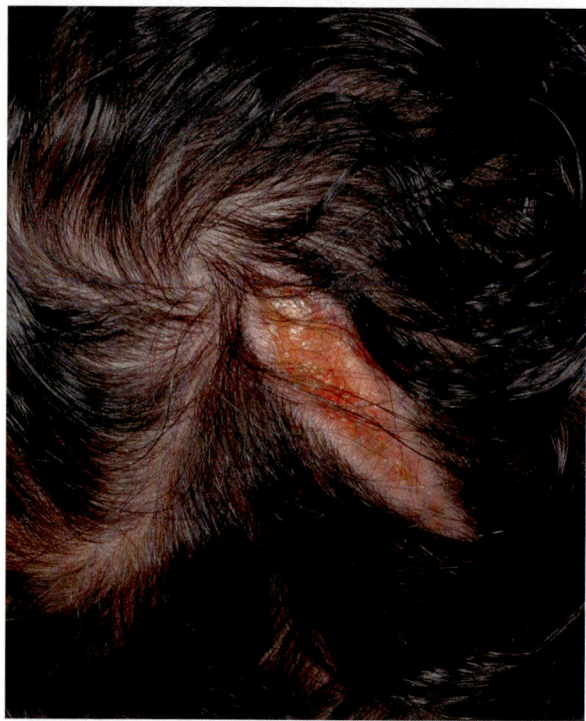

Figure 99.1. Stellate ulcer with overlying crust characteristic of aplasia cutis congenita.

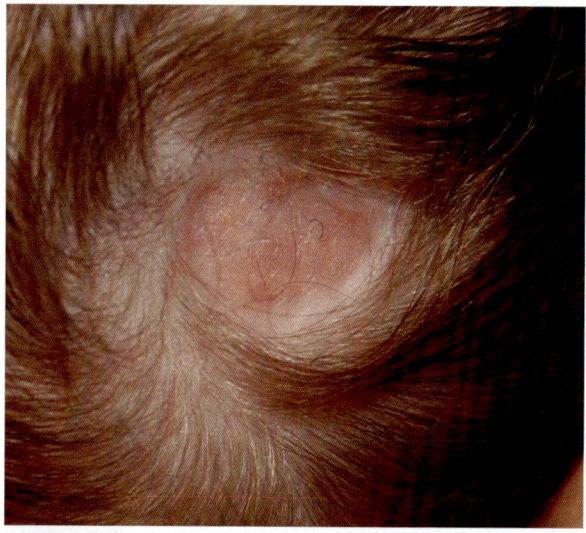

Figure 99.2. Aplasia cutis congenita presenting as an atrophic scar.

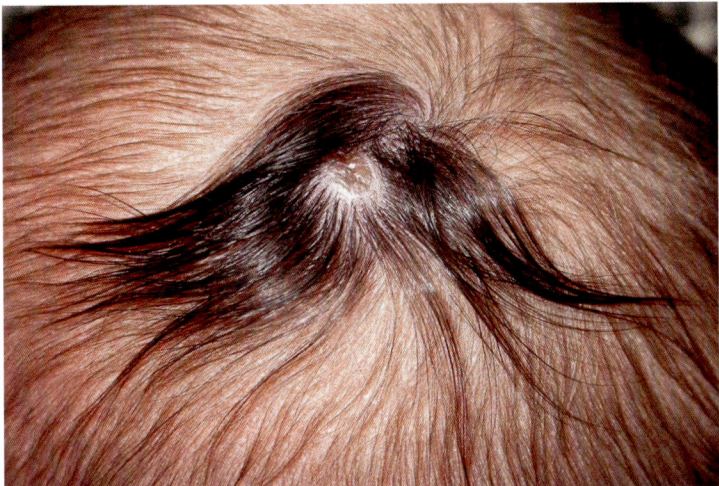

Figure 99.3. Aplasia cutis congenita in which a thin membrane is surrounded by long dark hairs (ie, the hair collar sign).

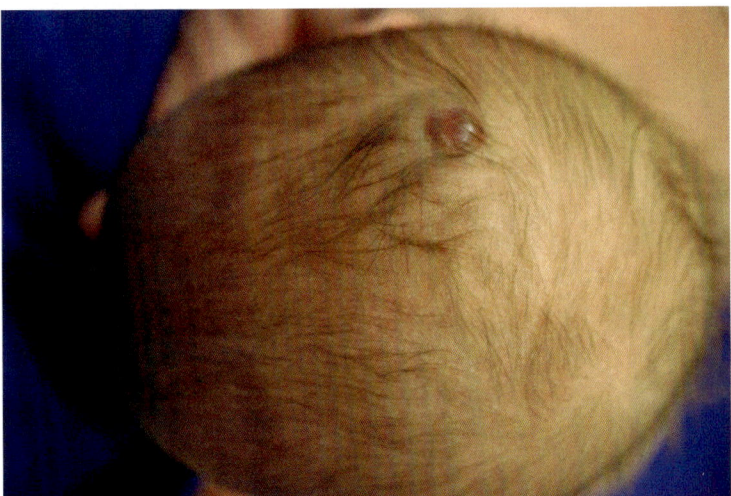

Figure 99.4. Bullous aplasia cutis congenita with a hair collar sign; surgical excision was performed (after imaging ruled out bony defect or tract to the central nervous system), and histologically this lesion was a cephalocele.

Look-alikes

Disorder	Differentiating Features
When Presenting as an Ulcer	
Herpes simplex virus infection	• Usually presents as clustered vesicles on an erythematous base (not a solitary large ulcer). • Lesions usually not present at birth.
Trauma from forceps	• May cause a scalp erosion (more superficial than an ulcer), and shape and location likely to be different than seen in aplasia cutis congenita (ACC).
Trauma from scalp electrode	• Usually produces an erosion (more superficial than an ulcer) and is typically smaller than ACC.
Epidermolysis bullosa	• Typically more superficial than ACC, with denudation and eroded patches. • Usually presents with multiple sites of involvement. • Oral mucosal involvement occasionally present.
When Presenting as a Scar	
Nevus sebaceus	• Usually presents as a verrucous (warty) plaque; however, some lesions are quite flat in neonates and may mimic a scar. • Often yellowish orange to tan. • If left untreated, becomes more elevated and verrucous in the peri-pubertal and postpubertal years.

How to Make the Diagnosis

▶ The diagnosis is usually made clinically based on lesion appearance.

Treatment

▶ For small ulcers, local wound care to prevent secondary bacterial infection is sufficient. Lesions presenting as scars require no treatment.
▶ Large lesions require plastic surgery consultation and imaging.

Prognosis

- Excellent for small lesions; atrophic scars will persist, and ulcers will heal with atrophic scars.
- Large lesions may be associated with underlying skull defects that may predispose to sagittal sinus hemorrhage or thrombosis, local infection, or meningitis. For such patients, plastic surgical consultation is recommended.

When to Worry or Refer

- Obtain plastic surgery consultation and consider imaging (for underlying central nervous system involvement) for patients with large lesions or deeper involvement. Also consider imaging for lesions accompanied by vascular stains or nodules or those with an associated hair collar sign (because of the risk of associated neural tube defect).

Resource for Families

- MedlinePlus: Information for patients and families sponsored by the US National Library of Medicine and National Institutes of Health. **https://medlineplus.gov/genetics/condition/nonsyndromic-aplasia-cutis-congenita/**

CHAPTER 100

Collodion Baby

Introduction/Etiology/Epidemiology

- *Collodion baby* is a term used for babies born with a membrane-like covering, which resembles collodion (a syrupy liquid that dries into a transparent film and is used as a topical protectant and in some topical medications), called a *collodion membrane.*
- This diagnostic term is not specific for any single disease state; most infants who are affected will have an autosomal recessive congenital ichthyosis (ARCI). The ARCIs include non-bullous congenital ichthyosiform erythroderma and classic lamellar ichthyosis.
- Approximately 5% of infants will shed their collodion membrane and eventually have typical skin; this has been termed *self-healing collodion baby.*
- Rarely, this presentation can be associated with syndromic forms of ichthyoses such as Conradi-Hünermann syndrome, Sjögren-Larsson syndrome, or trichothiodystrophy.

Signs and Symptoms

- Neonates present at birth with the skin surface covered in a parchment-like membrane; over time, this gradually sheds in sheets (Figure 100.1).
- Facial features may be distorted given the tautness of the membrane, and this may present as ectropion (eversion of the eyelids) (Figure 100.2), eclabium (eversion of the lips), and flattening of the ears.
- Digits on the extremities may reveal constriction.
- Inhibition of appropriate chest expansion by the membrane may result in respiratory distress and, when combined with the inability to suck properly, these infants may be at increased risk for aspiration pneumonia.

- ▶ Skin and systemic infection may occur given the impaired epidermal barrier (despite its thickness, the collodion membrane is ineffective in this regard).
- ▶ Excessive transcutaneous fluid losses may be associated with electrolyte imbalance, hypernatremic dehydration, and temperature instability.

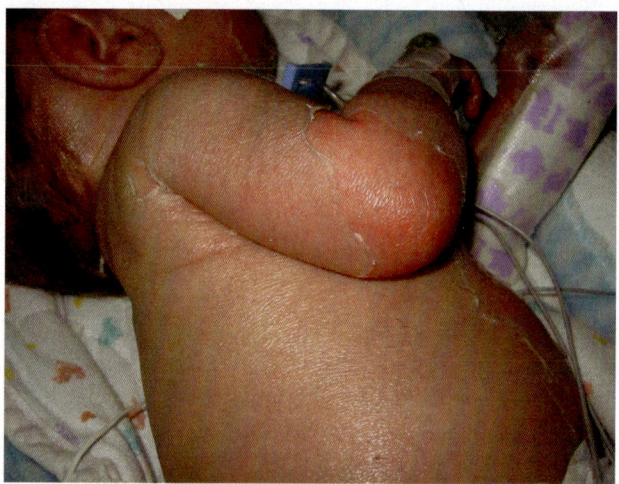

A

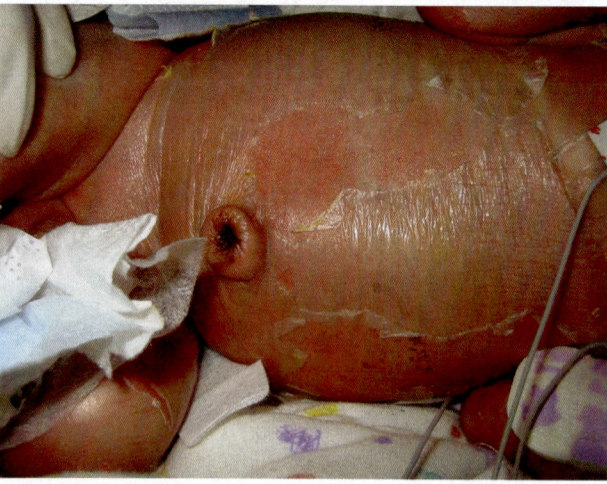

B

Figure 100.1. Collodion baby. This neonate was covered in a parchment-like membrane at birth. At 3 days of age, note the shedding of the membrane with peeling in sheets on the arm (A) and abdomen (B).

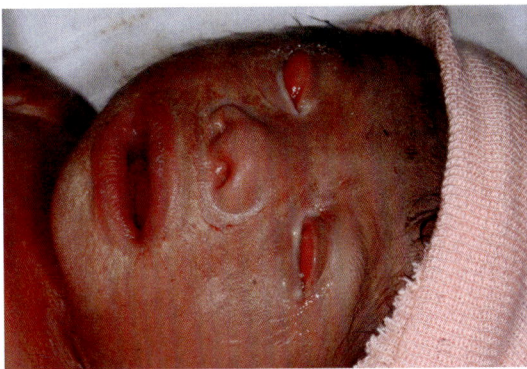

Figure 100.2. Eclabium (eversion of lips) and ectropion (eversion of eyelids) in a neonate with a collodion membrane. Note the taut facial skin with cracks and fissures.

Look-alikes

The collodion baby phenotype, with the combination of a parchment-like membrane and often the presence of digital contractures along with eclabium and/or ectropion, is quite characteristic and clinically diagnostic. Distinguishing between the various disorders that may present with a collodion membrane (such as lamellar ichthyosis, non-bullous congenital ichthyosiform erythroderma, or self-healing collodion baby) is often not possible during the neonatal period.

How to Make the Diagnosis

- As mentioned earlier, the constellation of presenting features often enables a rapid clinical diagnosis.
- Longitudinal follow-up of the baby with a collodion membrane will often help direct other diagnostic options, such as DNA-based molecular genetic testing; skin biopsy is rarely useful.
- If a pathogenic variant is identified, future DNA-based prenatal diagnosis will be an option for the parents with future pregnancies.

Treatment

- Supportive care is the mainstay of therapy for the newborn with a collodion membrane.
- Placement in a humidified incubator is recommended early on to minimize drying and cracking of the collodion membrane (which leads to further barrier instability) and to allow for gentle spontaneous debridement. Bland emollient therapy (such as petrolatum) is often recommended to assist in this process, but use of keratolytic agents should be avoided given the risk of absorption.

- ▶ Special attention should be given to temperature regulation, fluid and electrolyte status, and the risk for bacteremia and sepsis related to transcutaneously acquired infection.
- ▶ Antimicrobial therapy should be promptly instituted if infection is suspected.

Prognosis

- ▶ The prognosis for a collodion baby is good overall but depends on the associated underlying disorder, if any.
- ▶ Infants with an underlying ARCI may have a broad range of phenotypes and variable long-term severity.

When to Worry or Refer

- ▶ Consultation with a pediatric dermatologist and/or geneticist is desirable to assist with acute treatment and eventual diagnostic recommendations.

Resources for Families

- ▶ DermNet NZ: Collodion baby.
  https://dermnetnz.org/topics/collodion-baby
- ▶ Foundation for Ichthyosis and Related Skin Types: Collodion baby: a patient's perspective.
  https://www.firstskinfoundation.org/types-of-ichthyosis/collodion-baby#
- ▶ Ichthyosis Support Group: Collodion baby.
  https://www.ichthyosis.org.uk/faqs/collodion-baby

CHAPTER 101

Diaper Dermatitis

Introduction/Etiology/Epidemiology

▶ Diaper dermatitis is one of the most common skin disorders of infancy.

Signs and Symptoms

Table 101.1. Common Forms of Diaper Dermatitis

Condition	Cause	Clinical Features	Treatment
Irritant dermatitis (Figure 101.1)	• Moisture, friction, enzymes in stool.	• Erythematous patches that involve the lower abdomen, buttocks, and thighs. • Convex surfaces involved; inguinal folds often spared.	• Frequent diaper changes. • Topical barrier cream or ointment at all diaper changes. • Topical low-potency corticosteroid twice daily as adjunctive therapy.
Candidiasis (Figure 101.2)	• Infection with *Candida* species (primary or complicating existing irritant dermatitis).	• Erythematous patches that involve the convexities and inguinal creases. • Satellite papules and pustules. • Scaling at the margins of involved areas.	• Topical antifungal preparation (eg, nystatin, clotrimazole, or other azole antifungal agent).
Seborrheic dermatitis (Figure 101.3)	• Cause unknown. • Associated with sebaceous gland function. • May represent an inflammatory response to yeasts of the genus *Malassezia* (formerly *Pityrosporum*).	• Begins at 3 to 4 weeks of age and resolves by the end of the first year after birth. • Salmon-pink patches with greasy scale that involve the convexities and inguinal creases. • Involvement of the scalp, face, postauricular creases, umbilicus, or chest may be present.	• Skin: topical low-potency corticosteroid or antifungal preparation (eg, nystatin, clotrimazole, or other azole antifungal agent). • Scalp: oil massage and brushing or antiseborrheic shampoo (eg, containing pyrithione zinc or selenium sulfide).

(continued)

Table 101.1 (continued)

Condition	Cause	Clinical Features	Treatment
Bullous impetigo (Figure 101.4)	• Infection with *Staphylococcus aureus* that elaborates epidermolytic toxin.	• Flaccid blisters filled with clear or purulent fluid. • Blisters rupture rapidly, leaving round or oval crusted erosions with a rim of scale.	• Oral antistaphylococcal antibiotic (the agent selected depends on local antibiotic resistance patterns).
Folliculitis (Figure 101.5)	• Infection of hair follicles with *S aureus*.	• Pustules with surrounding erythema that are centered on hair follicles.	• Many lesions: oral antistaphylococcal antibiotic (the agent selected depends on local antibiotic resistance patterns). • Few lesions: topical antibiotic (eg, mupirocin, clindamycin, retapamulin, ozenoxacin). • Bleach baths (or cleansers containing sodium hypochlorite) may be useful for patients with persistent or recurrent infections.
Intertrigo (Figure 101.6)	• Rubbing of apposed skin surfaces complicated by heat and moisture.	• Erythema and superficial erosions located in the inguinal creases. • May become secondarily infected with *Candida* species or *Streptococcus pyogenes*, less commonly *S aureus*.	• Absorbent powder (to reduce moisture and friction). • Antifungal preparation (if candidal infection) or antibiotic (if bacterial infection).
Jacquet erosive diaper dermatitis (Figure 101.7)	• Multiple factors, including moisture, friction, enzymes in stool. Considered a variant of irritant dermatitis.	• Well-defined shallow ulcers or ulcerated nodules.	• Topical low-potency corticosteroid twice daily and barrier preparation at all diaper changes.

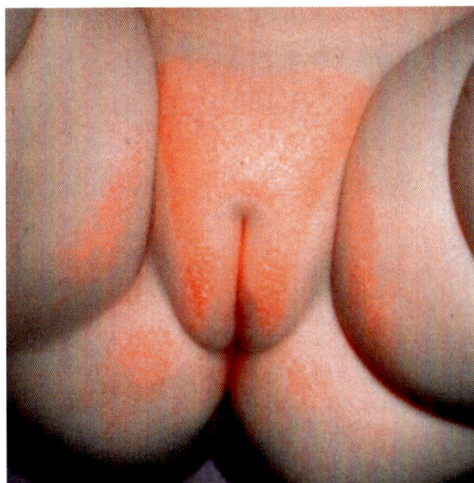

Figure 101.1. Irritant diaper dermatitis. Erythematous patches sparing the skinfolds.

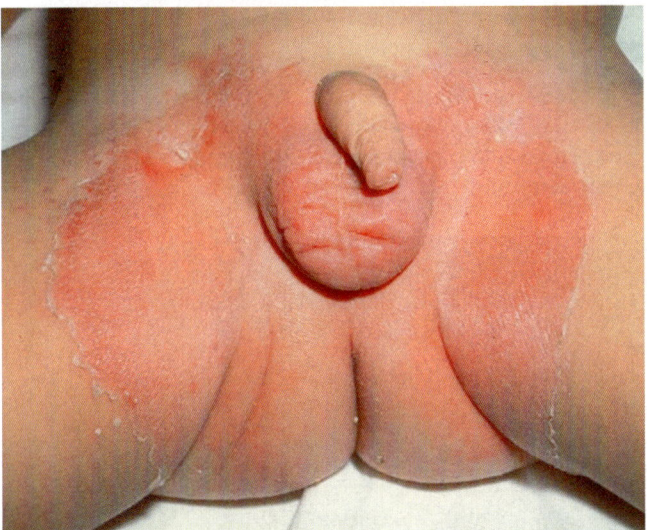

Figure 101.2. Erythematous patches that involve the creases and convexities are characteristic of candidal diaper dermatitis. Satellite lesions and scaling are present.

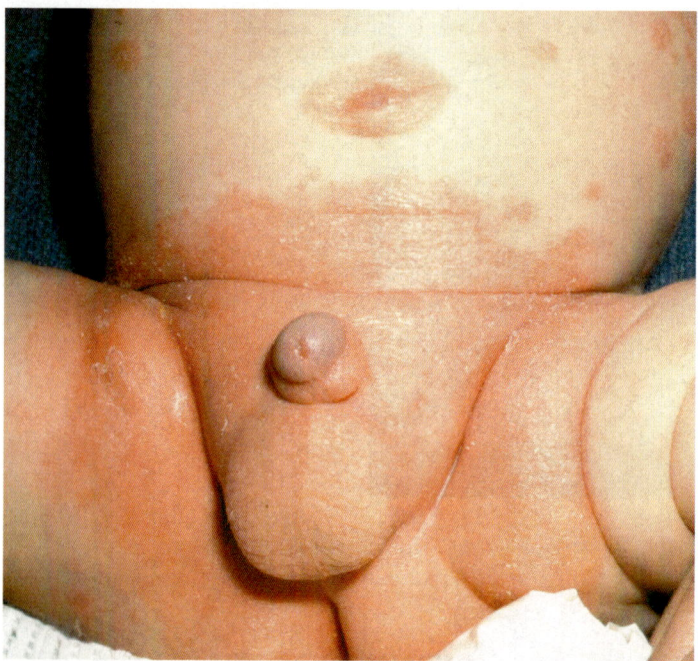

Figure 101.3. Salmon pink patches with greasy scale involve the creases and convexities in seborrheic dermatitis.

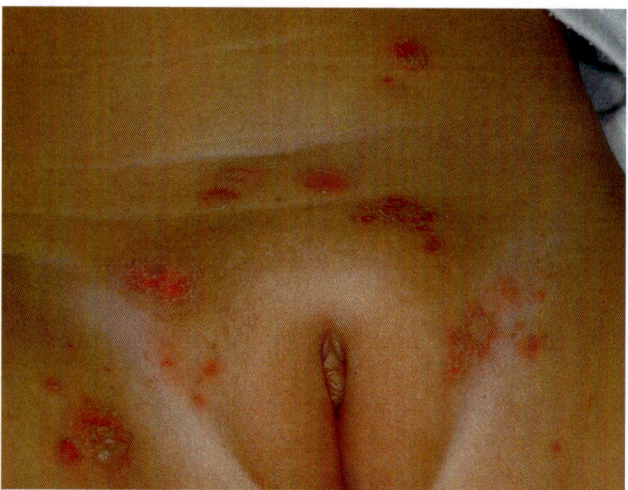

Figure 101.4. Flaccid bullae that rupture easily leaving round, crusted erosions occur in bullous impetigo.

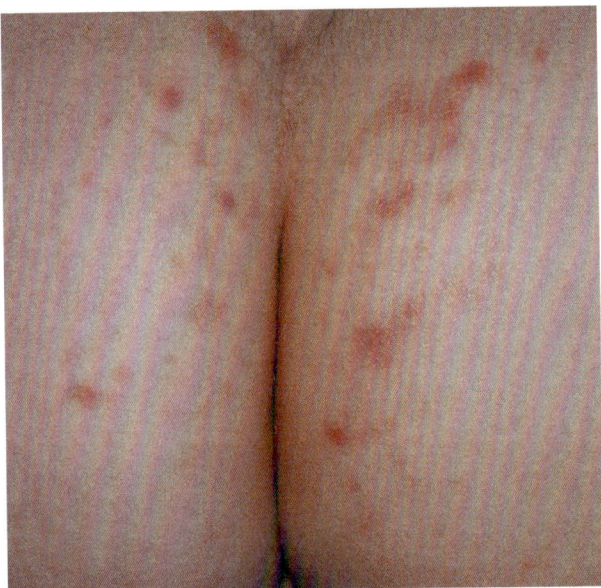

Figure 101.5. Folliculitis often involves the buttocks. There are erythematous papules centered on hair follicles. Frequently, patients also have pustules.

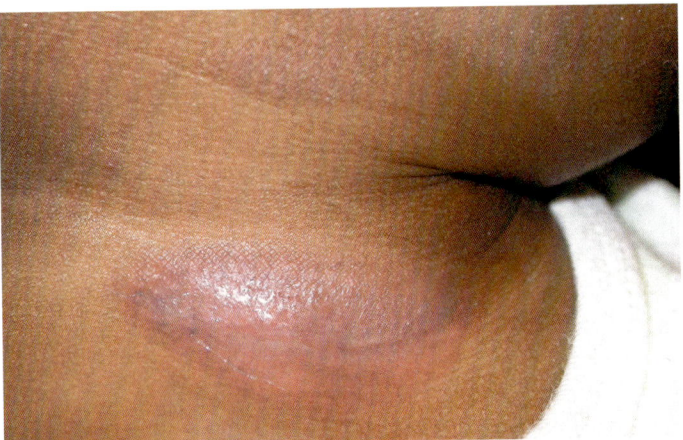

Figure 101.6. Intertrigo, shown here involving the neck, produces superficial erosions in areas where moist skin surfaces are in apposition.

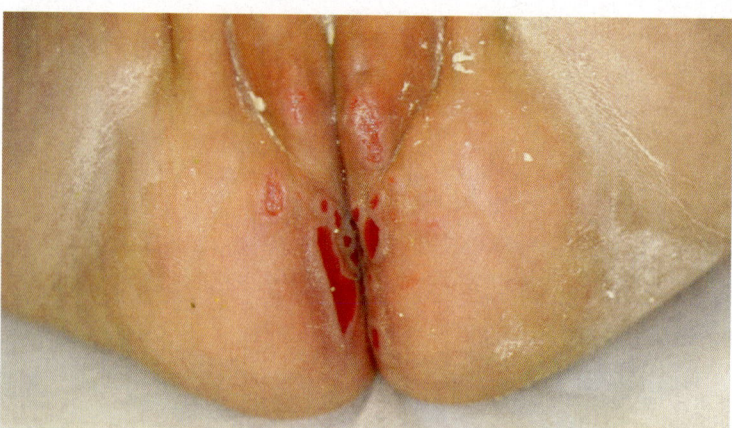

Figure 101.7. Jacquet erosive diaper dermatitis. Well-defined shallow ulcers and ulcerations with some healed areas.

Table 101.2. Uncommon Forms of Diaper Dermatitis

Condition	Cause	Clinical Features	Treatment
Psoriasis (Figure 101.8)	• Unknown.	• Erythematous scaling papules or plaques (scaling of the scalp and umbilicus may be present). • Lesions in the diaper area often lack scale characteristic of lesions located elsewhere. • May be difficult to distinguish from seborrheic dermatitis.	• Topical emollient and topical low-potency corticosteroid or calcineurin inhibitor.
Acrodermatitis enteropathica (Figure 101.9)	• Autosomal recessive disorder. • Defective transport protein causes impaired zinc absorption.	• Often begins when infants are weaned from human to cow milk formula. • Scaling, erosive erythematous eruption located around the mouth and in the diaper area. • Infants may have sparse hair, diarrhea, or failure to gain weight.	• Oral zinc supplementation. • Topical low-potency corticosteroid.
Langerhans cell histiocytosis (Figure 101.10)	• Rare disorder; Langerhans cells (antigen-processing cells in the skin) accumulate in skin or other organs.	• Lesion types: vesicles or pustules (often with a hemorrhagic crust); erythematous, orange, or yellowish brown papules or nodules; petechiae; erosions (in the diaper area). • Areas affected: scalp, palms and soles, skinfolds, diaper area. • Other features: infants may have hepatosplenomegaly, lymphadenopathy.	• Refer to pediatric dermatologist or pediatric oncologist for evaluation.
Congenital syphilis (Figure 101.11)	• Intrauterine infection with *Treponema pallidum*.	• Symptoms: rash, bloody diarrhea, rhinorrhea, irritability, pain with movement (Parrot pseudoparalysis). • Skin lesions: condylomata lata (ie, flat-topped papules and plaques located in the diaper area or at the angles of the mouth), scaling copper-colored papules and plaques on the trunk and extremities, or vesicles and bullae.	• Consult with a pediatric infectious disease specialist on evaluation and therapy.

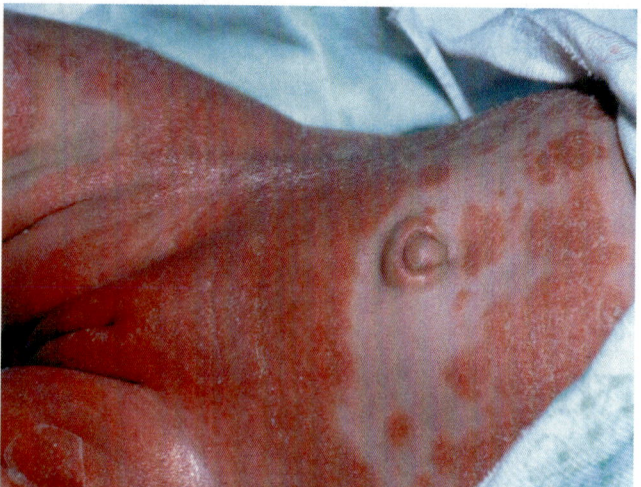

Figure 101.8. Psoriasis in the diaper area produces erythematous patches or plaques. Unlike lesions elsewhere, scale may be absent.

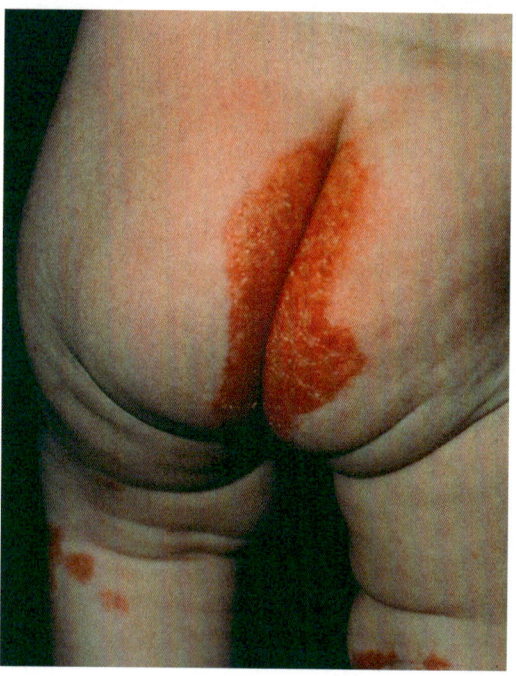

Figure 101.9. Acrodermatitis enteropathica causes erythematous patches in the diaper area and around the mouth.

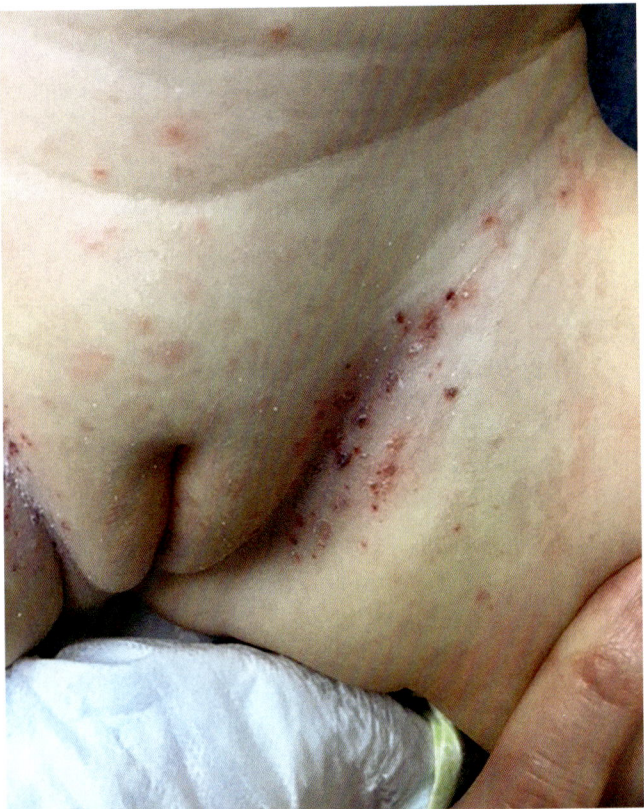

Figure 101.10. Eroded and crusted erythematous papules of Langerhans cell histiocytosis.

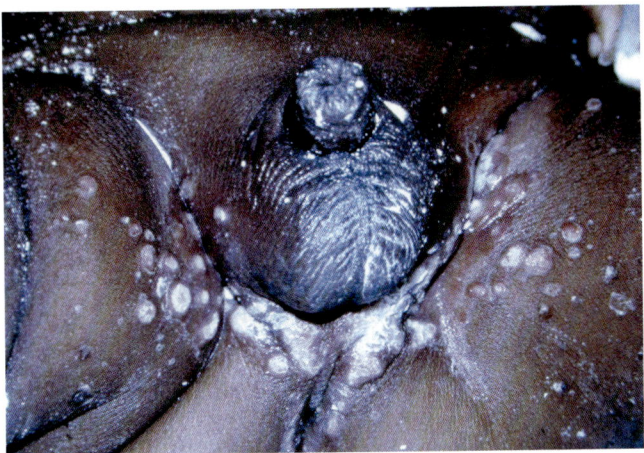

Figure 101.11. Condylomata lata, flat-topped papules and plaques, occur in the diaper area in congenital syphilis.

When to Worry or Refer

- Infants should be referred if appropriate therapy fails (to consider alternate diagnoses and possibly perform skin biopsy).
- Infants suspected of having Langerhans cell histiocytosis should be referred to a pediatric dermatologist or pediatric oncologist for evaluation.
- Consultation with a pediatric infectious disease specialist is warranted for infants suspected of having congenital syphilis.

Resources for Families

- American Academy of Pediatrics: HealthyChildren.org. **www.healthychildren.org/English/health-issues/conditions/infections/pages/Thrush-and-Other-Candida-Infections.aspx**
- Society for Pediatric Dermatology: Patient information on diaper care. **https://pedsderm.net/for-patients-families/patient-handouts/#DiaperCare**

CHAPTER 102

Eosinophilic Pustular Folliculitis

Introduction/Etiology/Epidemiology

- Rare disorder of unknown cause that usually begins during the first days or weeks after birth.

Signs and Symptoms

- Pruritic papules and pustules occur on the scalp (Figure 102.1) and occasionally the face, neck, and trunk.
- Crops of new lesions appear as others resolve, leading to a chronic relapsing course.

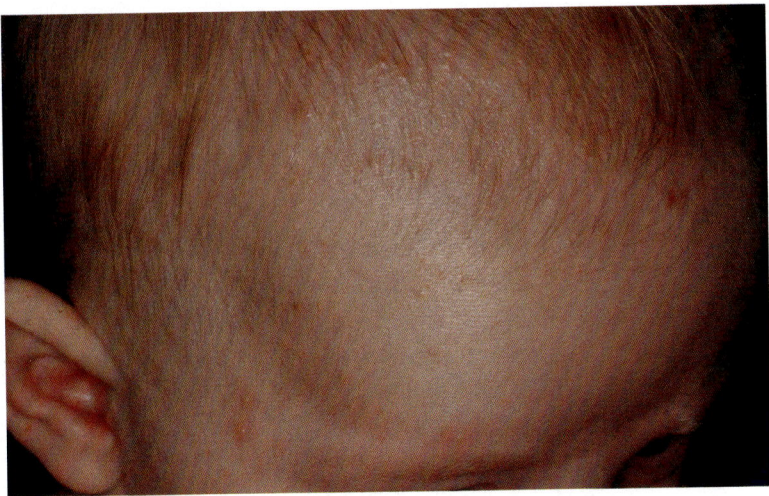

Figure 102.1. Follicular papules and pustules on the scalp and face of an infant with eosinophilic pustular folliculitis.

Look-alikes

Eosinophilic pustular folliculitis may be confused with infantile acropustulosis, erythema toxicum, and transient neonatal pustular melanosis, although its predominant distribution on the scalp helps to differentiate it from these disorders.

See Look-alikes in Chapter 103, Erythema Toxicum, to assist in differentiating eosinophilic pustular folliculitis from other disorders characterized by vesicles or pustules.

How to Make the Diagnosis

- The diagnosis may be suspected clinically and can be supported by finding a predominance of eosinophils on Wright stain of pustule fluid or skin biopsy specimen.

Treatment

- There is no specific treatment.
- A sedating oral antihistamine or topical corticosteroid may provide relief if pruritus is severe.

Prognosis

- Usually resolves spontaneously in several months to 5 years.

When to Worry or Refer

- Referral to pediatric dermatology generally is required to confirm the diagnosis.
- In some infants, eosinophilic pustular folliculitis may be a presenting feature of hyperimmunoglobulinemia E syndrome, which is characterized by immunodeficiency with very high immunoglobulin E levels, atopic dermatitis, bony variations, and recurrent cutaneous and sinopulmonary infections.

CHAPTER 103

Erythema Toxicum

Introduction/Etiology/Epidemiology

- Occurs in approximately 50% of newborns; rarely observed in preterm neonates.
- Cause is unknown.

Signs and Symptoms

- Usually begins 24 to 48 hours after birth; rarely, lesions may be present at birth or appear as late as 10 days after birth.
- Appears as discrete, blotchy erythematous macules or patches, each with a central papule, vesicle, or pustule (Figures 103.1 and 103.2).

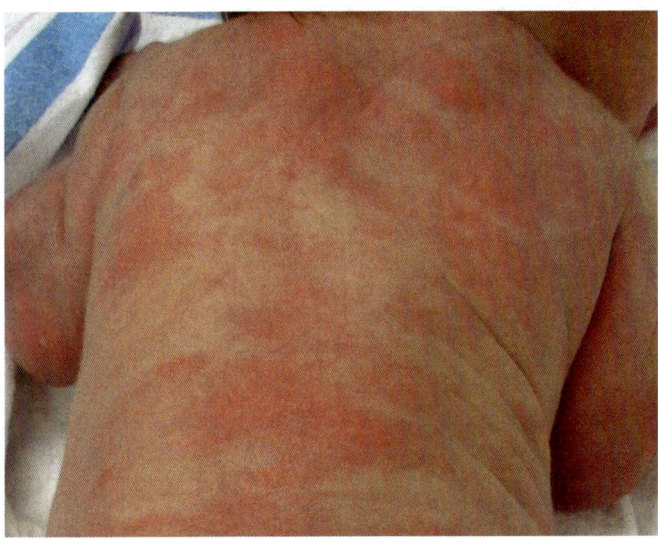

Figure 103.1. Erythematous macules, each with a central papule, are typical of erythema toxicum.

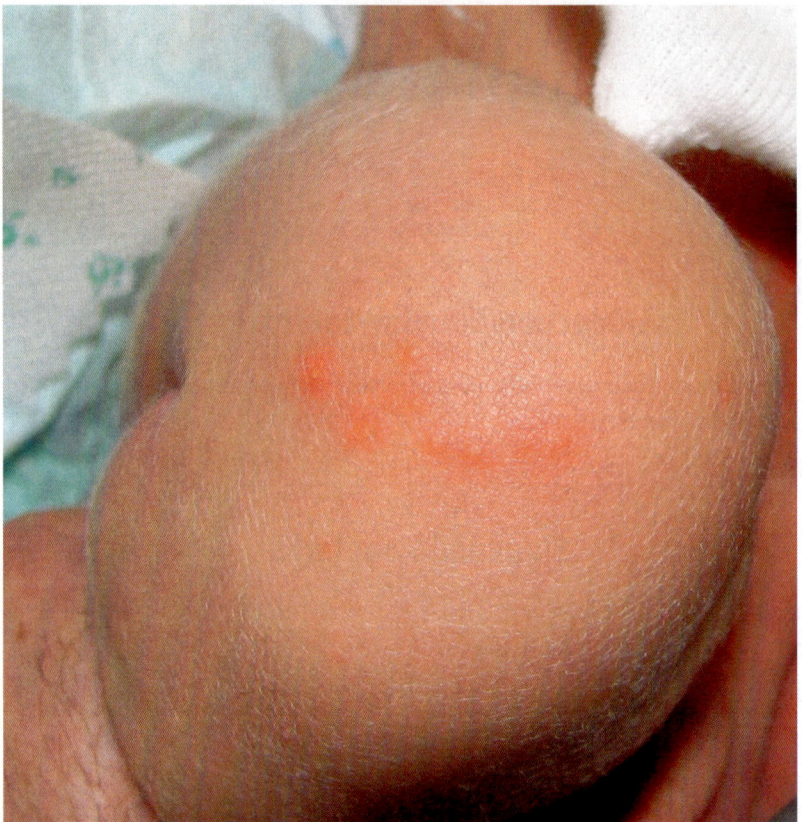

Figure 103.2. Erythematous papules of erythema toxicum located on the knee.

- Occasionally, there may be clusters of papules, vesicles, or pustules that form an erythematous plaque.
- Palms and soles are spared.
- New lesions appear for several days; the process lasts a week or less.

Look-alikes (in descending order of frequency of occurrence)

Disorder	Differentiating Features
Transient neonatal pustular melanosis	• Most often seen in Black newborns; rare in other racial groups. • Pustules (without erythema) or ruptured pustules that appear as small freckle-like hyperpigmented macules surrounded by a rim of scale. • Pustular fluid contains neutrophils.
Miliaria crystallina	• Fragile vesicles without surrounding erythema.
Neonatal acne (also termed *neonatal cephalic pustulosis*)	• Papules and pustules typically limited to face (some neonates may have lesions on scalp and upper chest).
Staphylococcal folliculitis	• White to slightly yellow pustules with surrounding rim of erythema. • Hair may be noted protruding centrally. • Gram stain and bacterial culture will reveal *Staphylococcus aureus*.
Bullous impetigo	• Flaccid bullae or ruptured bullae forming round or oval crusted erosions; vesicles occasionally present. • Gram stain and culture will reveal *S aureus*. • Occasionally presents as tense inflammatory pustules (referred to as *staphylococcal pustulosis*); pustules larger than seen in erythema toxicum and blotchy erythema absent.
Scabies	• Occurs rarely during the first month after birth. • Generalized eruption; may have vesicles but usually will be accompanied by erythematous papules or nodules and linear burrows. • Palmoplantar involvement common. • Mineral oil preparation of scrapings of papules will reveal mites, eggs, or fecal material.
Neonatal herpes simplex virus infection	• Typically, clustered vesicles on an erythematous base (although solitary vesicles occasionally occur). • Lesions concentrated on the head, particularly at sites of trauma (eg, that caused by a scalp electrode). • Neonates may have signs of sepsis (in disseminated disease) or seizures or coma (in central nervous system disease). • Tzanck test, direct fluorescence examination, viral culture, or polymerase chain reaction (cerebrospinal fluid) will confirm diagnosis.
Congenital candidiasis	• Widespread rash composed of many tiny erythematous papules and pustules and scaling. • Potassium hydroxide preparation of scale or a pustule roof will reveal pseudohyphae or spores. • Palmoplantar involvement common. • Nail changes (eg, yellow discoloration, ridging) may be present.

(*continued*)

Look-alikes (continued)

Disorder	Differentiating Features
Infantile acropustulosis	• Usually begins in first months (not in first days) after birth. • Vesicles or pustules limited to hands and feet, including palms, soles, wrists, and ankles. • Episodes last 5 to 10 days and reappear every 2 to 4 weeks.
Incontinentia pigmenti	• Vesicles on erythematous base appear at birth or within the first 2 weeks. • Arranged in linear fashion on extremities or in a swirled pattern on trunk (along Blaschko lines).
Eosinophilic pustular folliculitis	• Papules and pustules, typically located on scalp. • Exhibits chronic, intermittent course.

How to Make the Diagnosis

▶ The diagnosis is made clinically. If uncertainty exists, use of a Wright stain of vesicular fluid will reveal a predominance of eosinophils.

▶ Using a Tzanck smear, viral culture, direct fluorescence examination, polymerase chain reaction, Gram stain, or bacterial culture will assist in excluding infectious causes.

▶ Skin biopsy rarely is required to exclude incontinentia pigmenti.

Treatment

▶ No treatment is required.

Prognosis

▶ Resolves spontaneously; does not recur.

When to Worry or Refer

▶ Obtain consultation if presentation is atypical (eg, suggesting an alternate diagnosis such as herpes simplex virus infection, incontinentia pigmenti).

Resource for Families

▶ MedlinePlus: Information for patients and families (in English and Spanish) sponsored by the US National Library of Medicine and National Institutes of Health.
www.nlm.nih.gov/medlineplus/ency/article/001458.htm

CHAPTER 104

Infantile Acropustulosis

Introduction/Etiology/Epidemiology

- Uncommon disorder of unknown cause, although it is possible that, in some cases, it is a cyclical immune hyperreactivity to past scabies infestation.

Signs and Symptoms

- May be present at birth but most often begins during the first months after birth.
- Extremely pruritic, tense vesicles or pustules appear on the hands and feet (Figure 104.1), including the palms and soles and sides of the digits.
- Occasionally, a few lesions may be present on the trunk, proximal extremities, or scalp.
- Individual lesions last 5 to 10 days and then spontaneously resolve; the process recurs every 2 to 4 weeks.

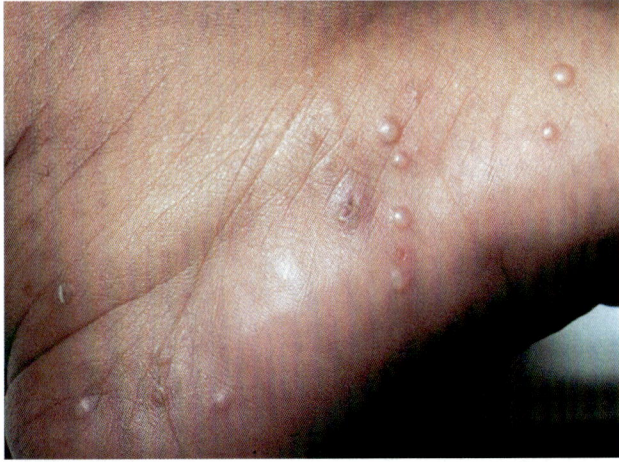

Figure 104.1. Tense vesicles or pustules on the foot in infantile acropustulosis.

Look-alikes

- Most often, infantile acropustulosis is confused with scabies; however,
  - In infants, scabies produces a generalized eruption that is not limited to the hands and feet and is unlikely to recur multiple times.
  - A mineral oil preparation of scrapings of pustules or burrows in scabies will reveal mites, eggs, or fecal material (scybala).
- Infantile acropustulosis may be confused with dyshidrotic eczema, but this condition rarely occurs in infancy. (This condition is characterized by recurring deep-seated vesicles concentrated on the lateral aspects of the digits.)
- See Look-alikes in Chapter 103, Erythema Toxicum, to assist in differentiating infantile acropustulosis from other disorders characterized by vesicles or pustules.

How to Make the Diagnosis

▶ The diagnosis usually is made clinically based on the history of recurrences and the location and appearance of lesions.

▶ If uncertainty exists, a Wright stain of vesicular fluid will reveal a predominance of neutrophils and eosinophils.

▶ Gram stain reveals no organisms, and a mineral oil preparation reveals no evidence of scabies.

Treatment

▶ If symptoms are mild, no therapy is required.

▶ If pruritus is severe, consider the following:
  - Potent topical corticosteroid applied to lesions twice daily during flares.
  - Oral sedating antihistamine to provide relief from pruritus.

▶ Dapsone may be used in severe cases (use with caution because of potential for hemolytic anemia and methemoglobinemia), although it is rarely indicated.

Prognosis

▶ Usually resolves within 1 to 2 years.

When to Worry or Refer

▶ Consider referral if diagnosis is uncertain or if severe pruritus does not respond to standard therapy.

CHAPTER
105

Intertrigo

Introduction/Etiology/Epidemiology

- Rubbing of moist skin surfaces results in superficial erosions.
- Often becomes secondarily infected with *Candida* species; also may be secondarily infected with *Streptococcus pyogenes* or, less commonly, *Staphylococcus aureus*.

Signs and Symptoms

- Erythema and superficial erosions located in the skinfolds (eg, anterior neck fold, axillae, inguinal creases) (Figure 105.1).
- If secondary candidal infection is present, the area often is bright red, and satellite lesions are present.
- Secondary *S pyogenes* (or, occasionally, *S aureus*) infection is suggested by persistent lesions that are superficially eroded, painful, and malodorous (Figure 105.2).

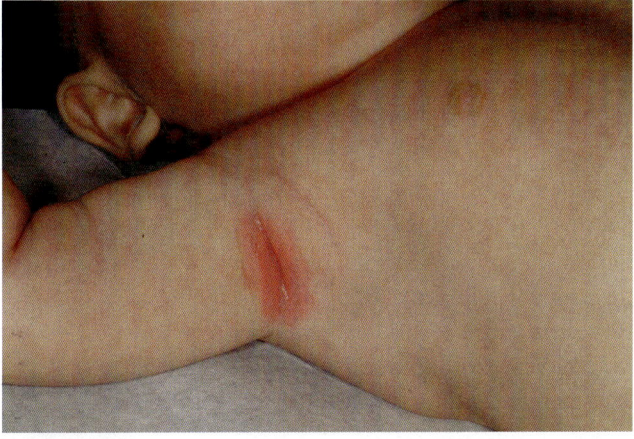

Figure 105.1. Intertrigo is characterized by erythematous superficial erosions located in the skinfolds.

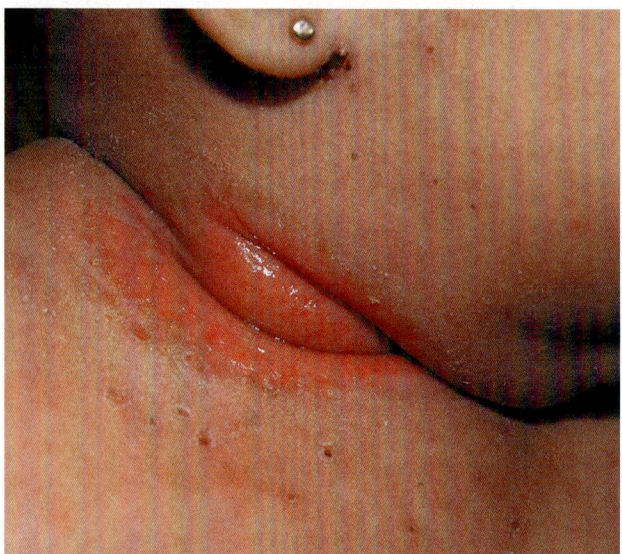

Figure 105.2. A superficially eroded area of intertrigo that was secondarily infected with *Streptococcus pyogenes*.

Look-alikes

Disorder	Differentiating Features
Seborrheic dermatitis	• Begins at 3 to 4 weeks and resolves by end of first year. • Salmon pink patches with greasy scaling. • Usually involves several sites (eg, scalp, postauricular folds, anterior neck fold, axillae, diaper area) symmetrically (not a single site, as in intertrigo).
Candidal diaper dermatitis	• Bright red, erythematous patches that involve inguinal creases, as well as convexities of the proximal thighs and lower abdomen. • Satellite lesions and scaling may be present. • Potassium hydroxide preparation will reveal pseudohyphae and spores.
Tinea cruris	• Erythematous patches involving proximal medial areas of the thighs and inguinal folds. • Border somewhat elevated and has associated scaling. • Potassium hydroxide preparation will reveal branching hyphae.
Erythrasma	• Erythematous to brown patches in skinfolds. • Coral red fluorescence at Wood lamp examination.

How to Make the Diagnosis

- The diagnosis is made clinically.

Treatment

- Apply an absorbent powder (to reduce moisture) or a greasy emollient (to reduce friction).
- For more severe cases, apply a low-potency topical corticosteroid.
- Treat with an antifungal preparation (if candidal infection suspected; this is often used in conjunction with a low-potency topical corticosteroid) or oral antibiotic (if streptococcal or staphylococcal infection suspected).

Prognosis

- Excellent.

When to Worry or Refer

- Patients should be referred if the diagnosis is uncertain or therapy fails.

Resources for Families

- MedlinePlus: Information for patients and families (in English and Spanish) sponsored by the US National Library of Medicine and National Institutes of Health.
  https://www.nlm.nih.gov/medlineplus/ency/article/003223.htm

CHAPTER
106

Miliaria

Introduction/Etiology/Epidemiology

- Obstruction of eccrine ducts. Three forms are recognized.
  - Miliaria rubra (prickly heat or heat rash): caused by deep intraepidermal obstruction of eccrine ducts accompanied by an inflammatory response.
  - Miliaria crystallina: caused by superficial obstruction that results in trapping of sweat.
  - Miliaria pustulosa: often considered a variant of miliaria rubra but with a more intense inflammatory response.
- Occurs in infants who are in warm environments, febrile, or dressed overly warmly.

Signs and Symptoms

- Miliaria rubra: erythematous papules located on the forehead, upper trunk, or flexural areas (eg, neck folds) or under clothing, bandages, or monitor leads (Figure 106.1).
- Miliaria crystallina: fragile, non-inflamed small vesicles filled with clear fluid (Figure 106.2).
- Miliaria pustulosa: pustules with surrounding erythema that are located in the areas described for miliaria rubra (Figure 106.3).

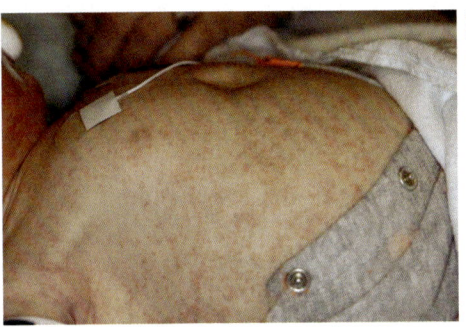

Figure 106.1. Numerous erythematous papules (miliaria rubra) on the trunk of an infant who was being over-swaddled and over-moisturized with emollients.

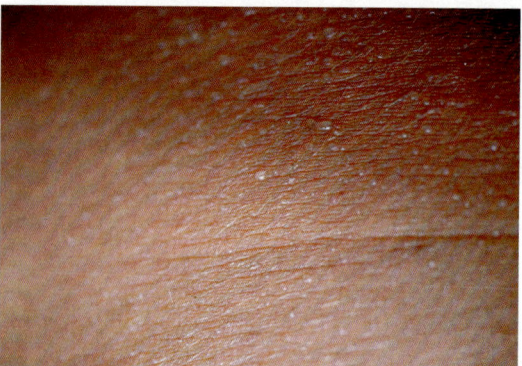

Figure 106.2. Miliaria crystallina is characterized by fragile superficial vesicles without surrounding erythema.

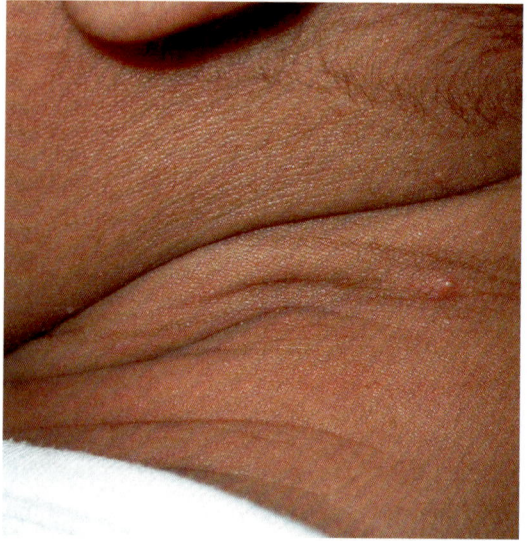

Figure 106.3. An infant with skin of color who has miliaria pustulosa. There are small pustules with surrounding erythema in the patient's neck folds.

Look-alikes

- Miliaria crystallina occasionally may be mistaken for herpes simplex virus infection; however, the lesions of miliaria crystallina have no associated erythema.
- Miliaria pustulosa and rubra may mimic staphylococcal folliculitis; however, a Gram stain of pustular contents would reveal no organisms, and a bacterial culture would be sterile.
- See Look-alikes in Chapter 103, Erythema Toxicum, to assist in differentiating miliaria from other disorders characterized by vesicles or pustules.

How to Make the Diagnosis

▶ The diagnosis is made clinically.

Treatment

▶ The best management is prevention. Avoid environmental overheating, overdressing infants, and overapplication of greasy or thick emollients that may obstruct eccrine ducts and contribute to the development of miliaria.
▶ For infants with established miliaria, provide an air-conditioned environment, if possible. Cool baths or sponge baths may be helpful.

Prognosis

▶ Resolves spontaneously.

When to Worry or Refer

▶ Referral is warranted only if diagnostic uncertainty exists.

Resource for Families

▶ American Academy of Pediatrics: HealthyChildren.org.
https://www.healthychildren.org/English/ages-stages/baby/bathing-skin-care/Pages/Heat-Rash.aspx

CHAPTER 107

Nevus Sebaceus (of Jadassohn)

Introduction/Etiology/Epidemiology

- Hamartoma of sebaceous and apocrine glands and epidermal elements present in 0.3% of newborns.
- Usually appears as an isolated finding; rarely associated with neurologic, ocular, or skeletal variations (ie, epidermal nevus or Schimmelpenning syndrome).

Signs and Symptoms

- Usually presents at birth as a solitary, well-circumscribed round or oval plaque.
- Typically located on the scalp, where it is associated with alopecia (Figures 107.1 and 107.2), or face (Figure 107.3).
- Lesions are yellow, yellowish brown, orange, or pink and have a velvety or verrucous (wartlike) texture. They are often linear or curvilinear.
- At puberty, androgenic stimulation causes lesions to become more elevated and verrucous, with development of a rough surface.

PEDIATRIC DERMATOLOGY

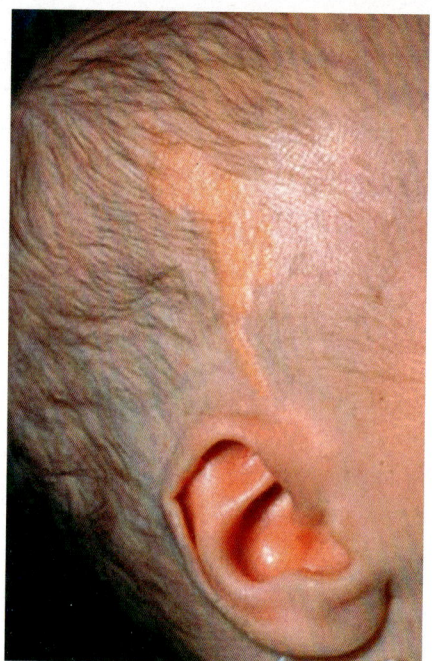

Figure 107.1. Nevus sebaceus. Yellowish tan hairless plaque located on the scalp.

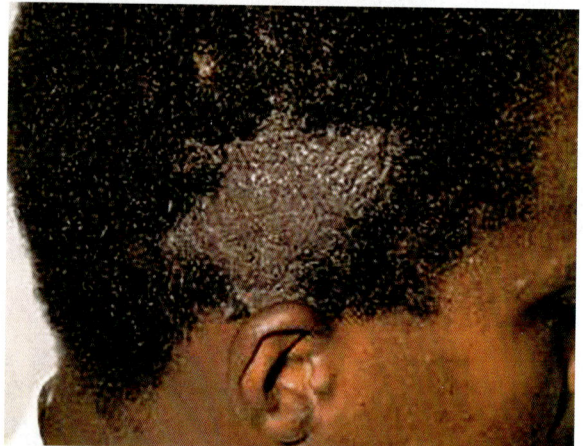

Figure 107.2. Large nevus sebaceus on the scalp of a young child with skin of color. Note the hairless pink to brown plaque. These lesions may not always appear yellowish orange in color, especially in those with darker skin tones. Reproduced with permission from DermNet NZ.

Chapter 107: Nevus Sebaceus (of Jadassohn)

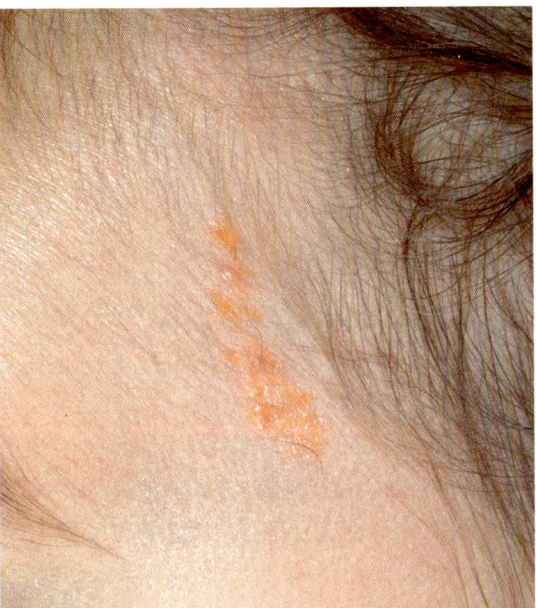

Figure 107.3. A linear nevus sebaceus located on the face.

Look-alikes

Disorder	Differentiating Features
Aplasia cutis congenita	• Presents at birth as an ulcer or scar. • Rarely is yellow; does not change at puberty.
Epidermal nevus	• May be difficult to differentiate from nevus sebaceus. • Often has rougher surface and is browner.
Juvenile xanthogranuloma	• One or more yellowish orange papules or dome-shaped non-verrucous plaques. • Usually acquired (not present at birth).

How to Make the Diagnosis

▶ The diagnosis may be suspected clinically and can be confirmed with skin biopsy.

Treatment

- No treatment is required during infancy or childhood.
- Because there is a small risk of developing basal cell carcinoma (and, rarely, other cutaneous malignancy) within the nevus after puberty, some advise elective excision before that time. Clinical observation is a reasonable alternative for lesions that are not psychosocially concerning and that remain stable. If secondary neoplasms develop within an existing nevus sebaceus, surgical excision with histopathologic analysis is strongly recommended.

Prognosis

- Most sebaceous nevi exhibit a benign course, although there is a small chance of secondary neoplasms (including malignant transformation), as discussed.

When to Worry or Refer

- Changes in a nevus sebaceus (eg, development of a nodule) should prompt referral to a dermatologist.
- If concern exists about epidermal nevus syndrome (eg, the nevus sebaceus is extensive or linear and associated with developmental delay, seizures, or ophthalmologic variations [eg, coloboma of the eyelid]), consultations with a pediatric dermatologist, neurologist, medical geneticist, and ophthalmologist should be sought, as indicated.

Resource for Families

- Society for Pediatric Dermatology: Patient information on nevus sebaceus. **https://pedsderm.net/for-patients-families/patient-handouts/#NevusSebaceus**

CHAPTER
108

Transient Neonatal Pustular Melanosis

Introduction/Etiology/Epidemiology

- Occurs in 5% of Black neonates; rare in other racial groups.
- Cause unknown.

Signs and Symptoms

- Present at birth.
- May present as pustules without surrounding erythema (Figure 108.1) or ruptured pustules that appear as small (several millimeters) hyperpigmented macules, often with a rim of surrounding scale (Figures 108.2 and 108.3).
- Lesions may occur at any location, but the forehead, chin, neck, and trunk most often are affected; the palms and soles occasionally are involved.
- Pustules resolve in several days; hyperpigmented macules resolve in 3 to 4 months.

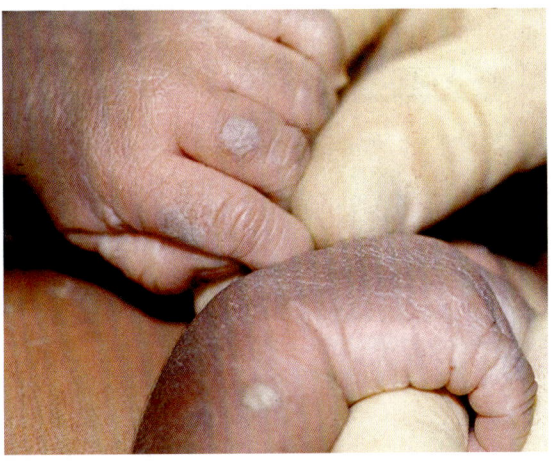

Figure 108.1. Pustules without surrounding erythema may be observed in neonates who have transient neonatal pustular melanosis.

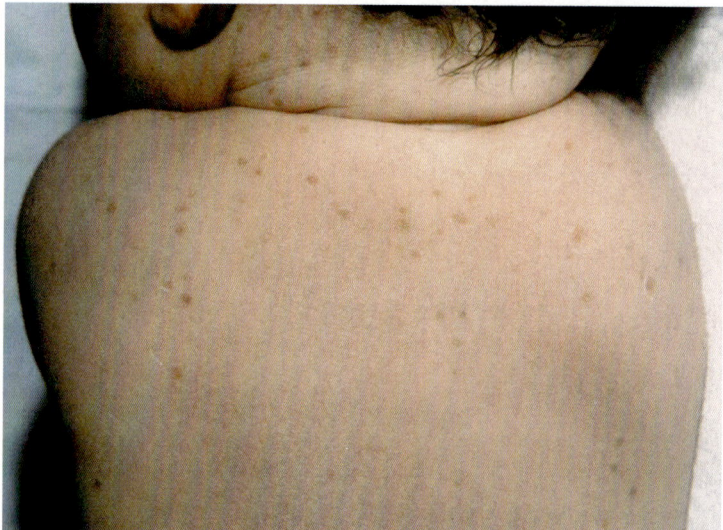

Figure 108.2. Hyperpigmented macules, some with a rim of scale, are seen in transient neonatal pustular melanosis.

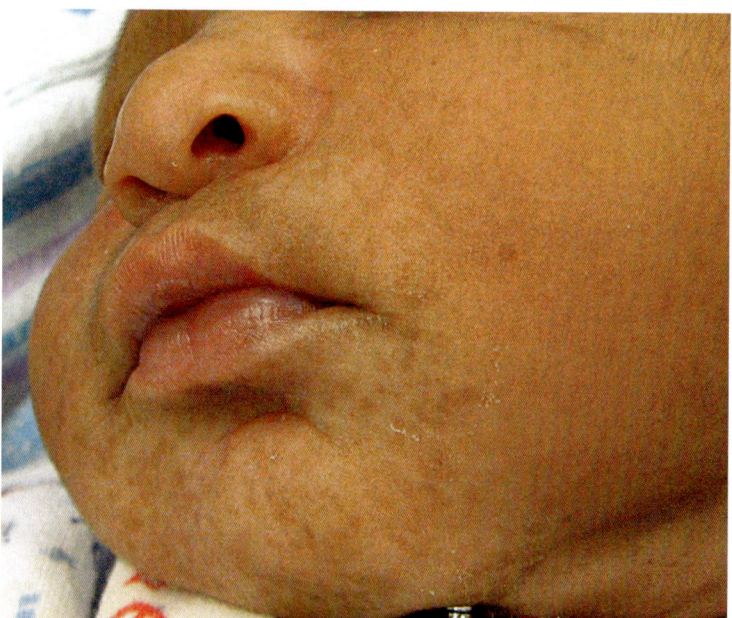

Figure 108.3. Transient neonatal pustular melanosis. Hyperpigmented macules on the chin. Note the collarettes of scale present in some areas.

Look-alikes

- The differential diagnosis includes miliaria, staphylococcal folliculitis, and congenital candidiasis (although these disorders produce lesions that exhibit erythema); infantile acropustulosis (lesions typically are pruritic and limited to the hands and feet); and congenital herpes simplex virus infection (lesions often are clustered, include erythema, and lack hyperpigmentation).
- See Look-alikes in Chapter 103, Erythema Toxicum, to assist in differentiating transient neonatal pustular melanosis from other disorders characterized by vesicles or pustules.

How to Make the Diagnosis

▶ The diagnosis is made clinically. If uncertainty exists, a Wright stain of vesicular fluid will reveal a predominance of neutrophils. Gram stain reveals no organisms.

▶ Gram stain and bacterial culture of pustular fluid will exclude staphylococcal folliculitis or pustulosis, the conditions with which transient neonatal pustular melanosis is most often confused. A potassium hydroxide preparation will exclude congenital cutaneous candidiasis.

Treatment

▶ No treatment is required.

Prognosis

▶ Resolves spontaneously; does not recur.
▶ Hyperpigmented macules may take 3 to 6 months to resolve.

When to Worry or Refer

▶ In view of the age of onset and typical clinical appearance, referral rarely is necessary.

Resource for Families

▶ DermNet NZ: Transient neonatal pustular melanosis. https://dermnetnz.org/topics/transient-neonatal-pustular-melanosis

CHAPTER
109

Subcutaneous Fat Necrosis (SFN)

Introduction/Etiology/Epidemiology

- ▶ Subcutaneous fat necrosis (SFN) is an uncommon, benign condition presenting as flesh-colored to erythematous, firm nodules and nodular plaques in the first few weeks after birth.
- ▶ This condition is a self-limited form of panniculitis, characterized by underlying inflammation of the fat, with necrosis.
- ▶ Although the exact etiology is unclear, most cases present in full-term neonates with history of perinatal stress or hypoxia.
  - Perinatal factors considered in the pathogenesis include hypothermia, mechanical trauma, ischemia, infection, and maternal preeclampsia and diabetes.
  - Because more saturated fatty acids are present in neonatal fat, some have proposed that this may predispose neonatal fat to crystallization at low temperatures, which may lead to inflammation and necrosis. This may account for its more common occurrence in neonates who receive cooling for hypoxic-ischemic encephalopathy.

Signs and Symptoms

- ▶ SFN typically presents in full-term, healthy neonates as well-demarcated, firm nodules and nodular plaques on the back, buttocks, or extremities (Figures 109.1 and 109.2). The face, particularly the cheeks, may also be involved.
- ▶ Nodules may appear as flesh-colored to erythematous to violaceous, often coalescing into indurated, larger plaques. Pain and tenderness may be noted in some infants. Rarely, ulceration may be present.
- ▶ Hypercalcemia is a rare associated complication; therefore, clinicians should be attentive to symptoms such as irritability, lethargy, hypotonia, poor feeding, constipation, and failure to thrive.

PEDIATRIC DERMATOLOGY

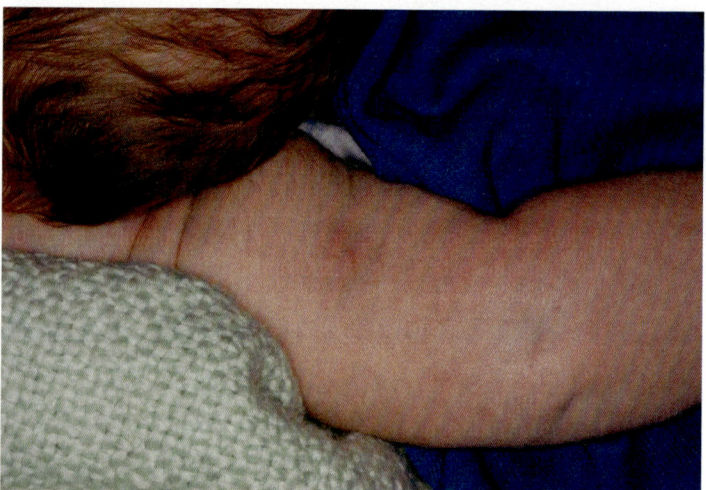

Figure 109.1. Subcutaneous fat necrosis. This 12-day-old developed red nodules and plaques on the extremities on the first day after birth and had associated hypercalcemia. The skin lesions and calcium elevation resolved over several months.

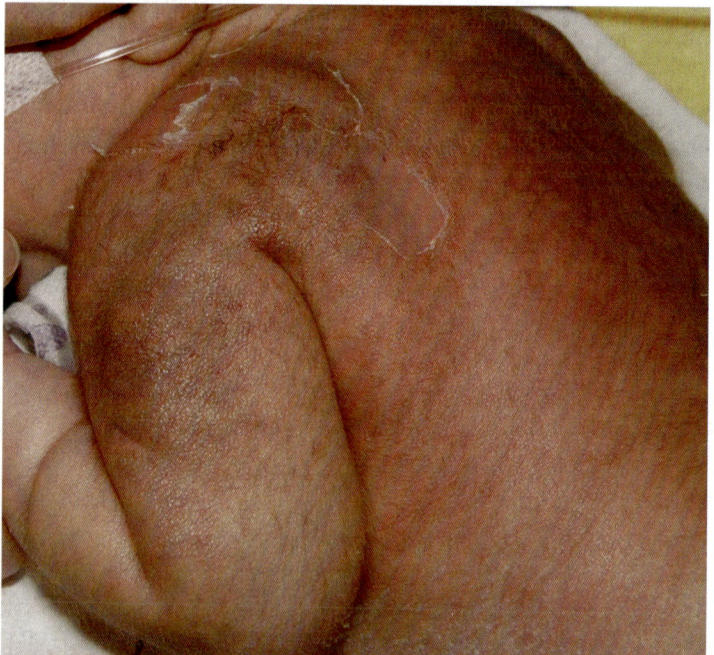

Figure 109.2. Erythematous nodular plaques on the left arm, shoulder, and upper back of a neonate with skin of color who has subcutaneous fat necrosis.

Look-alikes

Disorder	Differentiating Features
Cellulitis and erysipelas	• These infectious conditions may present with warmth, erythema, and tenderness similar to those of subcutaneous fat necrosis (SFN). • Multiple, firm indurated nodules and nodular plaques would be more suggestive of SFN. • Fever and leukocytosis often present. • Hypercalcemia not expected.
Sclerema	• Most often presents in neonates who are preterm and ill with underlying disease. • Prognosis is grave, as opposed to excellent prognosis in SFN. • Presents with diffuse involvement of more yellowish, waxy, firm bound-down skin.
Cold panniculitis	• Presents as symmetric indurated nodules and plaques with overlying erythema. • Lesions tend to be reproducible, usually within a few days of repeated cold exposure, with lesions localized to areas exposed to cold.
Malignancy	• Sarcomas and other malignancies may present with skin nodule(s) of various colors, often non-tender and without warmth. • These lesions are typically solitary, develop a few months after birth, and typically enlarge over time. • Histopathologic findings are diagnostic.
Myofibromatosis	• Can present in the neonatal period with skin nodules; various forms exist, including the more common solitary form. • Lesions may extend beyond the skin into the muscle or bone. • Lesions often persist for years. • Histopathologic findings are diagnostic.

How to Make the Diagnosis

▶ A clinical diagnosis can be made in many cases. When the diagnosis is unclear, a skin biopsy that includes the subcutaneous fat is often diagnostic.

▶ Histopathologic findings demonstrate fat necrosis, needle-shaped clefts, granulomatous inflammation, and possible calcification.

▶ Screening for hypercalcemia is strongly recommended. Blood ionized calcium levels should be checked periodically for the first several months after birth (can have a delayed onset). One such monitoring algorithm is shown in Figure 109.3. Some also suggest screening for thrombocytopenia and hyperlipidemia, which are very rare associations.

▶ In patients with persistent calcium elevation (>6 months), urinary system ultrasonography should be considered given risk for nephrocalcinosis.

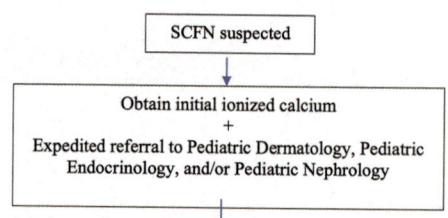

iCal < 1.4 mmol/L (5.61 mg/dl)	**Monitoring** Weekly until 1 month of age, then every other week until 3 months Can discontinue monitoring if normal at 3 months	**Care escalation** Symptomatic (fussiness, poor feeding, poor weight gain, irritability, constipation, vomiting, polyuria[1]) Referral to the emergency department for evaluation for inpatient management of hypercalcemia
iCal 1.41–1.5 mmol/L (5.65–6.01 mg/dl)	Twice weekly until stabilized or down trending, then weekly until normalized Once normalized, every other week until 3 months Evaluate for symptoms of hypercalcemia Hold vitamin D supplementation	
iCal 1.51–1.6 mmol/L (6.05–6.41 mg/dl)	Repeat in 1-2 days: If up trending consider referral to the emergency department If stable, follow 3 times weekly until less than 1.51 Hold vitamin D supplementation Evaluate for symptoms of hypercalcemia	Persistent calcium elevation after 6 months Consider obtaining urinary system ultrasound
iCal > 1.61 mmol/L (6.45 mg/dl)	Referral to the emergency department for hydration and evaluation for inpatient management of hypercalcemia Consider obtaining urinary system ultrasound	

Green: normal; Yellow: mild hypercalcemia, low risk for complications; Orange: mild hypercalcemia, increased risk for complications; Red: moderate hypercalcemia, high risk for complications.

Figure 109.3. Algorithm for monitoring of infants with subcutaneous fat necrosis. Abbreviations: iCal, ionized calcium; SCFN, subcutaneous fat necrosis. Adapted with permission from: Siegel LH, Alonso CF, Tuazon CFR, et al. Subcutaneous fat necrosis of the newborn: a retrospective study of 32 infants and care algorithm. *Pediatr Dermatol.* 2023;40(3):413–421.

Treatment

- Because SFN is self-limited, treatment of the skin nodules is not indicated.
- In patients with associated hypercalcemia, referral to an endocrinologist is indicated. If hypercalcemia treatment is necessary, options include intravenous fluids; diuretics; restriction of dietary calcium and vitamin D; and, rarely, systemic steroids, calcitonin, or etidronate.

Prognosis

- The prognosis is excellent, and in most cases the skin lesions resolve over weeks to months.
- Atrophy and scarring may rarely occur in some patients.
- Significant morbidity may result if severe hypercalcemia is present and left untreated.

When to Worry or Refer

- When the diagnosis is uncertain, consultation with a pediatric dermatologist is recommended.
- In patients with hypercalcemia or other metabolic changes, referral to a pediatric endocrinologist or other specialist experienced in the management of metabolic abnormalities is recommended.

Resources for Families

- DermNet NZ: Subcutaneous fat necrosis of the newborn.
  https://www.dermnetnz.org/topics/subcutaneous-fat-necrosis-of-the-newborn
- Medscape: Subcutaneous fat necrosis of the newborn.
  https://emedicine.medscape.com/article/1081910-overview

Acute Drug/Toxic Reactions

CHAPTER 110 — **Drug Hypersensitivity Syndrome** 701

CHAPTER 111 — **Erythema Multiforme (EM)** 707

CHAPTER 112 — **Exanthematous and Urticarial Drug Reactions** . . 713

CHAPTER 113 — **Fixed Drug Eruption** 719

CHAPTER 114 — **Serum Sickness–Like Reaction** 723

CHAPTER 115 — **Stevens-Johnson Syndrome (SJS),** ***Mycoplasma pneumoniae*****–Induced Rash and Mucositis (MIRM), and Reactive Infectious Mucocutaneous Eruption (RIME)** 729

CHAPTER 116 — **Toxic Epidermal Necrolysis (TEN)** 737

CHAPTER 117 — **Urticaria** 743

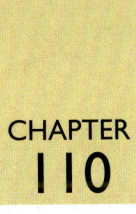

CHAPTER 110

Drug Hypersensitivity Syndrome

Introduction/Etiology/Epidemiology

- A severe cutaneous drug eruption in combination with systemic manifestations.
- Also known as *drug reaction with eosinophilia and systemic symptoms* (DRESS) and *drug-induced hypersensitivity syndrome.*
- Classic triad consists of fever, skin rash, and internal organ (usually liver) involvement.
- Occurs 1 to 8 weeks (most common: 2–6 weeks) after starting the drug.
- Most often occurs after initial exposure to the medication.
- Potentially life-threatening.
- Most common causative drugs include anticonvulsant agents (mainly the aromatic agents, including phenytoin, carbamazepine, and phenobarbital; also, lamotrigine), sulfonamides (mainly trimethoprim-sulfamethoxazole; rarely, furosemide), dapsone, minocycline, and allopurinol; nonsteroidal anti-inflammatory drugs also occasionally implicated.
- Etiology involves impaired detoxification of drug metabolites and may involve coinfection with human herpesvirus 6.
- May be a familial predisposition.

Signs and Symptoms

- Fever and malaise early.
- Rash begins as exanthematous eruption, becoming more edematous and erythematous and with confluence of lesions (Figure 110.1).
- Eruption may become vesicular, bullous, or purpuric; may simulate/progress to Stevens-Johnson syndrome or toxic epidermal necrolysis.
- Mucous membranes may be involved.
- Characteristic facial edema develops, especially periorbital (Figure 110.2).

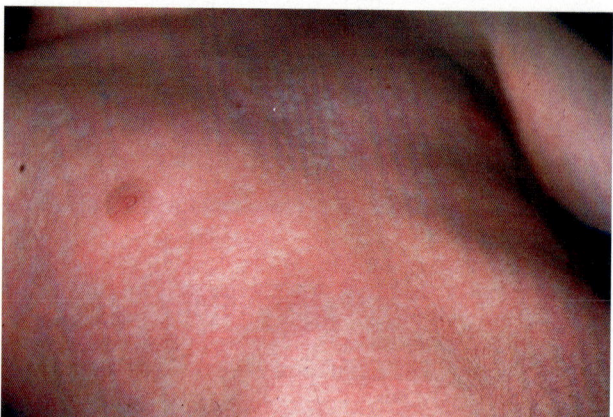

Figure 110.1. Drug hypersensitivity syndrome. This patient developed an eruption of erythematous macules and papules during the second week of carbamazepine therapy. Fever and hepatitis were also present.

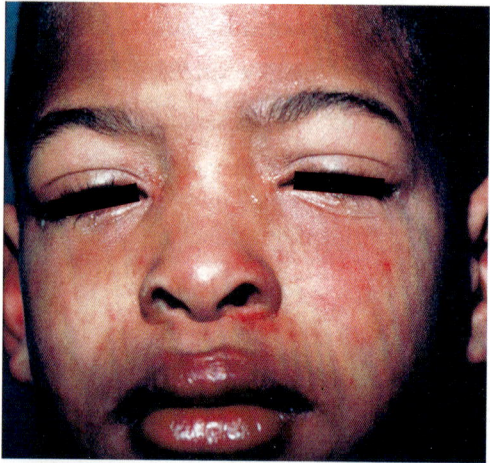

Figure 110.2. Drug hypersensitivity syndrome. Therapy with phenytoin resulted in a widespread skin eruption in this child, including facial involvement with prominent periorbital edema. The patient also had lip swelling, fever, lymphadenopathy, and hepatitis.

- ▶ Cervical lymphadenopathy is common.
- ▶ Liver is the most common extracutaneous site of involvement; may progress to fulminant hepatitis.
- ▶ Other involvement may include nephritis, pneumonitis, thyroiditis, pancreatitis, and myocarditis; thyroid involvement may be delayed, with hypothyroidism noted up to several months or years after the acute reaction.

Look-alikes

Disorder	Differentiating Features
Simple exanthematous drug eruption	• Typically earlier onset of symptoms; shorter latent period. • Lacks facial edema, lymphadenopathy, hepatitis, atypical lymphocytosis. • Fever less common.
Viral exanthem	• Less severe skin eruption. • Usually lacks facial edema, hepatitis. • Fever more commonly low-grade, transient. • History of drug ingestion lacking.
Cutaneous lymphoma	• Lacks facial edema, hepatitis. • Fever uncommon. • History of drug ingestion lacking. • Histopathologic features confirmatory.

How to Make the Diagnosis

- ▶ The diagnosis is suggested by fever and a severe rash in the presence of facial edema, lymphadenopathy, and a history of ingestion of an implicated drug.
- ▶ Supportive laboratory findings include atypical lymphocytosis and eosinophilia, as well as elevation of liver transaminases; thyroid testing should be performed at baseline and, if within reference range, screened routinely after DRESS; some authors suggest thyroid monitoring for at least 2 years after the diagnosis.
- ▶ Skin biopsy, when performed, reveals dense lymphocytic infiltrate with eosinophils in the dermis.
- ▶ Patch testing for drug allergy may be useful diagnostically, especially with carbamazepine and phenytoin, but exact sensitivity and specificity of this type of testing is unclear.
- ▶ Lymphocyte toxicity assays may be useful in confirming the triggering medication but are not readily available.

Treatment

- Offending agent should be immediately discontinued once the diagnosis has been recognized.
- Systemic corticosteroids are the most widely used and accepted treatment for severe or progressive disease, with a gradual and prolonged (3–6 month) taper to prevent rebound disease. Steroid-sparing therapies such as intravenous immunoglobulin have also been used with variable success.
- Antihistamines and topical corticosteroids may be useful for pruritus, and oral antipyretics may be useful in decreasing erythroderma and symptoms. Antipyretics should be used with caution in patients with liver involvement, especially when coadministered with systemic corticosteroids.

Treating Associated Conditions

- Hypothyroidism and other organ dysfunction should be treated appropriately, if present.

Prognosis

- Rapid recognition and prompt discontinuation of the causative agent may be associated with a better prognosis, although some patients will continue to progress.
- If the reaction is secondary to an aromatic anticonvulsant (eg, phenytoin, carbamazepine, phenobarbital, primidone), it is vital that substitution of another anticonvulsant from this group be avoided, given the high risk of cross-reactivity.
- The long-term outcome depends on the degree of extracutaneous involvement. Autoimmune conditions, including thyroiditis and type 1 diabetes, can develop months to years later.

When to Worry or Refer

- Consider drug hypersensitivity syndrome or dermatology consultation in the patient presenting with a severe skin eruption accompanied by fever and lymphadenopathy.
- If hepatitis or other organ dysfunction is noted, consultation with the appropriate specialties should be requested.

Resources for Families

- American Academy of Allergy, Asthma, and Immunology: Drug reaction with eosinophilia and systemic symptoms (DRESS). **www.aaaai.org/conditions-treatments/related-conditions/dress**
- DermNet NZ: Drug hypersensitivity syndrome. **https://dermnetnz.org/topics/drug-hypersensitivity-syndrome**
- DRESS Syndrome Foundation: **www.dresssyndromefoundation.org**

CHAPTER
111

Erythema Multiforme (EM)

Introduction/Etiology/Epidemiology

- Erythema multiforme (EM; previously called *erythema multiforme minor*) is a reactive inflammatory disorder of limited duration that may become recurrent.
- Causes include infection and medications, with infections the most common cause in children.
- Herpes simplex virus (HSV) infection is the most common cause of recurrent EM in children.

Signs and Symptoms

- Begins as erythematous, blanching, round or oval papules or plaques.
- Lesions then develop a target appearance, with central dusky to violaceous color (Figures 111.1 and 111.2) (sometimes with a central vesicle, bulla [Figures 111.3 and 111.4], or crust) surrounded by concentric white (sometimes) and red rings, the latter 2 representing vasoconstriction or vasodilation, respectively.
- A single mucosal surface (usually lips) may be involved.
- The disease lasts 7 to 10 days before resolving spontaneously.

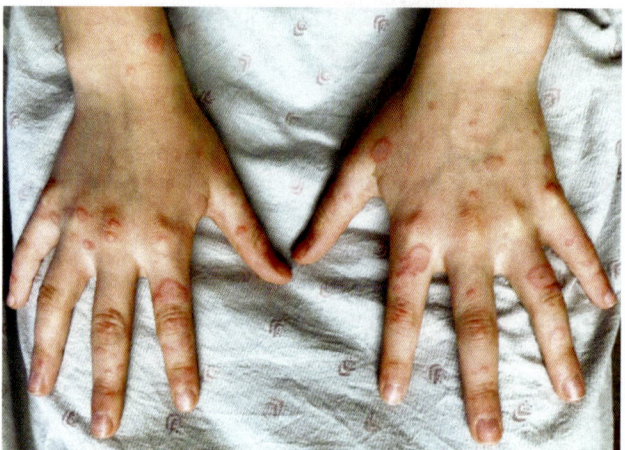

Figure 111.1. Erythema multiforme. Target lesions are papules or plaques that develop a central violaceous discoloration (or blister or crust), surrounded by a pale edematous zone and a peripheral red color.

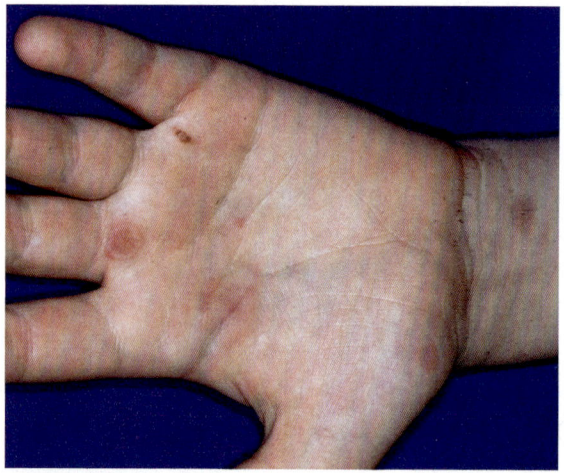

Figure 111.2. Erythema multiforme. Target lesions on the palm.

Chapter 111: Erythema Multiforme (EM)

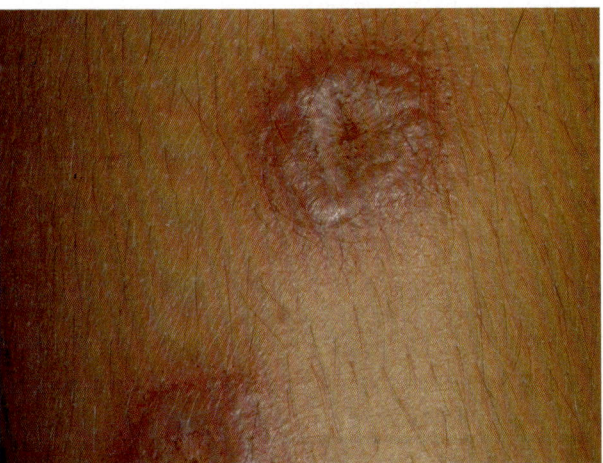

Figure 111.3. Target lesions may develop central bullae or vesicles.

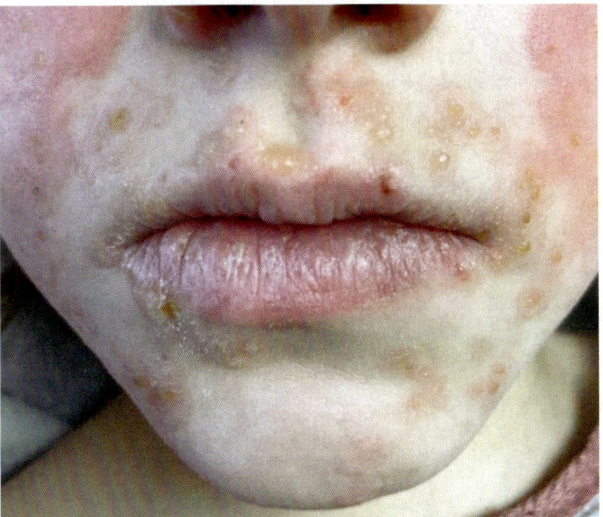

Figure 111.4. Target lesions on the face with central vesicles. This child had a preceding herpes simplex virus infection, as noted by the crusted papule on the left side of the upper lip.

Look-alikes

Disorder	Differentiating Features
Urticaria	• Erythematous blanching wheals that resolve or change in 24 hours or sooner. • Occasionally, lesions may become centrally dusky, but no vesicle or crust formation. • Although lesions may become annular, true target lesions do not occur. • In "urticaria multiforme," annular, polycyclic, and occasionally dusky urticarial papules and plaques occur and may be mistaken for erythema multiforme.
Stevens-Johnson syndrome (SJS)/toxic epidermal necrolysis (TEN)	• Prodromal symptoms (eg, fever, sore throat, malaise) precede appearance of rash by as much as 14 days. • Patients are systemically ill. • Target lesions may be few in number or atypical in their appearance (especially in TEN). • Erythematous macules or patches that develop bullae and erosions. • Extensive mucosal involvement with 2 or more sites affected. • TEN often associated with reaction to systemic drug.
Mycoplasma pneumoniae–induced rash and mucositis	• Newer classification for what once was referred to as "mucosal-predominant *M pneumoniae*–associated SJS." • Prominent erosions of 2 or more mucous membranes with more sparse skin lesions (target lesions and bullae). • Milder disease course than with SJS or TEN.
Serum sickness–like eruption	• Large, often purple, urticarial-appearing plaques present (has been termed "purple urticaria"). • Target lesions and blistering absent. • Fever, arthralgia, arthritis are common features. • Periarticular swelling often present. • Ambulatory children may refuse to walk during episode.

How to Make the Diagnosis

▶ The diagnosis of EM is made clinically and may be confirmed with skin biopsy.

▶ Presence of target lesions concentrated on the palms, soles, arms, and legs.

▶ Target lesions exhibit peeling, blistering, or crusting in the center of some lesions.

▶ Involvement of no more than 1 mucosal surface.

Treatment

- Consider antiviral prophylaxis for presumed HSV infection if EM is recurrent.
- If pruritus is significant, an antihistamine may be prescribed.
- Corticosteroid therapy is not indicated.

Prognosis

- EM resolves spontaneously, leaving only occasional postinflammatory hyperpigmentation.
- Recurrent EM may indicate HSV infection and reactivation. In such cases, antiviral prophylaxis may be required to prevent EM recurrences.

Resources for Families

- MedlinePlus: Information for patients and families (in English and Spanish) sponsored by the US National Library of Medicine and National Institutes of Health.
  https://www.nlm.nih.gov/medlineplus/ency/article/000851.htm
- WebMD: Autoimmune blistering disorders.
  https://www.webmd.com/skin-problems-and-treatments/autoimmune-blistering-disorders

CHAPTER 112

Exanthematous and Urticarial Drug Reactions

Introduction/Etiology/Epidemiology

- Drug reactions or eruptions may present in a variety of morphological forms.
- May include exanthematous (morbilliform), urticarial, pustular, and blistering presentations.
- Exanthematous form is the most common type of cutaneous drug eruption.
- Urticarial form is the second most common type of cutaneous drug eruption.
- Exanthematous eruptions may present anytime within first 2 weeks of starting the medication; urticarial eruptions tend to present more rapidly (ie, immediate reactions).
- These reactions are frequently responsible for premature discontinuation of treatment.
- Increased risk in patients receiving multiple medications and those with concomitant viral infection; classic example is the exanthematous eruption that occurs after ingestion of penicillin-class antibiotics in patients with acute Epstein-Barr virus infection (Figure 112.1).
- Most common cause of a drug eruption is an antimicrobial agent.
- Penicillin–cephalosporin cross-reactivity is generally overemphasized in the literature and classic teachings. Patients allergic to penicillin are at a very mildly (1%–3%) increased risk of reaction to first-generation cephalosporins (ie, cefadroxil, cefazolin, cephalexin, cephalothin, and cephaloridine) and to the second-generation cefamandole; there appears to be no increased risk associated with the use of other cephalosporins in these patients.

Signs and Symptoms

- Exanthematous eruption.
  - Generalized erythematous macules and papules (Figures 112.1 and 112.2).
  - May appear morbilliform (resembling measles) or scarlatiniform (resembling scarlet fever).
  - Often begins on the head and upper trunk, with cephalocaudal extension.
  - Lesions may become confluent and are often pruritic.
  - Rarely progresses to erythroderma or exfoliation.
  - Etiologies include antibiotics (especially β-lactams, sulfonamides), barbiturates, anticonvulsants, angiotensin-converting enzyme inhibitors, gold compounds, and nonsteroidal anti-inflammatory agents.

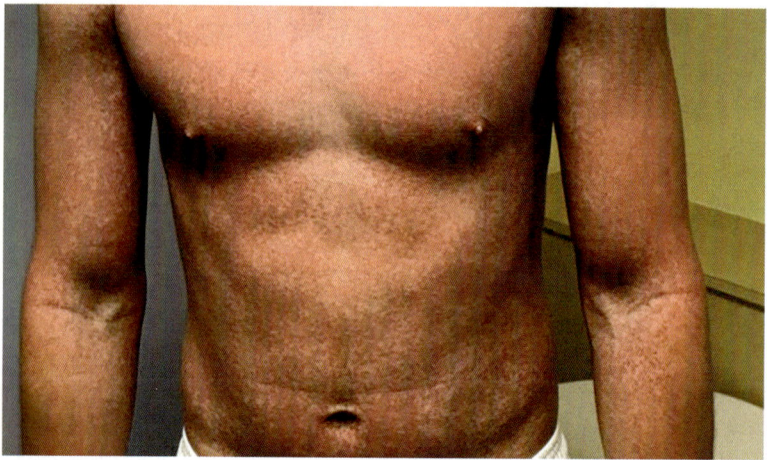

Figure 112.1. This erythematous eruption of macules and papules occurred after amoxicillin/clavulanic acid was administered in a patient who was later found to have infectious mononucleosis.

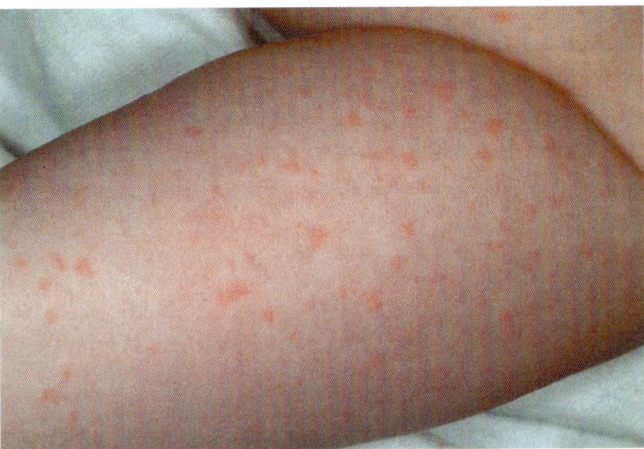

Figure 112.2. Exanthematous drug eruption. These erythematous macules and papules occurred during therapy with amoxicillin.

- Urticarial eruption.
    - Pruritic, edematous wheals of various sizes (Figure 112.3).
    - May appear annular, arcuate, or polycyclic.
    - Individual lesions last no longer than 24 hours, but new lesions may continue to develop.
    - When deeper subcutaneous or dermal tissues are involved (eg, lips, eyes, mucous membranes), it is termed *angioedema*.
    - Etiologies include antibiotics (especially sulfonamides, β-lactams), anticonvulsants, angiotensin-converting enzyme inhibitors, azole antifungal agents, narcotic analgesics, salicylates, and radiocontrast dye.

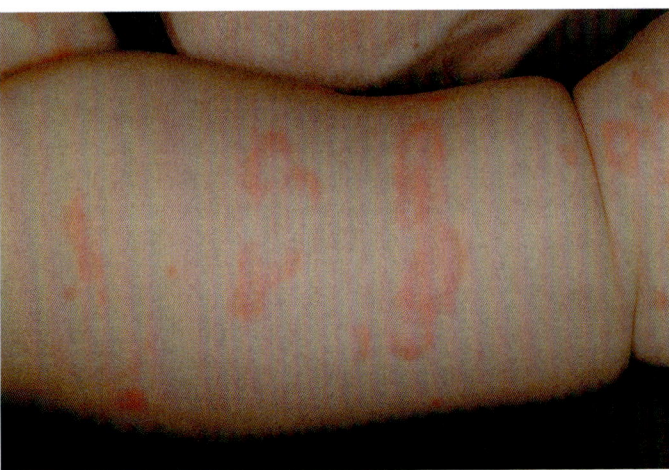

Figure 112.3. Urticarial drug eruption. These urticarial papules and plaques occurred 2 days after initiation of oral sulfonamide therapy.

Look-alikes

Disorder	Differentiating Features
Exanthematous Drug Eruption	
Viral exanthem	• Associated infectious symptoms. • Lack of preceding drug ingestion. • At times, the 2 may be indistinguishable.
Scarlet fever	• Accentuation of eruption in skinfolds. • Circumoral pallor. • Pharyngitis and strawberry tongue. • Rapid testing or culture result positive for *Streptococcus pyogenes*.
Miliaria rubra (prickly heat)	• Tends to predominate in occluded areas (eg, skinfolds). • Lack of preceding drug ingestion. • Often a history of overheating, swaddling, overapplication of greasy topical products (eg, petrolatum). • Resolves rapidly with cooling and avoidance of occlusion.
Drug hypersensitivity syndrome (also known as drug reaction with eosinophilia and systemic symptoms or DRESS)	• Marked facial edema with periorbital accentuation. • Cervical lymphadenopathy common. • Fever often present. • Atypical lymphocytosis, eosinophilia, and hepatitis on laboratory test results. • Later onset: classically develops 2 to 6 weeks after drug ingestion.
Graft-versus-host disease	• Susceptibility (eg, after stem cell transplant). • Palms, soles, posterior auricular scalp involved. • Associated diarrhea, bilirubin elevation. • Characteristic changes of graft-versus-host disease noted on skin biopsy samples.
Urticarial Drug Eruption	
Erythema multiforme	• True target lesions with 3 zones (central duskiness, surrounded by pallor, and then peripheral erythema). • Palm and sole involvement common. • Usually lack of preceding drug ingestion. • Occasional single mucous membrane involvement. • Commonly associated with recurrent herpes simplex virus infection in children.
Serum sickness–like eruption	• Purple appearance of urticarial lesions ("purple urticaria"). • Fever common. • Periarticular swelling and pain with ambulation. • Occasional proteinuria.
Kawasaki disease	• High fever common (for ≥5 days, to meet diagnostic criteria). • Conjunctival injection (non-purulent), oral mucosal hyperemia, lip fissuring, strawberry tongue present. • Cervical lymphadenopathy common. • May have accentuation of rash with desquamation in perineum. • Risk of coronary artery aneurysms.

How to Make the Diagnosis

- The diagnosis is assigned based on the cutaneous findings and presenting history.
- Development of a timeline of drug ingestion and development of the eruption may be useful in patients receiving multiple medications; often, however, the exact culprit may be difficult to confirm.
- Ruling out other potential explanations may be necessary with laboratory testing or medical imaging.
- Skin biopsy is occasionally helpful.

Treatment

- Withdrawal of the causative agent usually results in spontaneous resolution.
- Therapy is generally for symptoms and may include oral antihistamines and topical antipruritic preparations. The latter include topical corticosteroids, camphor and menthol preparations, calamine, and witch hazel; topical diphenhydramine is available but should be avoided, as it may result in contact sensitization (with allergic contact dermatitis).
- "Treating through" the cutaneous eruption may be considered for patients with an exanthematous drug eruption in whom the treatment is extremely important and when there is no satisfactory substitute; requires close clinical follow-up.
- Systemic corticosteroids are rarely indicated for exanthematous or urticarial drug eruptions.

Treating Associated Conditions

- In patients for whom an infectious exanthem cannot be excluded, appropriate examination, testing (when indicated), and parental education should be offered.

Prognosis

- Uncomplicated exanthematous and urticarial drug eruptions resolve completely and without permanent sequelae.

When to Worry or Refer

- Consider dermatology referral when:
  - Atypical cutaneous features are present.
  - The skin eruption is unusually severe or associated with extracutaneous findings.
  - The diagnosis is in question.

Resource for Families

- MedlinePlus: Information for patients and families (in English and Spanish) sponsored by the US National Library of Medicine and National Institutes of Health.
  https://www.nlm.nih.gov/medlineplus/ency/article/000819.htm

CHAPTER 113

Fixed Drug Eruption

Introduction/Etiology/Epidemiology

- Common drug eruption in children and adults.
- Characterized by recurrence of the eruption at same location on the body after repeat ingestion of etiologic medication.
- May involve skin or mucosal sites.
- May occur as a single lesion (Figure 113.1) or in a generalized form (Figure 113.2).
- Common causes include sulfonamides (typically trimethoprim-sulfamethoxazole), nonsteroidal anti-inflammatory agents, acetaminophen, salicylates, tetracycline, and pseudoephedrine; also reported in association with fluconazole, dextromethorphan, loratadine, sildenafil, metronidazole, ciprofloxacin, and phenylephrine.
- Latent period of 1 to 2 weeks after first exposure, 12 to 24 hours after subsequent exposures.
- "Fixed food eruption" has been described with similar clinical features in association with ingestion of licorice, asparagus, cashews, peanuts, lentils, quinine (in tonic water), and tartrazine (in artificially colored cheese crisps).

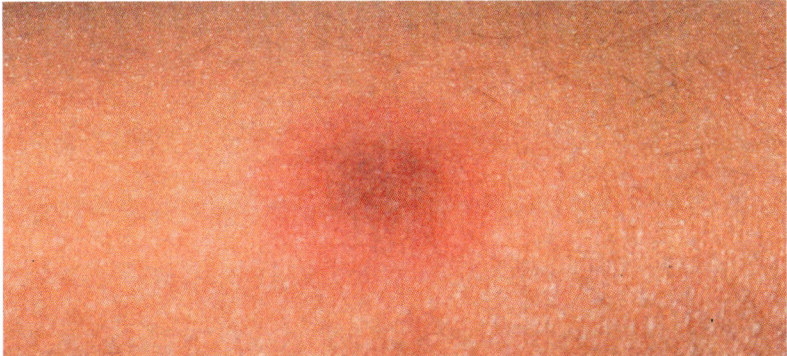

Figure 113.1. Fixed drug eruption. This single lesion occurred in response to sulfonamide ingestion.

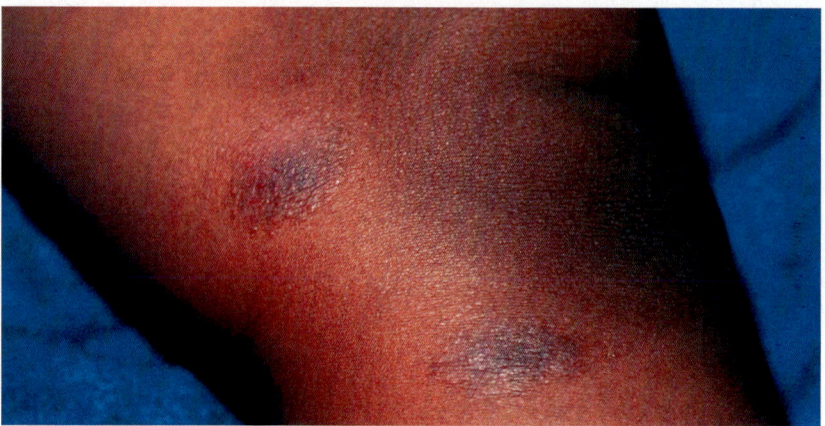

Figure 113.2 Fixed drug eruption. This child had multiple lesions, thought to be in response to acetaminophen or pseudoephedrine.

Signs and Symptoms

- Sharply demarcated, red to violaceous plaques.
- Occasionally, a central blister or erosion is present.
- Acute inflammation resolves over several days, leaving hyperpigmentation, which may persist for months to years.
- Sites of predilection include lips, face, extremities (especially hands), and genitalia.
- On repeat administration of the drug (or food), lesions recur in same location or locations (hence, the name).

Look-alikes

Disorder	Differentiating Features
Arthropod bite	• Usually pruritic. • Resolves without recurrence in same location. • History of preceding drug ingestion lacking.
Erythema multiforme	• Multiple lesions typical (less common with fixed drug eruption). • Symmetric palm and sole lesions common. • True "targetoid" lesions present. • May not always be able to distinguish.
Urticaria	• Rapid resolution of lesions over hours. • Persistent hyperpigmentation rare; when present, may suggest urticarial vasculitis. • Mixture of annular, solid, and arcuate patterns.
Herpes simplex virus infection	• May be considered in the differential diagnosis of genital fixed drug eruption. • Painful. • Blisters, erosions, or crusting consistently present. • History of sexual activity or concerns for sexual abuse present. • History of preceding drug ingestion lacking.

How to Make the Diagnosis

▶ Fixed drug eruption should be suspected clinically based on examination findings and drug ingestion history.

▶ History of recurrence with drug ingestion is supportive.

▶ Histologic findings (if skin biopsy performed) are confirmatory.

Treatment

▶ No treatment is necessary.

▶ Acute inflammation subsides over days, pigmentation over months to years.

▶ Drug can occasionally be readministered without exacerbation, although recurrence is likely.

▶ Avoidance of offending medication is key to prevention of future episodes.

Prognosis

- Fixed drug eruptions resolve completely, although the pigmentation may take months to years to fade.
- Fixed drug eruption is not indicative of a risk for more serious reactions to the offending agent.

When to Worry or Refer

- Consider referral when the diagnosis is in question.

CHAPTER 114

Serum Sickness–Like Reaction

Introduction/Etiology/Epidemiology

- Characterized by fever, rash, and arthralgias.
- More common in children.
- Usually occurs 1 to 3 weeks after starting implicated medication, occasionally earlier.
- Distinguished from "true" serum sickness by typical absence of immune complexes, hypocomplementemia, vasculitis, and kidney disease.
- Potential causes include cefaclor (classic description), other cephalosporins, penicillin, amoxicillin, tetracyclines, sulfonamides, clarithromycin and other macrolides, ciprofloxacin, griseofulvin, itraconazole, bupropion, and β-blockers; occasional reports in association with efalizumab, rituximab, infliximab, omalizumab, transfusions, and vaccinations against influenza, rabies, hepatitis B, and tetanus.
- Occasionally, presents without history of preceding drug ingestion; has been described in association with some infections including hepatitis B and C.

Signs and Symptoms

- Eruption may be morbilliform or, more commonly, urticarial (Figure 114.1).
- Classic feature is "purple urticaria," with violaceous hue in skin lesions (Figures 114.2 and 114.3).
- Periarticular swelling (especially knees and metacarpophalangeal joints) and pain with ambulation are common.
- Toddlers often refuse to bear weight on legs.
- Fever is often present, and lymphadenopathy is common.
- Other findings may include facial swelling, headache, and myalgias.

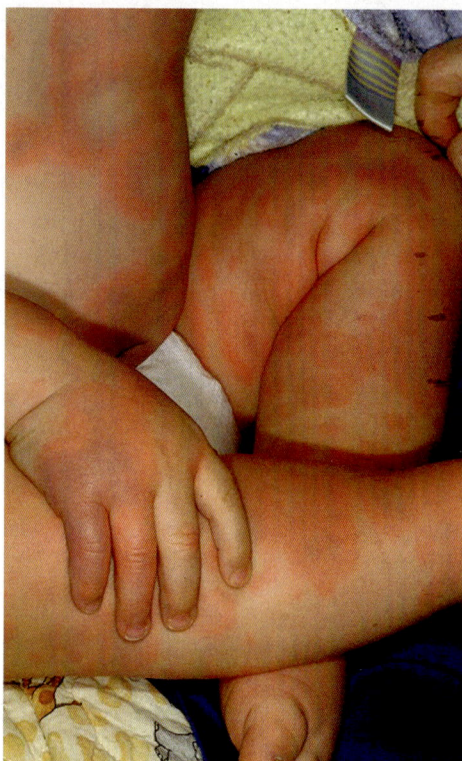

Figure 114.1. Serum sickness–like reaction. Urticarial papules and plaques with a purple hue ("purple urticaria") are seen in this 16-month-old, who also had marked periarticular swelling.

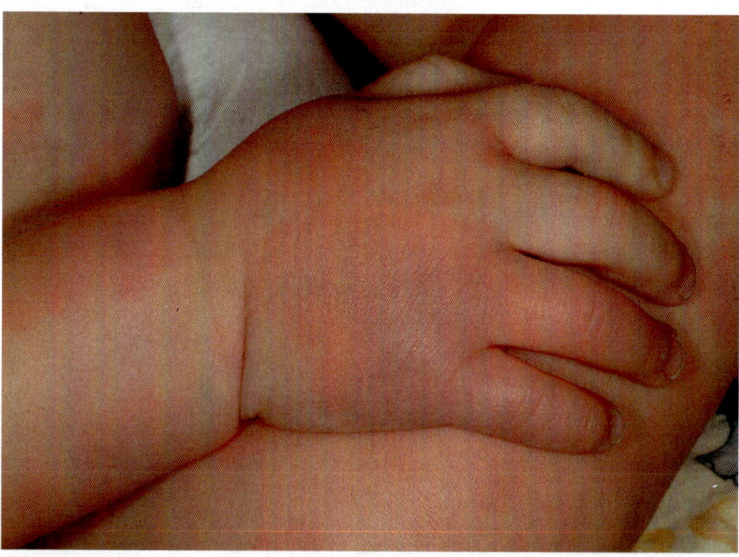

Figure 114.2. Serum sickness–like reaction. Hand swelling and urticarial plaques with a purple hue are seen in the same patient as in Figure 114.1.

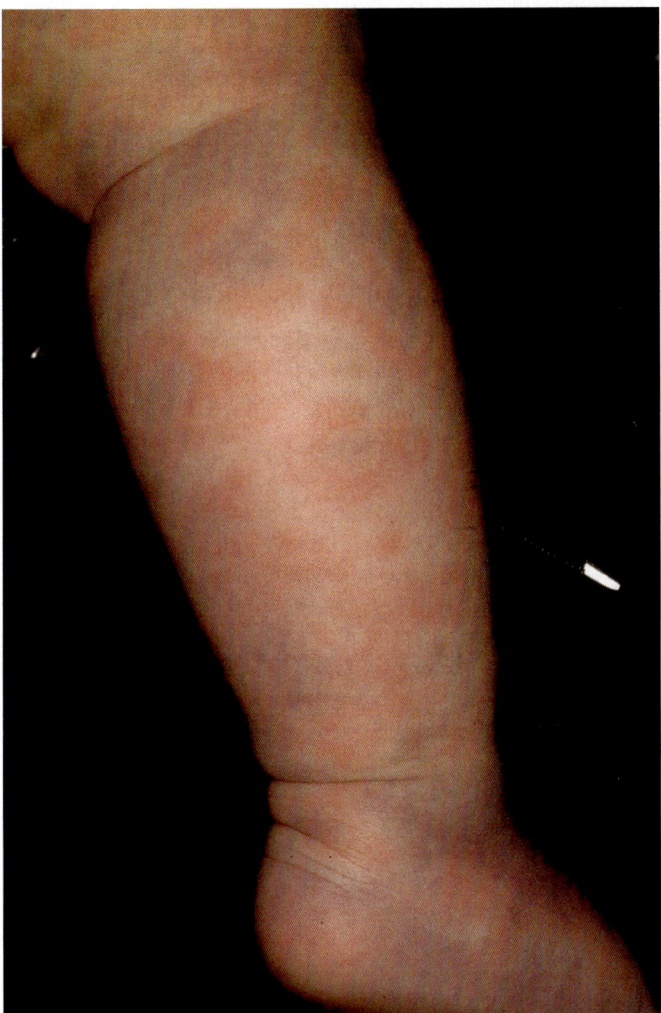

Figure 114.3. Serum sickness–like reaction. Purple urticaria is present on the lower extremity of this 15-month-old, who had been receiving amoxicillin-clavulanate therapy for otitis media.

Look-alikes

Disorder	Differentiating Features
Urticaria	• More transient, with individual lesions resolving within 24 hours. • Usually lacks violaceous appearance. • Pruritus more common. • Fever less common.
Urticaria multiforme	• Similar annular polycyclic plaques with purple discoloration, but individual lesions resolve within 24 hours. • Fever less common, of lower severity. • Pruritus more common.
Erythema multiforme	• Classic target lesions, with 3 zones of color: central duskiness (often with a vesicle or crust), surrounded by a pale ring and a peripheral red or purple ring. • Palm and sole involvement common. • Fever often absent. • Oral (occasionally other mucosal) blisters, erosions may be present. • Lack of preceding drug ingestion history. • May be recurrent, often in association with herpes simplex virus infection.
Kawasaki disease	• Conjunctival injection, oral mucosal hyperemia, lip fissuring usually present. • May have accentuation of rash with desquamation in perineum. • Cervical lymphadenopathy common. • Lack of preceding drug ingestion history.

How to Make the Diagnosis

- The diagnosis of serum sickness–like eruption should be considered in the febrile child presenting with purple urticaria and periarticular swelling after medication (especially antibiotic) ingestion.

Treatment

- The offending medication should be discontinued.
- Oral antihistamines and antipyretics may provide symptom relief.
- Nonsteroidal anti-inflammatory agents will offer relief of joint pain and may accelerate the resolution of swelling.
- In patients with severe symptoms, systemic corticosteroids may be helpful and should be tapered over 3 to 4 weeks to prevent a rebound in symptoms.
- Cross-reaction of the specific cephalosporin or penicillin with other β-lactams is unusual; avoidance of all β-lactam antibiotics is probably unnecessary but is recommended by some experts.

Prognosis

- Most patients with serum sickness–like eruption recover fully over several weeks, with no long-term sequelae.

When to Worry or Refer

- Consider dermatology referral when the diagnosis is in question or when symptoms are severe and therapy is being considered.

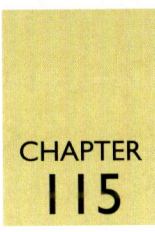

CHAPTER 115

Stevens-Johnson Syndrome (SJS), *Mycoplasma pneumoniae*–Induced Rash and Mucositis (MIRM), and Reactive Infectious Mucocutaneous Eruption (RIME)

Introduction/Etiology/Epidemiology

- Stevens-Johnson syndrome (SJS) (previously called *erythema multiforme* [EM] *major*) is a more serious condition that may not be related to EM. Many believe that SJS and toxic epidermal necrolysis (TEN) are variants of the same disease, differing in the extent of body surface involvement.
    - SJS is a delayed hypersensitivity-type systemic illness of acute onset, often triggered by infection (eg, with *Mycoplasma pneumoniae,* Epstein-Barr virus, cytomegalovirus, influenza B) or medications (eg, sulfonamides, antiepileptic drugs, acetaminophen, nonsteroidal anti-inflammatory drugs).
    - In the past, *M pneumoniae* was considered the leading infectious cause of SJS (and was termed "*Mycoplasma*-induced SJS"). Over time it became apparent that some patients have a distinctive clinical presentation with prominent mucosal involvement, a sparse bullous or targetoid skin eruption, and a milder disease course. This disease, which has been named "*M pneumoniae*–induced rash and mucositis (MIRM)," is believed to be an immune complex–mediated condition.
    - More recently it has been observed that many other infections can trigger the mucositis and rash that is seen in MIRM, so the umbrella term *reactive infectious mucocutaneous eruption* (RIME) is now favored. Although SJS and RIME/MIRM are considered distinct entities, they are discussed together because of their similar clinical presentations.
    - There are multiple known infectious triggers for RIME (aside from *M pneumoniae*), including *Chlamydophila* (formerly *Chlamydia*) *pneumoniae,* adenovirus, influenza A/B, enterovirus, rhinovirus, parainfluenza, human metapneumovirus, and SARS-CoV-2.

- Early in the course of the disease, SJS or RIME/MIRM may have a presentation similar to that of EM (eg, erythematous or targetoid lesions on extremities).
- The incidence of SJS is about 1 in 500,000 per year and can be seen in all ages, but RIME/MIRM is seen primarily in children and young adolescents.
- Recurrence of SJS may occur in up to 18% of patients and may be delayed for up to 7 years.
- RIME/MIRM can also recur and not necessarily in association with the same infectious trigger.

Signs and Symptoms

- Often begins with prodromal symptoms of fever, headache, cough, sore throat, arthralgias, or malaise that precede the onset of the rash by up to 14 days.
- Patients develop target lesions or areas of erythema that form blisters that rupture, leaving erosions (Figures 115.1 and 115.2). The skin may appear dull and dusky before the blistering phase begins. Skin lesions are less prominent in RIME/MIRM, and true target lesions are typically absent.
- Extensive mucosal surface erosions (involving ≥2 sites) are common; these may involve the eye (eyelids, conjunctiva, cornea), mouth/lips (Figure 115.3), nares, esophagus, anus, urethra, genitalia, or respiratory tract.

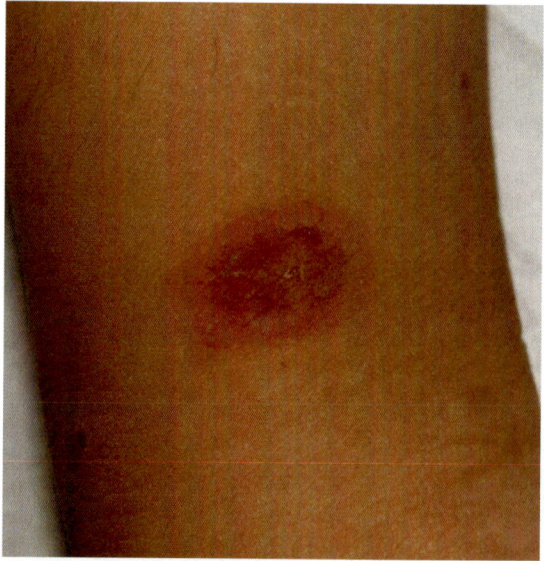

Figure 115.1. Target lesion in a patient who has Stevens-Johnson syndrome.

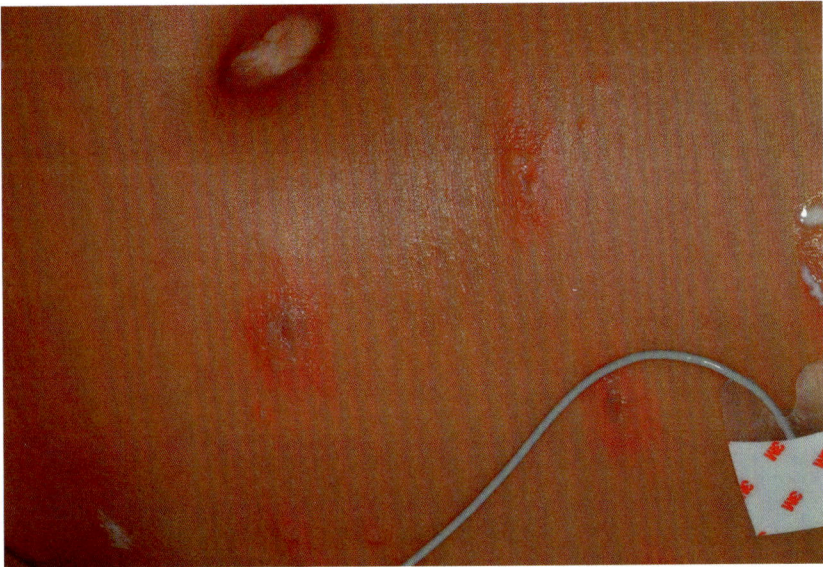

Figure 115.2. Erythematous erosions in a patient who has Stevens-Johnson syndrome.

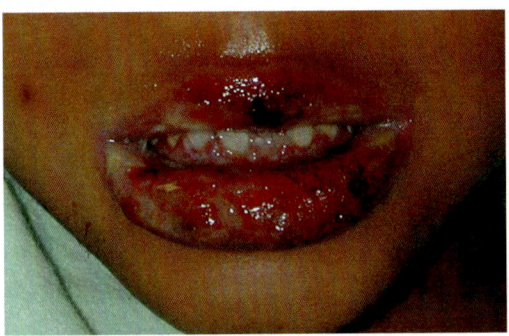

Figure 115.3. Extensive ulceration of the lips and oral mucosa are observed in Stevens-Johnson syndrome.

- While the mucosal and skin lesions of SJS and RIME/MIRM may be indistinguishable, RIME/MIRM tends to produce prominent mucous membrane involvement (Figure 115.4) and sparse cutaneous involvement that favors acral sites (Figure 115.5). Occasionally, patients with RIME/MIRM present with purely mucositis (without cutaneous involvement).
- Potential complications include interstitial pneumonitis, nephritis, and blindness. The severity of ocular sequelae is related to the severity of eye involvement early in the disease course.
- Dehydration from poor oral intake may be seen in patients with moderate to severe oral mucosal involvement.

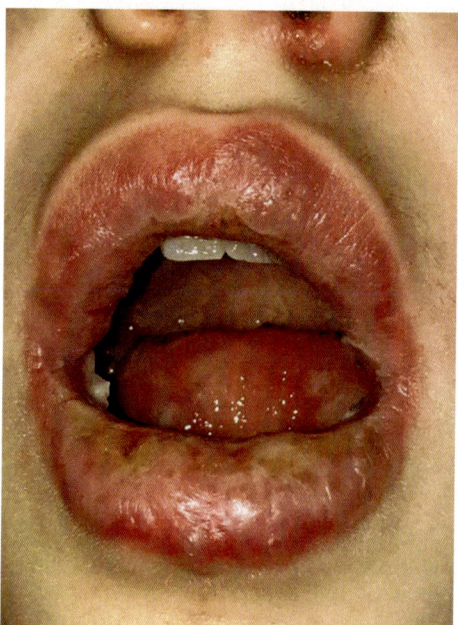

Figure 115.4. Prominent erosions of nasal and oral mucosa in a patient with *Mycoplasma pneumoniae*–induced rash and mucositis.

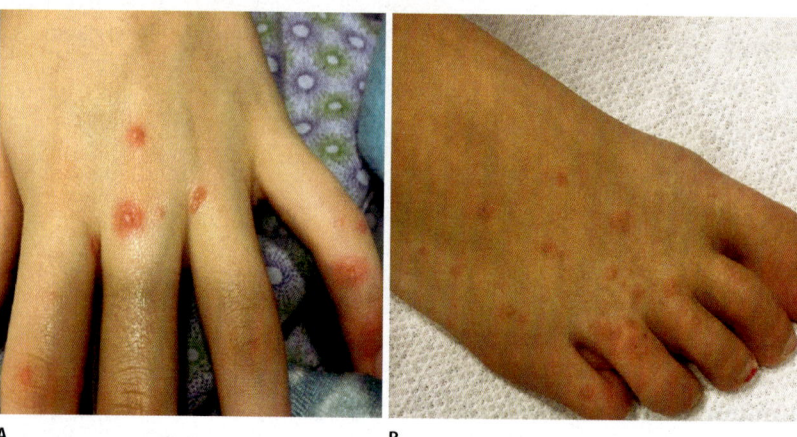

Figure 115.5. Small erythematous papules of the dorsal hand (A) and dorsal foot (B) of a patient with *Mycoplasma pneumoniae*–induced rash and mucositis.

Look-alikes

Disorder	Differentiating Features
Urticaria	• Erythematous blanching wheals that resolve or change in 24 hours or sooner. • Occasionally, lesions may become centrally dusky, but no vesicle or crust formation. • Although lesions may become annular, true target lesions do not occur. • Mucosal erosions do not occur.
Kawasaki disease	• Eruption typically morbilliform, without vesicles, bullae, or crusting. • Patients have non-purulent conjunctival injection, not purulent conjunctivitis as observed in SJS or RIME/MIRM. • Patients may have erythema and cracking of lips but not mucosal ulcers.
Serum sickness–like eruption	• Large, often purple, urticarial-appearing plaques present ("purple urticaria"). • Target lesions, blistering, mucosal erosions absent. • Fever, arthralgia, or arthritis are common features. • Periarticular swelling often present. • Ambulatory children may refuse to walk during episode.
Staphylococcal scalded skin syndrome	• Radial ("sunburst") erosions and crusting around mouth. • Sunburn-like erythema concentrated in skinfolds. • Superficial erosions develop but intact blisters uncommon (in contrast with SJS); Nikolsky sign present. • Oral erosions and ulcers absent. • Target lesions absent.
Toxic epidermal necrolysis (TEN)	• Target lesions may be present but also dusky erythematous patches that rapidly form bullae and erosions. • Widespread detachment of the epidermis usually present. • More extensive skin involvement in TEN (>30% of body surface area [BSA]); in SJS, less than 10% of BSA is involved, while in SJS-TEN overlap, 10% to 30% BSA is involved. • More often drug-related.

How to Make the Diagnosis

▶ Presence of prodromal symptoms.

▶ Target lesions, blisters, or erosions.

▶ Involvement of 2 or more mucosal surfaces.

▶ Infectious workup may include chest radiography, *M pneumoniae* titers, polymerase chain reaction panel for respiratory viruses, and additional testing based on clinical features or suspicion.

▶ Patients with SJS are systemically ill and may acutely decompensate.

Treatment

- Treatment is largely supportive.
- Identify and rapidly remove or treat the suspected precipitant (ie, medication); if infection with *M pneumoniae* or *C pneumoniae* is demonstrated or strongly suspected clinically, treat with an appropriate macrolide antibiotic.
- The role of systemic steroids for SJS and RIME/MIRM remains controversial, but occasionally used in more severe or recalcitrant cases.
- Patients who have SJS or RIME/MIRM may benefit from
  - Hospitalization (in a burn or other intensive care unit if there are extensive erosions) with careful attention to fluids, nutrition, and eye care (including consultation with ophthalmologist) and consideration for secondary bacterial infection.
  - Intravenous immunoglobulin administration.
  - Other treatments (ie, immunosuppressant or biologic agents such as cyclosporine, etanercept) occasionally used, but there is no consensus on their indications.
- Avoid repeat exposure to offending medications, when identified.

Prognosis

- SJS and RIME/MIRM usually last 1 to 2 weeks, but complicated cases may resolve more slowly. Severe ocular sequelae may result.
- Most pediatric patients with SJS or RIME/MIRM heal fully without permanent sequelae.
- The Score of TEN (SCORTEN) severity-of-illness scale has been used to predict mortality of SJS and TEN in adults and has also been shown to be useful in predicting morbidity in children when calculated within the first day of hospital admission.

When to Worry or Refer

- Ocular involvement in SJS or RIME/MIRM should prompt ophthalmologic consultation because patients may require amniotic membrane grafts.
- Widespread cutaneous blistering may require hospitalization in a burn or other intensive care setting.

Resources for Families

- Mayo Clinic: Stevens-Johnson syndrome.
  https://www.mayoclinic.org/diseases-conditions/stevens-johnson-syndrome/symptoms-causes/syc-20355936
- Stevens-Johnson Syndrome Foundation: Provides information, phone support, and referrals.
  www.sjsupport.org

CHAPTER 116

Toxic Epidermal Necrolysis (TEN)

Introduction/Etiology/Epidemiology

- Toxic epidermal necrolysis (TEN) is a severe, potentially life-threatening multisystem illness characterized by generalized tender erythema, widespread bulla formation, and loss of the epidermis.
- Most cases of TEN are caused by drugs. The most common offending agents are antibiotics, antiepileptics, sulfonamides, and nonsteroidal anti-inflammatory agents.
- The incidence is estimated to be 0.5 to 1.2 cases per million per year.

Signs and Symptoms

- Conjunctival injection, ocular foreign body sensation and itching, fever, skin tenderness, and constitutional symptoms (eg, malaise, myalgias, arthralgias, nausea, vomiting, diarrhea) often precede the eruption by several days.
- The onset is abrupt with generalized tender erythema, progressing rapidly to dusky gray with sloughing and development of large bullae (Figure 116.1).
- Sloughing skin removes the entire epidermis, including the pigmented layer, so the base is devoid of pigment (Figure 116.2).
- Glistening red and white patches resemble the base of a second-degree burn.
- Nikolsky sign is present (ie, gentle lateral pressure on an area of dusky erythema or the edge of a bulla leads to separation of the skin).
- Mucosal surfaces are tender, eroded, and crusted.
    - Oral mucosa is painful and ulcerated.
    - Conjunctivae erode and ulcerate.
    - Urethral involvement is common, occasionally leading to dysuria, urethral stricture.
    - Respiratory mucosa may be involved.

- Other organ systems involved include the following:
  - Renal (acute interstitial nephritis).
  - Gastrointestinal (mucosal sloughing and bleeding).
  - Pulmonary (tracheal and bronchial mucosal erosion, pneumonitis).

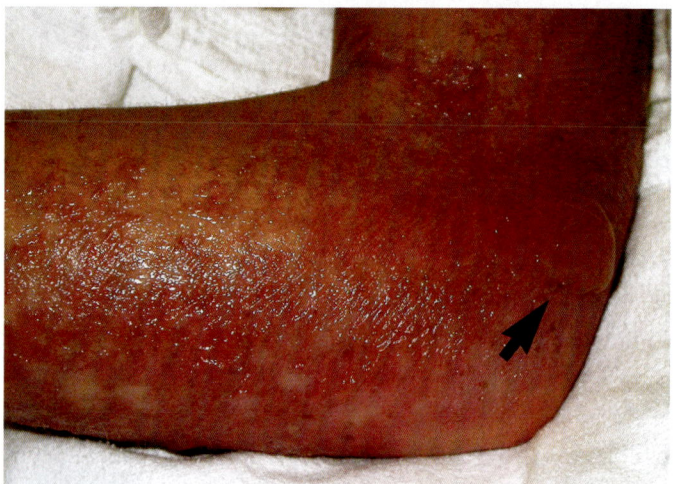

Figure 116.1. In toxic epidermal necrolysis, flaccid bullae (arrow) appear and rapidly rupture.

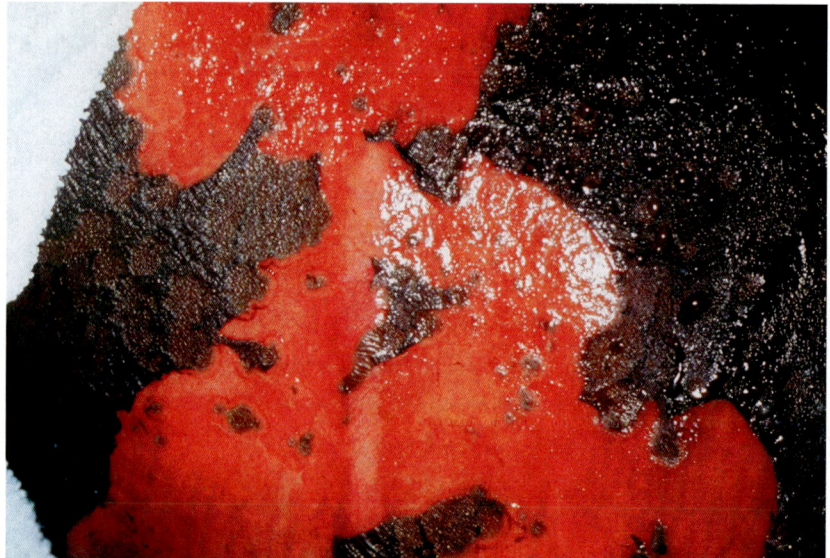

Figure 116.2. Toxic epidermal necrolysis is characterized by shedding of large areas of necrotic epidermis.

Look-alikes

Disorder	Differentiating Features
Stevens-Johnson syndrome (SJS)	• May have blister formation, but less severe than in toxic epidermal necrolysis (TEN; <10% of body surface area [BSA] is involved, whereas in TEN, >30% of BSA is affected); 10% to 30% BSA is considered SJS–TEN overlap. • More often related to infection than drugs in children.
Reactive infectious mucocutaneous eruption (RIME) and *Mycoplasma pneumoniae*–induced rash and mucositis (MIRM)	• Prominent erosions of 2 or more mucous membranes with more sparse skin lesions (erythematous papules, vesicles, bullae, and rarely target lesions). • Milder disease course typically seen compared with that of SJS or TEN. • Typical triggers include *M pneumoniae, Chlamydophila pneumoniae,* influenza A or B, adenovirus, enterovirus, rhinovirus, human metapneumovirus, parainfluenza, SARS-CoV-2.
Staphylococcal scalded skin syndrome	• Often begins with rhinorrhea and periorificial crusting. • Blisters form and rupture, leading to superficial exfoliation, but the pigmented epithelium is retained below the blister. • Constitutional symptoms milder and disease less severe. • Oral and conjunctival mucosae spared.
Kawasaki disease	• Eruption typically morbilliform, without presence of vesicles, bullae, or crusting. • Patients have non-purulent conjunctival injection but not the purulent conjunctivitis or erosions as seen in TEN. • Patients may have erythema and cracking of lips but not mucosal erosions. • Rash accentuated in flexural locations (especially the groin).
Toxic shock syndrome	• Patients exhibit diffuse erythema and may have superficial desquamation, but bullae and erosions absent. • Rash accentuated in flexural locations. • Nikolsky sign absent. • Hypotension required for definitive diagnosis.
Acute generalized exanthematous pustulosis	• Large areas of erythema with numerous superimposed small pustules. • Bullae and erosions absent.

How to Make the Diagnosis

- The diagnosis is suspected clinically based on the following:
  - Acute onset of a severe illness with rapid progression of generalized erythema to blistering and loss of the epidermis associated with mucosal and systemic features.
  - Presence of Nikolsky sign.
  - Loss of the pigmented epithelium with the blister roof.
- Skin biopsy or frozen section, as needed.

Treatment

- Admission to an intensive care or burn unit is imperative.
- Supportive care includes maintenance of fluid and electrolyte status, infection control, emollients over the denuded areas, and parenteral nutrition.
- Topical antibacterial ointments or creams are often useful, but beware the use of topical sulfa-based agents in patients whose TEN was triggered by sulfonamides.
- Remove the offending drug.
- Intravenous immunoglobulin should be considered; shown in some studies to be beneficial.
- Other treatments (eg, immunosuppressant or biologic agents) occasionally used, but there is no consensus on their indications.
- Systemic steroids are generally contraindicated owing to increased mortality risk in this patient population.

Treating Associated Conditions

- Monitor for and address renal, gastrointestinal, and pulmonary complications.
- Ophthalmologic consultation is indicated; aggressive lubrication is always recommended, and amniotic membrane transplant to the ocular surface is occasionally considered for aggressive ocular disease.
- Severe urethral involvement may cause urinary retention, requiring indwelling catheter placement.

Prognosis

- Mortality in drug-induced TEN is approximately 20%.
- Mortality in idiopathic TEN approaches 50%.
- Neutropenia, severe hypoproteinemia, and extensive surface area involvement are poor prognostic factors.
- Long-term complications affect the eyes (eg, keratoconjunctivitis sicca [dry eye syndrome], aberrant lashes, impaired tear production, corneal scarring, blindness), skin (eg, dyspigmentation), and nails (eg, deformities).

When to Worry or Refer

- All patients with TEN should be referred to an experienced burn center or intensive care unit.

Resource for Families

- WebMD: Information for families is contained in Skin Problems and Treatments.
  https://www.webmd.com/skin-problems-and-treatments/life-threatening-skin-rashes

CHAPTER 117

Urticaria

Introduction/Etiology/Epidemiology

- Acute urticaria (lasting <6 weeks) is a common condition of childhood; chronic urticaria (lasting ≥6 weeks) is uncommon.
- Erythema results from vasodilation, and wheals are produced by fluid leaking from blood vessels into the surrounding dermis.
- Histamine is the primary mediator in response to a variety of antigens (eg, infectious agents, drugs, foods, insect venom).
- Physical urticaria may be triggered by heat, cold, pressure, vibration, sunlight, water, or exercise.

Signs and Symptoms

- Lesions appear abruptly as pruritic, pink to red raised wheals of variable size and shape (eg, arcs, rings, plaques) in patients with lighter skin (Figures 117.1 and 117.2). In patients with darker skin tones, erythema may be subtle or inapparent.
- Lesions are transient, usually resolving in 0.5 to 3 hours, reappearing in other locations.
- Lesions may become large and annular (ie, central clearing occurs); referred to by some as *urticaria multiforme.*
- By definition, a lesion of urticaria must change or resolve within 24 hours of its appearance.

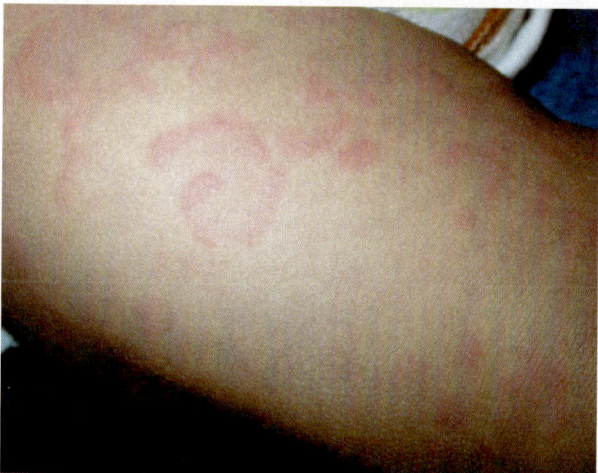

Figure 117.1. Urticaria. Erythematous wheals with multiple shapes, including papules and incomplete rings.

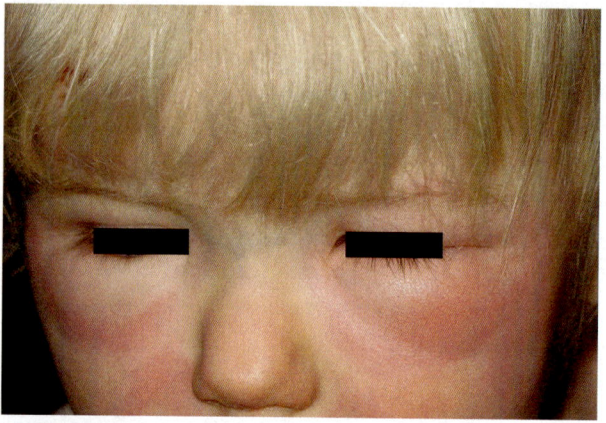

Figure 117.2. This child who has urticaria also exhibits angioedema, an indistinct swelling around the eyes.

Look-alikes

Disorder	Differentiating Features
Erythema multiforme (EM)	• Lesions of urticaria resolve or change shape in a few hours, whereas those of EM remain fixed in location for the duration of the illness (ie, 7–14 days). • Lesions of EM centrally dark and dusky and often develop a central blister or crust. • True target lesions present, consisting of central dusky area or vesicle or crust, a zone of pallor, and a peripheral zone of erythema. • Unlike the lesions of urticaria, those of EM often located on extremities (palmoplantar involvement very common) and face with relative sparing of trunk.
Urticaria multiforme	• Considered to be a variant of urticaria. • Annular, polycyclic, and occasionally dusky urticarial papules and plaques occur; may be mistaken for EM. • Lesions last less than 24 hours, but temporary duskiness may remain.
Henoch-Schönlein purpura	• Vasculitis, so lesions will remain fixed and become purpuric over time. • Generally confined to lower body and legs. • Abdominal pain, arthralgias, arthritis, or hematuria may accompany the cutaneous findings of Henoch-Schönlein purpura.
Serum sickness–like eruption	• Giant, often purple, urticarial plaques common ("purple urticaria"). • Fever, arthralgias, and arthritis common features. • Periarticular swelling often present. • Children who are ambulatory may refuse to walk during episode.
Papular urticaria	• Random pattern of urticarial-appearing papules, often with central puncta, that remain fixed in location for weeks and tend to recur in similar distribution pattern. • Vesiculation or trauma due to scratching common. • Often triggered by insect bite reactions.
Urticarial vasculitis	• Often associated with burning or pain. • Individual lesions last longer than 24 hours or may have a purpuric or hyperpigmented appearance. • May be associated with autoimmune disease, hepatitis, hypocomplementemia, or arthritis.

How to Make the Diagnosis

- The main discriminating features are erythematous wheals that resolve or change shape within 24 hours.
- Abrupt onset after exposure to specific triggers of histamine release.
- Identification of the trigger agent is usually difficult. Examples include infectious agents (eg, *Streptococcus pyogenes,* Epstein-Barr virus, adenovirus, parasites), drugs (eg, penicillin, opiates, nonsteroidal anti-inflammatory agents, insulin, blood products), foods (eg, peanuts, tree nuts, milk, eggs, shellfish), systemic diseases (eg, collagen vascular disease, inflammatory bowel disease, thyroiditis), and insect stings.
- If uncertainty about the diagnosis of urticaria exists, administration of subcutaneous epinephrine will cause lesions to resolve.

Treatment

- Oral antihistamines are effective in management of urticaria symptoms. First-generation agents, such as diphenhydramine hydrochloride (up to 5 mg/kg/d in 4 divided doses) or hydroxyzine hydrochloride (up to 2 mg/kg/d in 3–4 divided doses), are most commonly used.
- If sedation occurs or first-generation agents are ineffective, a second-generation (eg, cetirizine, loratadine) or third-generation (eg, desloratadine, fexofenadine, levocetirizine) antihistamine may be prescribed, reserving the first-generation agent for bedtime.
- Although controversial, the addition of an H_2 receptor antagonist (eg, cimetidine, ranitidine) may be effective when H_1 agents alone are ineffective.
- Systemic corticosteroids are second-line therapy for severe disease; steroids generally are not advisable given the risk of rebound flare on discontinuation and side effect profile when used for prolonged periods.
- Treatment should be maintained for 5 to 7 days after urticaria has resolved to prevent relapse; longer duration of antihistamine therapy may be necessary in chronic urticaria.
- If the offending trigger can be identified, avoidance or treatment is recommended.
- Omalizumab is a biologic therapy approved by the US Food and Drug Administration for patients aged 12 years or older with chronic spontaneous urticaria that does not respond to H_1 antihistamine treatment.

Treating Associated Conditions

- Subcutaneous extension of lesions (ie, angioedema) may occur.
  - Patients exhibit indistinct swelling of the eyelids, lips, extremities, or genitalia. Occasionally, there is involvement of the oral cavity or airway.
  - Management of uncomplicated angioedema associated with urticaria is as described in the preceding sections. Intramuscular epinephrine should be considered if there is evidence of respiratory compromise.
- Anaphylaxis.
  - Anaphylaxis is a medical emergency that occurs when massive histamine release causes airway edema, laryngospasm, profound hypotension, and cardiovascular collapse.
  - Airway compromise is responsible for most deaths.
  - Epinephrine must be administered emergently, along with antihistamines and, often, a corticosteroid.
- Heredity angioedema (caused by C1 esterase inhibitor deficiency) presents with swelling of the face, throat, or extremities or abdominal pain (without associated urticaria). Diagnosis is confirmed by measuring the C1 esterase inhibitor level.

Prognosis

- Acute urticaria often resolves within 1 to 2 weeks.
- Chronic urticaria may last for months to years, but it resolves spontaneously within 5 years in 30% to 55% of patients.

When to Worry or Refer

- Recurrent episodes of urticaria, chronic urticaria, or a single episode of anaphylaxis merit referral for allergy evaluation.

Resources for Families

- American Academy of Dermatology: Hives: diagnosis and treatment.
  https://www.aad.org/public/diseases/a-z/hives-treatment
- American Academy of Pediatrics: HealthyChildren.org.
  https://www.healthychildren.org/hives
- MedlinePlus: Information for patients and families (in English and Spanish) sponsored by the US National Library of Medicine and National Institutes of Health.
  https://www.nlm.nih.gov/medlineplus/ency/article/000845.htm
- Society for Pediatric Dermatology: Patient information on hives (urticaria).
  https://pedsderm.net/for-patients-families/patient-handouts/#Hives

Cutaneous Manifestations of Rheumatologic Diseases

CHAPTER 118 — **Juvenile Dermatomyositis (JDM)**............751

CHAPTER 119 — **Morphea (Localized Scleroderma)**............761

CHAPTER 120 — **Systemic Lupus Erythematosus (SLE)**..........777

CHAPTER 118

Juvenile Dermatomyositis (JDM)

Introduction/Etiology/Epidemiology

- Rare inflammatory vasculopathy primarily involving the skin and muscle with potential for multisystem compromise.
- A small subset of patients has no evidence of muscle disease; termed *dermatomyositis sine myositis* (or *amyopathic dermatomyositis*).
- Bimodal age peaks: childhood (5–10 years) and adulthood (45–55 years).
- Incidence of approximately 2 to 4 cases per 1 million children per year.
- Increased ratio of female to male patients in children and adults.
- Overlap with scleroderma, juvenile dermatomyositis (JDM) or other connective tissue disease may occur in a minority of patients.
- Although dermatomyositis in adult patients may be a marker for occult malignancy, this association is not seen in children.
- Etiology and pathogenesis of JDM are poorly understood; believed to be autoimmune in nature, and patients may have familial, genetic predisposition.

Signs and Symptoms

Cutaneous

- JDM has pathognomonic skin changes that may vary greatly in severity; characteristic inflammatory and telangiectatic skin findings are seen in the vast majority of children who are affected.
- Pink to violet discoloration of eyelids (heliotrope) and cheeks in malar distribution with or without associated edema of affected skin (Figures 118.1 and 118.2).
- Erythema may be present on the extensor aspects of the extremities (especially over elbows and knees), neck, over shoulders, and hairline.

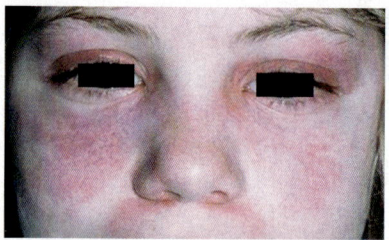

Figure 118.1. Heliotrope rash and telangiectatic erythema of the cheeks in a school-aged child with juvenile dermatomyositis.

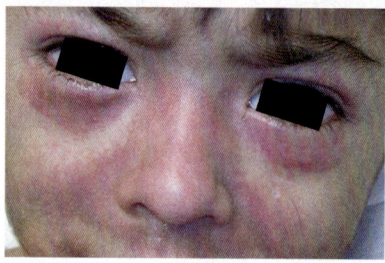

Figure 118.2. More pronounced erythematous to violaceous patches in juvenile dermatomyositis on the face of a child with a darker skin tone than the patient shown in Figure 118.1.

- A malar facial rash, similar to that seen in systemic lupus erythematosus, may occur.
- Photosensitivity is common, with relative sparing of sun-protected sites.
- Gottron sign or papules: pink to red telangiectatic macules (Gottron sign) or flat-topped lichenoid papules (Gottron papules), most often located over the proximal interphalangeal and metacarpophalangeal joints; less often involve the distal interphalangeal joints (Figures 118.3, 118.4, 118.5, and 118.6). These lesions may appear hypopigmented in darker skin tones.
  - May be scaly.
  - Occasionally appear symmetrically over the extensor aspects of the extremities (elbows, knees) and may resemble lesions of psoriasis (Figure 118.7).
- Dilated capillaries (telangiectasias) of the proximal nail folds (may need magnification with ophthalmoscopy or dermatoscopy to visualize) (Figure 118.8). May also see areas of capillary dropout within these areas of capillary dilatation. These periungual changes appear to correlate with skin disease activity.

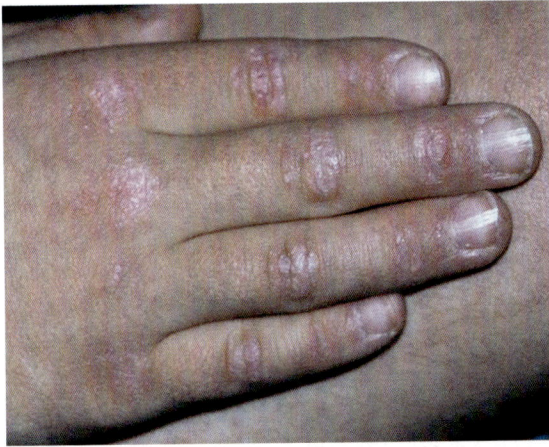

Figure 118.3. Typical Gottron papules (erythematous to violaceous flat-topped papules) overlying the knuckles in this 3-year-old with juvenile dermatomyositis. Note also the presence of dilated nail fold capillaries (see Figure 118.8).

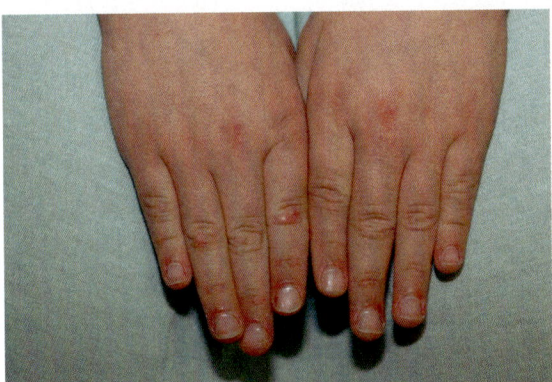

Figure 118.4. Gottron papules overlying knuckles in a child with juvenile dermatomyositis.

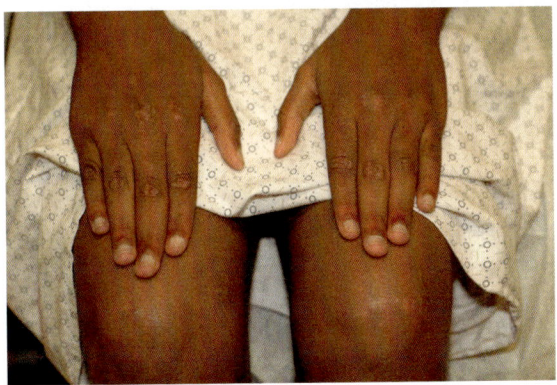

Figure 118.5. Juvenile dermatomyositis. Gottron papules on bilateral hands and knees.

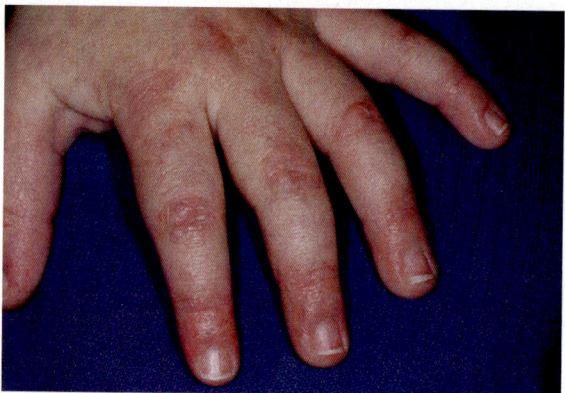

Figure 118.6. Numerous Gottron papules in a 2-year-old who has juvenile dermatomyositis.

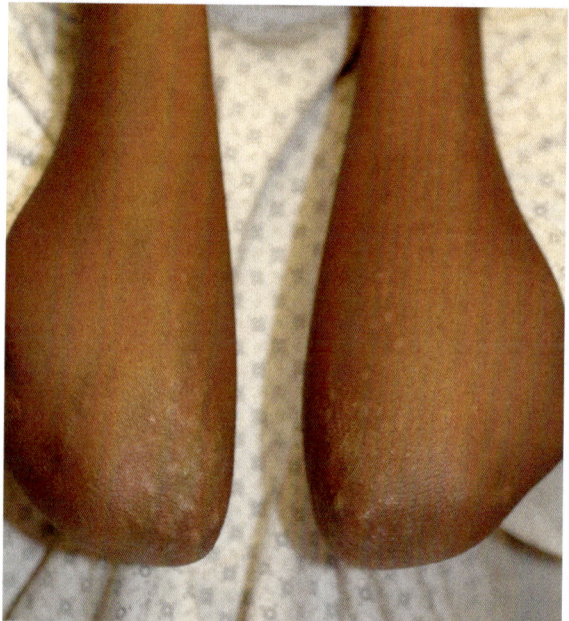

Figure 118.7. Erythematous xerotic papules on the elbows in a patient with juvenile dermatomyositis.

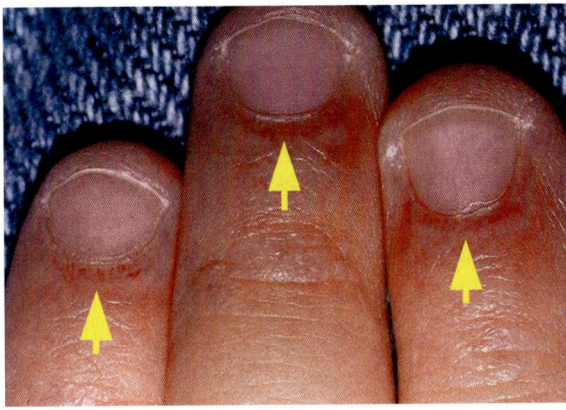

Figure 118.8. Dilated capillaries of the nail folds (arrows) in a child with juvenile dermatomyositis.

- Calcinosis cutis occurs in 30% to 50% of children who are affected. Variably sized calcium deposits can present as firm skin-colored to white or yellow papules or nodules, usually located over the joints of the elbows or knees and the buttocks, but may occur anywhere (Figure 118.9).
  - More common in pediatric than in adult patients.
  - Usually a later finding; rarely seen at time of initial presentation.
  - Occasionally become secondarily infected.
  - Can become disabling if extensive.
  - Severity of calcinosis seems to correlate with severity of inflammation and overall disease severity.
  - Seen less frequently with aggressive and early therapy.

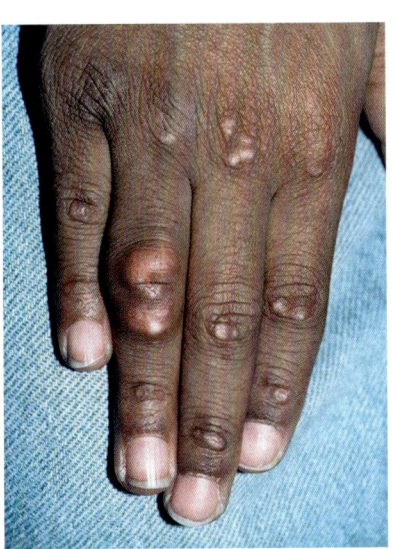

Figure 118.9. Calcinosis cutis of the fourth finger as well as Gottron papules on the knuckles in this patient with a long history of juvenile dermatomyositis.

- Widespread edema of the skin may be seen in more severe cases.
- Poikilodermatous changes (ie, atrophy, telangiectasias, and hypopigmentation and hyperpigmentation within same region of skin) may be seen in chronic disease; often, there is a distinct violaceous discoloration of the skin.
- Localized or widespread ulcerations may occur; extensive ulcerations believed to be associated with poor prognosis.
- Inflammation of the scalp with associated scarring or non-scarring alopecia seen occasionally in children with JDM; more often seen in adults.
- Lipodystrophy may occasionally be seen in association with panniculitis (inflammation of subcutaneous fat); may be generalized or partial.
- Acanthosis nigricans (velvety hyperpigmentation of the neck, axillae) is occasionally seen in patients with JDM, especially those with lipodystrophy.

Systemic

- Symmetric proximal muscle weakness may precede, accompany, or follow skin changes.
  - Usually involves the anterior neck flexors, the hip and shoulder girdles, and core musculature.
  - May present with difficulty climbing stairs, raising arms to brush hair, or rising from lying to sitting and sitting to standing positions (also known as Gower sign).
  - May or may not have associated muscle pain or tenderness to palpation.
- May involve other striated muscle and result in symptoms of dysphagia, dysphonia, choking, or nasal speech.
- In severe disease, can progress to involve respiratory muscles and lead to restrictive or interstitial lung disease.
- Vasculopathy can occasionally lead to myocarditis, pericarditis, mucosal ulcerations of the gastrointestinal tract, or microscopic hematuria.
- Fatigue and loss of energy are reported in most patients at presentation.
- A nondestructive arthritis may occur in up to one-half of children who are affected.
- Kidney involvement is more common in adults, and presence should prompt evaluation for lupus.

Look-alikes

Disorder	Differentiating Features
Psoriasis	• Psoriatic lesions of knees and elbows may resemble those of juvenile dermatomyositis (JDM) but usually contain thicker, micaceous (silvery white) scale. • May have associated nail changes (eg, pitting, onycholysis). • No dilated capillaries of nail folds. • No calcinosis cutis. • Facial involvement less common (but more common in pediatric psoriasis compared with that in adults). • Histologic findings distinctive. • Usually improves (rather than being exacerbated) with sun exposure.
Allergic contact dermatitis	• May have more marked edema of eyelids and affected skin. • More acute onset than JDM. • Severe pruritus usually present.
Systemic lupus erythematosus	• Usually less eyelid involvement. • Distinct systemic manifestations. • Photosensitivity a prominent feature, often with butterfly facial erythema (malar rash), with nasolabial sparing. • Erythema of the dorsal fingers usually spares the areas over joints. • Serological studies may help distinguish the 2 disorders.
Scleroderma or CREST syndrome (calcinosis, Raynaud phenomenon, esophageal involvement, sclerodactyly, telangiectasia)	• May have similar telangiectatic changes around the nails as in JDM. • May have symptoms of dysphagia in both conditions. • May also have calcinosis cutis in CREST syndrome. • Sclerodactyly (thickening and tightness of the fingers and toes) or generalized induration not typically seen in JDM. • Distinctive histologic changes at skin biopsy. • JDM and scleroderma can present together as an overlap syndrome in children.
Atopic dermatitis	• Often with earlier onset (infancy or toddler years). • Usually associated with more severe pruritus. • Predilection for neck and flexural aspects of extremities (extensor surfaces in infants).
Cutaneous T-cell lymphoma	• Rare in children. • Hypopigmented form most common in pediatric patients. • Poikilodermatous form seen mainly in adults. • Characteristic histologic features seen at skin biopsy.
Postinfectious myopathy/myositis	• No associated skin changes. • Usually self-limited, lasting days to weeks.
Collagen vascular disease–associated myositis or myopathy	• May or may not have associated dermatologic alterations. • Systemic lupus erythematosus–associated myositis generally does not have significant elevation of muscle enzymes. • May have other systemic alterations not typically seen in JDM.

How to Make the Diagnosis

- There is no single diagnostic test for JDM.
- The diagnosis is suggested clinically by the combined findings of pathognomonic skin changes and associated symmetric proximal muscle weakness.
- Supportive diagnostic evidence includes the following:
  - Elevated skeletal muscle enzymes.
    - Creatine phosphokinase.
    - Aldolase.
    - Aspartate aminotransferase, alanine aminotransferase, and lactate dehydrogenase; although generally characterized as liver enzymes, these may be elevated in dermatomyositis because they are released from damaged muscle tissue.
    - Elevated level of inflammatory markers (ie, erythrocyte sedimentation rate, C-reactive protein level) may be present, but does not necessarily correlate with disease activity and is nonspecific.
  - Characteristic histologic changes at skin biopsy (epidermal atrophy, interface dermatitis, mucin deposition).
  - Characteristic histologic findings from muscle biopsy (usually deltoid or quadriceps). Although this procedure has been largely replaced by magnetic resonance imaging, which reveals increased signal intensity on fat-suppressed T2-weighted images, it should be considered for patients in whom the clinical presentation is not classic or pathognomonic and may provide prognostic information; magnetic resonance imaging may be helpful in following the clinical course of muscle involvement.
  - Characteristic electromyographic findings.
  - Some myositis-specific antibodies may be present and may help in elucidating prognosis.

Treatment

- Most patients are treated by pediatric rheumatologists; pediatric dermatologists are often involved at diagnosis, when patients present with cutaneous signs and symptoms.
- Although muscle disease is usually quite responsive to therapy, cutaneous disease may be very resistant to multiple treatment modalities.
- Persistent cutaneous disease may be associated with long-term cardiovascular risk.

- Mainstays of treatment include the following:
  - Photoprotection.
    - Daily use of broad-spectrum sunscreen with sun protection factor 30 or higher.
    - Use of sun protective clothing (including wide-brimmed hats).
    - Avoidance of prolonged sun exposure.
  - Topical steroids or topical calcineurin inhibitors (eg, pimecrolimus, tacrolimus) may be helpful for any associated pruritus and erythema but rarely modify the course of cutaneous disease.
  - Systemic corticosteroids (oral or pulsed intravenous [IV]); specialists who treat JDM are increasingly using high-dose pulsed IV steroids.
  - Immunosuppressive therapy and steroid-sparing agents.
    - Methotrexate (oral or subcutaneous)
    - Hydroxychloroquine (low dose), often used for inflammatory skin disease (although effectiveness is controversial)
    - IV immunoglobulin
    - Cyclosporine
    - Mycophenolate mofetil
    - Tacrolimus
    - Pulsed cyclophosphamide
    - Rituximab
    - Tumor necrosis factor α antagonists including infliximab, adalimumab, and etanercept (although some patients appear to worsen with these therapies)
    - Abatacept (recombinant DNA–generated fusion protein)
    - Janus kinase inhibitors
  - Autologous stem cell transplant (in some severe cases).
  - Physical therapy.

Treating Associated Conditions

- Arthritis, gastrointestinal tract vasculopathy with ulceration or hemorrhage, malabsorption, and interstitial lung disease may occur and require specific evaluation as indicated.
- Calcinosis cutis is very difficult to treat; reported therapies include increasing systemic immunosuppression, bisphosphonates, sodium thiosulfate, surgery.

Prognosis

- The prognosis is variable but seems quite favorable for most children treated aggressively and early within the disease course. Many will become disease free after 2 to 4 years and remain so after therapy.
- Control of skin disease and muscle disease does not correlate well; muscle disease is usually quite responsive to corticosteroid therapy, whereas dermatologic manifestations often are recalcitrant and persistent despite good control of muscle disease.

When to Worry or Refer

- All patients with skin or muscle symptoms suggestive of JDM should be referred to a pediatric rheumatologist and dermatologist to confirm the clinical diagnosis and for ongoing treatment.
- Prompt and accurate diagnosis as well as aggressive systemic management are critical in the presence of muscle or systemic manifestations.

Resource for Families

- Cure JM Foundation: Provides information and support for patients who have JDM.
  https://www.curejm.org

CHAPTER 119

Morphea (Localized Scleroderma)

Introduction/Etiology/Epidemiology

- Also referred to as *localized scleroderma,* morphea is an uncommon autoimmune inflammatory sclerosing disorder of the skin and subcutaneous tissue.

- While the term *scleroderma* and the characteristic hardening (sclerosis) of the skin can be confused with systemic sclerosis, morphea does not progress to systemic disease. Rarely, though, morphea can coexist with systemic sclerosis. While it is variable, some clinicians prefer the term *morphea* over *localized scleroderma*.

- The occurrence is estimated to be 0.4 to 1 per 100,000 individuals, and the condition is 2 to 3 times more common in female than male patients; recent studies suggest morphea is more prevalent in white female patients.

- Mean age of onset in children is 5 to 8 years; however, morphea has been described in infants, and there are even case reports of congenital morphea.

- While most adults have disease limited to the skin and subcutaneous tissue, children have a higher risk for extra-cutaneous findings.

- Divided into several subtypes; clinical features vary depending on the subtype of morphea.

- Disease severity ranges from a solitary area of induration (hardening of skin) to severe, disfiguring and disabling disease affecting skin, subcutaneous tissue, underlying muscle and bone, and brain, ocular, and oral tissues. Involvement of the lung, heart, and gastrointestinal tract can also occur, but unlike with systemic sclerosis, this involvement is usually mild and nonprogressive.

- Occasionally observed in the setting of other connective tissue disorders, including juvenile idiopathic arthritis, systemic lupus erythematosus, systemic sclerosis, Sjögren syndrome, juvenile dermatomyositis, polymyositis, and eosinophilic fasciitis.

Signs and Symptoms

Skin Findings

- ▶ Begins insidiously as a gradual hardening of the skin and/or a change in skin color (eg, erythematous, violaceous).
- ▶ May begin with an inflammatory stage that presents with erythema or a violaceous discoloration of the skin (Figure 119.1); at times, this can resemble a port-wine stain (capillary malformation).
- ▶ With time, the redness fades and the affected area of skin becomes indurated and often ivory-colored and shiny in appearance (Figure 119.2).
- ▶ Over time, lesions become hyperpigmented and/or atrophic (see Figures 119.1 and 119.3). These changes usually evolve gradually over several months and are seen in older "burnt-out" lesions. However, these signs may coexist with active disease, so their presence does *not* completely exclude ongoing disease activity.
- ▶ Lesions can spontaneously soften over time.
- ▶ Overall clinical appearance varies depending on the subtype. There is no universally agreed-on classification of morphea, but a pediatric proposed classification system divides morphea into 5 subtypes:
  - Linear morphea (also called *linear scleroderma*)
  - Circumscribed (plaque) morphea
  - Generalized morphea
  - Pansclerotic morphea
  - Mixed morphea
- ▶ Linear morphea is the most common type of morphea in children and most often affects the face and/or extremities.
  - Hardening of the skin or subcutaneous tissue (as well as the associated hypopigmentation or hyperpigmentation) spreads in a linear distribution, most commonly over an extremity (Figure 119.4) or on the face (Figure 119.5). The distribution follows an embryonic pattern known as Blaschko lines.
  - Early findings of erythema and violaceous discoloration are more subtle in linear versus circumscribed (plaque) morphea; the early erythema can occasionally be confused with a port-wine stain.
  - When involving the forehead and scalp, referred to as *en coup de sabre* (cut of a saber) (Figures 119.6 and 119.7). Tends to have a unilateral distribution in most children; the skin gradually becomes more atrophic and develops a depressed, groove-like appearance. Can also affect underlying bone, causing disturbances to typical growth.

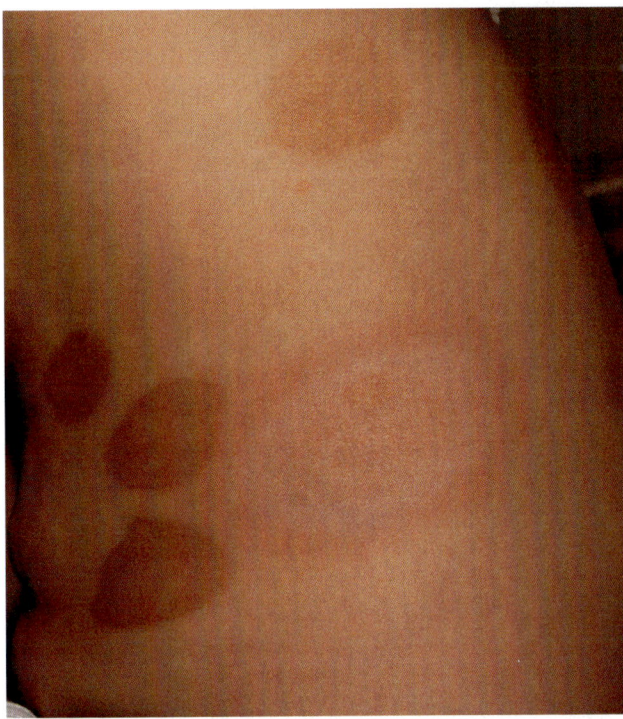

Figure 119.1. Circumscribed (plaque) morphea. There is a new lesion shown in the center of the photograph. It is an erythematous patch with a more intensely erythematous to violaceous border. Resolving lesions are seen as hyperpigmented patches.

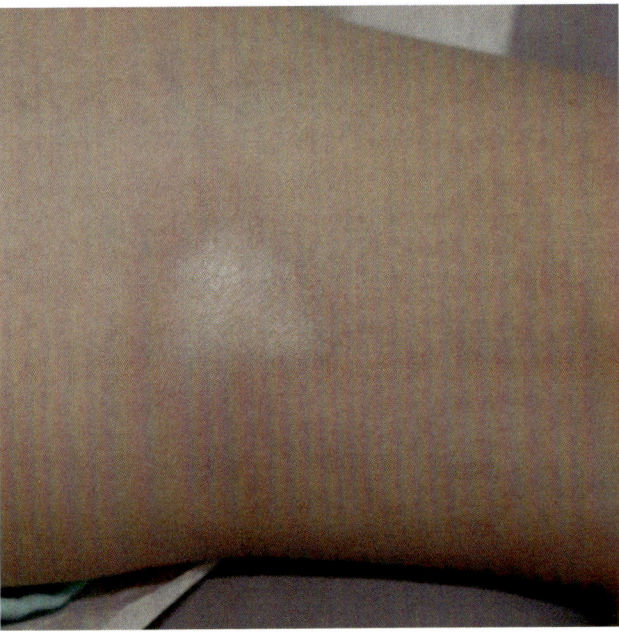

Figure 119.2. Morphea of the thigh. An ivory-colored indurated plaque with surrounding peripheral erythema.

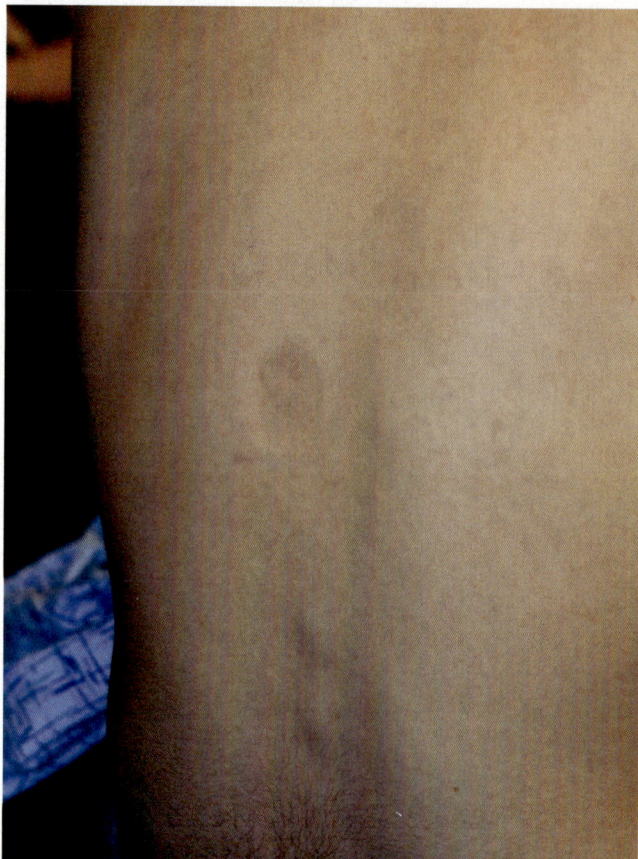

Figure 119.3. Localized morphea on the back of a teenager. This older lesion is characterized by an atrophic plaque.

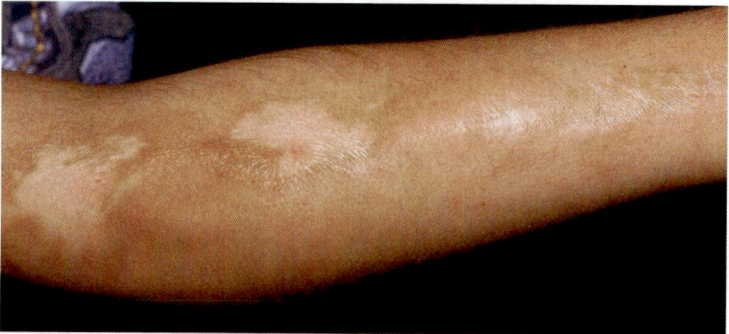

Figure 119.4. Linear morphea involving the arm. The lesions are ivory-colored and indurated. Hyperpigmentation is developing.

Chapter 119: Morphea (Localized Scleroderma)

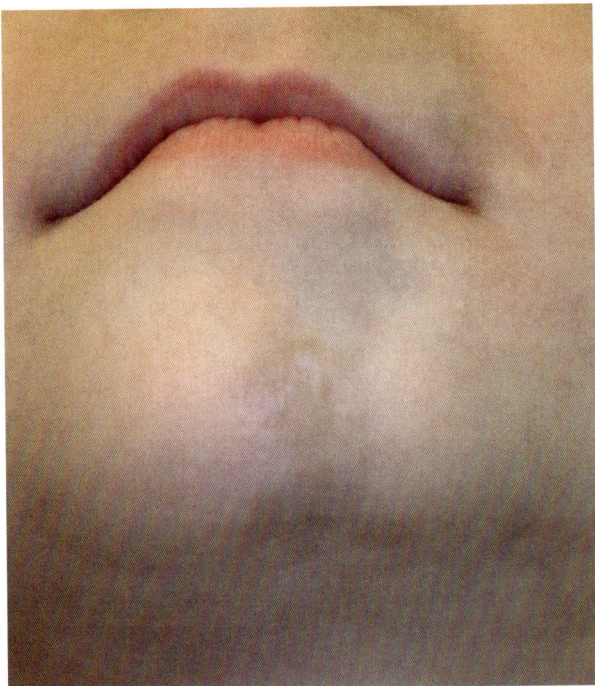

Figure 119.5. Linear morphea involving the face. Note the atrophy affecting the chin to the left of the midline.

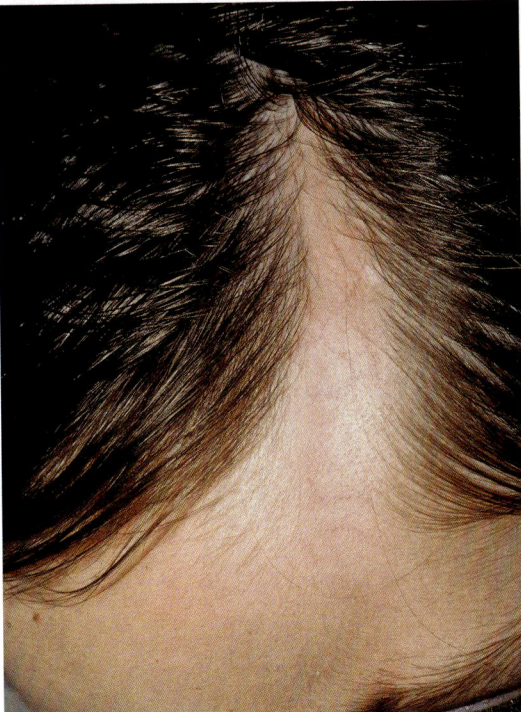

Figure 119.6. *En coup de sabre* (cut of a saber) form of linear morphea. There is a linear area of atrophy and alopecia involving the frontal scalp.

- More extensive hemifacial involvement may occur; it is termed *progressive facial hemiatrophy* (Parry-Romberg syndrome).
- Scalp involvement may be associated with alopecia (see Figure 119.6); can also spread inferiorly to involve the periorbital region (Figure 119.8), nose, and mouth; may become quite impacted as a result of marked atrophy.

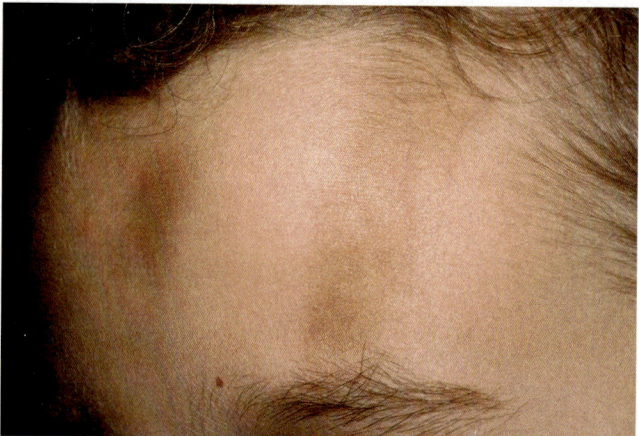

Figure 119.7. In this child with the *en coup de sabre* (cut of a saber) form of linear morphea, resolving lesions have become hyperpigmented.

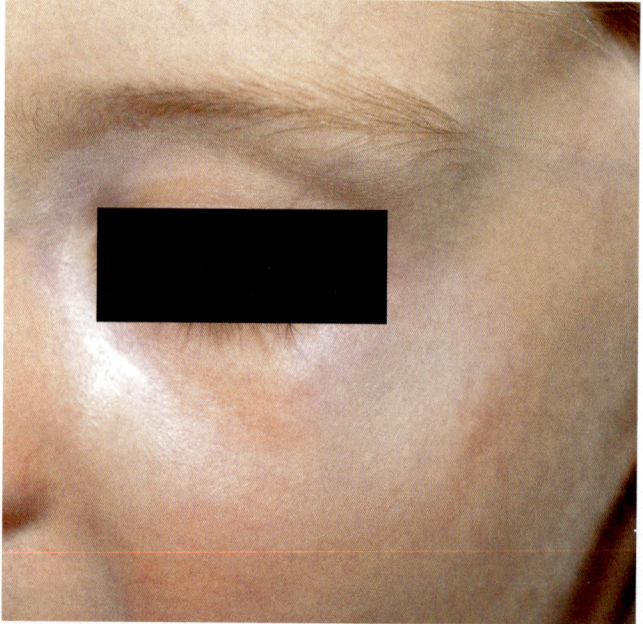

Figure 119.8. Patient with periorbital morphea in early stages.

- Morphea may be associated with significant atrophy of the skin and subcutaneous tissue; when involving a limb, this can result in circumferential and linear undergrowth of the affected extremity (Figures 119.9 and 119.10). Untreated, these problems can result in the need for orthopedic corrective surgery, which has included amputations in the past.
- When extending over a joint, morphea may result in contractures and impaired mobility or range of motion, which can be permanent.

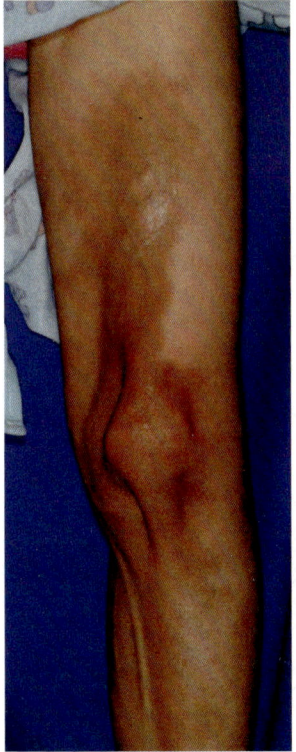

Figure 119.9. This 5-year-old had extensive morphea of the lower extremity, resulting in circumferential and linear size discrepancy with the unaffected side.

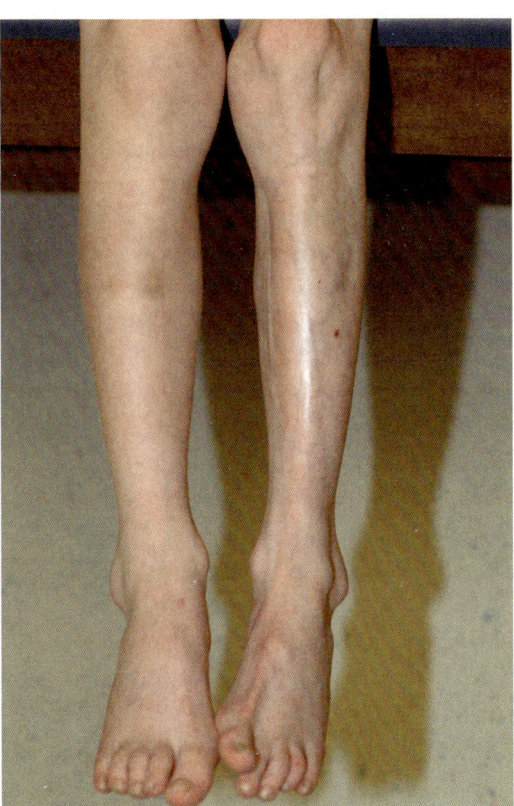

Figure 119.10. Patient with morphea of the left leg with leg length discrepancy and left foot hypoplasia.

- Circumscribed (plaque) morphea is the second most common subtype of morphea in children.
  - May present with one or more plaques of affected skin, most often located on the trunk. Affected skin usually begins with an oval or round circumscribed area of induration.
  - Often begins with erythematous or violaceous discoloration (see Figure 119.1), which gradually evolves to the characteristic ivory color with increasing induration; as the process progresses, the erythema or violet hue fades.
  - Circumscribed morphea can be further categorized as superficial or deep, depending on the depth of skin and soft-tissue involvement.
- Generalized morphea is defined by some experts as multiple plaques of morphea covering at least 30% of the body.
  - Classification defines generalized morphea as 4 or more individual plaques measuring more than 3 cm (which may become confluent), involving at least 2 of 7 anatomic sites (ie, head and neck, right or left arm, right or left leg, anterior trunk, posterior trunk) (Figure 119.11).

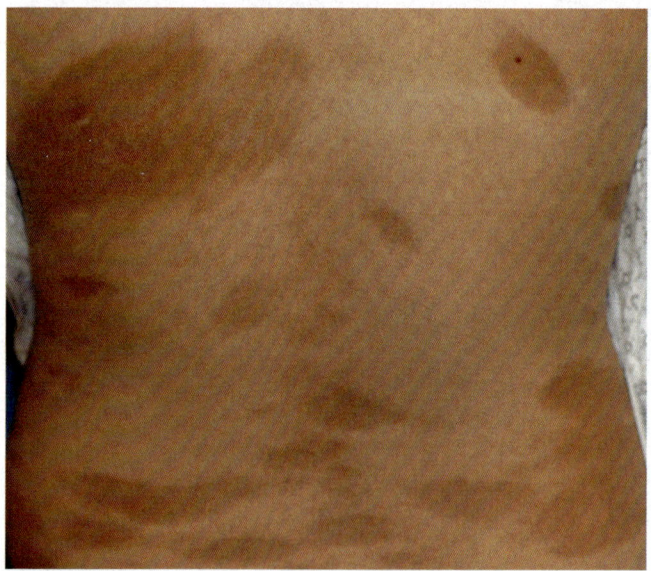

Figure 119.11. Generalized morphea. Multiple lesions involving the trunk have become hyperpigmented, and many are atrophic.

- Pansclerotic morphea is a rare subtype involving the skin, subcutaneous tissue, muscle, and bone, often on an extremity.
  - Usually results in circumferential involvement with significant cosmetic and functional compromise; skin may show pitting edema or diffuse painful areas with a puckered or peau d'orange texture.
    - This subtype can be life-threatening when rapidly progressive, as it can lead to widespread involvement with skin breakdown that not only puts the patient at risk for sepsis but also increases the risk for squamous cell cancer.
- Mixed morphea.
  - Some patients do not clearly have any of the subtypes of morphea because they have features of more than one subtype, most commonly a combination of linear and circumscribed (plaque) morphea.

Other Clinical Signs

It has become increasingly apparent that many patients with morphea experience associated extra-cutaneous involvement. A retrospective, multicenter international study of 750 patients with juvenile localized scleroderma (morphea) revealed that nearly one-quarter had extra-cutaneous features, while a more recent prospective, multicenter North American study of 86 patients identified a much higher extra-cutaneous frequency of 57%. Another study concluded that the risk for extra-cutaneous symptoms was greater among patients with disease onset before 10 years of age.

- Musculoskeletal findings are the most common type of extra-cutaneous problem, including contractures, arthralgias, arthritis, myalgia, myositis, weakness, and atrophy. Bony undergrowth has also been identified in about a quarter of the patients. Musculoskeletal manifestations are more common in those with linear scleroderma. Arthritis may affect joints with overlying skin lesions but also occurs remotely from the skin involvement in approximately 25% of patients.
- Neurologic problems have been reported, primarily with linear morphea of the upper face. Central nervous system manifestations include headaches, seizures, peripheral neuropathy, and behavioral or learning differences. Seizures can be complex and very difficult to control. Headaches appear to be the most common neurologic problem, and in some patients, they present as migraines, including status migrainosus. Changes seen at magnetic resonance imaging, including white matter lesions, intracerebral atrophy, and calcifications, have been reported in some patients. Rarely, vasculitis or vasculopathy has been found on brain biopsy specimens.

- Ocular manifestations may include episcleritis, uveitis, keratitis, xerophthalmia, glaucoma, and papilledema. Ophthalmologic evaluation is recommended for all patients with morphea at diagnosis, with routine follow-up screening recommended for those with craniofacial involvement.
- Vascular involvement (most commonly Raynaud phenomenon), gastroesophageal reflux or dysphagia, and involvement of the cardiac, pulmonary, and renal systems are infrequently associated with morphea. These problems are typically mild and nonprogressive, unlike the pattern found in systemic sclerosis.
- Extra-cutaneous involvement has been associated with more symptoms in the child (eg, trouble playing), poorer response to treatment (need for more treatments/longer treatment courses), and greater disease effects.
- Psychologic implications and functional impairment may result from this chronic disease. Outcome is improved by earlier treatment initiation, with use of systemic immunosuppressants recommended for patients with active disease who are at risk of experiencing poor outcome.

Look-alikes

Disorder	Differentiating Features
Capillary malformation (port-wine stain)	• May resemble early inflammatory stage of morphea. • Usually present at birth, unlike most morphea. • Usually stable during first several years after birth. • Flat and smooth, not firm or indurated, on palpation. • Some capillary malformations are associated with overgrowth (but not typically atrophy) of underlying tissues.
Lichen striatus	• May resemble early lesions of linear morphea. • Lichenoid skin-colored to pink papules that coalesce in a linear/band-like pattern; follows the lines of Blaschko. • No firmness or induration of affected skin. • Self-limited condition that often resolves spontaneously over 1–2 years. • May leave persistent hypopigmentation or hyperpigmentation, but no atrophy of affected skin.
Lichen sclerosus et atrophicus (LSA)	• May also show sclerotic white plaques with atrophy. • Most often involves the genitalia. • More likely to be associated with severe pruritus than morphea. • Extragenital LSA more likely to be associated with skin dryness than morphea. • Sclerotic white scar-like lesions usually smaller than those of morphea; may have guttate ("teardrop") pattern. • More likely to see telangiectasias or follicular plugging in LSA than with morphea. • Hemorrhagic blisters occasionally present.

Look-alikes

Disorder	Differentiating Features
Pasini-Pierini atrophoderma	• Considered by some clinicians to be a superficial variant of morphea. • Hyperpigmented (brown to gray to blue) patches seen most commonly on the back. • Lesions lack induration; preceding inflammatory phase always absent. • Face, hands, and feet usually spared. • Lesion borders are sharply defined; described as having "cliff-drop" borders ranging from 1–8 mm in depth. • Duration of many years to decades with benign course.
Linear atrophoderma of Moulin	• Atrophic plaques that are linear and may follow the lines of Blaschko. • Inflammation, induration, and pigmentary changes all absent.
Acrodermatitis chronica atrophicans	• Cutaneous manifestation of chronic Lyme disease. • Violaceous plaques of the distal extensor extremities that may become indurated, hyperpigmented, and atrophic. • Primarily seen in Europe, linked to *Borrelia* infection (connection between *Borrelia* infection and morphea remains controversial). • May have associated arthritis and neuropathy. • Primarily in adult women, occurring several months to years after initial infection. • Lyme antibody titer results may be positive.
Systemic sclerosis (scleroderma)	• Generalized disorder that may affect many organs in addition to the skin: lungs, kidneys, heart, gastrointestinal tract, and/or joints. • Much less common in children than adults. Very rare when younger than 5 years. • Nail fold capillary changes found in nearly all patients similar to those seen in juvenile dermatomyositis. • Early signs include Raynaud phenomenon, poor weight gain or weight loss, arthralgia, myalgia, and fatigue. Raynaud phenomenon can precede systemic sclerosis development by months to years. • Often associated with characteristic facial features: pinched nose, pursed lips, and small oral aperture. • Puffiness of the fingers (induration) is followed by sclerodactyly (shiny tapered fingertips with limited range of motion), with hand involvement found in most patients. • Other common features include arthralgias, decreased joint mobility, weight loss, fatigue, gastrointestinal symptoms, and shortness of breath with exertion. • Telangiectasias, calcification, and ulceration of the skin may occur (rarely seen in morphea). • Skin involvement is bilateral, symmetric, and diffuse, different from the linear or circumscribed lesions of morphea.

(continued)

Look-alikes (continued)

Disorder	Differentiating Features
Chronic graft-versus-host disease, sclerodermatous type	• History of preceding at-risk procedure (ie, bone marrow or stem cell transplant) and immunosuppression in host. • Widespread sclerodermatous plaques may be seen, similar to those of systemic sclerosis or generalized morphea. • May be associated with cutaneous ulceration, nail dystrophy, scarring alopecia, and joint contractures. • Erosions of the oral mucous membranes often present. • Systemic manifestations may include gastrointestinal, hepatic, pulmonary, cardiac, or hematologic aberrations. • Skin biopsy usually shows interface dermatitis in addition to dermal sclerosis.
Eosinophilic fasciitis	• Generalized infiltration/induration of skin of the trunk and/or extremities; classically spares hands, feet, and face (although hands and feet occasionally involved). • Abrupt onset of painful skin swelling. • Cobblestoned or puckered appearance of the skin may be present. • Usually responds well to systemic steroids. • Usually not well circumscribed or linear in distribution. • Associated with striking peripheral eosinophilia (but may rapidly correct on administration of systemic steroids), elevated erythrocyte sedimentation rate, and hypergammaglobulinemia.
Nephrogenic systemic fibrosis (nephrogenic fibrosing dermopathy)	• Usually seen in patients with renal insufficiency and exposure to gadolinium-based contrast media. • Often associated with a hypercoagulable state. • Poorly defined, indurated plaques usually distributed symmetrically on the extremities. • Frequently associated with joint contractures, pain, and decreased mobility. • May develop fibrosis of the heart, lungs, and skeletal muscle.
Progeria	• Very rare premature aging syndrome. • Diagnosis should be considered in young infants who present with widespread sclerodermatous plaques. • Other characteristic features include thin and beaked nose, midfacial duskiness and hypoplasia, micrognathia, and slow growth. • Prominent skin vasculature, especially over the scalp, develops over time. • Small face with birdlike appearance. • High-pitched voice. • Prominent eyes with incomplete closure of eyelids. • Caused by variation in *LMNA* gene.

How to Make the Diagnosis

- In most children, the diagnosis of morphea is based on clinical features. Skin biopsy can be helpful to confirm a clinical diagnosis when uncertain.
- Blood analyses may be used to screen for associated systemic autoimmune or rheumatologic disease but are not helpful in diagnosing morphea. In some patients, they may help with monitoring disease activity.
- Patients with rapidly progressive skin disease, more extensive skin or deeper tissue disease, or extra-cutaneous involvement or risk for extra-cutaneous involvement (eg, craniofacial involvement, all subtypes except for circumscribed superficial morphea) would benefit from comprehensive physical and laboratory evaluation by a pediatric rheumatologist.

Treatment

- Patients with morphea are usually treated by a pediatric dermatologist and/or pediatric rheumatologist; collaborative care between both specialists is optimal and recommended if possible.
- Clinical follow-up is challenging, and there is no consistently used tool to measure improvement or deterioration in disease; photographic comparisons, ultrasonography, thermography, and other imaging have all been used with variable consistency and utility; the Localized Scleroderma Cutaneous Assessment Tool (LoSCAT) and modified LoSCAT have been found useful in evaluating patient disease progression and in conducting clinical trials. However, LoSCAT assesses only skin involvement.
- Damage and extra-cutaneous involvement occur early, with children at risk of developing a serious problem because of the early onset of the disease and long duration. The best strategy to minimize severe damage is through early identification and treatment initiation.
- Treatment modality depends primarily on the severity of the patient's morphea and may vary from close clinical observation to multidisciplinary management with the use of topical and systemic agents.
    - Patients with mild, localized superficial morphea without extra-cutaneous involvement are most frequently treated with topical corticosteroids, calcipotriene (vitamin D analogue), or topical calcineurin inhibitors (tacrolimus ointment or pimecrolimus cream).
    - Patients with deeper, more extensive disease with or at risk for extra-cutaneous involvement are treated with systemic immunosuppressive

therapies, most commonly methotrexate with or without oral or intravenous corticosteroid pulse therapy. Mycophenolate mofetil is the next most commonly used systemic immunosuppressant. Several other treatments have been reported, including abatacept, tocilizumab, rituximab, Janus kinase inhibitors, and hydroxychloroquine, with combination therapy often used to control treatment-resistant disease.
- Phototherapy and photochemotherapy (particularly psoralen plus light from UV-A or UV-A1) has been used with success in the treatment of morphea, especially in adults. There is less experience with light therapy in the treatment of childhood morphea.

Treating Associated Symptoms

▶ Careful history and physical examination should be performed in all patients with morphea to screen for associated clinical symptoms or physical findings. While morphea is confined to the skin and subcutaneous tissues in many patients, children are at increased risk for deep tissue and severe extracutaneous manifestations compared to those with adult-onset disease.

▶ Extra-cutaneous involvement may be musculoskeletal, neurologic (primarily in patients with *en coup de sabre* distribution), ocular, oral, and, less commonly, vascular, gastrointestinal, pulmonary, or of another internal organ system. Early identification of deep tissue and extra-cutaneous tissue involvement is critical for reducing the risk for poor outcome, so early evaluation by a pediatric rheumatologist is recommended. Patients should be treated as necessary by a pediatric rheumatologist, pediatric dermatologist, pediatric ophthalmologist, or another appropriate subspecialist depending on the nature and extent of involvement.

▶ Physical and occupational therapy referrals should be initiated as indicated.

Prognosis

▶ Most adults with morphea have active disease for 3 to 5 years, but children have been found to have longer disease durations (13–13.5 years). Children also experience a higher relapse frequency than adults. Unlike with systemic sclerosis, most patients will go into spontaneous remission. The goal of treatment is to control activity to minimize damage, thereby reducing the risk for psychosocial and functional impairment and effects on quality of life.

- A minority of affected children may continue to have morphea during adulthood, and another subset may experience relapse of active disease even after several years of remission.
- Patients with limited plaque morphea usually do well with spontaneous remission after several years of disease activity. However, lesions of morphea can leave permanent pigmentary changes and atrophy of the affected skin, even after the active disease subsides.
- Severe linear morphea can result in limited range of motion and atrophy of affected extremities, resulting in discrepancies in length and circumference between affected and unaffected limbs.

When to Worry or Refer

- Children suspected of having cutaneous manifestations of morphea should be referred to a dermatologist or pediatric dermatologist for confirmation of the diagnosis and potential treatment.
- Patients with facial involvement, widespread skin lesions, aggressive disease progression, pansclerotic morphea, linear scleroderma, and mixed morphea should be referred to a pediatric rheumatologist to be evaluated for extracutaneous involvement and the need for systemic immunomodulators.
- Patients with severe morphea are often co-treated by pediatric dermatology and rheumatology specialists.

Resource for Families

- Mayo Clinic: Morphea.
  https://www.mayoclinic.org/diseases-conditions/morphea/symptoms-causes/syc-20375283

CHAPTER 120

Systemic Lupus Erythematosus (SLE)

Introduction/Etiology/Epidemiology

- A multisystem autoimmune disorder with protean skin manifestations resulting from immune complex deposition and end-organ damage.
- More common in female than male patients; approximately 80% of children and adults with systemic lupus erythematosus (SLE) are female; however, in prepubescent children, the male-to-female ratio may be more equal.
- Presents most often in postpubertal female patients (20% of cases are diagnosed in the first 2 decades after birth), especially African-American, Asian, Hispanic, and Native American patients.
- Median age of onset in childhood SLE is 11 to 12 years.
- Exact cause remains poorly understood; believed to be related to genetic and environmental factors; hormonal factors may also play a role.
- Extra-cutaneous targets most commonly include joints, hematologic system, lungs, heart, kidneys, and central nervous system.
- Approximately 80% of patients with SLE will have skin involvement at some point in their course and often as the presenting feature.
- Advances in early diagnosis and treatment have improved survival and quality of life for individuals who are affected; nevertheless, SLE can lead to significant morbidity and even mortality.

Signs and Symptoms

- Malar erythema often seen; redness occurs in a butterfly distribution over the cheeks, sparing the nasolabial folds, and often appears after sun exposure.
  - Edema often present along with facial erythema.
  - Occasionally, rash has a papular component.
  - Malar skin eruption usually transient and non-scarring.

- Erythematous patches and papules over the dorsal aspect of the fingers may occur and usually spare the areas overlying joints (in contrast with juvenile dermatomyositis).
- Discoid lupus erythematosus (DLE) lesions are a cutaneous manifestation seen in approximately 10% of children with SLE; DLE lesions are seen more commonly in adult SLE.
  - Lesions usually are located on face (Figure 120.1), on or around ears, or on the scalp and are usually round or coin shaped, annular (central clearing present), hyperpigmented, and often scaly (Figures 120.2 and 120.3).
  - Central atrophy may be present.
  - Lesions vary in size, usually 1 to 3 cm.
  - Often, lesions resolve with chronic pigmentary change (hypopigmentation or hyperpigmentation) and scarring (Figure 120.4).
  - Approximately 25% to 30% of children with DLE will eventually progress to SLE, with the greatest risk being within the first year after the DLE diagnosis.
- Non-scarring alopecia (hair loss) is commonly seen in SLE but is nonspecific; it most often presents as thinning of the hair in the temporal scalp regions.
- Nasal, oral, and palatal ulcerations (Figure 120.5); dilated nail fold capillaries (telangiectasias); petechial or purpuric lesions; livedo reticularis; erythema nodosum; photosensitivity; and small ice pick–like scars of the fingertips are other cutaneous features of SLE.

Other Clinical Findings

- Fever, malaise, weight loss, and arthralgias or arthritis are common in children with SLE.
- Additional signs and symptoms include fatigue, abdominal pain, muscle weakness, lymphadenopathy, hepatosplenomegaly, anorexia, weight loss, night sweats, and Raynaud phenomenon (blanching of fingertips with cold exposure followed by cyanosis and a reactive hyperemia on rewarming).
- Pulmonary (most often pleuritis) and cardiac (including pericarditis, myocarditis, valvular disease, and coronary artery vasculitis) manifestations may also occur in children with SLE.

Lupus Variants

Discoid Lupus Erythematosus (DLE)

- ▶ Discoid lesions may be seen in the setting of SLE or in patients with skin disease only.
- ▶ DLE is also known as chronic cutaneous lupus erythematosus.
- ▶ Skin lesions present as annular, scaly plaques with pigmentary change and atrophy (see Figures 120.1–120.4). Early discoid lesions may occasionally be confused with tinea corporis (ringworm).
- ▶ Scarring may occur.
- ▶ Lesions of DLE are often exacerbated by sun exposure.

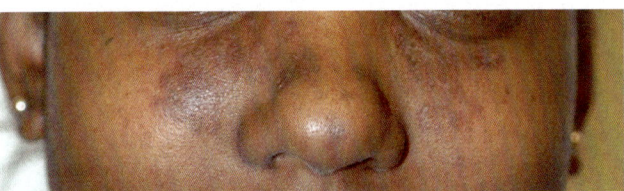

Figure 120.1. Teenage patient with systemic lupus erythematosus and facial lesions of discoid lupus erythematosus with erythema, atrophy, and hyperpigmentation.

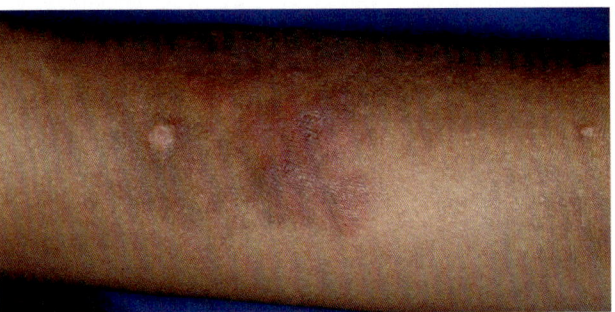

Figure 120.2. Lesions of active discoid lupus erythematosus on the arm in addition to areas of postinflammatory hyperpigmentation and scarring in sites of previous lesions.

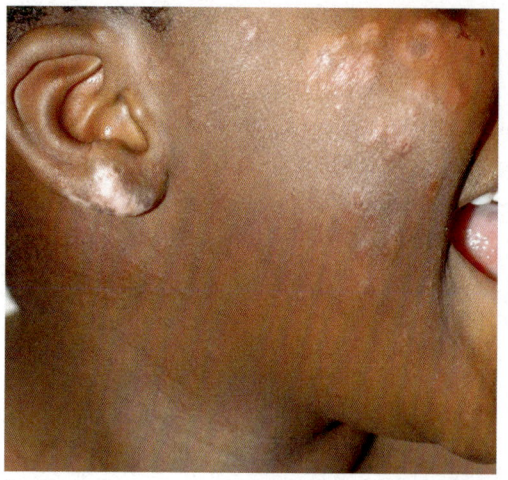
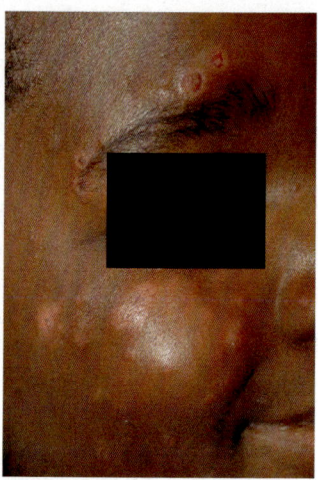

Figure 120.3. (A) Multiple erythematous papules and plaques on the face of a boy with chronic cutaneous (discoid) lupus erythematosus. Note the cutaneous atrophy of several lesions, particularly on the earlobe, a characteristic location for lupus lesions. (B) Erythematous papules on the cheek of the same patient with discoid lupus erythematosus shown in Figure 120.3A.

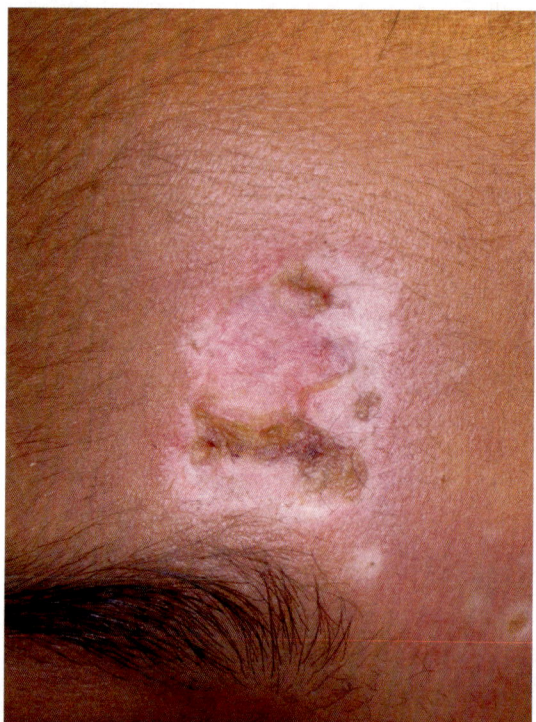

Figure 120.4. Atrophic crusted ulcerations on the face of an adolescent who has discoid and systemic lupus erythematosus.

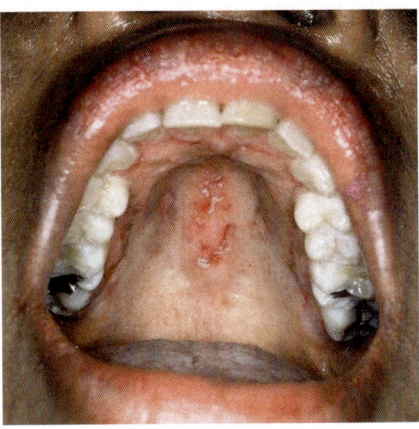

Figure 120.5. Palatal ulcerations in this young adult with systemic lupus erythematosus.

Subacute Cutaneous Lupus Erythematosus (SCLE)

▶ Subacute cutaneous lupus erythematosus (SCLE) is a subtype of lupus characterized by significant photosensitivity; it only occasionally occurs in children.

▶ Lesions usually appear in a sun-exposed distribution, and, in most, the condition is milder in severity than SLE.

▶ Lesions are often annular or psoriasis-like in configuration (Figure 120.6).

▶ Postinflammatory pigmentary changes are common, but scarring does not occur.

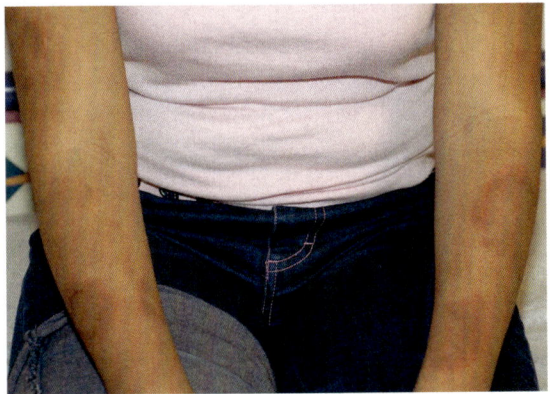

Figure 120.6. Large edematous, erythematous, arcuate, and annular plaques on the arms of this teenager with subacute cutaneous lupus erythematosus.

- Most patients have positive anti–SS-A (anti-Ro) antibody, which is associated with photosensitivity; pregnant women with anti–SS-A antibody (whether or not they have overt SLE or SCLE) are at risk of having a neonate with neonatal lupus erythematosus (NLE); anti–SS-B (anti-La) antibody is also associated with SCLE.
- Approximately 15% of patients with SCLE develop significant systemic disease with time; in general, though, patients with SCLE may have a better prognosis than those who have SLE.

Neonatal Lupus Erythematousus (NLE)

- A distinct type of lupus seen in newborns and young infants that results from transplacentally acquired autoantibodies, most often anti–SS-A (anti-Ro) antibody or anti–SS-B (anti-La) antibody, potentially in association with congenital heart block.
- Antibodies to U1 ribonucleoprotein (RNP) may also be associated with NLE and are usually not associated with congenital heart block.
- Most common target organs in NLE are the skin and heart.
- Approximately one-half of patients with NLE have cutaneous manifestations.
- NLE is the most common cause of congenital heart block; unfortunately, it often results in third-degree heart block requiring pacemaker placement.
- Skin lesions usually develop between birth and 8 weeks of age and are distributed most commonly on the face and head; parents often report exacerbation or appearance after sun exposure.
- Skin lesions are usually annular and erythematous or telangiectatic; they are often mildly scaly and may resemble lesions of tinea corporis (Figure 120.7), seborrheic dermatitis, or atopic dermatitis. Mild atrophy may be present.
- Although some infants with NLE have lesions in photodistribution (in areas of sun exposure), others may have more generalized eruptions involving skin that was never exposed to the sun (Figure 120.8).
- There may be a distinct periorbital accentuation, termed the "raccoon eyes" appearance.
- Lesions of NLE are self-limited and usually resolve by 6 months of age without scarring.
- Approximately 10% of infants may develop hepatic or hematologic alterations (usually self-limited).
- Fewer than one-half of mothers have a known diagnosis of autoimmune disease; mothers are most likely to have (or eventually develop) SCLE, SLE, or Sjögren syndrome.

- Infants with cutaneous findings suggestive of NLE should be evaluated for cardiac, hematologic, or hepatic abnormalities; serological studies usually confirm the diagnosis and should be performed in infant and mother.
- Skin biopsy is rarely indicated.
- Mothers who do not have symptoms but have infants with NLE should undergo comprehensive rheumatologic evaluation and be followed up closely for connective tissue disease.
- There is an increased risk of having another infant with NLE in subsequent pregnancies.

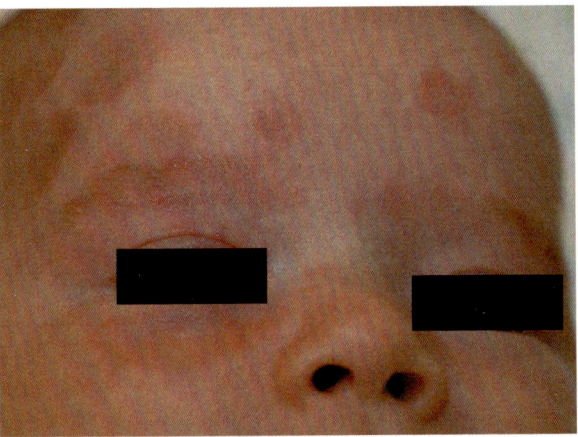

Figure 120.7. Multiple annular plaques with dusky atrophic centers on the face and scalp of this 1-month-old with neonatal lupus erythematosus. The mother had no previous history of connective tissue disease but later received a diagnosis of systemic lupus erythematosus. Her subsequent pregnancy resulted in a second child with cutaneous neonatal lupus erythematosus.

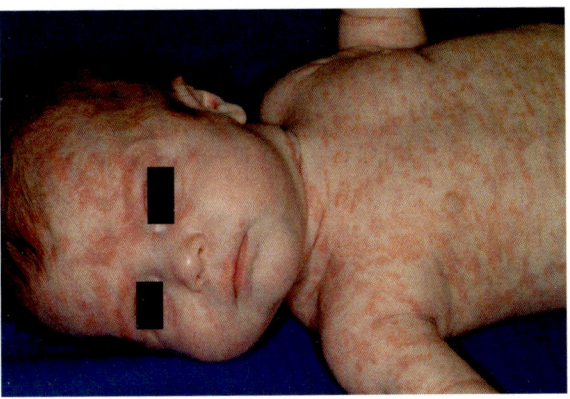

Figure 120.8. Young infant with widespread erythematous, slightly atrophic patches and plaques secondary to neonatal lupus erythematosus. Note the prominent involvement of the periorbital region, forehead, and scalp.

Look-alikes

Disorder	Differentiating Features
Systemic Lupus Erythematosus	
Juvenile idiopathic arthritis, systemic subtype	• Evanescent hive-like lesions. • Usually no malar erythema. • High-spiking fevers common, often correlate with the presence of skin eruption. • Skin findings may exhibit Koebner phenomenon.
Juvenile dermatomyositis	• Proximal muscle weakness in most patients; less common in systemic lupus erythematosus. • Arthritis usually absent. • Distribution of cutaneous lesions over extensor surfaces of arms and legs. • Heliotrope rash (periorbital distribution). • May have malar rash, which often does not spare nasolabial folds. • Skin changes often show lilac color. • Calcinosis cutis can occur in some patients. • Gottron sign (erythema) or papules (lichenoid papules) present over the knuckles and occasionally elbows, knees, and ankles.
Drug hypersensitivity syndrome (sulfa, minocycline, aromatic anticonvulsants, lamotrigine) (also known as drug reaction with eosinophilia and systemic symptoms [DRESS])	• Usually classic triad of fever, rash, and lymphadenopathy. • History of drug ingestion, usually preceding syndrome by 3 to 8 weeks. • Increased eosinophils and atypical lymphocytes on complete blood cell count. • Histologic findings distinct from those of lupus. • Sudden onset of diffuse cutaneous eruption; distinct facial or periorbital edema often present. • Eventual exfoliation; some patients with generalized exfoliative erythroderma. • Frequent liver involvement; occasionally fulminant hepatitis.
Rosacea	• No systemic abnormalities. • Often more prominent in the nasolabial folds and over medial aspect of the cheeks. • Inflammatory papules and pustules may be present. • Facial telangiectasias common. • May involve the eyes (ocular rosacea). • Chronic waxing and waning course. • Exacerbated by sunlight, heat, alcohol, hot beverages, spicy foods.
Polymorphous light eruption	• Lacks systemic associations. • Typically presents in late spring with initial sun exposure of the season. • Edema and erythema of the face, ears, arms, and dorsal aspect of the hands.

Look-alikes

Disorder	Differentiating Features
Subacute Cutaneous Lupus Erythematosus	
Psoriasis	• Most often occurs on knees, elbows, scalp, umbilicus, gluteal crease. • Lesions are plaques, typically thicker than subacute cutaneous lupus erythematosus lesions, and have silvery to white (micaceous) adherent scale. • May have associated nail findings. • Typically improves (rather than worsens) in sunlight. • Negative serological study results for lupus erythematosus.
Tinea corporis	• Plaques usually have more scaling and may have central clearing. • Inflammatory papules or pustules may be present. • No accentuation in sun-exposed sites. • Positive potassium hydroxide preparation or fungal culture results. • Negative serological study results for lupus erythematosus.
Granuloma annulare	• Annular smooth plaques that lack scale and are not exacerbated by sunlight. • Most often distributed on dorsal aspect of feet, ankles, wrists, and legs. • No systemic abnormalities in most patients. • Negative serological study results for lupus erythematosus. • Resolves spontaneously over 2 to 4 years.
Neonatal Lupus Erythematosus (None of the following conditions are associated with increased risk of congenital heart block, and in each of them, serological study results for neonatal lupus erythematosus would be negative.)	
Seborrheic dermatitis	• May also have scalp dermatitis, usually with greasy, adherent yellow scaling. • Erythema and maceration may occur in the neck, inguinal and axillary folds, and umbilicus (and, less often, the popliteal and antecubital fossae). • Onset in early infancy. • Usually self-limited with spontaneous clearing by 6 to 12 months of age.
Tinea corporis or faciei	• Positive potassium hydroxide preparation or fungal culture results. • May have more scale or inflammatory papules or pustules. • No accentuation in sun-exposed areas. • No periorbital accentuation. • History of known exposure may be present.
Psoriasis	• Facial involvement less common. • Often shows significant diaper and umbilical involvement in infant. • No accentuation in sun-exposed sites. • Typically improves (rather than worsening) with sun exposure.
Atopic dermatitis	• Pruritus very common. • No typical accentuation in sun-exposed areas. • Associated excoriations or crusting may be present. • Lichenification (thickening of skin in chronically rubbed sites) often present. • Lesions not typically annular. • Atopic diathesis often present.

How to Make the Diagnosis

- A thorough history, review of systems, and physical examination are critical in the accurate diagnosis of lupus. Helpful physical findings in SLE include the following:
  - Malar erythema
  - Nasal or oral ulcerations
  - Diffuse non-scarring alopecia
  - Raynaud phenomenon
  - Periungual telangiectasia
  - Vasculitis (red or purple macules and papules on hands or small ulcerations of the fingertips)
  - Lymphadenopathy
  - Erythema of the palms

- When a diagnosis of SLE is suspected, the following laboratory evaluations should be considered:
  - Antinuclear antibody profile (including anti-dsDNA, anti-Sm, anti–SS-A [anti-Ro], anti–SS-B [anti-La], anti-RNP antibodies)
  - Antiphospholipid antibody and lupus anticoagulant panels
  - Complete blood cell count with differential and platelet counts
  - Chemistries to include liver and renal function
  - Complement levels (C3, C4, total hemolytic complement)
  - Erythrocyte sedimentation rate (less commonly, C-reactive protein level)
  - Urinalysis with microscopic examination and first-morning spot ratio of protein to creatinine

- Serological studies may aid in confirming the diagnosis of lupus and may also help with categorization of subtype and prognosis.
  - Antinuclear antibody almost always positive in SLE but is also positive in 5% to 10% of the general population.
    - Five distinct staining patterns
      - Speckled: least specific (may be seen with Scl-70, Smith, RNP, SS-A, and SS-B antibodies)
      - Homogeneous: associated with anti-nucleoprotein antibodies
      - Shaggy or peripheral: associated with anti-dsDNA antibodies
      - Centromere: associated with CREST syndrome (*c*alcinosis, *R*aynaud phenomenon, *e*sophageal dysmotility, *s*clerodactyly, and *t*elangiectasias; also known as limited cutaneous systemic sclerosis)
      - Nucleolar: often seen in diffuse or limited cutaneous systemic sclerosis (scleroderma)

- If high clinical suspicion of lupus, check for anti–native dsDNA antibodies; these are highly specific for SLE and present in approximately one-half of patients; often associated with renal disease.
- Antibodies against small nuclear RNPs.
    - Anti-Smith: specific for SLE; present in 20% of patients with SLE; associated with higher risk for renal disease.
    - Anti-RNP: may be seen in SLE, scleroderma, NLE, or mixed connective tissue disease.
    - Anti–SS-A (anti-Ro): seen in approximately 30% of patients with SLE and approximately one-half of patients with Sjögren syndrome, as well as in patients with SCLE and NLE; strong association with photosensitivity.
    - Anti–SS-B (anti-La): positive in approximately 10% patients with SLE; often seen in association with anti–SS-A (anti-Ro) antibody; also seen in SCLE and NLE.
- Antiphospholipid antibody: occurs in 30% to 50% of adult patients with lupus and can also occur in patients with antiphospholipid antibody syndrome; associated with higher incidence of thrombotic events; skin findings may include livedo reticularis or cutaneous ulcerations.
- Patients with SLE should meet the new 2019 European League Against Rheumatism/American College of Rheumatology classification criteria for SLE according to the following weighted scoring system:

Table 120.1. The 2019 European League Against Rheumatism/American College of Rheumatology Classification Criteria

Additive Criteria	
Clinical domains and criteria	**Weight**
Constitutional Fever	2
Hematologic Leukopenia Thrombocytopenia Autoimmune hemolysis	3 4 4
Neuropsychiatric Delirium Psychosis Seizure	2 3 5

(continued)

Table 120.1. The 2019 European League Against Rheumatism/American College of Rheumatology Classification Criteria *(continued)*	
Mucocutaneous	
Non-scarring alopecia	2
Oral ulcers	2
Subacute lupus OR discoid lupus	4
Acute cutaneous lupus	6
Serosal	
Pleural or pericardial effusion	5
Acute pericarditis	6
Musculoskeletal	
Joint involvement	6
Renal	
Proteinuria >0.5 g/24 h	4
Renal biopsy Class II or V lupus nephritis	8
Renal biopsy Class III or IV lupus nephritis	10
Immunology domains and criteria	**Weight**
Antiphospholipid antibodies	
Anticardiolipin antibodies OR	
Anti-β2GP1 antibodies OR	2
Lupus anticoagulant	
Complement proteins	
Low C3 OR low C4	3
Low C3 AND low C4	4
Systemic lupus erythematosus–specific antibodies	
Anti-dsDNA antibody OR	
Anti-Smith antibody	6
Systemic lupus erythematosus classification requires antinuclear antibodies at a titer of 1:80 or greater, at least 1 clinical criterion, and >10 points. Adapted from Aringer M, Costenbader K, Daikh D, et al. 2019 European League Against Rheumatism/American College of Rheumatology classification criteria for systemic lupus erythematosus. *Arthritis Rheumatol.* 2019;71(9):1400–1412.	

- Traditional clinical and laboratory criteria that were used to diagnose SLE are listed here (American College of Rheumatology 1997 revised criteria for classification of SLE); SLE criteria are met if the patient has at least 4 of the 11 following:
  1. Malar rash
  2. Discoid rash
  3. Photosensitivity
  4. Oral ulcerations
      a. Oral or nasopharyngeal ulcers, usually painless

5. Arthritis
    a. Two or more joints
    b. Nonerosive arthritis
6. Serositis (pleuritis or pericarditis)
7. Renal disease (persistent proteinuria or cellular casts)
8. Neurologic manifestations (seizures, psychosis)
9. Hematologic disorder (≥1 of the following findings on >1 occasion):
    a. Hemolytic anemia
    b. Leukopenia ($<4,000/mm^3$)
    c. Lymphopenia ($<1,500/mm^3$)
    d. Thrombocytopenia ($<100,000/mm^3$)
10. Immunologic disorder (≥1 of the following):
    a. Anti-DNA antibody to native DNA in abnormal titer.
    b. Anti-Sm antibody.
    c. Positive finding of antiphospholipid antibodies on the basis of an abnormal serum level of immunoglobulin G or immunoglobulin M anticardiolipin antibodies, a positive test result for lupus anticoagulant according to a standard method, or a false-positive serological test result for syphilis known to be positive for at least 6 months and confirmed with *Treponema pallidum* immobilization or fluorescent treponemal antibody absorption test.
11. Antinuclear antibody (in absence of drugs known to cause drug-induced lupus).

Treatment

▶ Patients who have SLE should be followed up closely by a pediatric rheumatologist, and a multidisciplinary approach should be used for those who have significant systemic disease.

▶ Cutaneous manifestations may be managed in conjunction with a pediatric or adult dermatologist.

▶ Treatment of cutaneous disease may include (depending on severity and response to treatment) the following:
  - Photoprotection
    – Avoidance of excessive sun exposure, especially between 10:00 am and 4:00 pm.
    – Sun protective clothing (clothing with ultraviolet protection factor 50 rating, wide-brimmed hats, ultraviolet-protective sunglasses).
    – Daily broad-spectrum sunscreen use with high sun protection factor (≥30); products containing titanium dioxide or zinc oxide are optimal.

- Topical or intralesional corticosteroids
- Topical calcineurin inhibitors (tacrolimus, pimecrolimus)
- Systemic agents for more severe skin disease
    - Hydroxychloroquine (alone or in combination with quinacrine)
    - Retinoids
    - Corticosteroids
    - Dapsone
    - Methotrexate
    - Mycophenolate mofetil
    - Thalidomide
    - Azathioprine

▶ Treatment of systemic disease usually requires one or a combination of the following systemic medications:
- Corticosteroids
- Azathioprine
- Mycophenolate mofetil
- Methotrexate
- Cyclophosphamide
- Rituximab
- Belimumab, an anti–B-lymphocyte stimulator antibody
- Intravenous immunoglobulin

▶ In addition, nonsteroidal anti-inflammatory agents can be used for musculoskeletal symptoms and serositis but should not be used in patients with nephritis.

Treating Associated Conditions

▶ Patients with SLE are likely to need concurrent care from multiple specialists depending on the degree of end-organ involvement.

▶ Those with significant renal disease often benefit from collaborative care with a nephrologist.

▶ Those with neuropsychiatric disease may require specialty care directed at central nervous system complications.

▶ Because of the chronic and potentially disabling nature of lupus, the disorder can be associated with significant psychologic morbidity, and care from an appropriate specialist may be very beneficial.

Prognosis

- The prognosis for patients with SLE is quite variable and depends on the organ systems involved.
- Patients who have diffuse proliferative glomerulonephritis and associated hypertension often have a poorer prognosis.
- Infection is a major cause of death and is usually related to use of systemic corticosteroids or other immunosuppressive agents.
- Children with DLE generally have a good prognosis; however, these patients may go on to develop systemic disease (SLE) and should be followed up clinically and with intermittent laboratory evaluations.
- Infants with NLE have a good overall prognosis; those with congenital heart block often require pacemaker placement.

When to Worry or Refer

- Children suspected of having cutaneous or systemic manifestations of lupus should be referred to a rheumatologist or dermatologist for confirmation of diagnosis and management.
- If a patient with SLE acutely develops cytopenia and fever, the diagnosis of macrophage activation syndrome should be considered and is often accompanied by hyperferritinemia and hypertriglyceridemia; these patients should immediately be evaluated by a pediatric rheumatologist.
- Infants suspected of having NLE should undergo immediate cardiac evaluation, including electrocardiography, to assess for congenital heart block; mothers of these infants should be referred for rheumatologic evaluation.

Resources for Families

- Lupus Foundation of America: Provides information, support, and links for patients and families.
  www.lupus.org
- Lupus Initiative: Provides information and support for patients, families, and medical professionals. Sponsored by the American College of Rheumatology.
  www.thelupusinitiative.org
- Lupus Research Alliance: Provides information and support for patients and families.
  https://www.lupusresearch.org

Nutritional Dermatoses

CHAPTER 121 — **Acrodermatitis Enteropathica (AE)** 795

CHAPTER 122 — **Kwashiorkor** 801

CHAPTER 121

Acrodermatitis Enteropathica (AE)

Introduction/Etiology/Epidemiology

- Acrodermatitis enteropathica (AE) is an autosomal recessive disorder that results in a characteristic acral and periorificial eruption, diarrhea, and alopecia.
  - AE is caused by variations in the *SLC39A4* gene that encodes an intestinal transporter required for zinc absorption from the small intestine.
- Acquired zinc deficiency (eg, due to excessive losses [eg, chronic diarrhea], dietary restriction, administration of total parenteral nutrition with inadequate zinc supplementation) results in symptoms and signs analogous to those of AE. An unusual form of acquired zinc deficiency may occur in infants who are breastfed whose mothers produce zinc-deficient milk.

Signs and Symptoms

- In neonates and infants who are fed formula, the symptoms of AE typically appear days to weeks after birth when zinc stores become depleted. In infants who are breastfed, AE becomes manifest shortly after weaning. This delay in onset is thought to be the result of enhanced bioavailability of zinc in human milk.
- Rash is often the first sign of disease.
  - The rash of AE is acral (ie, on the extremities) and periorificial (ie, around the mouth, nose, eyes, and anus) (Figures 121.1–121.4). The digits may be involved with periungual erythema and swelling.
  - Lesions are erythematous patches with well-defined borders. Scaling, erosions, crusting, vesicles, and bullae may occur.
- The most common associated symptoms are alopecia and diarrhea. Others include anorexia, behavioral changes (eg, irritability, apathy), failure to thrive, ocular symptoms (eg, blepharitis, conjunctivitis), and recurring bacterial or fungal infections.

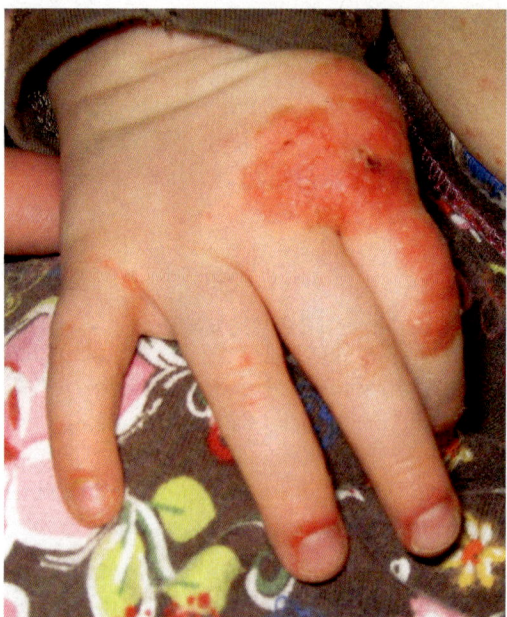

Figure 121.1. Acrodermatitis enteropathica. Erythema, scaling, and crusting on the hand.

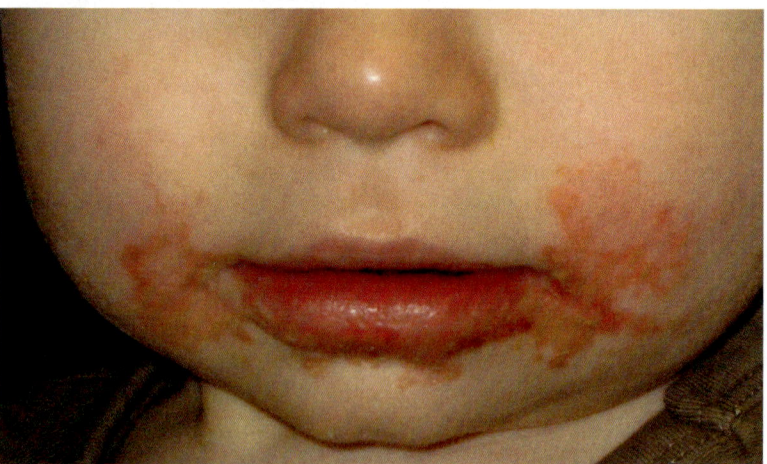

Figure 121.2. Acrodermatitis enteropathica. Erythema and crusting around the mouth of the patient shown in Figure 121.1.

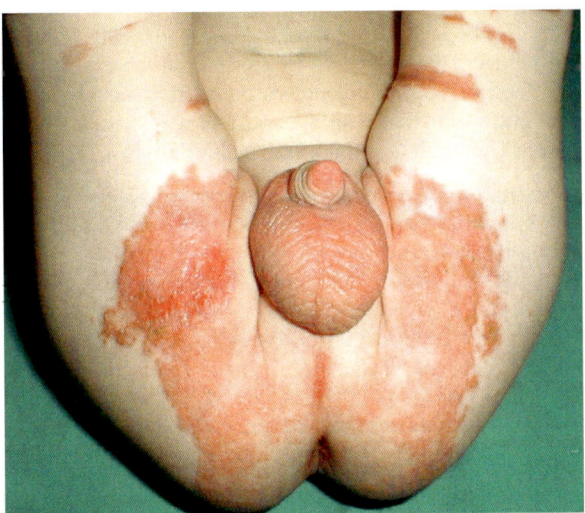

Figure 121.3. Erythema and crusting in the diaper area of an infant who has acrodermatitis enteropathica.

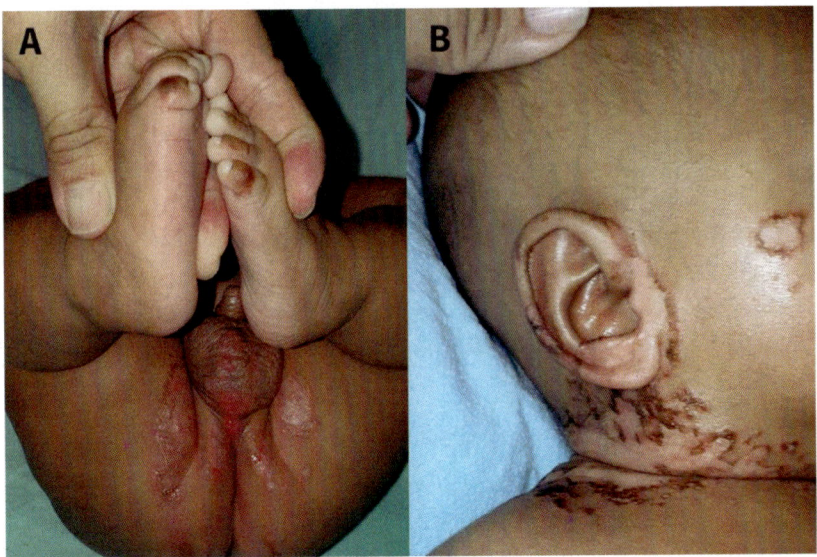

Figure 121.4. Acrodermatitis enteropathica. (A) Multiple well-demarcated erosions and patches in a 3-month-old, involving the toes and genital and perineal areas. (B) Well-defined, crusted erosions on the neck and right auricle. Patchy alopecia of the scalp is also visible. Used with permission from Leung AKC, Leong KF, Lam JM. Acrodermatitis enteropathica in a 3-month-old boy. *CMAJ.* 2021;193(7):E243.

Look-alikes

Kwashiorkor, essential fatty acid deficiency (including the rash seen in cystic fibrosis), vitamin B_{12} deficiency, isoleucine deficiency, certain organic acid disorders, and biotin deficiency may produce an eruption similar to that of AE. The acral and periorificial distribution of the rash of AE may help to distinguish it from other disorders.

Disorder	Differentiating Features
Atopic dermatitis	• Diaper area usually spared. • Trunk often affected in infants (uncommon in acrodermatitis enteropathica [AE]). • Facial involvement (eg, cheeks) occurs frequently, but perioral and periorbital involvement uncommon. • Pruritus usually present.
Crusted impetigo	• Distribution usually not as extensive as AE. • Lesions appear as erosions with a yellow crust; erythematous patches are typically absent.
Irritant diaper dermatitis	• Rash limited to the diaper area.
Psoriasis	• Diaper area involvement may mimic that of AE, but typical psoriatic lesions (ie, erythematous papules and plaques with thick scale) may be present elsewhere. • Erosive changes absent.
Seborrheic dermatitis	• Scalp involvement common (ie, cradle cap). • Skin lesions often have greasy scale. • Perioral and periorbital involvement uncommon. • Erosive changes absent.

How to Make the Diagnosis

▶ The presence of AE is suggested by the acral and periorificial distribution of the erosive rash and the presence of lesions with well-defined borders.

▶ A serum zinc level 50 mcg/dL or lower supports the clinical diagnosis; care should be exercised to collect blood in correct tubes, given potential zinc contamination of some materials.

▶ Low serum alkaline phosphatase level is often present.

▶ Rapid response of the rash and other symptoms to zinc supplementation supports the diagnosis.

Treatment

- Oral zinc supplementation (usually lifelong in AE). Supplementation should be provided at a dose of 1 to 3 mg/kg per day of elemental zinc. Several formulations exist, but zinc sulfate is the preferred oral agent; the dose is 5 to 15 mg/kg per day. This may be divided twice or 3 times a day and is best administered 1 to 2 hours before a feeding or meal.
- Irritability, anorexia, diarrhea, and the rash improve within days (Figure 121.5).
- Monitor zinc level periodically (every 3–6 months) and adjust dose accordingly.
- Adverse effects include the following:
  - Zinc may cause nausea or vomiting.
  - Because zinc may interfere with the absorption of copper, some recommend periodic measurement of the serum copper concentration.

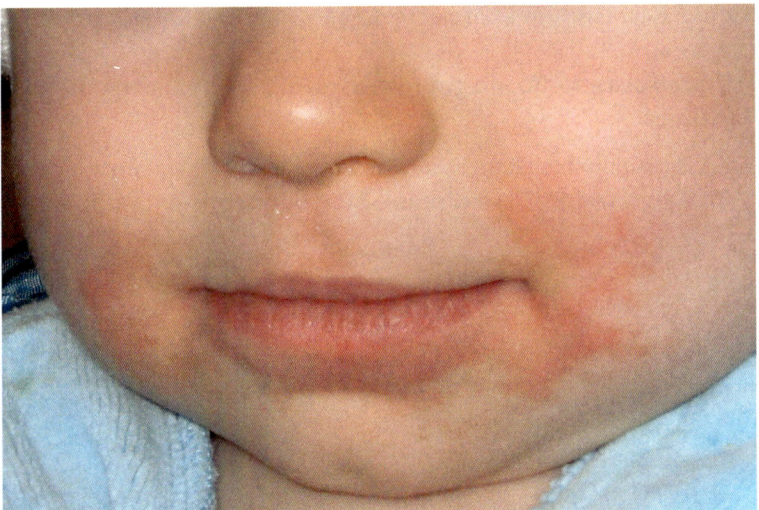

Figure 121.5. The patient shown in Figure 121.2 10 days after beginning zinc supplementation. The perioral eruption has improved greatly.

Prognosis

- Excellent, although lifelong zinc supplementation generally is required for neonates or infants who have AE.
- In patients who are zinc deficient due to defective mammary zinc secretion, discontinuation of zinc supplementation is typically possible at the time of weaning.

When to Worry or Refer

- Consider consultation or referral if the zinc therapy fails. If the patient has an acquired form of zinc deficiency, identification and treatment of the underlying cause are necessary.

Resources for Families

- Genetic and Rare Diseases Information Center: Acrodermatitis enteropathica.
  https://rarediseases.info.nih.gov/diseases/5723/acrodermatitis-enteropathica
- National Organization for Rare Disorders: Acrodermatitis enteropathica.
  http://rarediseases.org/rare-diseases/acrodermatitis-enteropathica

CHAPTER
122

Kwashiorkor

Introduction/Etiology/Epidemiology

- Kwashiorkor is a disorder characterized by insufficient protein intake in the setting of adequate caloric intake. The typical skin findings include a "flaky paint" rash and alopecia.
- It usually is considered a disease of children residing in areas of famine. However, the disease has been reported in higher-income countries when children are fed protein-deficient diets or have malabsorption or failure to thrive owing to neglect. Some examples include the following:
  - Infants fed rice milk by parents in an attempt to manage food allergies.
  - Infants fed protein-deficient diets to treat underlying diseases (eg, nonketotic hyperglycemia, glutaricaciduria type I).
  - Infants who have diseases characterized by malabsorption (eg, Crohn disease, cystic fibrosis).
  - Infants fed diluted formula by caregivers in an attempt to make the formula last longer or intentionally limit calories.
  - Infants fed inappropriately by their caregivers because of mental illness or unusual feeding practices or beliefs.

Signs and Symptoms

- Systemic symptoms include fatigue, lethargy, and irritability. As protein deprivation continues, individuals exhibit growth failure, generalized edema, and a protuberant abdomen due to hepatomegaly (from fatty infiltration) or ascites.
- The diffuse rash of kwashiorkor is composed of well-defined erythematous patches with overlying scale; in patients with skin of color, lesions may appear hyperpigmented. The scale edges are elevated, an appearance similar to that of peeling paint chips (Figures 122.1–122.4). This finding has led to the term *flaky paint dermatosis*.
- Other cutaneous variations include loss of skin pigment and thinning and diminished pigmentation of the hair.

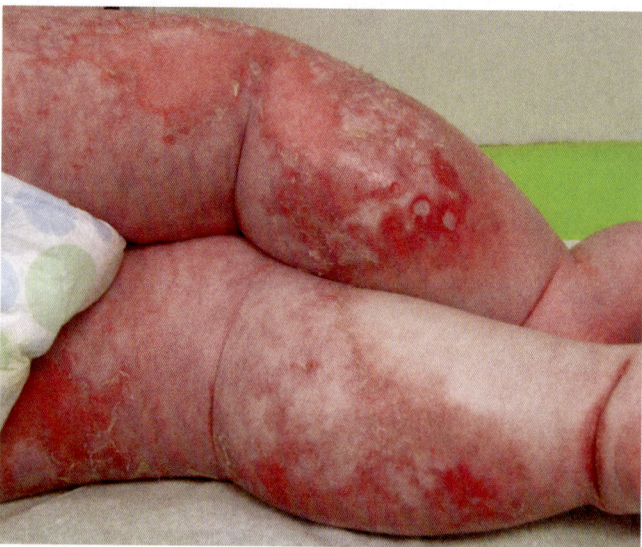

Figure 122.1. Toddler who had kwashiorkor and zinc deficiency. There are well-defined erythematous erosive patches.

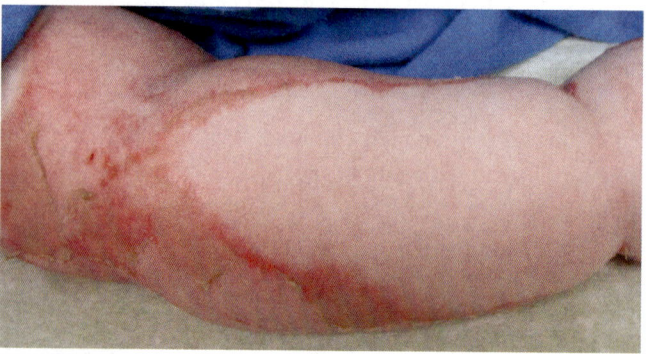

Figure 122.2. Sharply marginated patches with "flaky paint" scale (ie, scale with a well-defined raised edge) are present in the same patient as shown in Figure 122.1.

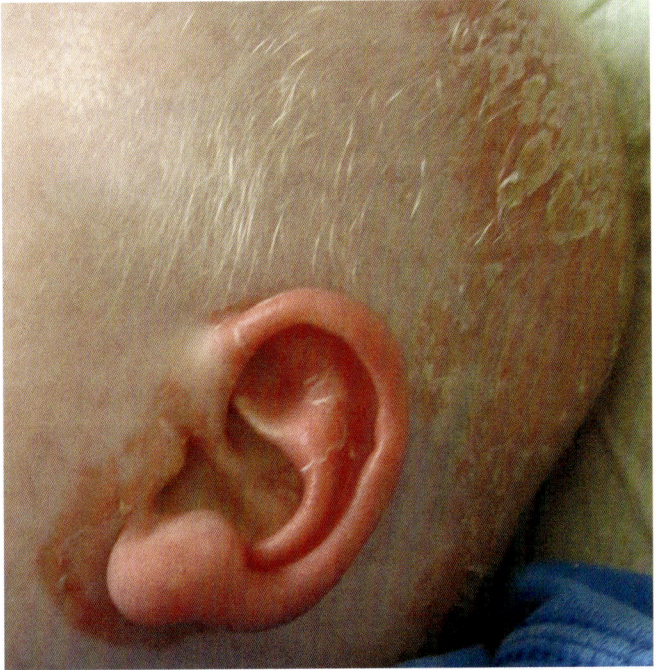

Figure 122.3. Scalp involvement in kwashiorkor with a prominent "flaky paint" appearance (ie, scale with a well-defined raised edge).

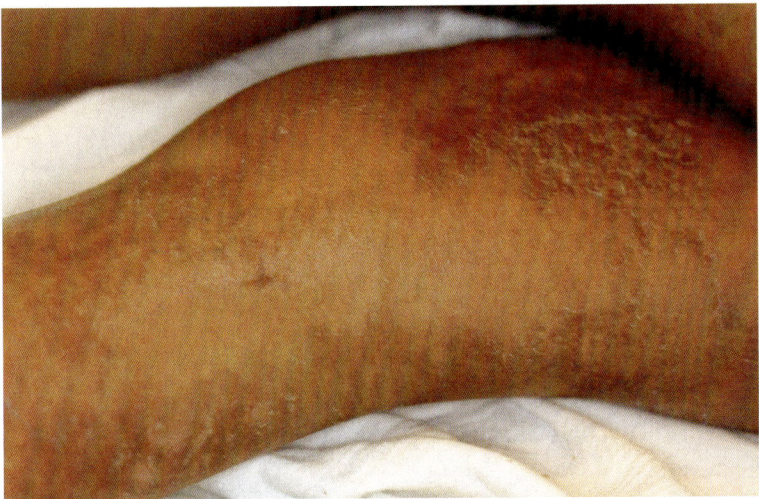

Figure 122.4. In patients with skin of color, the lesions of kwashiorkor may appear hyperpigmented. However, the "flaky paint" appearance (ie, scale with a well-defined raised edge) is present.

Look-alikes

The presence of edema, hypoproteinemia, and hypoalbuminemia helps to differentiate kwashiorkor from other disorders that may produce a similar eruption, including those characterized by nutritional deficiency (eg, of essential fatty acids, vitamin B_{12}, isoleucine, zinc, biotin).

Disorder	Differentiating Features
Acrodermatitis enteropathica	• It may be difficult to distinguish acrodermatitis enteropathica from kwashiorkor clinically, and the 2 entities may coexist. • Periorificial and acral involvement common (unlike kwashiorkor). • Edema, hypoproteinemia, hypoalbuminemia absent. • Serum zinc concentration reduced.
Atopic dermatitis	• Edema, hypoproteinemia, hypoalbuminemia absent. • "Flaky paint" appearance of scale absent. • Characteristic distribution by age.
Crusted impetigo	• Distribution usually not as extensive as in kwashiorkor. • Edema, hypoproteinemia, hypoalbuminemia absent. • Flaky paint appearance of scale absent.
Psoriasis	• Edema, hypoproteinemia, hypoalbuminemia absent. • Typical psoriatic lesions (ie, papules and plaques with thick adherent scale) usually present (scale does not have the flaky paint appearance), although diaper involvement may reveal minimal scaling. • Preference for scalp, umbilicus, diaper region in infants.
Seborrheic dermatitis	• Edema, hypoproteinemia, hypoalbuminemia absent. • Flaky paint appearance of scale absent (scale often characterized as greasy). • Preference for scalp, umbilicus, diaper region in infants.

How to Make the Diagnosis

▶ The diagnosis is suspected clinically based on the appearance of the rash and presence of edema.

▶ The presence of hypoproteinemia and hypoalbuminemia supports the diagnosis.

Treatment

- Institution of a diet or parenteral nutrition containing appropriate amounts of protein is paramount. Depending on the underlying cause of protein deficiency, this may require consultation with colleagues in nutrition, gastroenterology, or other disciplines.
- Investigation for coexisting nutritional deficiencies (eg, acrodermatitis enteropathica) may be appropriate.

Prognosis

- Treatment early in the course of the disease is associated with excellent prognosis.
- In severe cases, death may occur, caused by electrolyte disturbances or immunodeficiency resulting in infection.

When to Worry or Refer

- If kwashiorkor is suspected, prompt laboratory evaluation and initiation of nutritional restitution are vital.
- If abuse or neglect is suspected, a referral to child protective services should be made.

Resource for Families

- MedlinePlus: Information for patients and families (in English and Spanish) sponsored by the US National Library of Medicine and National Institutes of Health.
www.nlm.nih.gov/medlineplus/ency/article/001604.htm

Other Disorders

CHAPTER 123 — **Erythema Nodosum** 809

CHAPTER 124 — **Henoch-Schönlein Purpura** 813

CHAPTER 125 — **Kawasaki Disease** 821

CHAPTER 126 — **Langerhans Cell Histiocytosis** 829

CHAPTER 127 — **Lichen Sclerosus et Atrophicus (LSA)** 837

CHAPTER 128 — **Polymorphous Light Eruption** 843

CHAPTER 129 — **Confluent and Reticulated Papillomatosis (CARP)** 849

CHAPTER 130 — **Hyperhidrosis** 853

CHAPTER 123

Erythema Nodosum

Introduction/Etiology/Epidemiology

- Erythema nodosum (EN) is a reactive inflammatory disorder of the subcutaneous fat (ie, panniculitis) that has a limited duration and resolves spontaneously.
- Potential triggers include infections (*Streptococcus pyogenes* is most common trigger in children; others include *Mycoplasma pneumoniae, Yersinia enterocolitica,* tuberculosis, and cutaneous fungal infections), medications (estrogen in oral contraceptives, sulfonamides), and inflammatory disorders such as inflammatory bowel disease or sarcoidosis.
- EN is the most common panniculitis in all age groups. It is rare in those younger than 2 years. Incidence increases with age, with peaks in teens and young adults. Among children with EN, there is a slight female predominance.

Signs and Symptoms

- Red, tender, 1- to 3-cm nodules and plaques often start on the shins (Figures 123.1 and 123.2).
- In children, lesions may also develop on thighs; arms; face; trunk; and, very rarely, palms or soles.
- Lesions do not ulcerate or leave scars.
- May turn violaceous before resolution.
- Approximately 10% of children with EN may have arthralgias.
- Lasts up to 6 weeks and may recur intermittently for a few months.
- Recurrences after resolution are unusual.

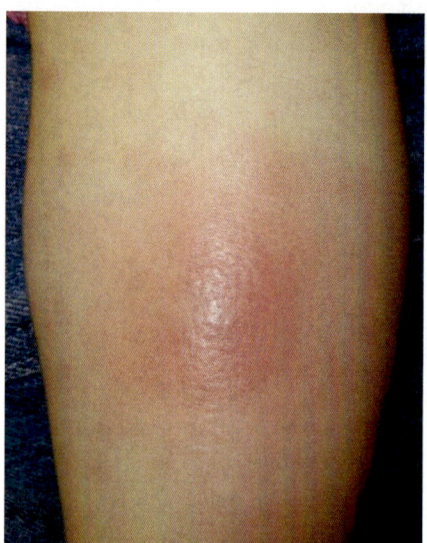

Figure 123.1. A tender red nodule on the shin characteristic of erythema nodosum.

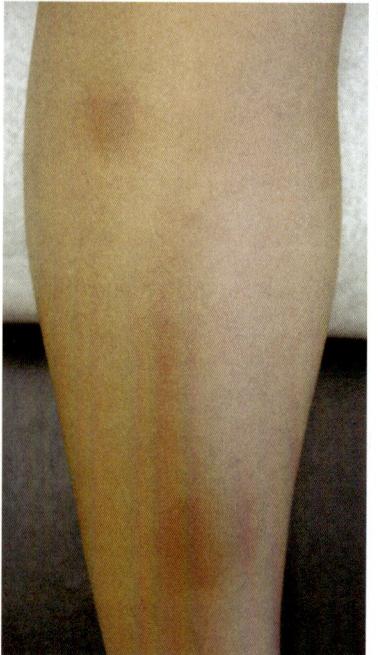

Figure 123.2. Two tender erythema nodosum nodules on the shin with less pronounced erythema.

Look-alikes

Disorder	Differentiating Features
Eccrine hidradenitis	• Confined to palms and soles. • Mainly occurs in summer; teens and preteens. • No history of antecedent infection.
Bruises, ecchymoses	• Often a history of trauma. • Typically undergo color evolution from purple to green and yellow before resolving completely.
Cellulitis	• Usually unifocal. • Associated fever often present. • Less nodular, usually more of a patch or thin plaque.
Arthropod bites	• Rarely tender; usually very pruritic. • Often see small puncta at bite site.
Vasculitis	• Palpable purpura with no blanching. • Often progressive. • Lesions range from small petechiae to larger ecchymotic or purpuric papules or nodules.

How to Make the Diagnosis

▶ EN can usually be diagnosed clinically but may be confirmed with skin biopsy if uncertainty exists.

▶ If the patient is healthy and a cause is not immediately apparent, consider screening tests, including measurement of antistreptolysin O or anti-deoxyribonuclease B titers, complete blood cell count, serum calcium level, stool hemoccult testing, chest radiography, and testing for tuberculosis (ie, purified protein derivative or interferon-γ receptor assay [QuantiFERON-TB Gold]).

Treatment

▶ Treat or remove underlying cause, if identified.

▶ If pain is significant, advise rest, leg elevation, and a nonsteroidal anti-inflammatory agent.

▶ Persistent cases may require a brief oral corticosteroid course; other reported therapies include colchicine, salicylates, and potassium iodide.

Prognosis

- Excellent. EN usually resolves spontaneously in 2 to 6 weeks, with rare long-term recurrence risk.

When to Worry or Refer

- Atypical, prolonged, or severe course.
- Concern exists for a systemic illness precipitating EN (eg, inflammatory bowel disease).

Resources for Families

- MedlinePlus: Information for patients and families (in English and Spanish) sponsored by the US National Library of Medicine and National Institutes of Health.
  https://www.nlm.nih.gov/medlineplus/ency/article/000881.htm
- WebMD: Information for families is contained in Skin Problems and Treatments.
  www.webmd.com/skin-problems-and-treatments/erythema-nodosum

CHAPTER 124

Henoch-Schönlein Purpura

Introduction/Etiology/Epidemiology

- Henoch-Schönlein purpura (HSP) is a systemic small-vessel vasculitis with immunoglobulin (Ig) A immune complexes. It is the most common vasculitis of childhood.
- Etiology of HSP is unknown, but frequent occurrence after acute infections (especially upper respiratory tract infection or streptococcal pharyngitis) suggests infectious triggers. Immunizations and medications have been implicated, although less often.
- Most commonly seen between 2 and 11 years of age, with a mean age of 6 years; slight male predominance.
- Incidence is estimated to be 10 to 30 cases per 100,000 per year in those younger than 17 years.

Signs and Symptoms

- Classic tetrad of nonthrombocytopenic palpable purpura, arthralgias, abdominal pain, and renal involvement.
- Skin.
  - Rash begins as urticarial macules and plaques on legs and buttocks, progressing to palpable purpura (Figures 124.1 and 124.2); petechiae may be present.
  - Forearms, elbows, trunk (Figure 124.3), and face (ears) may be involved in younger children or more severe cases, along with hand and foot edema. The rash often involves pressure points or dependent areas.
  - Occasional oral and nasal mucosal involvement.
  - Lesions develop in crops, with newer urticarial lesions intermixed with older palpable purpura.
  - Occasionally, patients may develop blisters, ulcers, or necrosis (Figures 124.4 and 124.5).

- Renal involvement occurs in 20% to 50% of patients.
  - Spectrum of disease ranges from microscopic hematuria or minimal proteinuria to nephritic or nephrotic syndrome (5%); 2% to 5% of patients progress to end-stage renal failure.
  - May not appear until weeks after the onset of disease but usually within 3 months of onset; therefore, blood pressure monitoring and serial urine evaluations recommended for several months (typically every 1–2 weeks initially, then monthly for up to 3–6 months) after the diagnosis.
- Gastrointestinal involvement occurs in 50% to 70% of children.
  - Colicky abdominal pain, vomiting, and gross or occult bleeding are most common.
  - Intussusception in 2% to 4%, usually involving the small bowel; more common in boys.
- Musculoskeletal.
  - Arthralgias occur in 60% to 80% of children with HSP; rarely true arthritis.
  - Ankles and knees most commonly affected.
- Other.
  - Rarely, central nervous system (eg, headache, seizures, behavioral changes) or lung involvement (ie, infiltrates or diffuse alveolar hemorrhage) may occur.
  - Infrequent scrotal involvement with purpura (Figure 124.6) or pain that may mimic testicular torsion.

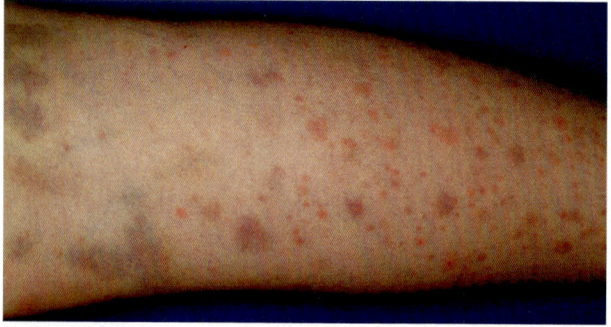

Figure 124.1. A mixture of urticarial, violaceous, and purpuric plaques on the legs is typical of Henoch-Schönlein purpura.

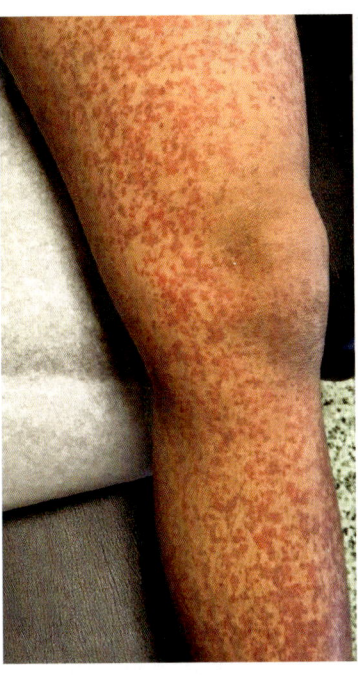

Figure 124.2. Lesions became progressively more confluent and purpuric in this patient with Henoch-Schönlein purpura.

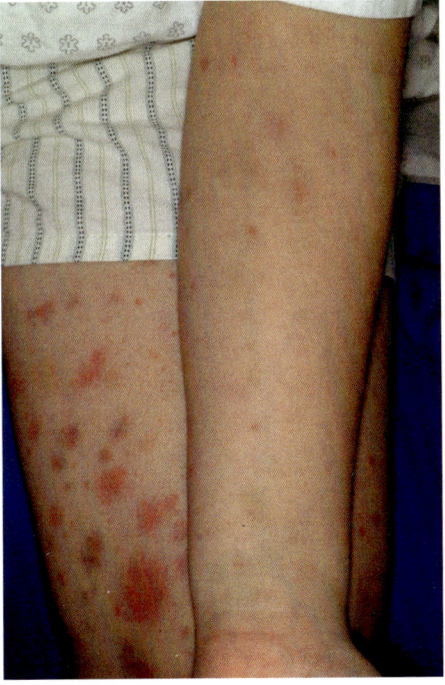

Figure 124.3. In more extensive cases of Henoch-Schönlein purpura, lesions can be seen on the upper extremities as well as more classic sites like the lower extremities; both were present in this patient.

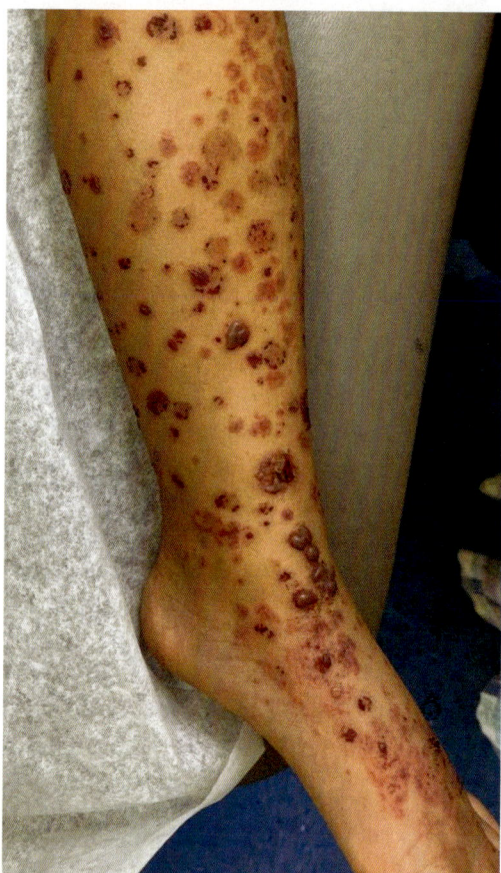

Figure 124.4. This child had numerous Henoch-Schönlein purpura lesions, with a mix of palpable purpura and bullae.

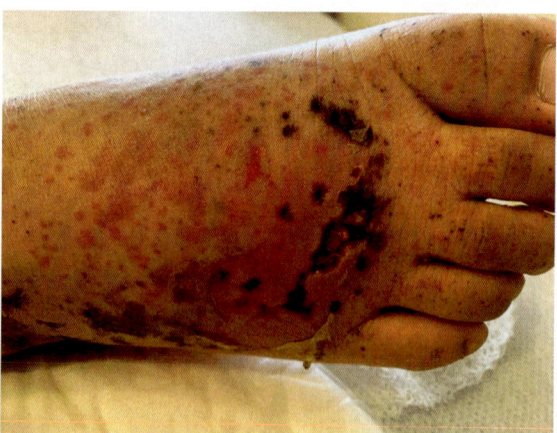

Figure 124.5. This severe case of Henoch-Schönlein purpura resulted in ulcers with necrosis on the dorsal aspect of the feet, which ultimately healed with scarring.

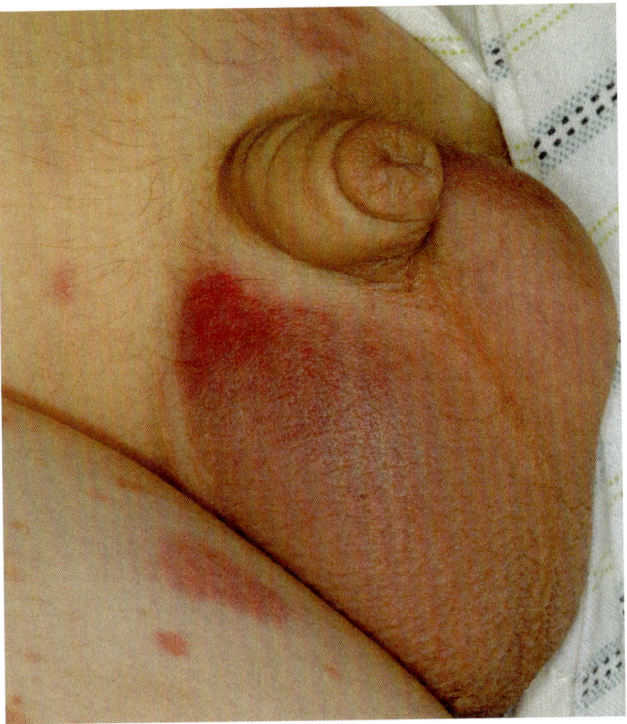

Figure 124.6. Purpura involving the scrotum in a patient with Henoch-Schönlein purpura and scrotal pain.

Look-alikes

Disorder	Differentiating Features
Acute hemorrhagic edema of infancy	• Younger children (4 months–3 years). • Cockade (medallion-like) purpura. • Facial, hand, and foot edema. • No systemic features. • Immunoglobulin A deposition usually absent at histologic evaluation of skin biopsy specimen. • Benign self-limited course.
Septic vasculitis	• Febrile and often appears toxic; shock may be present. • Progressive course. • Often a more widespread distribution. • Multisystem disease.
Hypersensitivity vasculitis	• Often induced by medication. • Lesions often more widespread. • Often presents with petechiae and small purpuric papules.
Ecchymoses, benign	• Usually no renal, gastrointestinal, or joint concerns. • Skin lesions typically fewer in number. • Usually limited to areas overlying bony prominences (eg, anterior tibial surfaces).
Ecchymoses associated with child abuse	• Usually no renal, gastrointestinal, or joint associations. • Skin lesions typically fewer in number. • Historical context important. • Other features of abuse may be present (eg, retinal hemorrhage, bony fractures).
Urticaria	• May mimic early Henoch-Schönlein purpura. • Purpura absent. • Lesions usually widespread and transient (resolving within 24 hours).

How to Make the Diagnosis

▶ The clinical presentation is usually highly suggestive, especially when the classic tetrad (ie, lower body purpura, arthralgias, abdominal pain, renal involvement) is present.

▶ No laboratory tests are specific to HSP, making it largely a clinical diagnosis.

▶ Skin biopsy (when necessary) is usually confirmatory at histologic and immunofluorescence study (demonstrating hypersensitivity vasculitis with IgA1 deposits and neutrophil infiltration of small blood vessel walls).

▶ Renal biopsy, if needed, reveals proliferative glomerulonephritis with IgA1 deposition.

Treatment

- Most patients require only supportive care.
- If severe joint or abdominal pain or with severe skin involvement, consider oral corticosteroid therapy.
- Must assess renal function and urinalysis in the long term, given possible delayed presentation of renal disease in HSP.
- Treatment of renal involvement depends on severity. In patients with significant nephritis or nephrosis, consultation with a pediatric nephrologist is warranted.
- Some evidence exists that treatment with systemic corticosteroids may reduce intussusception risk or renal disease progression. Steroid use does not prevent recurrence.

Prognosis

- Excellent in most. Typically resolves in 4 to 6 weeks.
- Recurrences in one-third of patients, usually within 3 to 4 months.
- Severity of nephritis predicts outcome.

When to Worry or Refer

- Renal insufficiency or rapidly progressive kidney disease, nephritic or nephrotic syndrome.
- Concern for intussusception.
- Acute scrotal pain or swelling (when concern exists for testicular torsion).
- Central nervous system involvement (eg, change in mental status or behavior, seizures).
- Hemoptysis.

Resources for Families

- MedlinePlus: Information for patients and families (in English and Spanish) sponsored by the US National Library of Medicine and National Institutes of Health.
  https://www.nlm.nih.gov/medlineplus/ency/article/000425.htm
- WebMD: Information for families is contained in Skin Problems and Treatments.
  www.webmd.com/skin-problems-and-treatments/henoch-schonlein-purpura-causes-symptoms-treatment#1

CHAPTER 125

Kawasaki Disease

Introduction/Etiology/Epidemiology

- Also known as acute febrile mucocutaneous lymph node syndrome.
- Acute multisystem vasculitis of children, usually younger than 5 years; involves small and medium muscular arteries.
- Most common cause of acquired heart disease in children in high-income countries.
- Etiology remains unknown; research has focused on infectious and environmental factors, abnormal immune responses, and genetic predisposition.
- A marked seasonality has been observed (more cases during winter and spring).
- No single diagnostic test exists.
- Coronary artery aneurysms may develop in up to 25% of patients who are untreated (2%–4% with appropriate therapy).

Signs and Symptoms

- Diagnosis is based on fulfillment of diagnostic criteria, which consist of fever for at least 5 days and 4 of the following 5 clinical features:
  - Bilateral bulbar conjunctival injection (non-exudative), classically with perilimbic sparing (Figure 125.1).
  - Oral mucosa changes, including erythematous, fissured lips (Figure 125.2); strawberry tongue (Figure 125.3); pharyngeal erythema.
  - Nonsuppurative cervical lymphadenopathy (at least 1.5 cm and often unilateral).
  - Edema and erythema of the hands and feet (early) (Figure 125.4); periungual desquamation in subacute phase.
  - Polymorphous rash.

- Fevers are usually high (≥39 °C [102.2 °F]).
- Irritability is common and may reflect cerebral vasculitis or aseptic meningitis.
- Rash may be exanthematous (macular, papular), urticarial, scarlet fever–like, erythrodermic, or erythema multiforme–like in character; pustular presentations have also been observed.
- Accentuation of skin eruption frequently noted in perineal and genital regions (Figure 125.5); may be desquamative and is considered an important clue to the diagnosis.
- Bacille Calmette-Guérin vaccination site erythema and induration may be noted.
- Vesicles, bullae, and purpura are usually not seen; peripheral gangrene may rarely occur (Figure 125.6).
- A psoriasis-like skin eruption may be present, especially during the convalescent phase.
- In addition to coronary artery aneurysms, other cardiac complications may include myocarditis, valvulitis, pericardial effusion, pericarditis, and myocardial infarction.
- Other features may include gastrointestinal symptoms, lethargy, uveitis, arthralgias, gangrene.
- Incomplete or atypical Kawasaki disease may occur, especially in infants, in which patients do not fulfill classic diagnostic criteria; in a child with unexplained fever and some diagnostic features, this diagnosis should be considered.

Chapter 125: Kawasaki Disease

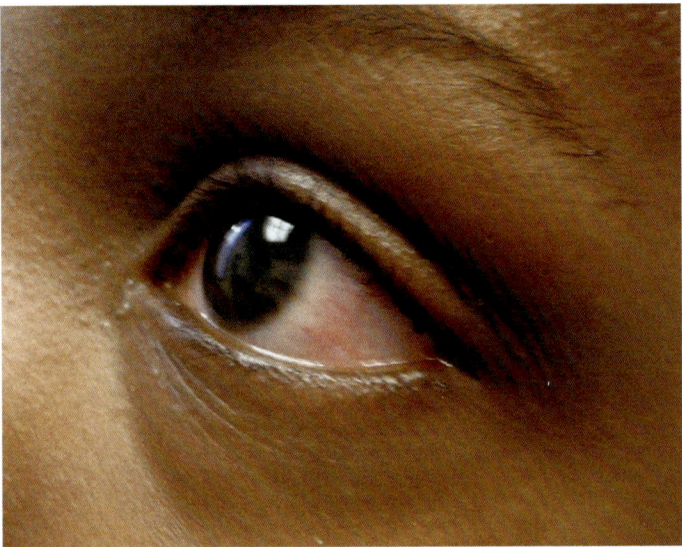

Figure 125.1. In Kawasaki disease, non-exudative conjunctival injection is present, often with perilimbic sparing.

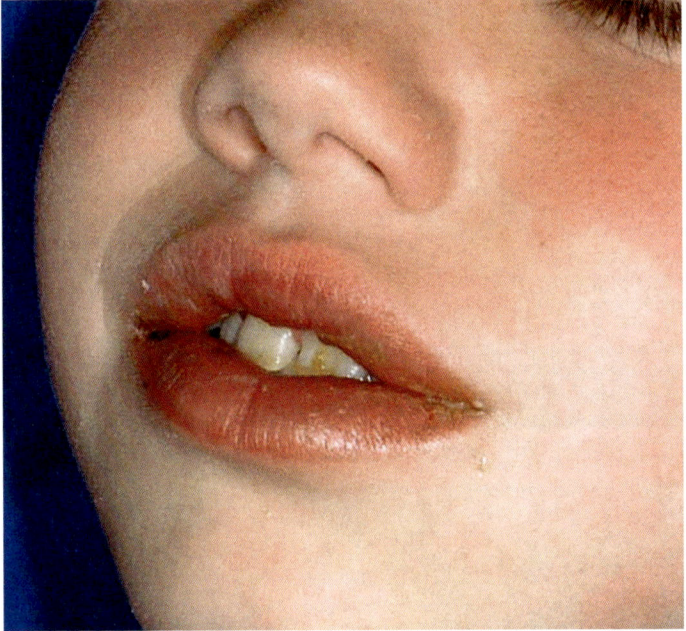

Figure 125.2. Kawasaki disease. Hyperemia, edema, and fissuring of the lips.

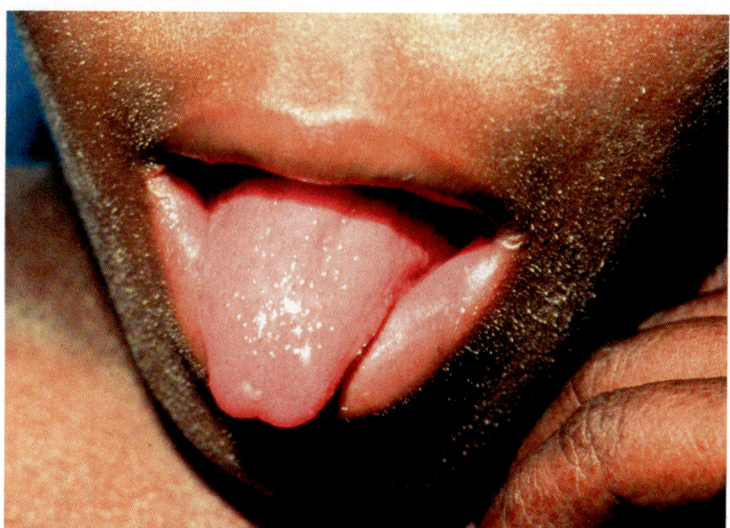

Figure 125.3. Kawasaki disease. Strawberry tongue was present in this child with severe coronary artery aneurysms.

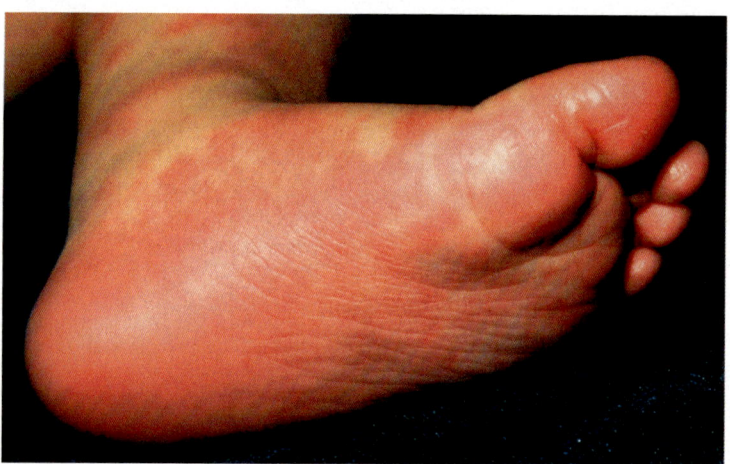

Figure 125.4. Kawasaki disease. Erythematous patches and plaques with foot swelling.

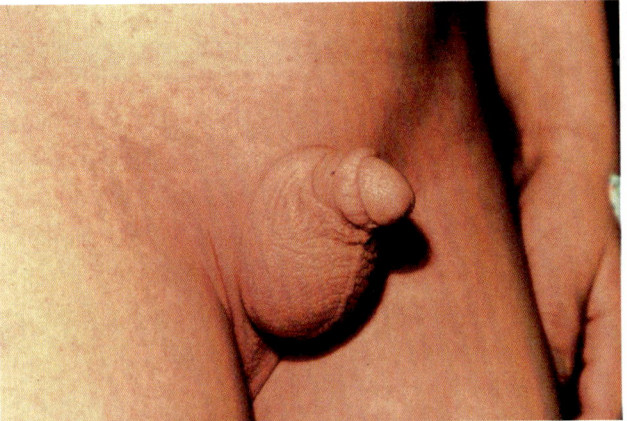
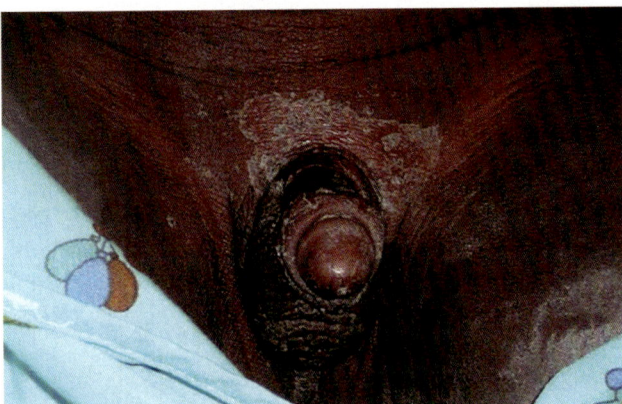

Figure 125.5. Perineal accentuation in Kawasaki disease. (A) Accentuation of erythema in the perineum and genital region is a frequent finding, as seen in this young child. (B) Erythema was followed by thick desquamation in this 5-year-old with skin of color who had diagnostic features of Kawasaki disease.

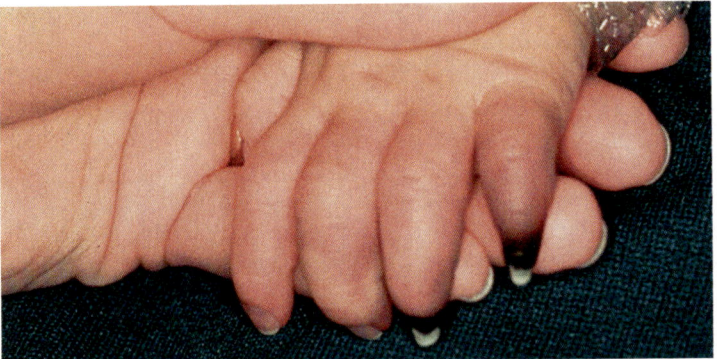

Figure 125.6. Kawasaki disease. Peripheral gangrene involving the fourth and fifth digits occurred in this toddler.

Look-alikes

Disorder	Differentiating Features
Serum sickness–like eruption	- History of preceding drug ingestion. - Mucous membrane and eye findings usually absent. - Purple urticaria most characteristic skin finding, in conjunction with periarticular swelling.
Viral exanthem (ie, adenovirus, measles)	- Exudative conjunctivitis, Koplik spots, severe cough present (measles). - Rash begins behind ears, does not accentuate in perineum (measles). - Conjunctivitis does not spare perilimbic area. - Inflammatory marker levels (eg, C-reactive protein) minimally elevated (measles and adenovirus).
Scarlet fever	- Exudative pharyngitis present. - Conjunctivae normal. - When facial rash present, circumoral pallor is often present. - Positive test result for *Streptococcus pyogenes*.
Toxic shock syndrome (TSS)	- Hypotension present. - Renal involvement (elevated serum creatinine level), elevation of creatine phosphokinase level. - Disseminated intravascular coagulopathy and adult respiratory distress syndrome–like illness may be present (streptococcal TSS). - Rash appears as diffuse erythema. - Primary focus of *Staphylococcus aureus* or streptococcal infection may be present. - Note: Kawasaki disease shock syndrome may present with hypotension and shock and is differentiated from TSS by echocardiographic findings suggestive of Kawasaki disease, higher platelet counts, and more severe anemia.
Systemic-onset juvenile idiopathic arthritis	- Hepatosplenomegaly often present. - Rash is evanescent, salmon colored; often correlates with presence of fever. - Quotidian (daily) or double quotidian (twice daily) fever curve with relative wellness between spikes.
Stevens-Johnson syndrome (SJS)/ *Mycoplasma pneumoniae*–induced rash and mucositis (MIRM), reactive infectious mucocutaneous eruption (RIME)	- Skin blisters, denudation (SJS > MIRM or RIME). - Mucosal blistering and erosions (mouth, eyes, genitals) (MIRM or RIME > SJS). - MIRM classically associated with *M pneumoniae* infection; RIME associated with several potential etiologic agents (*Chlamydia pneumoniae*, influenza, parainfluenza, others); SJS often triggered by drug exposure but may also be associated with infection.

How to Make the Diagnosis

- The diagnosis is suggested by the presence of prolonged fever and other diagnostic criteria; incomplete Kawasaki disease is diagnosed when patient has fever for 5 or more days and 2 or 3 diagnostic criteria together with other supportive findings.
- Elevation of inflammatory marker levels (eg, erythrocyte sedimentation rate, C-reactive protein) is nearly universal in Kawasaki disease; conversely, normal levels of inflammatory markers argue strongly against this diagnosis.
- Other laboratory findings that support diagnosis include sterile pyuria, elevation of serum transaminase levels, cerebrospinal fluid pleocytosis, and increased N-terminal pro–brain natriuretic peptide levels.
- Thrombocytopenia, anemia, and hypoalbuminemia may be present during the acute phase; thrombocytosis develops during the second to third week of disease.
- White blood cell count may be normal to elevated, with a neutrophil predominance.
- Cardiac imaging with 2-dimensional echocardiography is recommended; other investigative modalities include multisection spiral computed tomography and coronary magnetic resonance angiography.
- Patients with fever for 5 days or longer and fewer than 4 principal features can have Kawasaki disease diagnosed when coronary artery disease is detected with 2-dimensional echocardiography or coronary angiography.

Treatment

- Treatment is most effective at decreasing risk of development of coronary artery aneurysms when administered within the first 10 days of the illness.
- Intravenous immunoglobulin (IVIG), 2 g/kg as a single infusion over 10 to 12 hours.
- Moderate-dose (30–50 mg/kg per day) or high-dose (80–100 mg/kg per day) aspirin (divided into 4 doses) during acute phase.
- After 14 days or minimum of 3 days of patient being afebrile, dose of aspirin reduced (3–5 mg/kg once daily); if no echocardiographic variations present, aspirin is discontinued when laboratory study results are appropriate (usually 4–6 weeks).

- Some recommend a second infusion of IVIG for those in whom it did not work the first time (or those with only transient improvement). Systemic steroids and infliximab are typically the next steps in the United States if 2 rounds of IVIG have failed. These treatments should be performed in consultation with a Kawasaki disease expert.
- Other options for refractory Kawasaki disease can be considered via consultation with an infectious diseases or Kawasaki disease expert and may include plasmapheresis, interleukin-1 inhibitors (anakinra and canakinumab), interleukin-6 inhibitors (tocilizumab), methotrexate, and the anti-CD20 monoclonal antibody rituximab.

Prognosis

- If the disease is untreated, 20% to 25% of patients develop coronary artery aneurysms; giant lesions entail the greatest risk of long-term morbidity.
- Prognosis in those with coronary artery aneurysms is variable, and patients require lifelong follow-up.
- Patients receiving a diagnosis when younger than 6 months or older than 9 years appear to have poorer outcomes.
- Patients with a history of Kawasaki disease may have a more adverse cardiovascular risk profile, predisposing them to premature atherosclerosis. Consultation with a Kawasaki disease specialist or center is recommended to determine optimal long-term cardiac monitoring and disease management.

When to Worry or Refer

- Referral to an experienced Kawasaki disease specialist or center should be considered for any patient presenting who has prolonged fever and clinical features that are on the diagnostic spectrum and for whom an alternative diagnosis cannot be confirmed.

Resources for Families

- American Academy of Pediatrics: HealthyChildren.org.
  https://www.healthychildren.org/kawasaki
- American Heart Association: Kawasaki disease.
  https://www.heart.org/en/health-topics/kawasaki-disease
- Kawasaki Disease Foundation: Provides information, including a pamphlet and newsletter, for patients and families.
  https://kdfoundation.org

CHAPTER 126

Langerhans Cell Histiocytosis

Introduction/Etiology/Epidemiology

- One of the histiocytoses, a group of disorders that share in common the atypical proliferation of histiocytes (a bone marrow progenitor cell). Langerhans cells are 1 type of histiocyte; others include dermal dendrocytes and macrophages.

- Langerhans cell histiocytosis (LCH) is the contemporary umbrella term for the disorder known in the past variably as histiocytosis X, eosinophilic granuloma, Letterer-Siwe disease, and Hand-Schüller-Christian disease; severities of presentation include unifocal, multifocal, and disseminated disease.

- LCH may occur at any age but has a peak incidence in children aged between 1 and 4 years.

- The exact pathogenesis remains unclear; proposed etiologies include infection, somatic variation, or immune dysregulation; somatic variations in the *BRAF V600E* gene have been identified in some patients with LCH; other reported variations include *MAP2K1, MAP3K1,* and *ARAF.*

- The neoplastic versus reactive nature of LCH continues to be debated.

Signs and Symptoms

- Multiple organ systems may be involved (the most important from the standpoint of prognosis are bone marrow, liver, spleen, and lung); skin and bone are the most common.

- Bone involvement presents as pain, with or without swelling, that affects (in order of decreasing frequency) the skull, long bones of the extremities, and flat bones (eg, pelvis, vertebrae, ribs); radiographs reveal unifocal or multifocal lytic lesions.

- Skin involvement presents with scaly red papules and plaques, with a predilection for the scalp, posterior ear folds (Figure 126.1), axillae, groin (especially inguinal folds) (Figure 126.2) and neck folds; at times, LCH may mimic seborrheic dermatitis (Figure 126.3), although other features listed in this chapter often help distinguish the conditions.
- Papules are often red to brown and may be accompanied by punctate erosions, crusting (Figure 126.4), and hemorrhage or petechiae (Figure 126.5); they may occasionally be lichenoid (flat-topped lesions).
- Crusted papules on the palms (Figure 126.6) and soles are common, as is lymphadenopathy.

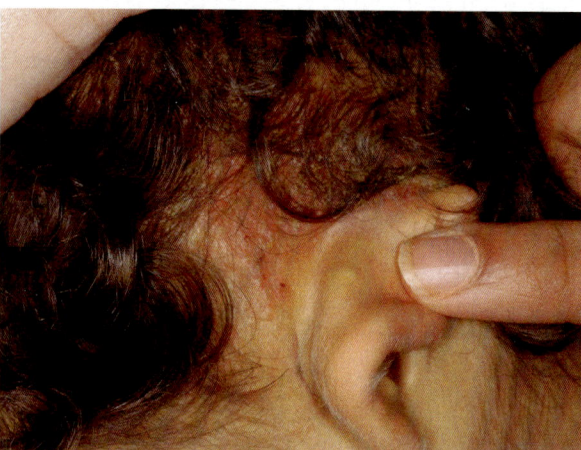

Figure 126.1. Erythema and scaling with some associated hemorrhage in the posterior auricular fold of a child with multisystem Langerhans cell histiocytosis.

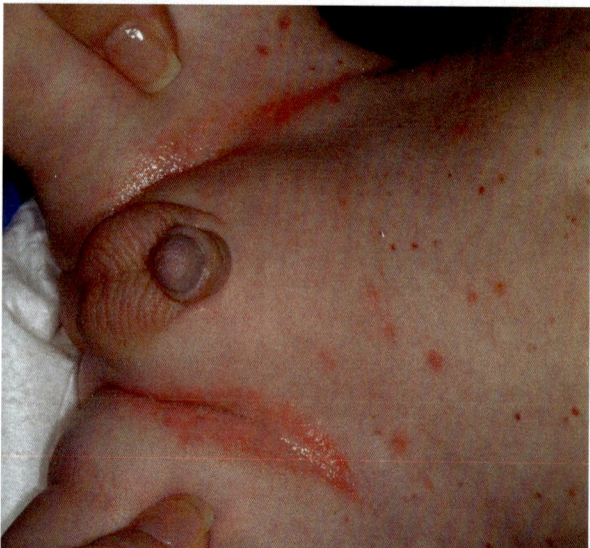

Figure 126.2. Erythema of the inguinal creases with scattered lichenoid, hemorrhagic papules.

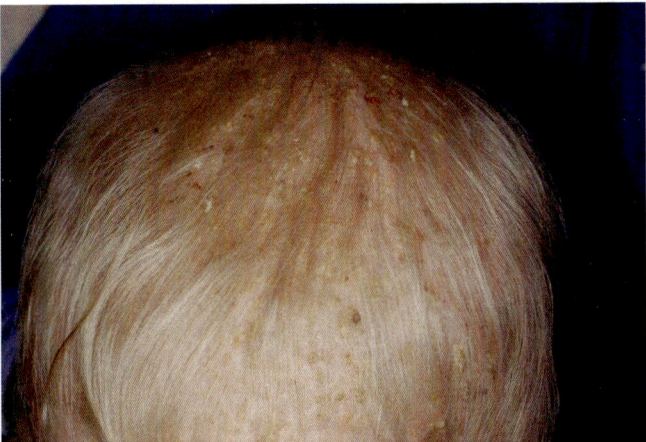

Figure 126.3. Greasy, scaly plaques (mimicking seborrheic dermatitis) admixed with hemorrhagic and crusted papules on the scalp of a 10-month-old with multisystem Langerhans cell histiocytosis.

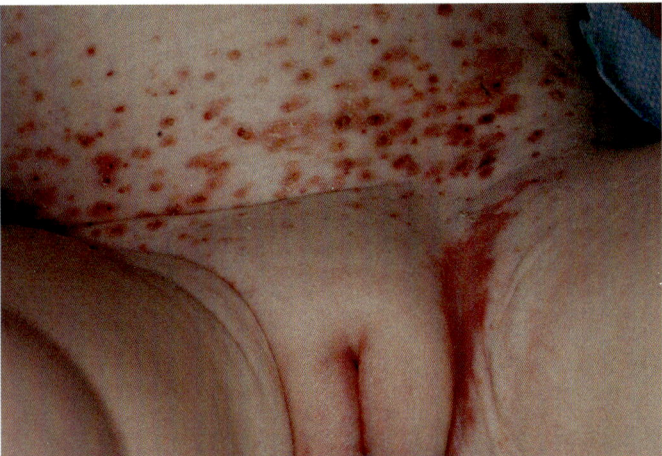

Figure 126.4. Eroded, crusted papules on the lower abdomen and suprapubic area; note the associated involvement of the inguinal crease.

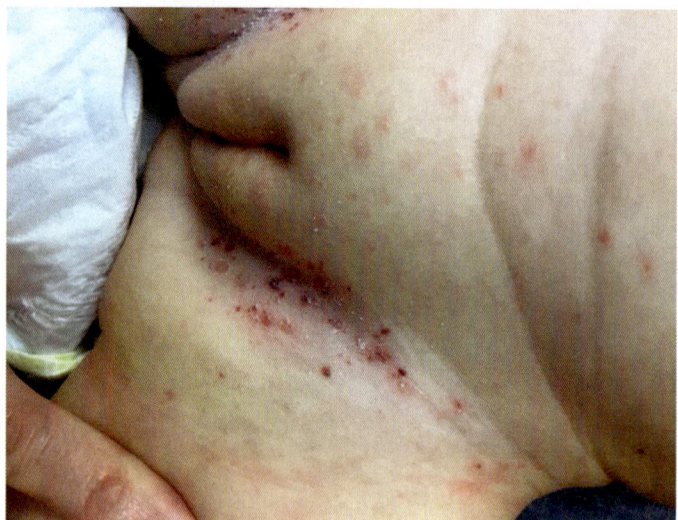

Figure 126.5. Langerhans cell histiocytosis. Hemorrhagic papules and erosions in the inguinal crease of a 10-month-old girl.

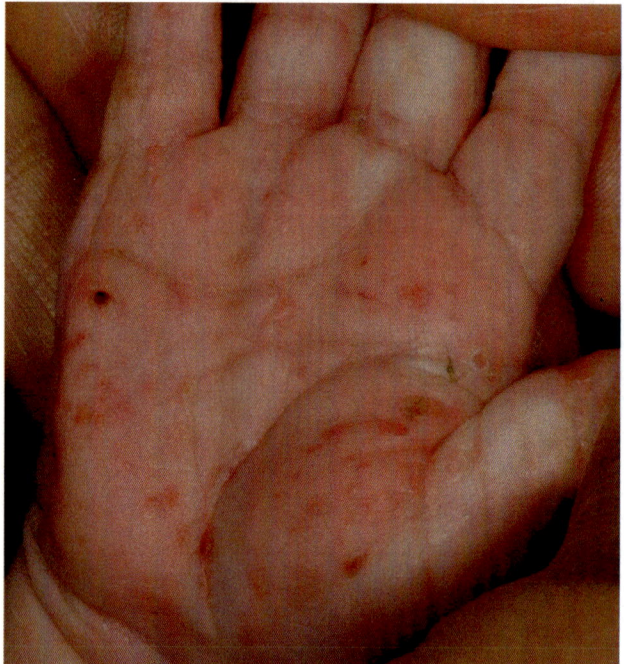

Figure 126.6. Scaly and hemorrhagic papules on the palm of this child with Langerhans cell histiocytosis, who was initially treated for presumed scabies infestation.

- In neonates with LCH, lesions may appear more vesicular or vesiculopustular and may mimic neonatal herpes or varicella; these vesicular lesions often become hemorrhagic or crusted.
- Mucosal involvement may include erosive gingivitis; hemorrhage; and, in infants, premature eruption of deciduous teeth (also known as natal teeth).
- Involvement of the external auditory canal may result in chronic otitis externa.
- Nail involvement may rarely be seen and may present as hemorrhage, pustules, paronychia, or nail plate changes (eg, grooves, pitting).
- The classic triad (formerly Hand-Schüller-Christian disease, now termed *multifocal LCH*) consists of skull lesions, diabetes insipidus (caused by posterior pituitary involvement), and exophthalmos.
- Aside from mucocutaneous and bone, other involvement may include lymph nodes, liver, spleen, lungs, gastrointestinal tract, thymus, and bone marrow; constitutional symptoms may include fever, malaise, anorexia, and weight loss.
- Central nervous system involvement may include hypothalamic-pituitary infiltration (diabetes insipidus is the most classic presentation), cranial nerve variations, ataxia, seizures, hydrocephalus, and neuropsychologic defects.

Look-alikes

Disorder	Differentiating Features
Seborrheic dermatitis	• Most often limited to scalp (cradle cap), face, umbilicus, or diaper region. • Lacks papules, erosions, crusting, and hemorrhage.
Scabies	• Burrows usually present. • Severe pruritus common. • Close contacts often report pruritus or skin lesions. • Mineral oil examination of skin lesion scrapings reveals mites, feces, and eggs.
Atopic dermatitis	• Diaper area spared. • Skin lesions more often plaques with lichenification, rather than papules. • In infants, involvement more likely to be on extensor surfaces (rather than flexural). • Lacks hemorrhage. • Other atopic disorders (eg, keratosis pilaris, ichthyosis vulgaris, allergic rhinoconjunctivitis, asthma, food allergies) or family history of such is often present.

(continued)

Look-alikes (continued)

Disorder	Differentiating Features
Intertrigo	• Although there is erythema in skinfolds, papules, crusting, and hemorrhage are usually absent. • When secondarily infected with yeast (ie, *Candida*), presents as beefy red color with peripheral satellite papules and pustules. • When secondarily infected with bacteria (eg, *Streptococcus pyogenes*, *Staphylococcus aureus*), erosive change may be present but is usually diffuse, rather than the punctate erosions seen in Langerhans cell histiocytosis.
Diaper dermatitis	• In irritant contact dermatitis, red patches involve lower abdomen, buttocks, and thighs with sparing of the inguinal folds. • Papules, crusting, erosions, and hemorrhage usually absent. • In diaper candidiasis, erythema may involve inguinal creases, but crusting, erosions, and hemorrhage are usually absent. • Satellite (peripheral to the primary erythema) papules and pustules may be noted when candidal infection present. • In Jacquet erosive diaper dermatitis, well-defined shallow ulcers or ulcerated nodules are present but most often limited to the perianal region.

How to Make the Diagnosis

▶ Skin biopsy reveals typical histologic changes of a Langerhans cell infiltrate into the epidermis and dermis.

▶ Diagnostic confirmation is achieved with positive immunostaining with S100, CD1a, or langerin.

▶ Electron microscopy (rarely used in the current era) reveals a characteristic organelle, Birbeck granules, within Langerhans cells.

▶ Other recommended evaluations may include complete blood cell count, hepatic function testing, coagulation studies, inflammatory markers, urine osmolality, radiographic skeletal survey, and chest radiography; more specific studies are performed as clinically indicated.

Treatment

▶ Therapy depends on the extent of disease.

▶ With skin-limited LCH, observation alone is often appropriate; when severe, however, therapies for more extensive involvement are often used.

▶ Unifocal bone lesions may be treated with observation, curettage, excision, or intralesional steroid injection.

- Multifocal and multisystem disease (as well as unifocal lesions in some special sites) requires systemic therapy; first-line treatment includes vinblastine, etoposide, and prednisone.
- Second-line therapies include clofarabine, cytarabine, cyclosporine A, and cladribine (2-chlorodeoxyadenosine).
- Bone marrow or cord blood transplant is occasionally indicated; targeted therapies (ie, *BRAF* and *MEK* inhibitors) are an area of active study.

Prognosis

- Prognosis for LCH depends on extent of involvement, degree of organ dysfunction, and initial response to therapy.
- Delayed sequelae may include skeletal defects, dental issues, growth failure and other endocrinopathies (most often diabetes insipidus), hearing loss, and neurodegenerative central nervous system dysfunction.

When to Worry or Refer

- If the diagnosis of cutaneous LCH is being considered, the patient should be referred to a pediatric dermatologist for evaluation and skin biopsy or other specialist (eg, orthopedic surgeon, oncologist) as applicable.
- A pediatric oncologist performs treatment and long-term follow-up in patients with LCH.

Resources for Families

- Histiocytosis Association: Langerhans cell histiocytosis in children. **www.histio.org/lchinchildren**
- MedlinePlus: Information for patients and families sponsored by the US National Library of Medicine and National Institutes of Health. **https://medlineplus.gov/genetics/condition/langerhans-cell-histiocytosis/**
- National Organization for Rare Disorders: Langerhans cell histiocytosis. **https://rarediseases.org/rare-diseases/langerhans-cell-histiocytosis/**

CHAPTER 127

Lichen Sclerosus et Atrophicus (LSA)

Introduction/Etiology/Epidemiology

- Uncommon chronic inflammatory disease of unknown cause that most frequently involves the anogenital region.
- More common in female patients (approximately 8:1), especially prepubertal and postmenopausal female patients (5%–15% of cases occur in children).
- Approximately 70% of prepubertal cases begin before age 7 years.
- Overall prevalence estimated at 1 in 900 female patients.

Signs and Symptoms

- Presents as small, pink to white, minimally raised macules and papules that coalesce into patches and plaques with eventual atrophy and small follicular plugs of the surface.
- Anogenital involvement presents as shiny, pink to ivory-colored, hypopigmented atrophic plaques of the vulvar or perianal region in female patients with a figure 8 or hourglass distribution (ie, affected area surrounds the vulva, perineum, and anus) (Figures 127.1 and 127.2).
  - Associated pruritus (50%) or discomfort of genital region and painful urination or defecation often present. Excoriations may be present. Painful defecation may lead to constipation.
  - Erythema with bullae (occasionally hemorrhagic) may be present before hypopigmentation and atrophy are seen; wrinkling is another clinical feature that may be present.
  - Older or inactive lesions often appear hypo- and/or hyperpigmented.
  - Other symptoms may include pain with urination, bleeding, and vaginal discharge.

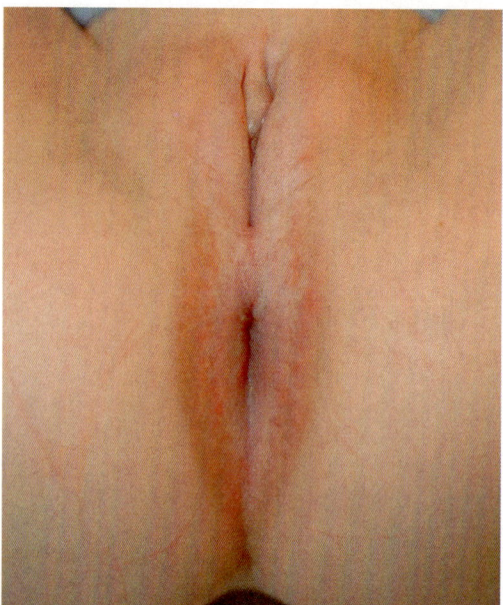

Figure 127.1. Circumferential hypopigmented atrophic patches in a figure 8 configuration characteristic of lichen sclerosus.

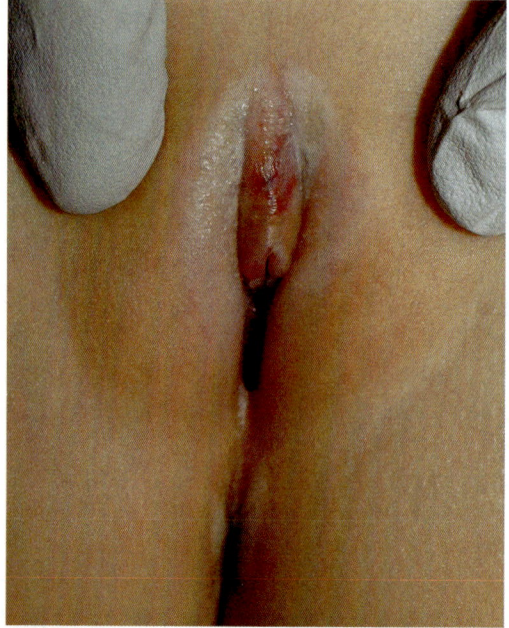

Figure 127.2. Characteristic shiny, hypopigmented, atrophic plaques of the vulvar region with associated ecchymosis.

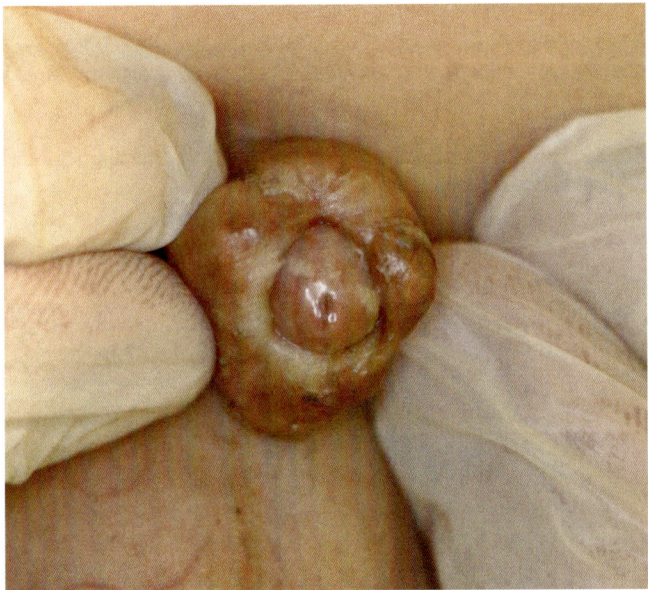

Figure 127.3. Balanitis xerotica obliterans. This 9-year-old with buried penis and phimosis presented with pain, adhesions, and hypo- and hyperpigmentation of the glans penis and foreskin.

- In male patients, the prepuce becomes sclerotic and difficult to retract (phimosis); the glans may appear shiny and blue-white in color (Figure 127.3).
  - Involvement in male patients has been termed *balanitis xerotica obliterans*.
  - Unlike in female patients, lichen sclerosus et atrophicus (LSA) in male patients almost always spares the perianal region, and there is rarely involvement of the penile shaft or scrotum.
  - Male patients may experience purpura and hemorrhagic bullae after the trauma of intercourse or masturbation.
  - Many male patients with balanitis xerotica obliterans receive a diagnosis after undergoing circumcision for recurrent phimosis and finding the characteristic histopathologic features at pathologic examination.
- Genital LSA may have associated fissures, erosions, hemorrhagic bullae, or purpura of the affected skin; these lesions may be predominant in many female patients, often involving the labia minora and clitoral hood.
- Long-standing LSA can lead to scarring and architectural changes within the anogenital region (in female patients) and phimosis (in male patients).
- Extragenital LSA usually is asymptomatic and most commonly occurs in the inframammary region, shoulders, back, neck, and flexural extremities.

Look-alikes

Disorder	Differentiating Features
Erosive lichen planus	• Typical extragenital lesions present (purple, polygonal, flat-topped papules). • White, reticulated patches often present on buccal mucosae (Wickham striae). • May involve vagina. • Less commonly seen in children than lichen sclerosus et atrophicus (LSA).
Cicatricial pemphigoid	• Rare in children; an autoimmune blistering disorder. • Usually blisters/erosions of mucosal surfaces of eyes, mouth. • Distinct histologic findings (subepidermal bullae).
Childhood sexual abuse	• Ivory/shiny atrophic plaques in figure 8 distribution are usually not observed. • May see other physical evidence of physical/sexual abuse. • May have similar findings of purpura, telangiectasias. • Possible to have coexistent LSA and abuse.
Psoriasis	• Well-demarcated erythematous plaques with predilection for intergluteal and hair-bearing regions (may have postinflammatory hypopigmentation after treatment). • Presence of characteristic nongenital lesions (erythematous scaling papules and plaques) or nail changes. • Frequently associated with positive family history.
Vitiligo	• Occasionally confused with the hypopigmentation of lichen sclerosus. • Lacks the atrophy, wrinkling, bullae, hemorrhage. • Vitiligo is usually depigmented (versus the hypopigmentation of LSA); can sometimes be verified with a Wood lamp examination. • Depigmented patches in other sites (especially periorbital and over bony prominences) often present.
Irritant dermatitis or vulvovaginitis	• Severe pruritus often present. • Lack of hypopigmentation, atrophy, bullae, hemorrhage. • Usually no pain with defecation. • Irritant exposure may be elicited by history (eg, bubble baths, harsh soaps).
Pinworm infestation	• Nighttime/early morning perianal, vaginal itching. • Eggs may be identified at microscopic examination of debris collected with tape ("tape test"). • Flashlight examination of perianal region may reveal worms, which appear small, white, and threadlike.

How to Make the Diagnosis

- The diagnosis is usually straightforward based on clinical examination.
- If clinical diagnosis is uncertain, a skin biopsy may be helpful for confirmation (rarely necessary).
- Characteristic histologic findings include thinned epidermis, interface dermatitis, and dermal sclerosis.

Treatment

- There is no known cure for LSA.
- First-line treatment usually includes medium- to high-potency topical corticosteroid; many clinicians treat initially or during disease flares with ultra-potent topical steroid (group 1; see Chapter 3) for several weeks and then gradually taper frequency of medication use or potency of topical steroid as condition improves.
- Generous use of barrier protection, such as zinc oxide–containing products or petrolatum-based emollients, may improve symptoms of pruritus as well as pain with urination or defecation.
- Avoid fragrance-containing soaps, bubble baths, or skin care products.
- Topical calcineurin inhibitors (eg, tacrolimus ointment, pimecrolimus cream) have been proven effective in the initial treatment of LSA and often are used to maintain remission after initial therapy with a topical corticosteroid.
- Topical testosterone or estrogen products were used frequently in the past; however, untoward side effects make them less desirable in children.

Treating Associated Conditions

- Secondary bacterial or candidal infections must be recognized and treated, as indicated. Maintain a high index of suspicion during disease flares and obtain skin cultures for confirmation.
- Surgical intervention may rarely be necessary to correct narrowing of introitus or reverse burying of clitoris. Male patients may require circumcision if they develop significant phimosis.

Prognosis

- Data are conflicting on the spontaneous involution rate of pediatric LSA at puberty.
- Relapses are common, and retreatment with more potent topical preparations may be necessary.
- Increased risk of squamous cell carcinoma, as documented in adult cases, not established in pediatric disease.

When to Worry or Refer

- Consider referral to a pediatric dermatologist for confirmation of diagnosis or management of the condition.
- Consider referral to a child abuse specialist for full evaluation if any clinical suspicion of abuse is present.

Resources for Families

- Genetic and Rare Diseases Information Center: Lichen sclerosus.
  https://rarediseases.info.nih.gov/diseases/6905/lichen-sclerosus
- Lichen Sclerosus Support Network.
  https://lssupportnetwork.org
- Society for Pediatric Dermatology: Patient Handout.
  https://pedsderm.net/site/assets/files/1028/40_spd_lichen_sclerosus_web_v1.pdf
- WebMD: Information for families is contained in Skin Problems and Treatments.
  www.webmd.com/skin-problems-and-treatments/lichen-sclerosus

CHAPTER 128

Polymorphous Light Eruption

Introduction/Etiology/Epidemiology

- Polymorphous light eruption (PMLE) is the most common type of photodermatitis in children; it is estimated to occur in 5% to 15% of the population.
- Occurs more often in individuals who are fair skinned but may occur in all skin types; it occurs more commonly in female than in male patients (4:1).
- Usually presents in the second or third decade after birth; however, 20% of patients present in childhood.
- Occasionally referred to as *sun poisoning* or *sun allergy,* the exact etiology of PMLE remains unclear; it is believed to be an immune-mediated delayed hypersensitivity reaction to UV radiation (290–480 nm wavelength).
- Genetic factors may play a role, and an autosomal dominant form has been described.

Signs and Symptoms

- The skin lesions are polymorphous or variable in appearance, as the name suggests; however, the appearance tends to be quite monomorphous in individual patients.
- Characteristic findings include small papules or vesicles, urticarial plaques (Figure 128.1), and eczematous eruptions; in some patients, the appearance may mimic erythema multiforme.
- The most commonly involved areas include the face (most prominent), lateral aspects of the neck, and sun-exposed areas of the hands and arms.
- The lesions of PMLE tend to be quite pruritic; they typically appear 24 to 48 hours after sun exposure and last for 1 to 2 weeks.
- PMLE is most common in the spring and early summer and often improves

over the summer months (the phenomenon of hardening from continued UV exposure); it tends to recur yearly in the spring and early summer in individuals who are affected.

▶ Juvenile spring eruption may be a subtype of PMLE and is characterized by self-limited recurrent outbreaks of papules and papulovesicles, usually localized to the sun-exposed areas of the helices (Figure 128.2); it is seen primarily in young boys, especially those with short hair and larger or protruding ears.

▶ Juvenile spring eruption recurs in the spring and early summer, although there are reports of the disorder in the cold winter months as well.

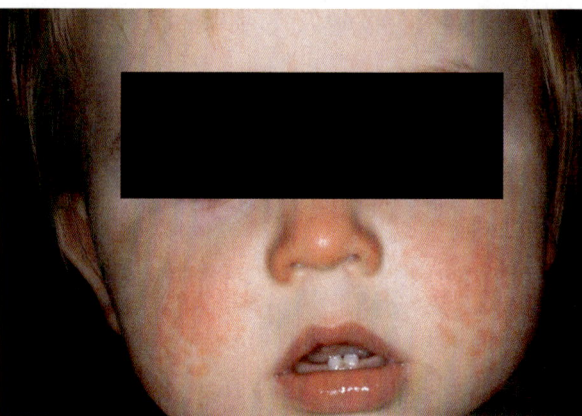

Figure 128.1. Polymorphous light eruption. Urticarial papules and plaques in a toddler after intense sun exposure.

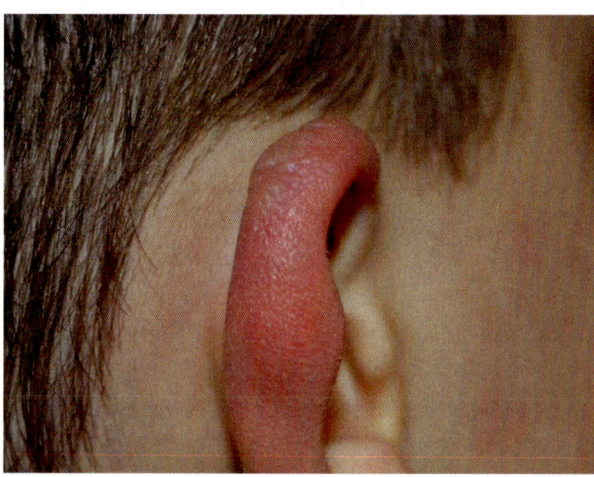

Figure 128.2. Juvenile spring eruption. Erythema of the superior helix with multiple vesicles in a 4-year-old after the first significant sun exposure of the spring.

Look-alikes

Disorder	Differentiating Features
Systemic lupus erythematosus	• Malar or butterfly eruption (involves cheeks and, classically, the nasal bridge). • May have other characteristic skin findings, including discoid lesions, oral ulcerations, livedo reticularis, bright red to purple papules and plaques on the dorsal aspect of the hands (often sparing the areas over joints), or panniculitis (inflammation of the fat). • Arthritis, fever, malaise may be present. • Other extra-cutaneous targets include the hematologic system, lungs, heart, kidneys, and central nervous system. • Positive serological study results, elevated inflammatory marker levels, and decreased complement levels may help distinguish systemic lupus erythematosus from polymorphous light eruption.
Solar urticaria	• Redness and itching of the skin occurs during or within 30 minutes of sun exposure. • Initial reaction is followed by urticarial lesions in areas of sun exposure. • Lesions typically resolve within hours. • Rare in children; usually presents in third or fourth decade after birth.
Actinic prurigo	• Most often affects Indio and Mestizo populations of Mexico and Central and South America. • Red, itchy papules and plaques of the face and arms, but legs, knees, and sun-protected sites (eg, buttocks) may also be involved. • Oral and ocular mucosae are commonly involved; individuals who are affected often have associated conjunctivitis, photophobia, or cheilitis. • Excoriations and scarring may be present. • More likely than polymorphous light eruption to persist into winter months.
Hydroa vacciniforme	• Very rare condition; usually beginning in childhood. • Eruption characterized by edematous papules, vesicles, or bullae that occur hours to days after sun exposure and last for several days. • Heals with characteristic varioliform scarring.

Juvenile dermatomyositis	• Characteristic skin findings include the following:
	  – Pink to violet discoloration of the eyelids (heliotrope).
	  – Pink to red macules or papules overlying knuckles, especially proximal interphalangeal and metacarpophalangeal joints (Gottron sign or papules).
	  – Dilated capillaries of the proximal nail folds (may need magnification to see).
	  – Calcium deposits over joints (knees, elbows) known as calcinosis cutis.
	• Less common skin findings may include lipoatrophy, poikiloderma (ie, hyperpigmentation, hypopigmentation, telangiectasias, and atrophy), ulcerations.
	• Patients often present with fatigue and loss of energy.
	• Usually associated with proximal muscle weakness (muscle enzyme levels often elevated); may have associated dysphagia, dysphonia, choking, nasal speech.

How to Make the Diagnosis

- PMLE is usually diagnosed based on clinical features and timing of skin eruption.
- Diagnosis can be confirmed with phototesting, if necessary.
- Because clinical features of PMLE may be indistinguishable from lupus erythematosus, serological testing should be considered.
- Skin biopsy is usually not helpful because the histologic features are nonspecific and depend on the clinical morphology of the lesion on which the biopsy is performed.

Treatment

- Treatment of PMLE is largely aimed at prevention.
- Sun protection measures should include broad-spectrum sunscreen (with good UV-A protection; SPF) and sun protection clothing, as well as avoidance of significant midday sun exposure.
- Severe cases may benefit from oral hydroxychloroquine therapy.
- Use of UV therapy (usually narrowband UV-B or psoralen plus UV-A) 2 to 3 times weekly for several weeks may help to harden or desensitize the skin.
- Use of oral beta-carotene may be helpful in some patients.
- Topical or, rarely, systemic steroids may help treat the acute eruption and relieve associated symptoms.

Prognosis

- The condition tends to recur each spring and early summer; in some patients, PMLE may improve or even resolve over time.
- Although the condition may significantly affect quality of life, PMLE is not associated with any significant long-term morbidity or mortality.

When to Worry or Refer

- Consider referral to a pediatric dermatologist or rheumatologist if there are concerns about potential lupus erythematosus.
- Consider referral to a pediatric dermatologist for confirmation of diagnosis or management.

Resources for Families

- British Association of Dermatologists: Patient information leaflet on polymorphic light eruption.
  https://www.bad.org.uk/pils/polymorphic-light-eruption/
- Skin Cancer Foundation: Information on sun protection measures.
  https://www.skincancer.org/skin-cancer-prevention/sun-protection

Chapter 129

Confluent and Reticulated Papillomatosis (CARP)

Introduction/Etiology/Epidemiology

- Confluent and reticulated papillomatosis (CARP; also known as Gougerot-Carteaud syndrome) is an uncommon disorder of unknown cause.
  - In the past it has been linked to insulin resistance, disordered keratinization, UV light, and an abnormal host response to the yeast *Malassezia furfur.*
  - Some have suggested that CARP may be the result of follicular infection with *Dietzia papillomatosis,* a gram-positive bacterium. This association is intriguing because the organism implicated appears to be sensitive to tetracyclines and erythromycin.
- CARP typically has its onset during puberty, and girls are affected more often than boys.
- Most often, CARP occurs sporadically, but familial cases have been reported.

Signs and Symptoms

- CARP presents as hyperpigmented patches and thin papules and plaques, most often involving the intermammary region, epigastrium, and upper back. The face, neck, and shoulders occasionally are involved.
- Papules coalesce becoming confluent centrally and reticulated peripherally (Figures 129.1 and 129.2).
- The eruption usually is asymptomatic, but mild pruritus may be present.

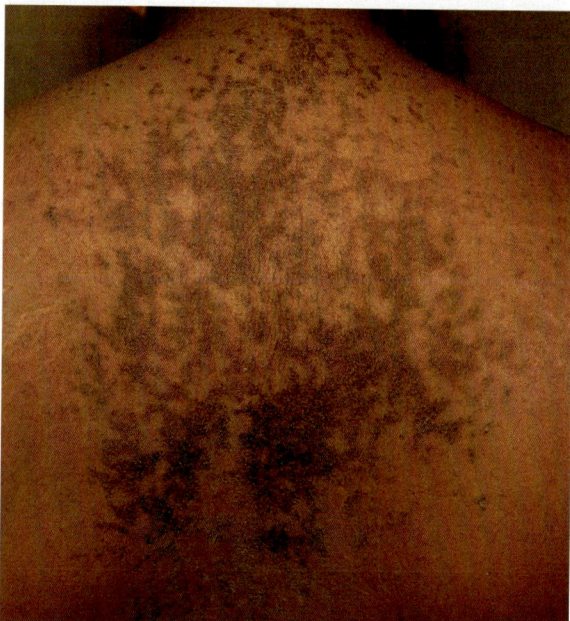

Figure 129.1. The eruption of confluent and reticulated papillomatosis is confluent centrally and reticulated peripherally.

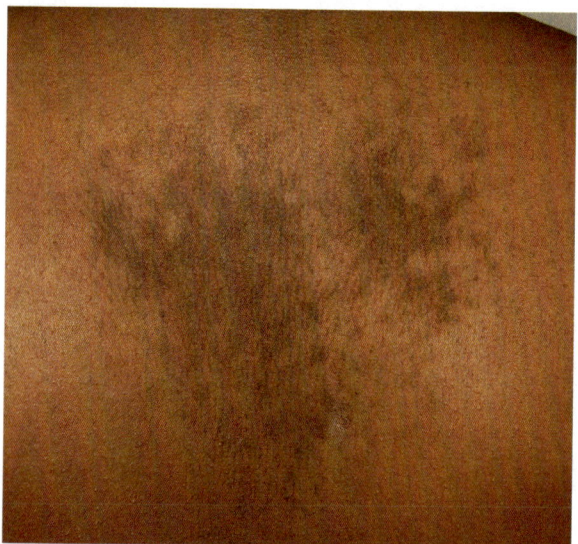

Figure 129.2. Confluent and reticulated papillomatosis often affects the upper back. In this patient, there are 2 distinct patches (left larger than right) that are confluent centrally and reticulated peripherally.

Look-alikes

Several eruptions are concentrated on the trunk and may mimic CARP. The majority of these do not typically have central confluence and peripheral reticulation.

Disorder	Differentiating Features
Acanthosis nigricans	• Velvety thickening of the skin often located at the nape or sides of the neck and in the axillae. • Considered a marker for insulin resistance.
Tinea versicolor (hyperpigmented form)	• Lesions are hyperpigmented scaling macules that often coalesce into patches. • Reticulated appearance absent.
Pityriasis rosea	• Typical lesions are thin oval plaques with long axes oriented parallel to lines of skin stress. • Initial larger lesion (herald patch) presents before the secondary smaller lesions. • Reticulated appearance absent.
Pityriasis lichenoides chronica	• Rash more generalized (not limited to the trunk). • Involvement of the buttocks is common. • Surface scaling with thin crusts common. • Reticulated appearance absent.
Prurigo pigmentosa	• Recurrent crops of pruritic erythematous papules and reticulate hyperpigmentation. • Similar distribution with preference for neck, chest, and back. • Most common in young Asian women. • Typically reported in association with ketosis (and conditions such as fasting, diabetes, ketogenic diets). • Treated with dietary modification and systemic antibiotics.

How to Make the Diagnosis

▶ The diagnosis is made clinically on the basis of the typical appearance and distribution of the rash.

Treatment

▶ Treating CARP may be challenging because no treatment is universally effective and the eruption may recur after withdrawal of treatment.

▶ Treatment with minocycline (or doxycycline) orally for 1 to 2 months is considered the most effective option. Some clinicians recommend adding a topical emollient containing α-hydroxy acids (most commonly lactic acid or ammonium lactate) to the treatment regimen.

- Other treatments that have variable efficacy include topical selenium sulfide, topical or oral antifungal agents, and topical keratolytics alone.

Prognosis

- The prognosis generally is good, although no treatment is universally effective, and recurrences are possible.

When to Worry or Refer

- Consider referral to a dermatologist when the diagnosis is in doubt or when disease does not respond to treatment.

CHAPTER
130

Hyperhidrosis

Introduction/Etiology/Epidemiology

- ▶ Hyperhidrosis (ie, excessive sweating) is characterized by the secretion of sweat that is greater than what is typically needed for thermoregulation.
- ▶ Primary hyperhidrosis is idiopathic and chronic. It usually presents between 14 and 25 years of age and can be familial.
- ▶ Focal, primary hyperhidrosis is usually palmoplantar and/or axillary. Sweating tends to be bilateral and symmetric; involvement is rarely generalized.
- ▶ The face, scalp, inguinal folds, and inframammary regions can also be involved.
  - Heat and emotional stimuli can make sweating worse.
  - Quality of life and mood can be affected depending on the severity and individual.

Signs and Symptoms

- ▶ Moist skin or visible droplets of sweat may be seen at examination (Figures 130.1 and 130.2).
- ▶ There may be erythema, unpleasant odor, or skin maceration in involved regions.
- ▶ Patients may keep hands in pockets, keep wiping hands on their pants, or wear layers of clothing to avoid sweat being visible.

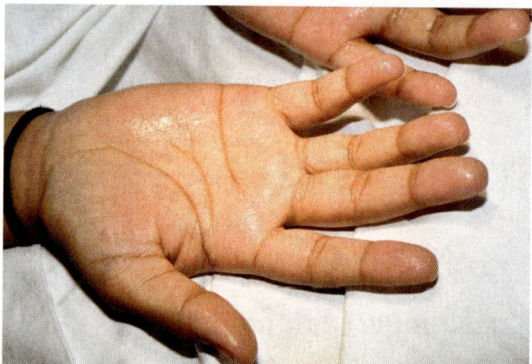

Figure 130.1. Excessive palmar and fingertip sweating in a teenager with hyperhidrosis.

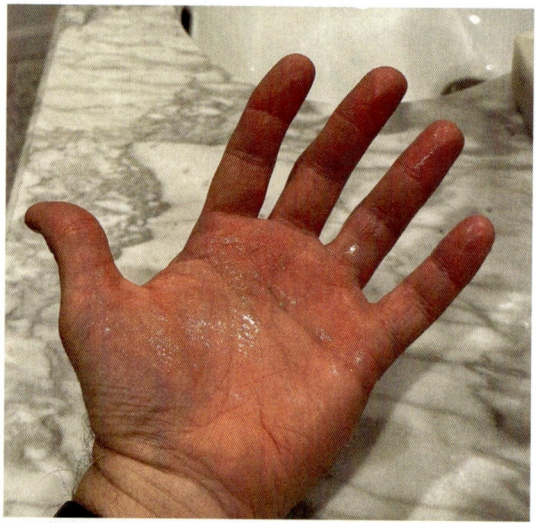

Figure 130.2. Palmar hyperhidrosis. Note the excessive sweating of the palm and fingers.

Look-alikes (secondary forms of hyperhidrosis)

Disorder	Differentiating Features
Drug-induced hyperhidrosis (cholinergic agonists, antidepressants, sympathomimetics, hypoglycemic agents, others)	• Generalized sweating that may also include component of flushing. • Commencement of sweating when medication was started.
Malignancy (lymphoma, solid tumors)	• Generalized sweating. • Fever, enlarged lymph nodes, unintentional weight loss.
Infection (tuberculosis, HIV, malaria, tick-borne illnesses, bacterial, others)	• Generalized sweating. • History of infected contacts or risk factors for infection. • Fever, weight loss, cough may be present.
Endocrine disorders (carcinoid syndrome, insulinoma, pheochromocytoma, hyperthyroidism)	• Generalized sweating, usually with flushing. • Tachycardia, weight changes, diarrhea, wheezing. • Sweating may occur when asleep.
Neurologic (spinal cord injury and syringomyelia)	• Localized or generalized sweating, usually with flushing. • Fever, muscle spasticity, bowel/urinary continence dysfunction, changes in blood pressure.

How to Make the Diagnosis

▶ The history and physical examination are typically sufficient to make the diagnosis of primary idiopathic hyperhidrosis.

▶ Further investigations should be considered if there are clinical concerns for an underlying associated disorder.

▶ Generalized hyperhidrosis warrants special attention.

Treatment

▶ First-line treatments.
  - Topical antiperspirants such as aluminum chloride, aluminum sesquichlorohydrate, or formaldehyde typically are considered first-line agents for focal hyperhidrosis.
  - Glycopyrrolate wipes are available and may be effective, but cost may be a limiting factor. May cause blurry vision if product gets into eye.

- Oral anticholinergics such as glycopyrrolate and oxybutynin may be useful if other therapies fail or hyperhidrosis is more severe; adverse effects of these medications may limit their use (including, for example, dry mouth, tachycardia).
- Tap water iontophoresis may be useful for recalcitrant hyperhidrosis that does not respond to other therapies (hands, axilla, feet).

▶ Other treatments.
- Botulinum toxin A or B injections to the affected areas.
- Rarely, other systemic agents such as oral clonidine, benzodiazepines, and calcium channel blockers.
- Thoracic sympathectomy is rarely recommended as a last resort for severe, debilitating cases (and may be complicated by postoperative compensatory hyperhidrosis).
- Microwave technology can be used to treat axillary hyperhidrosis, but it is not approved in children.

Prognosis

▶ Hyperhidrosis is a chronic condition. In addition to the treatments mentioned herein, referral to a mental health professional may be helpful in more severe cases.

When to Worry or Refer

▶ Refer to a dermatologist when hyperhidrosis is severe, unresponsive to first-line therapies, and/or affecting daily activities or quality of life.

Resources for Families

▶ International Hyperhidrosis Society.
https://www.sweathelp.org

▶ Society for Pediatric Dermatology: Patient handout on hyperhidrosis.
https://pedsderm.net/for-patients-families/patient-handouts/#Hyperhidrosis

INDEX

Italicized page numbers indicate a figure or table.

A

Abametapir, 312
ABCDE criteria, 475, 485
Abscesses, 4
    compared to tinea capitis, 274
Acanthosis nigricans
    compared to confluent and reticulated papillomatosis (CARP), 851
    compared to lichenification, 469
    compared to postinflammatory hyperpigmentation, 469
    diagnosis, 469
    introduction/etiology/epidemiology, 467
    prognosis, 470
    resources, 470
    signs and symptoms, 467–469, *468*
    treatment, 469
    when to worry or refer, 470
ACC. *See* Aplasia cutis congenita (ACC)
ACD. *See* Allergic contact dermatitis (ACD)
Acne
    acne vulgaris, 67–78
    compared to folliculitis/furunculosis/carbunculosis, 188
    compared to tuberous sclerosis complex (TSC), 595
    with darker skin tones, *11*
    distribution of lesions, 6
    neonatal and infantile, 79–82
Acne rosacea, compared to acne vulgaris, 70
Acne vulgaris
    compared to acne rosacea, 70
    compared to angiofibromas, 70
    compared to flat warts, 70
    compared to gram-negative folliculitis, 70
    compared to keratosis pilaris, 70
    compared to *Malassezia* folliculitis, 70
    compared to miliaria rubra, 70
    compared to molluscum contagiosum, 70
    compared to periorificial dermatitis, 70, 85
    compared to steroid acne, 70
    diagnosis, 71
    factors that exacerbate, 68
    introduction/etiology/epidemiology, 67
    multifactorial pathogenesis, 67–68
    pathophysiology, 67
    periorificial dermatitis, 85
    prognosis, 77
    resources, 78
    signs and symptoms, 68–70
    treatment, *71–73, 71–76, 74, 77*
    when to worry or refer, 77
Acquired epidermolysis bullosa
    compared to childhood dermatitis herpetiformis, 548
    compared to epidermolysis bullosa (EB), 557
    compared to linear immunoglobulin A dermatosis, 564
Acquired melanocytic nevi
    compared to café au lait macules, 474
    compared to ephelides, 474
    compared to lentigines, 474
    diagnosis, 474
    introduction/etiology/epidemiology, 471
    prognosis, 475
    resources, 476
    signs and symptoms, 471–474, *472–473*
    treating associated conditions, 474
    treatment, 474
    when to worry or refer, 475
Acrocyanosis, compared to pernio/chilblains, 414
Acrodermatitis chronica atrophicans, compared to morphea, 771
Acrodermatitis enteropathica (AE), 5
    compared to atopic dermatitis, 798
    compared to candidal diaper dermatitis, 252
    compared to crusted impetigo, 798
    compared to irritant diaper dermatitis, 798
    compared to kwashiorkor, 804
    compared to psoriasis, 798
    compared to seborrheic dermatitis, 798
    diagnosis, 798
    diaper dermatitis, *665–666*
    introduction/etiology/epidemiology, 795
    prognosis, 800
    resources, 800
    signs and symptoms, 795–798, *796–797*
    treatment, *799, 799*
    when to worry or refer, 800

Acropustulosis of infancy, compared to
    scabies, 328
Actinic prurigo, compared to polymorphous
    light eruption (PMLE), 845
Acute febrile mucocutaneous lymph node
    syndrome. *See* Kawasaki
    disease
Acute generalized exanthematous pustulosis,
    compared to toxic epidermal
    necrolysis (TEN), 739
Acute hemorrhagic edema of infancy,
    compared to Henoch-
    Schönlein purpura (HSP),
    818
Acute paronychia
    compared to blistering distal dactylitis,
        175, 178
    compared to chronic paronychia, 175,
        256
    compared to felon, 175
    compared to herpes simplex virus
        infection, 175
    compared to psoriasis, 175
    compared to trauma, 175
    diagnosis, 175
    introduction/etiology/epidemiology,
        173
    prognosis, 176
    resources, 176
    signs and symptoms, 173–175, *174*
    treatment, 176
    when to worry or refer, 176
Acyclovir, 102
Adams-Oliver syndrome, 387, 649
Addison disease, compared to melanonychia
    striata, 499
Adverse effects
    moisturizers, 26
    topical corticosteroids, 24
AE. *See* Acrodermatitis enteropathica (AE)
Albinism
    compared to piebaldism, 443
    compared to vitiligo, 443
    compared to Waardenburg syndrome,
        443
    diagnosis, 443
    introduction/etiology/epidemiology, 441
    prognosis, 444
    resources, 444
    signs and symptoms, 441–443, *442*
    treating associated conditions, 444
    treatment, 443
    when to worry or refer, 444
Alclometasone dipropionate, *22*

Allergic contact dermatitis (ACD). *See also*
    Irritant contact dermatitis
    arrangement of lesions, 7, *7*
    compared to asteatotic eczema, 50
    compared to atopic dermatitis, 57
    compared to cercarial dermatitis, 335
    compared to cutaneous larva migrans,
        307
    compared to hand, foot, and mouth
        disease (HFMD), 138
    compared to herpes simplex, 95
    compared to herpes zoster, 57, 101
    compared to irritant contact dermatitis,
        57
    compared to juvenile dermatomyositis
        (JDM), 757
    compared to periorificial dermatitis, 85
    compared to seborrheic dermatitis, 57
    diagnosis, 57
    introduction/etiology/epidemiology, 53
    prognosis, 58
    resources, 59
    signs and symptoms, 53–57, *54–56*
    treatment, 58
    when to worry or refer, 58
Allylamine, 285, 289
Alopecia, 271
Alopecia areata
    compared to androgenetic alopecia, 610,
        617
    compared to loose anagen syndrome,
        610, 625
    compared to telogen effluvium, 610, 632
    compared to tinea capitis, 274, 610
    compared to traction alopecia, 610, 637
    compared to trichotillomania, 610, 644
    diagnosis, 611
    introduction/etiology/epidemiology, 605
    prognosis, 613
    resources, 613
    signs and symptoms, 605–610, *606,
        608–609*
    treating associated conditions, 612
    treatment, 611–612
    when to worry or refer, 613
Aluminum acetate solution, 102
Amcinonide, *21*
Amoxicillin, 228
Ampicillin, 214
Anabolic steroids and acne vulgaris, 68, 70
Analgesics, for herpes simplex, 97
Androgenetic alopecia
    compared to alopecia areata, 610, 617
    compared to scarring alopecia, 617

compared to telogen effluvium, 617
diagnosis, 617
introduction/etiology/epidemiology, 615
prognosis, 618
resources, 618
signs and symptoms, 615–617, *616*
treatment, 617
when to worry or refer, 618
Angiofibromas, compared to acne vulgaris, 70
Angioma serpiginosum, 421
diagnosis, 424
signs and symptoms, 422
treatment, 425
Angular cheilitis/perlèche
compared to contact dermatitis, 248
compared to lip-licking dermatitis, 248
compared to localized trauma, 248
compared to secondary syphilis, 248
diagnosis, 248, *248*
introduction/etiology/epidemiology, 247
prognosis, 249
resources, 249
signs and symptoms, *247*, 247–248
treating associated conditions, 249
treatment, 249
when to worry or refer, 249
Anhidrotic ectodermal dysplasia, 599, *600–601*
Annular arrangement of lesions, 7, *8*
Lyme disease, *206*
Anogenital warts, 114
Anthralin, 611
Antibiotics
for acne vulgaris, 74, *74*, 74–76
for acute paronychia, 176
for atopic dermatitis, 42
for blistering distal dactylitis, 179
for infantile acne, 82
for meningococcemia, 214
for periorificial dermatitis, 86
for pityriasis lichenoides, 357
for Rocky Mountain spotted fever (RMSF), 220
for toxic shock syndrome (TSS), 241
for varicella, 168
Anticholinergics, 856
Antifungals
for angular cheilitis/perlèche, 249
for tinea capitis, 276–277, *278*
for tinea corporis, 285
for tinea cruris, 289
for tinea pedis, 294
for tinea versicolor, 300

Antihistamines
for atopic dermatitis, 42
for cutaneous mastocytosis, 514
for Gianotti-Crosti syndrome, 130
for insect bites, 322
for urticaria, 746
Antiperspirants, 855
Antiphospholipid antibodies, 415, 787, 789
Antipruritics
for herpes zoster, 102
for insect bites, 322
Antivirals, for herpes zoster, 102
Aphthous stomatitis, compared to herpes simplex, 95
Aphthous ulcer
compared to herpangina, 138
compared to herpes simplex, 95
Aplasia cutis congenita (ACC)
compared to epidermolysis bullosa, 652
compared to herpes simplex virus infection, 652
compared to nevus sebaceus, 652, 687
compared to trauma from forceps, 652
compared to trauma from scalp electrode, 652
diagnosis, 652
introduction/etiology/epidemiology, 649
prognosis, 653
resources, 653
signs and symptoms, 649–652, *650–651*
treatment, 652
when to worry or refer, 653
Arcanobacterium haemolyticum infection, compared to scarlet fever, 227
ARCI. *See* Autosomal recessive congenital ichthyosis (ARCI)
Arteriovenous malformation
compared to infantile hemangioma, 400
signs and symptoms, 430, *430*
treatment, 433
Arthropod bite reaction. *See also* Insect bite reaction
compared to cercarial dermatitis, 335
compared to childhood dermatitis herpetiformis, 547
compared to cutaneous mastocytosis, 513
compared to erythema nodosum (EN), 811
compared to fixed drug eruption, 721
compared to Lyme disease, 207
compared to scabies, 328
Asteatotic eczema, 48, *49*
compared to nummular eczema, 50
treatment, 52

Ataxia-telangiectasia, 421
  diagnosis, 424
  prognosis, 425
  signs and symptoms, 422–423
  treatment, 425
Atopic dermatitis
  compared to acrodermatitis
    enteropathica (AE), 798
  compared to allergic contact dermatitis
    (ACD), 57
  compared to asteatotic eczema, 50
  compared to contact dermatitis, 39
  compared to juvenile dermatomyositis
    (JDM), 757
  compared to kwashiorkor, 804
  compared to Langerhans cell
    histiocytosis (LCH), 833
  compared to neonatal lupus
    erythematosus (NLE), 785
  compared to periorificial dermatitis, 85
  compared to pityriasis rubra pilaris
    (PRP), 375
  compared to psoriasis, 39
  compared to scabies, 39, 328
  compared to seborrheic dermatitis, 39,
    380
  compared to tinea corporis, 39
  daily measures, 40–41
  with darker skin tones, 10, *11–13*
  diagnosis, 40
  distribution of lesions, 6
  flares, 42, *43*
  infections due to, 42, *43*
  introduction/etiology/epidemiology, 33
  lichenification with, 9
  prognosis, 45
  resources, 46
  signs and symptoms, 33–38, *34–39*
  treating associated conditions, 45
  treatment, 40–45
  when to worry or refer, 46
Atrophy, 9
Atypical measles, 142
  compared to Rocky Mountain spotted
    fever (RMSF), 219
Atypical nevi, 473, *473*
Augmented betamethasone dipropionate, *21*
Auspitz sign, 370
Autoimmune blistering disorders, compared
    to hand, foot, and mouth
    disease (HFMD), 138
Autosomal recessive congenital ichthyosis
    (ARCI), 655
Azithromycin, 228

B

Bacillary angiomatosis, compared to eruptive
    pseudoangiomatosis, 138
Bacille Calmette-Guérin vaccination, 822
Bacteremias
  compared to meningococcemia, 213
  compared to Rocky Mountain spotted
    fever (RMSF), 219
Bacterial abscess, compared to tinea capitis,
    274
Bacterial folliculitis, compared to tinea
    capitis, 274
Balanoposthitis, 197, *198*
Barrier repair agents, 25–26
  atopic dermatitis, 44
Becker melanosis
  compared to congenital melanocytic nevi
    (CMN), 484
  compared to pigmentary mosaicism,
    hyperpigmented, 505
Bedbugs, 318–319, *319*, 323
Benign cephalic histiocytosis
  compared to flat warts, 115
  compared to periorificial dermatitis, 85
Benzodiazepines, 855
Benzoyl peroxide, 81–82
Berdazimer, 109
Betamethasone valerate, *21–22*
Biotin-dependent multiple carboxylase
    deficiency, 50
Blanching of lesions, 8
Blaschko lines, 502, *504*, 579
Blistering distal dactylitis
  compared to acute paronychia, 175, 178
  compared to bullous impetigo, 178
  compared to burn, 178
  compared to chronic paronychia, 256
  compared to epidermolysis bullosa, 178
  compared to hand, foot, and mouth
    disease, 178
  compared to herpes simplex, 95, 178
  diagnosis, 178
  introduction/etiology/epidemiology,
    177
  prognosis, 179
  resources, 179
  signs and symptoms, *177*, 177–178
  treatment, 179
  when to worry or refer, 179
Bloom syndrome, 480
  compared to neurofibromatosis (NF),
    587
Blue nevi, compared to congenital dermal
    melanocytosis, 494

Blue rubber bleb nevus syndrome, compared to vascular malformations, 435
Borrelia burgdorferi. *See* Lyme disease
Botulinum toxin, 855
Branchial cleft cyst, compared to pilomatricoma, 536
Brown recluse spider bite, compared to ecthyma, 183
Bruising
 from birth trauma, vascular malformations, 431
 compared to congenital dermal melanocytosis, 494
 compared to erythema nodosum (EN), 811
Bullae, 4, 5
 crusting of, 9
 hand, foot, and mouth disease (HFMD), *134*
 staphylococcal scalded skin syndrome (SSSS), 231, *232*
 tinea pedis, *292*
Bullous congenital ichthyosiform erythroderma, compared to epidermolysis bullosa (EB), 556
Bullous impetigo
 compared to blistering distal dactylitis, 178
 compared to cutaneous mastocytosis, 513
 compared to epidermolysis bullosa (EB), 556
 compared to erythema toxicum, 673
 compared to hand, foot, and mouth disease (HFMD), 138
 compared to herpes simplex, 95
 compared to insect bites, 321
 compared to irritant contact dermatitis, 50
 compared to linear immunoglobulin A dermatosis, 563
 compared to staphylococcal scalded skin syndrome (SSSS), 233
 diaper dermatitis, 660, 662
Bullous insect bite reaction. *See* Insect bite reaction
Bullous lupus erythematosus
 compared to childhood dermatitis herpetiformis, 547
 compared to linear immunoglobulin A dermatosis, 563
Bullous mastocytoma, compared to herpes simplex, 95

Bullous pemphigoid
 compared to childhood dermatitis herpetiformis, 547
 compared to epidermolysis bullosa (EB), 557
 compared to insect bites, 321
 compared to linear immunoglobulin A dermatosis, 563
Burns
 compared to blistering distal dactylitis, 178
 compared to herpes simplex, 95
 compared to staphylococcal scalded skin syndrome (SSSS), 233

C

Café au lait macules, *2*
 compared to acquired melanocytic nevi, 474
 compared to congenital melanocytic nevi (CMN), 479, 484
 compared to cutaneous mastocytosis, 513
 compared to ephelides, 479, 488
 compared to lentigines, 479, 491
 compared to neurofibromatosis (NF), 587
 compared to postinflammatory hyperpigmentation, 479
 diagnosis, 479
 introduction/etiology/epidemiology, 477
 prognosis, 480
 signs and symptoms, *477–478*, 477–479
 treating associated conditions, 479–480
 treatment, 479
 when to worry or refer, 480
Calcineurin inhibitors, 86
 for alopecia areata, 611
 for lichen sclerosus et atrophicus (LSA), 841
 for vitiligo, 462
Calcipotriene, 371, 773
Calcium channel blockers, 855
Callus, 115
Candida
 introduction/etiology/epidemiology, 245
 resources, 245
Candidal diaper dermatitis
 compared to acrodermatitis enteropathica, 252
 compared to intertrigo, 252, 678
 compared to irritant dermatitis, 252
 compared to Langerhans cell histiocytosis, 252
 compared to psoriasis, 252

Candidal diaper dermatitis, *continued*
   compared to seborrheic dermatitis, 252
   diagnosis, 252, *253*
   introduction/etiology/epidemiology, 251
   prognosis, 253
   resources, 258
   signs and symptoms, *251*, 251–252, *659, 661*
   treating associated conditions, 253
   treatment, 253
   when to worry or refer, 258
Candidiasis, 16, *17*
   acute paronychia and, 173
   angular cheilitis/perlèche and, 247
   compared to chronic paronychia, 256
   compared to erythema toxicum, 673
   compared to irritant contact dermatitis, 50
   compared to onychomycosis, 268
   compared to perianal bacterial dermatitis, 199
   compared to tinea cruris, 289
   neonatal/congenital, 249–262
Canker sores, 95, 138
Cantharidin, 109
Capillary malformation. *See* Vascular malformations
Capillary malformation-arteriovenous malformation (CM-AVM) syndrome, compared to vascular malformations, 434, *435–436*
Carbunculosis. *See* Folliculitis/furunculosis/carbunculosis
CARP. *See* Confluent and reticulated papillomatosis (CARP)
Ceftriaxone, 214
Cellulitis
   compared to erythema nodosum (EN), 811
   compared to staphylococcal scalded skin syndrome (SSSS), 233
   compared to subcutaneous fat necrosis (SFN), 695
Cephalexin, 176, 228
Cercarial dermatitis
   compared to allergic contact dermatitis, 335
   compared to arthropod bite reactions, 335
   compared to nonspecific viral exanthem, 335

   compared to *Pseudomonas* folliculitis, 335, *336*
   compared to seabathers eruption, 335, *336*
   diagnosis, 337
   introduction/etiology/epidemiology, 333
   prognosis, 337
   resources, 338
   signs and symptoms, 333–335, *334*
   treating associated conditions, 337
   treatment, 337
   when to worry or refer, 337
Chédiak-Higashi syndrome, 442
Chemical sunscreens, 28
Cherry angioma, compared to telangiectasias, 424
Cheyletiella, 318
Chickenpox. *See* Varicella
Chilblains. *See* Pernio/chilblains
Child abuse, 818, 840
Childhood dermatitis herpetiformis
   compared to acquired epidermolysis bullosa, 548
   compared to arthropod bites and papular urticaria, 547
   compared to bullous lupus erythematosus, 547
   compared to bullous pemphigoid, 547
   compared to epidermolysis bullosa, 548
   compared to herpes simplex virus infection, 547
   compared to linear immunoglobulin A dermatosis, 547
   compared to pityriasis lichenoides et varioliformis acuta, 547
   compared to scabies, 547
   diagnosis, 548
   introduction/etiology/epidemiology, 545
   prognosis, 549
   resources, 549
   signs and symptoms, *545–546*, 545–548
   treating associated conditions, 549
   treatment, 548
   when to worry or refer, 549
Christ-Siemens-Touraine syndrome, 599
Chronic bullous disease of childhood. *See* Linear immunoglobulin A dermatosis
Chronic graft-versus-host disease, sclerodermatous type, compared to morphea, 772
Chronic mucocutaneous candidiasis, compared to chronic paronychia, 256

Chronic paronychia
  compared to acute paronychia, 175, 256
  compared to blistering dactylitis, 256
  compared to chronic mucocutaneous candidiasis, 256
  compared to herpetic whitlow, 256
  compared to tinea unguium, 256
  diagnosis, 257
  introduction/etiology/epidemiology, 255
  prognosis, 257
  signs and symptoms, 255–256, *255–256*
  treating associated conditions, 257
  treatment, 257
Cicatricial pemphigoid, compared to lichen sclerosus et atrophicus (LSA), 840
CIE. *See* Congenital ichthyosiform erythroderma (CIE), signs and symptoms
Cigarette burns
  compared to ecthyma, 183
  compared to impetigo, 194
Cimetidine, 117
Cimex lectularius, 318
Citronella, 323
Clarithromycin, 228
Classic rubella, 155–160
  signs and symptoms, 155–156, *156*
Clindamycin, 81–82, 176, 228, 241
Clobetasol propionate, *21*
Clonidine, 855
Closed comedones, 68, *69*
  compared to molluscum contagiosum, 108
Clotrimazole, 249
Clouston syndrome, 600
CMN. *See* Congenital melanocytic nevi (CMN)
CMTC. *See* Cutis marmorata telangiectatica congenita (CMTC)
Cold panniculitis, compared to subcutaneous fat necrosis (SFN), 695
Cold sore, 92, *93*
Collagen vascular disease–associated myositis or myopathy, compared to juvenile dermatomyositis (JDM), 757
Collodion baby
  diagnosis, 657
  introduction/etiology/epidemiology, 655
  prognosis, 658
  resources, 658
  signs and symptoms, 655–657, *656–657*
  treatment, 657–658
  when to worry or refer, 658
Color of lesions, 8
  in skin of color, 10, *11–13*
Common warts, 111, *112*
  compared to epidermal nevi, 115
  compared to granuloma annulare, 115
  compared to knuckle pads, 115
Compound nevi, 471, *472*
Condylomata acuminata, *114*
  compared to warts, 115
Condylomata lata, 115
  diaper dermatitis, *667*
Confluent and reticulated papillomatosis (CARP)
  compared to acanthosis nigricans, 851
  compared to pityriasis lichenoides chronica, 851
  compared to pityriasis rosea, 851
  compared to prurigo pigmentosa, 851
  compared to tinea versicolor, 299, 851
  diagnosis, 851
  introduction/etiology/epidemiology, 849
  prognosis, 851
  signs and symptoms, 849–851, *850*
  treatment, 851–852
  when to worry or refer, 851
Congenital candidiasis, compared to erythema toxicum, 673
Congenital cutaneous candidiasis, 5
Congenital dermal melanocytosis
  compared to blue nevus, 494
  compared to bruise, 494
  compared to minocycline hyperpigmentation, 494
  compared to nevus of Ito, 494
  compared to nevus of Ota, 494
  diagnosis, 495
  introduction/etiology/epidemiology, 493
  prognosis, 495
  resources, 495
  signs and symptoms, 493–494, *493–494*
  treatment, 495
  when to worry or refer, 495
Congenital generalized phlebectasia. *See* Cutis marmorata telangiectatica congenita (CMTC)
Congenital ichthyosiform erythroderma (CIE), signs and symptoms, 572, *573*

Congenital melanocytic nevi (CMN)
  compared to Becker melanosis, 484
  compared to café au lait macules, 479, 484
  compared to ephelides, 484
  compared to lentigines, 484
  compared to plexiform neurofibroma, 484
  diagnosis, 484
  introduction/etiology/epidemiology, 481
  prognosis, 485
  resources, 486
  signs and symptoms, 481–484, *482–483*
  treating associated conditions, 485
  treatment, 484
  when to worry or refer, 485
Congenital rubella, 155–160
Congenital syphilis
  compared to rubella, 158
  diaper dermatitis, *665, 667*
Congenital thrombocytopenia, compared to rubella, 158
Conradi-Hünermann syndrome, 655
Contact dermatitis
  compared to angular cheilitis/perlèche, 248
  compared to atopic dermatitis, 39
  compared to impetigo, 194
  compared to juvenile plantar dermatosis, 61
  compared to scabies, 328
  compared to tinea pedis, 293
  compared to unilateral laterothoracic exanthem (ULE), 164
  irritant, 47–52
Contraceptives and acne vulgaris, 68
Cornelia de Lange syndrome, 619
Corticosteroids
  acne vulgaris and, 68
  angular cheilitis/perlèche and, 249
  for infantile hemangioma, 402
  intralesional, 611
  periorificial dermatitis and, 83
  systemic. *See* Systemic corticosteroids
  topical. *See* Topical corticosteroids
Corynebacterium, Wood lamp examination for, 20
COVID-19
  compared to measles, 144
  compared to pernio/chilblains, 414
Creams
  moisturizer, 25
  topical corticosteroids, 23

CREST syndrome, compared to juvenile dermatomyositis (JDM), 757
Cromolyn sodium, 514
Crusted (Norwegian) scabies, 327
Crusted impetigo
  compared to acrodermatitis enteropathica (AE), 798
  compared to kwashiorkor, 804
Crusting, 9
  acrodermatitis enteropathica (AE), *796, 796–797*
  atopic dermatitis, *35–36*
  ecthyma, *182*
  impetigo, *192*
  incontinentia pigmenti, *578*
  staphylococcal scalded skin syndrome (SSSS), 231
Cryotherapy, 27
  for molluscum contagiosum, 109
  for warts, 116
Cryptococcosis, compared to molluscum contagiosum, 108
Cushing syndrome, acne vulgaris and, 68
Cutaneous anthrax, compared to ecthyma, 183
Cutaneous bronchogenic cyst
  compared to dermoid cysts, 519
  compared to pilomatricoma, 536
Cutaneous herpes simplex virus infection, compared to cutaneous mastocytosis, 513
Cutaneous larva migrans
  compared to allergic contact dermatitis, 307
  compared to other nematode infestations, 307
  compared to phytophotodermatitis, 307
  compared to scabies, 307
  compared to tinea corporis, 307
  diagnosis, 307
  introduction/etiology/epidemiology, 305
  prognosis, 308
  resources, 308
  signs and symptoms, 305–307, *306*
  treating associated conditions, 308
  treatment, 308
  when to worry or refer, 308
Cutaneous lymphoma, compared to drug hypersensitivity syndrome, 703
Cutaneous mastocytosis
  compared to arthropod bites, 513
  compared to bullous impetigo, 513
  compared to café au lait macules, 513

compared to cutaneous herpes simplex
virus infection, 513
compared to juvenile xanthogranuloma,
513
compared to melanocytic nevus, 513
compared to nevus sebaceus, 513
compared to nodular scabies, 513
compared to urticaria, 513
diagnosis, 514
introduction/etiology/epidemiology, 509
prognosis, 515
resources, 515
signs and symptoms, 509–513, *510–512*
treatment, 514
when to worry or refer, 515
Cutaneous T-cell lymphoma, compared
to juvenile dermatomyositis
(JDM), 757
Cutaneous vasculitis, compared to papular-
purpuric gloves-and-socks
syndrome (PPGSS), 149
Cutibacterium acnes, 68
Cutis marmorata
compared to cutis marmorata
telangiectatica congenita
(CMTC), 386, 390
compared to erythema infectiosum, 386
compared to livedo reticularis, 386
compared to port-wine stain, 386
diagnosis, 386
introduction/etiology/epidemiology, 385
prognosis, 386
signs and symptoms, *385,* 385–386
treating associated conditions, 386
treatment, 386
when to worry or refer, 386
Cutis marmorata telangiectatica congenita
(CMTC)
compared to cutis marmorata, 386, 390
compared to Klippel-Trénaunay
syndrome, 390
compared to livedo reticularis, 390
compared to persistent cutis marmorata,
390
compared to reticulated port-wine stain,
390
diagnosis, 390
introduction/etiology/epidemiology, 387
prognosis, 391
resources, 391
signs and symptoms, 387–390, *388–389*
treating associated conditions, 390
treatment, 390
when to worry or refer, 391

Cystic fibrosis, 50
Cysts, 4
Cytomegalovirus infection, compared to
rubella, 158

D

Dapsone, 548, 564
Darker skin tones. See Skin of color
DEET, 322–323
Demodex, folliculitis and, 185
Depigmented lesions, 8. See also Vitiligo
Wood lamp examination for, 20
Depressed lesions, 4
Dermacentor variabilis, 217
Dermatitis herpetiformis
compared to epidermolysis bullosa (EB),
557
compared to linear immunoglobulin A
dermatosis, 563
Dermatomal arrangement of lesions, 7, 8
Dermatomyositis, compared to psoriasis, 370
Dermoid cysts
compared to cutaneous bronchogenic
cyst, 519
compared to infantile hemangioma, 519
compared to milia, 519
compared to other epithelial cysts, 519
compared to pilomatricoma, 519, 536
diagnosis, 519
introduction/etiology/epidemiology, 517
prognosis, 520
resources, 520
signs and symptoms, 517–519, *518*
treatment, 519
when to worry or refer, 520
Desonide, *22*
Diagnosis
acanthosis nigricans, 469
acne vulgaris, 71
acquired melanocytic nevi, 474
acrodermatitis enteropathica (AE), 798
acute paronychia, 175
albinism, 443
allergic contact dermatitis (ACD), 57
alopecia areata, 611
androgenetic alopecia, 617
angular cheilitis/perlèche, 248, *248*
aplasia cutis congenita (ACC), 652
atopic dermatitis, 40
blistering distal dactylitis, 178
café au lait macules, 479
candidal diaper dermatitis, 252, *253*
cercarial dermatitis, 337
childhood dermatitis herpetiformis, 548

Diagnosis, *continued*
  chronic paronychia, 257
  collodion baby, 657
  confluent and reticulated papillomatosis (CARP), 851
  congenital dermal melanocytosis, 495
  congenital melanocytic nevi (CMN), 484
  cutaneous larva migrans, 307
  cutaneous mastocytosis, 514
  cutis marmorata, 386
  cutis marmorata telangiectatica congenita (CMTC), 390
  dermoid cysts, 519
  drug hypersensitivity syndrome, 703
  ecthyma, 184
  ectodermal dysplasia, 601
  eosinophilic pustular folliculitis, 670
  ephelides, 488
  epidermal nevi, 523
  epidermolysis bullosa (EB), 557
  erythema infectiosum/human parvovirus B19 infection (fifth disease), 124
  erythema multiforme (EM), 710
  erythema nodosum (EN), 811
  erythema toxicum, 674
  exanthematous and urticarial drug reactions, 717
  fixed drug eruption, 721
  folliculitis/furunculosis/carbunculosis, 188
  Gianotti-Crosti syndrome, 130
  granuloma annulare, 527
  hand, foot, and mouth disease (HFMD), 137
  head lice, 311, *311*
  Henoch-Schönlein purpura (HSP), 818
  herpes simplex, 96, *96*
  herpes zoster, 101–102
  hyperhidrosis, 855
  hypertrichosis and hirsutism, 621
  ichthyosis, 574
  impetigo, 195
  incontinentia pigmenti, 580, *581*
  infantile acropustulosis, 676
  infantile hemangioma, 400–401
  insect bites, 321
  intertrigo, 679
  irritant contact dermatitis, 51
  juvenile dermatomyositis (JDM), 758
  juvenile xanthogranuloma (JXG), 531
  Kasabach-Merritt phenomenon (KMP), 409
  Kawasaki disease, 827
  kwashiorkor, 804
  Langerhans cell histiocytosis (LCH), 834
  lentigines, 491
  lichen nitidus, 343
  lichen planus (LP), 347
  lichen sclerosus et atrophicus (LSA), 841
  lichen striatus, 351
  linear immunoglobulin A dermatosis, 564
  loose anagen syndrome, 625, *626*
  Lyme disease, 208
  measles, 145
  melanonychia striata, 499
  meningococcemia, 213
  miliaria, 683
  molluscum contagiosum, 109
  morphea, 773
  Mycoplasma pneumoniae–induced rash and mucositis (MIRM), 733
  neonatal/congenital candidiasis, 262
  neurofibromatosis (NF), 587
  nevus sebaceus, 687
  onychomycosis, 269
  papular-purpuric gloves-and-socks syndrome (PPGSS), 149
  perianal bacterial dermatitis, 200
  periorificial dermatitis, 85
  pernio/chilblains, 415
  pigmentary mosaicism
    hyperpigmented, 505
    hypopigmented, 448–449
  pilomatricoma, 536
  pityriasis alba, 452
  pityriasis lichenoides, 357
  pityriasis rosea, 361
  pityriasis rubra pilaris (PRP), 375
  polymorphous light eruption (PMLE), 846
  postinflammatory hypopigmentation, 456
  psoriasis, 370
  pyogenic granuloma, 419
  reactive infectious mucocutaneous eruption (RIME), 733
  Rocky Mountain spotted fever (RMSF), 220
  roseola infantum (exanthem subitum), 153
  rubella, 159
  scabies, 329, *329*
  scarlet fever, 228
  seborrheic dermatitis, 381
  serum sickness–like reaction, 727
  Spitz nevus, 542

staphylococcal scalded skin syndrome (SSSS), 234
Stevens-Johnson syndrome (SJS), 733
subcutaneous fat necrosis (SFN), 695, 696
systemic lupus erythematosus (SLE), 786–789
telangiectasias, 424
telogen effluvium, 632–633
thrush, 264
tinea capitis, 275, *275–276*
tinea corporis, 284, *285*
tinea cruris, 289
tinea pedis, 293
tinea versicolor, 299, *300*
toxic shock syndrome (TSS), 240
traction alopecia, 637
transient neonatal pustular melanosis, 691
trichotillomania, 644
tuberous sclerosis complex (TSC), 596
unilateral laterothoracic exanthem (ULE), 164
urticaria, 746
varicella, 168
vascular malformations, 431–432
vitiligo, 462
Diagnostic and Statistical Manual of Mental Disorders, 639
Diagnostic techniques
　fungal culture, 17–18, *18*
　KOH preparation, 15–16, *16–17*
　mineral oil preparation for scabies, 18, *19*
　Wood lamp examination, 20, *20*
Diaper dermatitis. *See also* Irritant diaper dermatitis
　common forms, *659–664*
　compared to Langerhans cell histiocytosis (LCH), 834
　introduction/etiology/epidemiology, 659
　resources, 668
　signs and symptoms, *659–667*
　uncommon forms, *665–667*
　when to worry or refer, 668
Dietary therapy
　atopic dermatitis, 44
　gluten sensitivity, 548–549
　ichthyosis, 574–575
Dietzia papillomatosis, 849
Diffuse cutaneous mastocytosis, 509–515
Diflorasone diacetate, *21*
Discoid lupus erythematosus (DLE), 778–779, *779–781*
Disseminated herpes zoster, compared to varicella, 167
Disseminated intravascular coagulation, 211–212, *212*
Dowling-Meara type of epidermolysis bullosa (EB), 552
Doxycycline, 176, 220
DRESS. *See* Drug reaction with eosinophilia and systemic symptoms (DRESS)
Drug hypersensitivity syndrome
　compared to cutaneous lymphoma, 703
　compared to exanthematous drug reaction, 716
　compared to simple exanthematous drug eruption, 703
　compared to systemic lupus erythematosus (SLE), 784
　compared to viral exanthem, 703
　diagnosis, 703
　introduction/etiology/epidemiology, 701
　prognosis, 704
　resources, 705
　signs and symptoms, 701–703, *702*
　treating associated conditions, 704
　treatment, 704
　when to worry or refer, 704
Drug-induced hyperhidrosis, 855
Drug-induced hypersensitivity syndrome, 701
Drug reaction with eosinophilia and systemic symptoms (DRESS), 701
　compared to systemic lupus erythematosus (SLE), 784
Dry skin dermatitis, 38
Dust mite avoidance, 45
Dysproteinemias, compared to pernio/chilblains, 414
Dystrophic epidermolysis bullosa (EB), 551, 554, *555–556*

E

EB. *See* Epidermolysis bullosa (EB)
Ecchymoses
　compared to erythema nodosum (EN), 811
　compared to Henoch-Schönlein purpura (HSP), 818
Eccrine hidradenitis, compared to erythema nodosum (EN), 811
Eclipse nevi, 473, *473*
Ecthyma
　compared to brown recluse spider bite, 183
　compared to cigarette burns, 183

Ecthyma, *continued*
  compared to cutaneous anthrax, 183
  compared to ecthyma gangrenosum, 183
  compared to impetigo, 183, 194
  compared to tinea corporis, 284
  compared to vasculitis, 183
  diagnosis, 184
  introduction/etiology/epidemiology, 181
  prognosis, 184
  resources, 184
  signs and symptoms, 181–183, *182*
  treatment, 184
  when to worry or refer, 184
Ecthyma gangrenosum, compared to ecthyma, 183
Ectodermal dysplasia
  compared to keratosis-ichthyosis-deafness syndrome, 601
  compared to loose anagen syndrome, 625
  compared to pachyonychia congenita, 601
  diagnosis, 601
  introduction/etiology/epidemiology, 599
  prognosis, 602
  resources, 602
  signs and symptoms, 599–601, *600–601*
  treatment, 602
  when to worry or refer, 602
Eczema
  asteatotic, 48, *49,* 50, 52
  compared to granuloma annulare, 527
  compared to pityriasis rosea, 361
  compared to tinea corporis, 284
  compared to unilateral laterothoracic exanthem (ULE), 164
  coxsackium, *135*
  herpeticum, 94, *94,* 138
  nummular, *35,* 50, 284, 361, 527
Edema, papular-purpuric gloves-and-socks syndrome (PPGSS), *148*
Elevated lesions, 1
EM. *See* Erythema multiforme (EM)
EN. *See* Erythema nodosum (EN)
Endocrine disorders and sweating, 855
Enterococcus faecium, bedbugs and, 318
Enteroviral exanthems. *See* Hand, foot, and mouth disease (HFMD)
Enteroviral infection, compared to rubella, 158
Eosinophilic fasciitis, compared to morphea, 772
Eosinophilic pustular folliculitis
  compared to erythema toxicum, 674
  compared to incontinentia pigmenti, 580

  compared to neonatal/congenital candidiasis, 261
  diagnosis, 670
  introduction/etiology/epidemiology, 669
  prognosis, 670
  signs and symptoms, *669,* 669–670
  treatment, 670
  when to worry or refer, 670
Ephelides
  compared to acquired melanocytic nevi, 474
  compared to café au lait macules, 479, 488
  compared to congenital melanocytic nevi (CMN), 484
  compared to lentigines, 488, 491
  compared to melanocytic nevi, 488
  diagnosis, 488
  introduction/etiology/epidemiology, 487
  prognosis, 488
  signs and symptoms, *487,* 487–488
  treatment, 488
  when to worry or refer, 488
Epidermal nevi
  compared to common warts, 115
  compared to incontinentia pigmenti, 523
  compared to inflammatory linear verrucous epidermal nevus, 523
  compared to lichen striatus, 523
  compared to nevus sebaceus, 687
  compared to verruca vulgaris, 523
  diagnosis, 523
  introduction/etiology/epidemiology, 521
  prognosis, 524
  resources, 524
  signs and symptoms, 521–523, *522*
  treatment, 524
  when to worry or refer, 524
Epidermolysis bullosa (EB)
  compared to acquired epidermolysis bullosa, 557
  compared to aplasia cutis congenita (ACC), 652
  compared to blistering distal dactylitis, 178
  compared to bullous congenital ichthyosiform erythroderma, 556
  compared to bullous impetigo, 556
  compared to bullous pemphigoid, 557
  compared to childhood dermatitis herpetiformis, 548
  compared to dermatitis herpetiformis, 557

compared to erythema multiforme
major, 557
compared to herpes simplex virus
infection, 556
compared to incontinentia pigmenti,
556
compared to linear immunoglobulin A
dermatosis, 557, 563
dermatitis herpetiformis, 557
diagnosis, 557
introduction/etiology/epidemiology, 551
prognosis, 558–559
resources, 559
signs and symptoms, *552–556, 552–557*
treating associated conditions, 558
treatment, 558
when to worry or refer, 559
Epidermolytic ichthyosis, signs and
symptoms, 573, *574*
Epidermophyton floccosum, 291
Erosions, *4, 5*
impetigo, *192, 192–193*
intertrigo, 677
staphylococcal scalded skin syndrome
(SSSS), *232*
tinea pedis, *292*
Erosive lichen planus, compared to lichen
sclerosus et atrophicus (LSA),
840
Eruptive pseudoangiomatosis, 131–132
compared to bacillary angiomatosis, 138
compared to infantile hemangioma, 138
compared to pyogenic granuloma, 138
signs and symptoms, 136
Erythema infectiosum/human parvovirus
B19 infection (fifth disease)
compared to cutis marmorata, 386
compared to exanthematous drug
eruption, 124
compared to exanthem of juvenile
idiopathic arthritis, 124
compared to livedo reticularis, 124
compared to measles, 144
compared to nonspecific viral exanthem,
124
compared to scarlet fever, 124, 227
compared to urticaria, 124
diagnosis, 124
introduction/etiology/epidemiology, 121
prognosis, 125
resources, 125
signs and symptoms, 121–124, *122–123*
treatment, 124
when to worry or refer, 125

Erythema migrans, arrangement of lesions, 7
Erythema multiforme (EM)
compared to epidermolysis bullosa (EB),
557
compared to fixed drug eruption, 721
compared to Lyme disease, 207
compared to *Mycoplasma pneumoniae*-
induced rash and mucositis,
710
compared to serum sickness–like
eruption, 710
compared to serum sickness–like
reaction, 726
compared to Stevens-Johnson syndrome
(SJS), 710
compared to urticaria, 710, 745
compared to urticarial drug eruption,
716
diagnosis, 710
introduction/etiology/epidemiology, 707
prognosis, 711
resources, 711
signs and symptoms, 707–710, *708–709*
treatment, 711
Erythema nodosum (EN)
compared to arthropod bites, 811
compared to bruises, ecchymoses, 811
compared to cellulitis, 811
compared to eccrine hidradenitis, 811
compared to vasculitis, 811
diagnosis, 811
introduction/etiology/epidemiology, 809
prognosis, 812
resources, 812
signs and symptoms, 809–811, *810*
treatment, 811
when to worry or refer, 812
Erythematous cheeks, *123*
Erythematous lesions, *8*
acrodermatitis enteropathica (AE), 795,
796, 796–797
atopic dermatitis, *34, 36*
cutis marmorata, *385*
with darker skin tones, 10, *11*
juvenile plantar dermatosis, *62*
molluscum contagiosum, *107–108*
papular-purpuric gloves-and-socks
syndrome (PPGSS), *148*
perianal bacterial dermatitis, *198*
roseola infantum (exanthem subitum),
152
rubella, *156*
systemic lupus erythematosus (SLE), 778
tinea pedis, *292–293*

Erythema toxicum
  compared to bullous impetigo, 673
  compared to congenital candidiasis, 673
  compared to eosinophilic pustular folliculitis, 674
  compared to incontinentia pigmenti, 580, 674
  compared to infantile acropustulosis, 674
  compared to miliaria crystallina, 673
  compared to neonatal acne, 673
  compared to neonatal/congenital candidiasis, 261
  compared to neonatal herpes simplex virus infection, 673
  compared to scabies, 673
  compared to staphylococcal folliculitis, 673
  compared to transient neonatal pustular melanosis, 673
  diagnosis, 674
  introduction/etiology/epidemiology, 671
  prognosis, 674
  resources, 674
  signs and symptoms, *671–672,* 671–674
  treatment, 674
  when to worry or refer, 674
Erythrasma
  compared to intertrigo, 678
  compared to tinea cruris, 289
  compared to tinea pedis, 293
  Wood lamp examination for, 20
Erythromycin, 81–82, 228
Exanthematous and urticarial drug reactions
  compared to drug hypersensitivity syndrome, 716
  compared to erythema infectiosum/human parvovirus B19 infection, 124
  compared to erythema multiforme, 716
  compared to graft-versus-host disease, 716
  compared to Kawasaki disease, 716
  compared to measles, 144
  compared to miliaria rubra, 716
  compared to rubella, 158
  compared to scarlet fever, 716
  compared to serum sickness–like eruption, 716
  compared to viral exanthem, 716
  diagnosis, 717
  introduction/etiology/epidemiology, 713
  prognosis, 717
  resources, 718
  signs and symptoms, *714–715,* 714–716
  treating associated conditions, 717
  treatment, 717
  when to worry or refer, 718
Exanthem of juvenile idiopathic arthritis, 124
Exanthem subitum. *See* Roseola infantum (exanthem subitum)
Excess body hair, 621
Excoriation, 9

F
Famciclovir, 97, 102
Felon, 175
Fifth disease. *See* Erythema infectiosum/human parvovirus B19 infection (fifth disease)
Finasteride, 617
Fissuring
  juvenile plantar dermatosis, 61, *62*
  tinea pedis, *292*
Fixed drug eruption
  compared to arthropod bite, 721
  compared to Lyme disease, 207
  diagnosis, 721
  introduction/etiology/epidemiology, 719, *719–720*
  prognosis, 722
  signs and symptoms, 720–721
  treatment, 721
  when to worry or refer, 722
Flaky paint dermatosis, 801, *803*
Flat lesions, 1
Flat warts, 114, *114*
  compared to acne vulgaris, 70
  compared to benign cephalic histiocytosis, 115
  compared to lichen nitidus, 115, 342
  compared to lichen planus, 115
  compared to molluscum contagiosum, 108, 115
  compared to periorificial dermatitis, 85
Fleas, 316, *317,* 323
Fluconazole, 257, 264, 269, 277, *278,* 301
Fluid-filled lesions, 4
Fluocinolone acetonide, *21–22*
Fluocinonide, *21*
Fluticasone propionate, *21–22*
Folliculitis/furunculosis/carbunculosis
  compared to acne nodule, 188
  compared to hidradenitis suppurativa, 188
  compared to impetigo, 194
  compared to insect bites, 188

compared to irritant contact dermatitis,
    50
  compared to tinea capitis, 274
  compared to viral exanthem, 188
  diagnosis, 188
  diaper dermatitis, *660, 663*
  introduction/etiology/epidemiology, 185
  prognosis, 190
  resources, 190
  signs and symptoms, *186–187,* 186–188
  treatment, 188–190
  when to worry or refer, 190
Forceps trauma, 652
Freckles, 441, 479, *487,* 489. *See also*
    Ephelides
Frictional lichenoid dermatitis, compared to
    molluscum contagiosum, 108
Frostbite, compared to pernio/chilblains, 414
Fungal culture, 17–18, *18*
Furunculosis. *See* Folliculitis/furunculosis/
    carbunculosis

G

Gels, corticosteroid, 23
Generalized essential telangiectasia, 421
  signs and symptoms, 422
Genital HSV infection, 92
Geographic tongue, 264
Gianotti-Crosti syndrome
  compared to insect bites, 129, 321
  compared to lichenoid drug eruption,
    129
  compared to lichen planus, 129
  compared to molluscum contagiosum,
    129
  compared to papular atopic dermatitis,
    129
  compared to pityriasis lichenoides, 356
  compared to unilateral laterothoracic
    exanthem (ULE), 164
  diagnosis, 130
  introduction/etiology/epidemiology, 127
  prognosis, 130
  resources, 130
  signs and symptoms, 127–129, *128–129*
  treatment, 130
Glomerulonephritis, 228
Gluten sensitivity, 545–549
Glycemic index and acne vulgaris, 68
Glycopyrrolate wipes, 855
Gnathostoma spinigerum, 307
Goltz syndrome, compared to pigmentary
    mosaicism, hypopigmented,
    448

Gonococcemia
  compared to meningococcemia, 213
  compared to Rocky Mountain spotted
    fever (RMSF), 219
Gougerot-Carteaud syndrome, 299
Graft-versus-host disease, compared to
    exanthematous drug reaction,
    716
Gram-negative folliculitis, 185
  compared to acne vulgaris, 70
Granuloma annulare
  arrangement of lesions, 7
  compared to common warts, 115
  compared to nummular eczema, 527
  compared to rheumatoid nodules, 527
  compared to sarcoidosis, 527
  compared to soft-tissue malignancy, 527
  compared to subacute cutaneous lupus
    erythematosus (SCLE), 785
  compared to tinea corporis, 284, 527
  diagnosis, 527
  introduction/etiology/epidemiology, 525
  prognosis, 528
  resources, 528
  signs and symptoms, *525–526,* 525–527
  treating associated conditions, 528
  treatment, 527
  when to worry or refer, 528
Granulomatous periorificial dermatitis, 83,
    84
Griseofulvin, 269, 276, *278*
Group A β-hemolytic streptococci (GABHS)
  ecthyma and, 181
  scarlet fever and, 223
Grouped arrangement of lesions, 7, *7*
Guttate psoriasis
  compared to pityriasis lichenoides, 356
  compared to pityriasis rosea, 361

H

Hair
  alopecia areata, 605–613
  androgenetic alopecia, 615–618
  excess body, 621
  hypertrichosis and hirsutism, 619–622
  loose anagen syndrome, 623–627
  products, debris, 310
  shaft abnormalities, 625
  telogen effluvium, 629–634
  traction alopecia, 635–638
  trichotillomania, 639–646
Hair casts, 310
Hair collar sign, 651
Halobetasol propionate, *21*

Halo nevi, 471, *472*
Hand, foot, and mouth disease (HFMD)
  compared to allergic contact dermatitis, 138
  compared to autoimmune blistering disorders, 138
  compared to blistering distal dactylitis, 178
  compared to bullous impetigo, 138
  compared to eczema herpeticum, 138
  compared to herpes simplex, 95
  compared to papular-purpuric gloves-and-socks syndrome (PPGSS), 149
  compared to pernio/chilblains, 414
  compared to varicella, 138, 167
  diagnosis, 137
  introduction/etiology/epidemiology, 131–132
  prognosis, 139
  resources, 139
  signs and symptoms, 132–133, *133–136*
  when to worry or refer, 139
Head lice
  compared to hair casts, 310
  compared to hair products, 310
  compared to piedra, 310
  compared to psoriasis, 310
  compared to seborrheic dermatitis, 310
  diagnosis, 311, *311*
  introduction/etiology/epidemiology, 309
  prognosis, 313
  resources, 314
  signs and symptoms, 309–310, *310*
  treating associated conditions, 313
  treatment, 312–313
  when to worry or refer, 314
Hemangioma. *See* Infantile hemangioma
Henoch-Schönlein purpura (HSP)
  compared to acute hemorrhagic edema of infancy, 818
  compared to ecchymoses, benign, 818
  compared to ecchymoses associated with child abuse, 818
  compared to hypersensitivity vasculitis, 818
  compared to meningococcemia, 213
  compared to Rocky Mountain spotted fever (RMSF), 219
  compared to septic vasculitis, 818
  compared to urticaria, 745, 818
  diagnosis, 818
  introduction/etiology/epidemiology, 813
  prognosis, 819
  resources, 820
  signs and symptoms, 813–818, *814–817*
  treatment, 819
  when to worry or refer, 819
Hereditary hemorrhagic telangiectasia (HHT), 421
  diagnosis, 424
  prognosis, 425
  signs and symptoms, 422
  treatment, 425
Herlitz type, JEB, 553, *553*
Hermansky-Pudlak syndrome, 442
Herpangina, 131
  compared to aphthous ulcer, 138
  compared to herpes gingivostomatitis, 138
  compared to herpes simplex, 95
  compared to thrush, 264
  signs and symptoms, 136
Herpes gingivostomatitis
  compared to herpangina, 95
  compared to thrush, 264
Herpes gladiatorum, 92
Herpes labialis, 92, *93*
Herpes simplex virus infection. *See also* Neonatal herpes simplex virus infection
  arrangement of lesions, 7, *7*
  compared to acute paronychia, 175
  compared to allergic contact dermatitis, 95
  compared to aphthous stomatitis, 95
  compared to aplasia cutis congenita (ACC), 652
  compared to blistering distal dactylitis, 95, 178
  compared to bullous impetigo, 95
  compared to bullous mastocytoma, 95
  compared to childhood dermatitis herpetiformis, 547
  compared to cutaneous mastocytosis, 513
  compared to epidermolysis bullosa (EB), 556
  compared to fixed drug eruption, 721
  compared to hand, foot, and mouth disease, 95
  compared to herpangina, 95
  compared to herpes zoster, 95, 101
  compared to impetigo, 194
  compared to linear immunoglobulin A dermatosis, 563
  compared to rubella, 158
  compared to thermal burn, 95
  compared to varicella, 167
  compared to vascular malformations, 431

diagnosis, 96, *96*
erythema multiforme (EM) and, 707
introduction/etiology/epidemiology,
   89–90, *90*
neonatal. *See* Neonatal herpes simplex
   virus
prognosis, 97
resources, 98
signs and symptoms, 91–95, *92–94*
treatment, 97
when to worry or refer, 97–98
Herpes zoster
   arrangement of lesions, 7, *8*
   compared to allergic contact dermatitis
      (ACD), 57, 101
   compared to herpes simplex, 95, 101
   compared to varicella, 167
   diagnosis, 101–102
   introduction/etiology/epidemiology, 99
   resources, 103
   signs and symptoms, 99–101, *100*
   treatment, 102
   when to worry or refer, 102
Herpetic whitlow, 92
   compared to acute paronychia, 175
   compared to chronic paronychia, 256
HFMD. *See* Hand, foot, and mouth disease
   (HFMD)
Hidradenitis suppurativa, compared to
   folliculitis/furunculosis/
   carbunculosis, 188
Hidrotic ectodermal dysplasia, 600
Hirsutism. *See* Hypertrichosis and hirsutism
Histoplasmosis, compared to molluscum
   contagiosum, 108
HSP. *See* Henoch-Schönlein purpura (HSP)
Human herpesvirus (HHV). *See* Roseola
   infantum (exanthem subitum)
Human parvovirus B19. *See* Erythema
   infectiosum/human
   parvovirus B19 infection (fifth
   disease)
Hutchinson sign, 497
Hydroa vacciniforme, compared to
   polymorphous light eruption
   (PMLE), 845
Hydrocortisone, *22*
Hydrocortisone valerate, *21–22*
Hydroxychloroquine, 415
Hypercalcemia, 693, 695, 697
Hyperhidrosis, 855
   compared to drug-induced
      hyperhidrosis, 855
   compared to endocrine disorders, 855

compared to infection, 855
compared to malignancy, 855
compared to neurologic injuries and
   illnesses, 855
diagnosis, 855
introduction/etiology/epidemiology,
   853
prognosis, 855
resources, 855
signs and symptoms, 853–855, *854*
treatment, 855–856
when to worry or refer, 855
Hyper-linearity, atopic dermatitis, 38
Hyperpigmented lesions, 8
   acanthosis nigricans, 467–470
   acquired melanocytic nevi, 471–476
   café au lait macules, 477–480
   confluent and reticulated papillomatosis
      (CARP), 849–852
   congenital dermal melanocytosis,
      493–495
   congenital melanocytic nevi (CMN),
      481–485
   with darker skin tones, 10, *11–12*
   ephelides, 487–488
   incontinentia pigmenti, *579*
   lentigines, 489–492
   lichen planus (LP), *346*
   melanonychia striata, 497–500
   pigmentary mosaicism, 501–506
   tinea corporis, *282*
   tinea versicolor, *298*
Hypersensitivity vasculitis, compared to
   Henoch-Schönlein purpura
   (HSP), 818
Hypertrichosis and hirsutism, *620*, 620–621
   compared to excess body hair as
      biological variant, 621
   diagnosis, 621
   introduction/etiology/epidemiology,
      619
   prognosis, 622
   resources, 622
   signs and symptoms, *620*, 620–621
   treatment, 621–622
   when to worry or refer, 622
Hypopigmented lesions, 8
   atopic dermatitis, *34*, 38, *38*
   with darker skin tones, 10
   pigmentary mosaicism, 445–449
   postinflammatory, 455–457
   tinea versicolor, 297
   Wood lamp examination for, 20

I

Ichthyosis
  diagnosis, 574
  introduction/etiology/epidemiology, 569
  prognosis, 575
  resources, 575
  signs and symptoms, 569–574, *570–574*
  treating associated conditions, 575
  treatment, 574–575
  when to worry or refer, 575
Ichthyosis vulgaris
  atopic dermatitis, 38, *39*, 45
  signs and symptoms, 569, *570*
Id reaction, *56*, 58
Imidazole, 257, 285, 289, 294
Imiquimod, 110, 117
Immunoglobulin
  for Kawasaki disease, 827–828
  for toxic shock syndrome (TSS), 241
Immunotherapy
  for alopecia areata, 611
  for molluscum contagiosum, 110
  for morphea, 773–774
Impetigo
  compared to acrodermatitis
    enteropathica (AE), 798
  compared to contact dermatitis, 194
  compared to ecthyma, 183, 194
  compared to folliculitis, 194
  compared to herpes simplex virus
    infection, 194
  compared to inflicted cigarette burns, 194
  compared to kwashiorkor, 804
  compared to scabies, 328
  compared to varicella-zoster virus
    infection, 194
  diagnosis, 195
  introduction/etiology/epidemiology, 191
  prognosis, 195
  resources, 196
  signs and symptoms, 191–194, *193–194*
  treating associated conditions, 195
  treatment, 195
  when to worry or refer, 196
Incontinentia pigmenti, 7
  compared to bullous impetigo, 580
  compared to eosinophilic pustular
    folliculitis, 580
  compared to epidermal nevi, 523
  compared to epidermolysis bullosa (EB),
    556
  compared to erythema toxicum, 580, 674
  compared to infantile acropustulosis, 580
  compared to miliaria crystallina, 580
  compared to neonatal/congenital
    candidiasis, 261
  compared to neonatal herpes simplex
    virus infection, 580
  compared to pigmentary mosaicism
    hyperpigmented, 505
    hypopigmented, 448
  compared to scabies, 580
  diagnosis, 580, *581*
  introduction/etiology/epidemiology, 577
  prognosis, 582
  resources, 582
  signs and symptoms, 577–580, *578–579*
  treating associated conditions, 582
  treatment, 581–582
  when to worry or refer, 582
Infantile acne
  compared to keratosis pilaris, 81
  introduction/etiology/epidemiology, 80
  prognosis, 82
  resources, 82
  signs and symptoms, 80, *80*
  treatment, 82
  when to worry or refer, 82
Infantile acropustulosis
  compared to erythema toxicum, 674
  compared to incontinentia pigmenti, 580
  compared to neonatal/congenital
    candidiasis, 261
  diagnosis, 676
  introduction/etiology/epidemiology, 675
  prognosis, 676
  signs and symptoms, *675*, 675–676
  treatment, 676
  when to worry or refer, 676
Infantile hemangioma, 10
  compared to arteriovenous
    malformation, 400
  compared to dermoid cysts, 519
  compared to eruptive
    pseudoangiomatosis, 138
  compared to kaposiform
    hemangioendothelioma, 400
  compared to Kasabach-Merritt
    phenomenon (KMP), 409
  compared to lymphatic malformation,
    400
  compared to port-wine stain, 400
  compared to pyogenic granuloma, 400,
    419
  compared to soft-tissue malignancy, 400
  compared to vascular malformations, 431
  compared to venous malformation, 400
  diagnosis, 400–401

introduction/etiology/epidemiology, 393
prognosis, 404
resources, 406
signs and symptoms, 393–400, *394–397,
	399*
treating associated conditions, 404
treatment, 401–404
when to worry or refer, 405, *405*
Infections and sweating, 855
Infectious mononucleosis
	compared to measles, 144
	compared to rubella, 158
	compared to scarlet fever, 227
Inflammation
	acne vulgaris, 67–69
	acute paronychia, *174*
	atopic dermatitis, 42
	tinea capitis, 271
Inflammatory linear verrucous epidermal
		nevus, compared to epidermal
		nevi, 523
Insect bite reaction. *See also* Arthropod bite
		reaction
	compared to bullous impetigo, 321
	compared to bullous pemphigoid, 321
	compared to folliculitis/furunculosis/
		carbunculosis, 188
	compared to Gianotti-Crosti syndrome,
		129, 167, 321
	compared to linear immunoglobulin A
		dermatosis, 564
	compared to lymphomatoid papulosis,
		321
	compared to pityriasis lichenoides, 321
	compared to urticaria, 321
	compared to varicella, 167
	diagnosis, 321
	introduction/etiology/epidemiology,
		315
	prognosis, 324
	resources, 324
	signs and symptoms, 315–321, *316–320*
	treating associated conditions, 323
	treatment, 322–323
	when to worry or refer, 324
Intertrigo
	compared to candidal diaper dermatitis,
		252, 678
	compared to erythrasma, 678
	compared to irritant contact dermatitis,
		50
	compared to Langerhans cell
		histiocytosis (LCH), 834
	compared to seborrheic dermatitis, 678

compared to tinea cruris, 289, 678
diagnosis, 679
diaper dermatitis, *660, 663*
introduction/etiology/epidemiology, 677
prognosis, 679
resources, 679
signs and symptoms, 677–678, *677–678*
treatment, 679
when to worry or refer, 679
Intradermal melanocytic nevus, compared to
		Spitz nevus, 541
Intradermal nevus, 471, *472*
Intralesional corticosteroids, 611
Ipsilateral limb hypoplasia, 387
Irritant contact dermatitis. *See also* Allergic
		contact dermatitis (ACD)
	compared to allergic contact dermatitis
		(ACD), 57
	compared to bullous impetigo, 50
	compared to candidal diaper dermatitis,
		252
	compared to candidiasis, 50
	compared to folliculitis, 50
	compared to intertrigo, 50
	compared to Jacquet erosive dermatitis,
		50
	compared to Langerhans cell
		histiocytosis, 50
	compared to nutrition or metabolic
		disorders, 50
	compared to perianal bacterial
		dermatitis, 50, 199
	compared to periorificial dermatitis, 85
	compared to seborrheic dermatitis, 50
	diagnosis, 51
	introduction/etiology/epidemiology, 47
	prognosis, 52
	signs and symptoms, 48, *48–50*
	treatment, 51–52
	when to worry or refer, 52
Irritant diaper dermatitis, 48, *48*. *See also*
		Diaper dermatitis
	compared to bullous impetigo, 50
	compared to candidiasis, 50
	compared to folliculitis, 50
	compared to intertrigo, 50
	compared to Jacquet erosive dermatitis,
		50
	compared to Langerhans cell
		histiocytosis, 50
	compared to lichen sclerosus et
		atrophicus (LSA), 840
	compared to nutrition or metabolic
		disorders, 50

Irritant diaper dermatitis, *continued*
   compared to perianal bacterial
      dermatitis, 50
   compared to seborrheic dermatitis, 50
   signs and symptoms, *659, 661*
   treatment, 51
Itraconazole, 269, 277, *278,* 301
Ivermectin, 312
Ixodes pacificus. See Lyme disease
Ixodes scapularis. See Lyme disease

J

Jacquet erosive dermatitis
   compared to irritant contact dermatitis, 50
   diaper dermatitis, *660, 664*
Janus kinase (JAK) inhibitors, 611–612
JDM. *See* Juvenile dermatomyositis (JDM)
Junctional epidermolysis bullosa (EB), 551, 553, *553–554*
Junctional nevi, 471, *472*
Juvenile dermatomyositis (JDM)
   compared to allergic contact dermatitis, 757
   compared to atopic dermatitis, 757
   compared to collagen vascular disease–associated myositis or myopathy, 757
   compared to cutaneous T-cell lymphoma, 757
   compared to polymorphous light eruption (PMLE), 845
   compared to postinfectious myopathy/myositis, 757
   compared to psoriasis, 757
   compared to scleroderma or CREST syndrome, 757
   compared to systemic lupus erythematosus (SLE), 757, 784
   cutaneous, 751–756, *752–755*
   diagnosis, 758
   introduction/etiology/epidemiology, 751
   prognosis, 760
   resources, 760
   signs and symptoms, 751–757, *752–755*
   systemic, 756
   treating associated conditions, 759
   treatment, 758–759
   when to worry or refer, 760
Juvenile idiopathic arthritis, systemic subtype, compared to systemic lupus erythematosus (SLE), 784

Juvenile plantar dermatosis
   compared to contact dermatitis, 61
   compared to pityriasis rubra pilaris, 61
   compared to psoriasis, 61
   compared to tinea pedis, 61, 293
   introduction/etiology/epidemiology, 61
   prognosis, 63
   signs and symptoms, 61, *62*
   treatment, 63
   when to worry or refer, 63
Juvenile xanthogranuloma (JXG)
   compared to cutaneous mastocytosis, 513
   compared to melanocytic nevus, 531
   compared to nevus sebaceus, 687
   compared to pyogenic granuloma, 419
   compared to solitary mastocytoma, 531
   compared to Spitz nevus, 531, 541
   diagnosis, 531
   introduction/etiology/epidemiology, 529
   prognosis, 532
   resources, 532
   signs and symptoms, 529–531, *530–531*
   treating associated conditions, 532
   treatment, 532
   when to worry or refer, 532
JXG. *See* Juvenile xanthogranuloma (JXG)

K

Kaposiform hemangioendothelioma
   compared to infantile hemangioma, 400
   Kasabach-Merritt phenomenon (KMP), *408,* 410
Kasabach-Merritt phenomenon (KMP)
   compared to infantile hemangioma, 409
   compared to soft-tissue malignancy, 409
   diagnosis, 409
   infantile hemangioma and, 404
   introduction/etiology/epidemiology, 407
   prognosis, 410
   resources, 410
   signs and symptoms, 407–409, *408*
   treating associated conditions, 410
   treatment, 409
   when to worry or refer, 410
Kawasaki disease
   compared to measles, 144
   compared to *Mycoplasma pneumoniae*–induced rash and mucositis (MIRM), 733, 826
   compared to reactive infectious mucocutaneous eruption (RIME), 733, 826
   compared to scarlet fever, 227, 826

compared to serum sickness–like
reaction, 726, 826
compared to staphylococcal scalded skin
syndrome (SSSS), 233
compared to Stevens-Johnson syndrome
(SJS), 733, 826
compared to systemic-onset juvenile
idiopathic arthritis, 826
compared to toxic epidermal necrolysis
(TEN), 739
compared to toxic shock syndrome
(TSS), 240, 826
compared to urticarial drug eruption, 716
compared to viral exanthem, 826
diagnosis, 827
introduction/etiology/epidemiology, 821
prognosis, 828
resources, 828
signs and symptoms, 821–826, *822–825*
treatment, 827–828
when to worry or refer, 828
Keratosis-ichthyosis-deafness syndrome,
compared to ectodermal
dysplasia, 601
Keratosis pilaris, *38*
atopic dermatitis, 38, 45
compared to acne vulgaris, 70
compared to infantile acne, 81
compared to lichen nitidus, 342
compared to lichen planus (LP), 347
compared to tuberous sclerosis complex
(TSC), 595
Kerion, 271, *273, 274,* 277, 279
Ketoconazole, 277, 300
Klipper-Trénaunay syndrome
compared to cutis marmorata
telangiectatica congenita
(CMTC), 390
compared to vascular malformations,
433, *435*
KMP. *See* Kasabach-Merritt phenomenon
(KMP)
Knuckle pads, 115
Koebner type of epidermolysis bullosa (EB),
552
Koganbyo. *See* Cercarial dermatitis
KOH preparation, 15–16, *16–17*
for angular cheilitis/perlèche, 248, *248*
for tinea corporis, 284, *285*
for tinea pedis, 293
for tinea versicolor, 299, *300*
Koplik spots, 142, *143*
compared to thrush, 264

Kwashiorkor
compared to acrodermatitis
enteropathica, 804
compared to atopic dermatitis, 804
compared to crusted impetigo, 804
compared to psoriasis, 804
compared to seborrheic dermatitis, 804
diagnosis, 804
introduction/etiology/epidemiology, 801
prognosis, 805
resources, 805
signs and symptoms, 801–804, *802–803*
treatment, 805
when to worry or refer, 805

L

Labial melanotic macule, *491*
compared to lentigines, 491
LAMB syndrome, 490
Lamellar ichthyosis, 571, *571–572*
Langerhans cell histiocytosis (LCH)
compared to atopic dermatitis, 833
compared to candidal diaper dermatitis,
252
compared to diaper dermatitis, 834
compared to intertrigo, 834
compared to irritant contact dermatitis,
50
compared to scabies, 328, 833
compared to seborrheic dermatitis, 380,
833
diagnosis, 834
diaper dermatitis, *665, 667*
introduction/etiology/epidemiology, 829
prognosis, 835
resources, 835
signs and symptoms, 829–834, *830–832*
treatment, 834–835
when to worry or refer, 835
Laugier-Hunziker syndrome, compared to
melanonychia striata, 499
LCH. *See* Langerhans cell histiocytosis
(LCH)
Lentigines
compared to acquired melanocytic nevi,
474
compared to café au lait macules, 479,
491
compared to congenital melanocytic nevi
(CMN), 484
compared to ephelides, 488, 491
compared to labial melanotic macule, 491
compared to melanocytic nevi, 491
diagnosis, 491

Lentigines, *continued*
   introduction/etiology/epidemiology, 489
   prognosis, 492
   signs and symptoms, 489–491, *490*
   treatment, 492
   when to worry or refer, 492
Lentiginosis, 489
LEOPARD syndrome, 489, *490*
Lesions
   appearance differences in skin of color, 10, *11–13*
   arrangement of, 7, *7–8*
   color of, 8
   depressed, 4
   distribution of, 6
   elevated, 1
   flat, 1
   fluid-filled, 4
   secondary changes with, 9
   types of primary, 1, *2–6*, 4
Leukocytoclastic vasculitis, compared to pernio/chilblains, 414
Lichenification, 9, *9*
   atopic dermatitis, *34, 36*, 38
   compared to acanthosis nigricans, 469
Lichen nitidus
   compared to flat warts, 115, 342
   compared to keratosis pilaris, 342
   compared to lichen planus (LP), 342, 347
   compared to lichen spinulosus, 342
   compared to lichen striatus, 351
   compared to molluscum contagiosum, 342
   compared to papular atopic dermatitis, 342
   diagnosis, 343
   introduction/etiology/epidemiology, 341
   prognosis, 343
   resources, 343
   signs and symptoms, 341–342, *341–342*
   treatment, 343
   when to worry or refer, 343
Lichenoid drug eruption, compared to Gianotti-Crosti syndrome, 129
Lichen planus (LP)
   compared to flat warts, 115
   compared to Gianotti-Crosti syndrome, 129
   compared to keratosis pilaris, 347
   compared to lichen nitidus, 342, 347
   compared to lichen sclerosus et atrophicus (LSA), 840
   compared to lichen striatus, 347, 351
   compared to onychomycosis, 268
   compared to pityriasis lichenoides, 356
   compared to psoriasis, 347, 370
   diagnosis, 347
   introduction/etiology/epidemiology, 345
   prognosis, 348
   resources, 348
   signs and symptoms, 345–347, *346–347*
   treatment, 348
   when to worry or refer, 348
Lichen sclerosus et atrophicus (LSA)
   compared to childhood sexual abuse, 840
   compared to cicatricial pemphigoid, 840
   compared to erosive lichen planus, 840
   compared to irritant dermatitis or vulvovaginitis, 840
   compared to morphea, 770
   compared to perianal bacterial dermatitis, 199
   compared to pinworm infestation, 840
   compared to psoriasis, 840
   compared to vitiligo, 840
   diagnosis, 841
   introduction/etiology/epidemiology, 837
   prognosis, 842
   resources, 842
   signs and symptoms, 837–840, *838–839*
   treating associated conditions, 841
   treatment, 841
   when to worry or refer, 842
Lichen spinulosus, compared to lichen nitidus, 342
Lichen striatus
   arrangement of lesions, 7
   compared to epidermal nevi, 523
   compared to lichen nitidus, 351
   compared to lichen planus (LP), 347, 351
   compared to linear epidermal nevus, 351
   compared to morphea, 770
   compared to pigmentary mosaicism, hypopigmented, 448
   compared to psoriasis, 351
   diagnosis, 351
   introduction/etiology/epidemiology, 349
   prognosis, 352
   resources, 352
   signs and symptoms, 349–351, *350–351*
   treatment, 351
   when to worry or refer, 352
Lindane, 312
Linear arrangement of lesions, 7, *7*
Linear atrophoderma of Moulin, compared to morphea, 771
Linear epidermal nevus, compared to lichen striatus, 351

Linear immunoglobulin A dermatosis, 5
    compared to acquired epidermolysis, 564
    compared to bullous impetigo, 563
    compared to bullous insect bites, 564
    compared to bullous lupus
        erythematosus, 563
    compared to bullous pemphigoid, 563
    compared to childhood dermatitis
        herpetiformis, 547
    compared to dermatitis herpetiformis,
        563
    compared to epidermolysis bullosa (EB),
        557, 563
    compared to herpes simplex virus
        infection, 563
    compared to Stevens-Johnson syndrome,
        563
    diagnosis, 564
    introduction/etiology/epidemiology, 561
    prognosis, 565
    resources, 565
    signs and symptoms, 561–564, *562*
    treating associated conditions, 564
    treatment, 564
    when to worry or refer, 565
Linezolid, 241
Lip-licking dermatitis, 248
Liquid nitrogen, 27
Livedo reticularis, 124
    compared to cutis marmorata, 386
    compared to cutis marmorata
        telangiectatica congenita
        (CMTC), 390
Localized scleroderma. *See* Morphea
Loose anagen syndrome
    compared to alopecia areata, 610, 625
    compared to ectodermal dysplasia, 625
    compared to hair shaft abnormalities, 625
    compared to telogen effluvium, 625, 632
    compared to trichotillomania, 625
    diagnosis, 625, *626*
    introduction/etiology/epidemiology, 623
    prognosis, 626
    signs and symptoms, 623–625, *624*
    treatment, 626
    when to worry or refer, 627
Lotions
    moisturizer, 25
    topical corticosteroid, 23
Louis-Bar syndrome, 422
LP. *See* Lichen planus (LP)
LSA. *See* Lichen sclerosus et atrophicus
    (LSA)

Lupus erythematosus, arrangement of
    lesions, 7
Lyme disease
    compared to arthropod bites, 207
    compared to erythema multiforme, 207
    compared to fixed drug eruption, 207
    compared to Southern tick-associated
        rash illness (STARI), 207
    compared to tinea corporis, 207
    compared to urticaria, 207
    diagnosis, 208
    introduction/etiology/epidemiology, 205
    prognosis, 209
    resources, 209
    signs and symptoms, 205–207, *206*
    ticks and, 319
    treating associated conditions, 209
    treatment, 208
    when to worry or refer, 209
Lymphatic malformation
    compared to infantile hemangioma, 400
    signs and symptoms, 428, *429*
    treatment, 432
Lymphomatoid papulosis, compared to
    insect bites, 321

M

Macrocephaly-capillary malformations, 387
    compared to vascular malformations, 434
Macrocystic lymphatic malformation, 430,
    430
    treatment, 432
Macules, 1
    café au lait, 2, *2*, 474, 477–480
    lichen sclerosus et atrophicus (LSA),
        837–840, *838–839*
    pernio/chilblains, *412*
    pityriasis alba, 451, *451–452*
    Rocky Mountain spotted fever (RMSF),
        218
    tinea versicolor, *298*
    tuberous sclerosis complex (TSC), 591,
        592
Maffucci syndrome, compared to vascular
    malformations, 435
Malar erythema, 777
Malassezia
    compared to acne vulgaris, 70
    confluent and reticulated papillomatosis
        (CARP) and, 849
    folliculitis and, 185
    tinea versicolor, 297
    Wood lamp examination for, 20
Malathion, 312

McCune-Albright syndrome, 479
  compared to neurofibromatosis (NF), 587
  compared to pigmentary mosaicism, hyperpigmented, 505
Measles
  compared to COVID-19, 144
  compared to erythema infectiosum, 144
  compared to exanthematous drug eruption, 144
  compared to infectious mononucleosis, 144
  compared to Kawasaki disease, 144
  compared to meningococcemia, 144
  compared to papular-purpuric gloves-and-socks syndrome, 144
  compared to Rocky Mountain spotted fever (RMSF), 144, 219
  compared to roseola, 144
  compared to rubella, 144, 158
  compared to thrush, 264
  diagnosis, 145
  introduction/etiology/epidemiology, 141
  prognosis, 145
  resources, 146
  signs and symptoms, 142–144, *143*
  treatment, 145
  when to worry or refer, 146
Melanocytic nevi
  compared to cutaneous mastocytosis, 513
  compared to ephelides, 488
  compared to juvenile xanthogranuloma (JXG), 531
  compared to lentigines, 491
Melanoma, 485
Melanonychia, physiologic, 499
Melanonychia striata
  compared to Addison disease, 499
  compared to Laugier-Hunziker syndrome, 499
  compared to onychomycosis, 499
  compared to Peutz-Jeghers syndrome, 499
  compared to physiologic melanonychia, 499
  diagnosis, 499
  introduction/etiology/epidemiology, 497
  prognosis, 500
  resources, 500
  signs and symptoms, 497–499, *498*
  treatment, 499–500
  when to worry or refer, 500
Meningococcemia
  compared to gonococcemia, 213
  compared to Henoch-Schönlein purpura, 213

  compared to measles, 144
  compared to other bacteremias, 213
  compared to papular-purpuric gloves-and-socks syndrome (PPGSS), 149
  compared to Rocky Mountain spotted fever (RMSF), 213, 219
  diagnosis, 213
  introduction/etiology/epidemiology, 211
  prognosis, 215
  resources, 215
  signs and symptoms, 211–213, *212*
  treating associated conditions, 214
  treatment, 214
  when to worry or refer, 215
Metabolic disorders, compared to irritant contact dermatitis, 50
Metastatic neuroblastoma, compared to pilomatricoma, 536
Methicillin-resistant *Staphylococcus aureus*
  blistering distal dactylitis and, 179
  folliculitis and, 185
  toxic shock syndrome (TSS) and, 241
Methotrexate, 357, 371
Miconazole, 249, 264
Microcystic lymphatic malformation, 7
  treatment, 432
Microsporum, 271, 275
Microsporum canis, 16
  Wood lamp examination for, 20, *20*
Microwave technology, 855
Milia
  compared to dermoid cysts, 519
  compared to molluscum contagiosum, 108
  compared to neonatal acne, 81
  compared to pilomatricoma, 536
Miliaria
  diagnosis, 683
  introduction/etiology/epidemiology, 681
  resources, 683
  signs and symptoms, *681–682*, 681–683
  treatment, 683
  when to worry or refer, 683
Miliaria crystallina
  compared to erythema toxicum, 673
  compared to incontinentia pigmenti, 580
  signs and symptoms, 681, *682*
Miliaria pustulosa, 81
  signs and symptoms, 681, *682*
Miliaria rubra
  compared to acne vulgaris, 70
  compared to exanthematous drug reaction, 716

compared to neonatal acne, 81
compared to neonatal/congenital
 candidiasis, 261
signs and symptoms, 681, *681*
Mineral oil preparation for scabies, 18, *19*
Minocycline hyperpigmentation, compared
 to congenital dermal
 melanocytosis, 494
Minoxidil, 611, 617
MIRM. *See Mycoplasma pneumoniae*-
 induced rash and mucositis
 (MIRM)
Mites, 317–318, *318*
Modified ABCD criteria, 475, 485
Modified measles, 142
Moisturizers
  adverse effects, 26
  frequency of application, 26
  selecting, 25–26
Molluscum contagiosum, 2
  arrangement of lesions, 7
  compared to acne vulgaris, 70
  compared to closed comedones, 108
  compared to condylomata acuminata, 115
  compared to cryptococcosis, 108
  compared to flat warts, 108, 115
  compared to frictional lichenoid
   dermatitis, 108
  compared to Gianotti-Crosti syndrome,
   129
  compared to histoplasmosis, 108
  compared to lichen nitidus, 342
  compared to milia, 108
  compared to tuberous sclerosis complex
   (TSC), 595
  compared to vascular malformations, 431
  compared to warts, 115
  diagnosis, 109
  introduction/etiology/epidemiology, 105
  resources, 110
  signs and symptoms, 105–108, *106–108*
  treatment, 109–110
  when to worry or refer, 110
Mometasone furoate, *21*
Monilethrix, 625
Morbilliform drug eruptions, 10
Morgan folds, 38
Morphea
  compared to acrodermatitis chronica
   atrophicans, 771
  compared to capillary malformation, 770
  compared to chronic graft-versus-host
   disease, sclerodermatous type,
   772

compared to eosinophilic fasciitis, 772
compared to lichen sclerosus et
 atrophicus (LSA), 770
compared to lichen striatus, 770
compared to linear atrophoderma of
 Moulin, 771
compared to nephrogenic systemic
 fibrosis, 772
compared to Pasini-Pierini
 atrophoderma, 771
compared to progeria, 772
compared to systemic sclerosis, 771
diagnosis, 773
introduction/etiology/epidemiology, 761
prognosis, 774–775
resources, 775
signs and symptoms, 762–772, *763–768*
treating associated symptoms, 774
treatment, 773–774
when to worry or refer, 775
Mosquitoes, 315, *316,* 323
Mottling, cutis marmorata telangiectatica
 congenita (CMTC), 387,
 388–389
Mucha-Habermann disease, 353
Multifactorial pathogenesis, acne vulgaris,
 67–68
Mupirocin, 176
Muscular dystrophy, epidermolysis bullosa
 (EB) with, 552
Mycoplasma pneumoniae–induced rash and
 mucositis (MIRM)
  compared to erythema multiforme (EM),
   710
  compared to Kawasaki disease, 826
  compared to linear immunoglobulin A
   dermatosis, 563
  compared to toxic epidermal necrolysis
   (TEN), 739
  erythema nodosum (EN), 809
  introduction/etiology/epidemiology,
   729–730
  prognosis, 734
  resources, 735
  signs and symptoms, *730–732,* 730–733
  treatment, 734
  when to worry or refer, 734
Myofibromatosis, compared to subcutaneous
 fat necrosis (SFN), 695

N

Nails
  acute paronychia and, 173–176
  chronic paronychia and, 255–262

Nails, *continued*
melanonychia striata and, 497–500
neonatal/congenital candidiasis and, 259, *260*
onychomycosis and, 267–270
NAME syndrome, 490
Neisseria meningitidis, 211
Neonatal acne
compared to erythema toxicum, 673
compared to milia, 81
compared to miliaria rubra or pustulosa, 81
compared to sebaceous hyperplasia, 81
compared to seborrheic dermatitis, 81
compared to staphylococcal pustulosis, 81
introduction/etiology/epidemiology, 79, *79*
prognosis, 82
resources, 82
signs and symptoms, 80, *80*
treatment, 81
when to worry or refer, 82
Neonatal cephalic pustulosis
compared to neonatal acne, 79
compared to neonatal/congenital candidiasis, 261
Neonatal/congenital candidiasis
compared to eosinophilic pustular folliculitis, 261
compared to erythema toxicum, 261
compared to incontinentia pigmenti, 261
compared to infantile acropustulosis, 261
compared to miliaria rubra, 261
compared to neonatal cephalic pustulosis, 261
compared to neonatal herpes simplex virus infection, 261
compared to scabies, 261
compared to staphylococcal folliculitis, 261
compared to transient neonatal pustular melanosis, 261
diagnosis, 262
introduction/etiology/epidemiology, 259
prognosis, 262
resources, 262
signs and symptoms, 259–261, *260–261*
treatment, 262
when to worry or refer, 262
Neonatal herpes simplex virus infection, 90, *90*, 97. *See also* Herpes simplex virus infection
compared to erythema toxicum, 673

compared to incontinentia pigmenti, 580
compared to neonatal/congenital candidiasis, 261
Neonatal lupus erythematosus (NLE), 782–783, *783*
compared to seborrheic dermatitis, 380
Nephrogenic systemic fibrosis, compared to morphea, 772
Neurofibromas, *3*, 479
compared to congenital melanocytic nevi (CMN), 484
compared to pigmentary mosaicism, hyperpigmented, 505
Neurofibromatosis (NF)
compared to Bloom syndrome, 587
compared to cutaneous mastocytosis, 513
compared to McCune-Albright syndrome, 587
compared to multiple café au lait macules without neurofibromatosis, 587
compared to Silver-Russell syndrome, 587
diagnosis, 587
introduction/etiology/epidemiology, 583
prognosis, 589
resources, 589
signs and symptoms, 583–587, *584–585*
treating associated conditions, 588
treatment, 588
when to worry or refer, 589
Neurofibromatosis type 1, *3*, 583
diagnosis, 587
signs and symptoms, 583, *584–585*, 586
treatment, 588
when to worry or refer, 589
Neurofibromatosis type 2, 583
diagnosis, 587
signs and symptoms, 586
treatment, 588
when to worry or refer, 589
Neurologic disorders and sweating, 855
Nevus anemicus, compared to tuberous sclerosis complex (TSC), 595
Nevus of Ito, compared to congenital dermal melanocytosis, 494
Nevus of Ota, compared to congenital dermal melanocytosis, 494
Nevus sebaceus
compared to aplasia cutis congenita (ACC), 652, 687
compared to cutaneous mastocytosis, 513
compared to epidermal nevus, 687

compared to juvenile xanthogranuloma, 687
diagnosis, 687
introduction/etiology/epidemiology, 685
prognosis, 688
resources, 688
signs and symptoms, 685–687, *686–687*
treatment, 688
when to worry or refer, 688
NF. *See* Neurofibromatosis (NF)
Nickel contact dermatitis, *54,* 55, *55–56*
Nifedipine, 415
Nikolsky sign, 231
Nitrogen, liquid, 27
NLE. *See* Neonatal lupus erythematosus (NLE)
Nodular scabies, compared to cutaneous mastocytosis, 513
Nodules, 1, *3*
  erythema nodosum (EN), 809, *810*
  rubella, *157*
  scabies, 325, *327*
  subcutaneous fat necrosis (SFN), 693–697
Non-corticosteroid Janus kinase inhibitors, 43
Non-corticosteroid phosphodiesterase inhibitors, 43
Non-corticosteroid topical calcineurin inhibitors, 43
Non-Herlitz type, JEB, 553
Nonspecific viral exanthem, 124. *See also* Viral exanthem
  compared to cercarial dermatitis, 335
Noonan syndrome, 626
Nummular eczema, *35*
  compared to asteatotic eczema, 50
  compared to granuloma annulare, 527
  compared to pityriasis rosea, 361
  compared to tinea corporis, 284
Nutritional disorders, compared to irritant contact dermatitis, 50
Nystatin, 249, 257, 264

O

Ocular HSV infection, 92
Oculocerebrocutaneous (Delleman) syndrome, 649
Oculocutaneous albinism (OCA). *See* Albinism
Oil-in-water emulsions, 25
Oil of lemon eucalyptus, 322
Ointments
  moisturizer, 25
  topical corticosteroid, 23
Omalizumab, 746

Onychomadesis, hand, foot, and mouth disease (HFMD), *136*
Onychomycosis. *See also* Tinea unguium, compared to chronic paronychia
  compared to candidiasis, 268
  compared to lichen planus, 268
  compared to melanonychia striata, 499
  compared to pachyonychia congenita, 268
  compared to psoriasis, 268
  compared to trachyonychia, 268
  diagnosis, 269
  introduction/etiology/epidemiology, 267
  prognosis, 270
  resources, 270
  signs and symptoms, 267–268, *267–268*
  treatment, 269
  when to worry or refer, 270
Open comedones, 68, *69*
Osler-Weber-Rendu disease, 422
Oxybenzone, 28–29

P

Pachyonychia congenita
  compared to ectodermal dysplasia, 601
  compared to onychomycosis, 268
PANDAS (Pediatric Autoimmune Neuropsychiatric Disorder Associated with Group A Streptococci), 229
PANS (Pediatric Acute-Onset Neuropsychiatric Syndrome), 229
Papular atopic dermatitis, compared to Gianotti-Crosti syndrome, 129
Papular eczema, compared to unilateral laterothoracic exanthem (ULE), 164
Papular-purpuric gloves-and-socks syndrome (PPGSS)
  compared to cutaneous vasculitis, 149
  compared to hand, foot, and mouth disease, 149
  compared to measles, 144
  compared to meningococcemia, 149
  compared to Rocky Mountain spotted fever, 149
  diagnosis, 149
  introduction/etiology/epidemiology, 147
  prognosis, 149
  signs and symptoms, 147–149, *148*
  treatment, 149
  when to worry or refer, 150

Papular urticaria
    compared to childhood dermatitis herpetiformis, 547
    compared to scabies, 328
    compared to urticaria, 745
    introduction/etiology/epidemiology, 315
    signs and symptoms, 320, *320*
Papules, 1
    allergic contact dermatitis (ACD), *56*
    atopic dermatitis, *37*, 38, *38*
    cercarial dermatitis, *334*
    with darker skin tones, 10, *12–13*
    eosinophilic pustular folliculitis, *669*, 669–670
    erythema toxicum, 671–672, *671–672*
    folliculitis/furunculosis/carbunculosis, 186–187
    Gianotti-Crosti syndrome, *128*, 128–129
    incontinentia pigmenti, *578*
    infantile acne, *80*
    juvenile xanthogranuloma (JXG), 529–531, *530–531*
    Langerhans cell histiocytosis (LCH), 830, *830–832*
    lichen nitidus, 341, *341*
    lichen planus (LP), 345, *346*
    lichen sclerosus et atrophicus (LSA), 837–840, *838–839*
    lichen striatus, 349, *350–351*
    linear arrangement of, *7*
    measles, *143*
    molluscum contagiosum, *2, 106*
    neonatal acne, *80*
    neonatal/congenital candidiasis, 259, *259*
    periorificial dermatitis, 83, *83, 83–84*
    pityriasis lichenoides, *354–355*
    pityriasis rosea, 359–361, *360–361*
    polymorphous light eruption (PMLE), 843–845, *844*
    psoriasis, 363–370, *364–369*
    pyogenic granuloma, *417–418*
    roseola infantum (exanthem subitum), 151, *152*
    scabies, 325, *326*
    scarlet fever, *224*
    tuberous sclerosis complex (TSC), 591, *592*
    unilateral laterothoracic exanthem (ULE), *162*
    warts, *112–113*
Papulonodular lesions, juvenile xanthogranuloma (JXG), 529–531, *530–531*

Papulopustules, periorificial dermatitis, 83, *83*
Paronychia
    acute. *See* Acute paronychia
    chronic. *See* Chronic paronychia
Parvovirus B19. *See* Erythema infectiosum/human parvovirus B19 infection (fifth disease)
Pasini-Pierini atrophoderma, compared to morphea, 771
Patches, 1
    atopic dermatitis, *34, 37*
    candidal diaper dermatitis, *251*
    kwashiorkor, *802*
    molluscum contagiosum, *107*
    port-wine stains, *2*
    thrush, 263, *263*
    tinea capitis, *272*
    tinea cruris, 287, *288*
    tuberous sclerosis complex (TSC), 591, *593*
Pathophysiology, acne vulgaris, 67
Pattern alopecia, 615
Pediculicides, 312
Penicillin-cephalosporin cross-reactivity, 713
Penicillin G, 214, 228
Penicillin V, 228
Pentoxifylline, 415
Perianal bacterial dermatitis, 50
    compared to candidiasis, 199
    compared to irritant contact dermatitis, 199
    compared to lichen sclerosus et atrophicus, 199
    compared to pinworm infestation, 199
    compared to psoriasis, 199
    compared to seborrheic dermatitis, 199
    compared to sexual abuse, 199
    diagnosis, 200
    introduction/etiology/epidemiology, 197
    prognosis, 200
    resources, 201
    signs and symptoms, 197–199, *198*
    treating associated conditions, 200
    treatment, 200
    when to worry or refer, 200
Periorificial dermatitis
    compared to acne vulgaris, 70
    compared to allergic contact dermatitis, 85
    compared to atopic dermatitis, 85
    compared to benign cephalic histiocytosis, 85
    compared to flat warts, 85

compared to irritant contact dermatitis, 85
compared to sarcoidosis, 85
compared to seborrheic dermatitis, 380
compared to tuberous sclerosis complex (TSC), 595
diagnosis, 85
introduction/etiology/epidemiology, 83
prognosis, 86
resources, 86
signs and symptoms, 83–85
when to worry or refer, 86
Periungual warts, 114
Perlèche. *See* Angular cheilitis/perlèche
Permethrin, 312, 323
Pernio/chilblains
   compared to acrocyanosis, 414
   compared to COVID-19 toes, 414
   compared to dysproteinemias, 414
   compared to frostbite, 414
   compared to hand, foot, and mouth disease, 414
   compared to leukocytoclastic vasculitis, 414
   compared to Raynaud phenomenon, 414
   diagnosis, 415
   introduction/etiology/epidemiology, 410
   prognosis, 415
   resources, 416
   signs and symptoms, 410–414, *412–413*
   treatment, 415
   when to worry or refer, 416
Persistent cutis marmorata, compared to cutis marmorata telangiectatica congenita (CMTC), 390
Peutz-Jeghers syndrome, 489, *490*
   compared to melanonychia striata, 499
Phakomatosis pigmentovascularis (PPV), compared to vascular malformations, 433
Photoprotection, 425, 443, 448–449, 759, 789
Phytophotodermatitis, compared to cutaneous larva migrans, 307
Picaridin, 322
Piebaldism
   compared to albinism, 443
   compared to pigmentary mosaicism, hypopigmented, 448
   compared to postinflammatory hypopigmentation, 456
   compared to tuberous sclerosis complex (TSC), 595
   compared to vitiligo, 462
Piedra, compared to head lice, 310

Pigmentary mosaicism
   hyperpigmented
      compared to Becker nevus, 505
      compared to incontinentia pigmenti, 505
      compared to McCune-Albright syndrome, 505
      compared to plexiform neurofibroma, 505
      diagnosis, 505
      introduction/etiology/epidemiology, 501
      prognosis, 506
      resources, 506
      signs and symptoms, 501–505, *502–504*
      treatment, 506
      when to worry or refer, 506
   hypopigmented
      compared to Goltz syndrome, 448
      compared to incontinentia pigmenti, 448
      compared to lichen striatus, 448
      compared to piebaldism, 448
      compared to vitiligo, 448
      diagnosis, 448–449
      introduction/etiology/epidemiology, 445
      prognosis, 449
      resources, 449
      signs and symptoms, 445–448, *446–447*
      treatment, 449
      when to worry or refer, 449
Pigmentary mosaicism–hypomelanosis of Ito type, compared to tuberous sclerosis complex (TSC), 595
Pigmentary mosaicism–nevus depigmentosus type, compared to tuberous sclerosis complex (TSC), 594
Pigmented purpura, compared to telangiectasias, 424
Pilomatricoma
   compared to branchial cleft cyst, 536
   compared to cutaneous bronchogenic cysts, 536
   compared to dermoid cysts, 519, 536
   compared to metastatic neuroblastoma, 536
   compared to milia, 536
   compared to other epithelial cysts, 536
   compared to thyroglossal duct cyst, 536
   compared to venous malformation, 536

Pilomatricoma, *continued*
  diagnosis, 536
  introduction/etiology/epidemiology, 533
  prognosis, 537
  resources, 537
  signs and symptoms, 533–536, *534–535*
  treatment, 536
  when to worry or refer, 537
Pimecrolimus, 514
Pinworm infestation
  compared to lichen sclerosus et atrophicus (LSA), 840
  compared to perianal bacterial dermatitis, 199
Pitted keratolysis, compared to tinea pedis, 293
Pityriasis alba
  atopic dermatitis, 38, *38,* 45
  compared to postinflammatory hypopigmentation, 456
  compared to tinea versicolor, 299, 452
  compared to tuberous sclerosis complex (TSC), 594
  compared to vitiligo, 452, 462
  diagnosis, 452
  introduction/etiology/epidemiology, 451
  prognosis, 453
  resources, 453
  signs and symptoms, 451–452, *451–452*
  treating associated conditions, 453
  treatment, 453
  when to worry or refer, 453
Pityriasis lichenoides
  compared to confluent and reticulated papillomatosis (CARP), 851
  compared to Gianotti-Crosti syndrome, 356
  compared to guttate psoriasis, 356
  compared to insect bites, 321
  compared to pityriasis rosea, 356, 361
  compared to secondary syphilis, 356
  compared to varicella, 356
  diagnosis, 357
  introduction/etiology/epidemiology, 353
  prognosis, 357
  resources, 358
  signs and symptoms, 353–356, *354–355*
  treatment, 357
  when to worry or refer, 358
Pityriasis lichenoides chronica (PLC). *See* Pityriasis lichenoides
Pityriasis lichenoides et varioliformis acuta (PLEVA). *See* Pityriasis lichenoides

Pityriasis rosea
  compared to confluent and reticulated papillomatosis (CARP), 851
  compared to guttate psoriasis, 361
  compared to nummular eczema, 361
  compared to pityriasis lichenoides, 356, 361
  compared to pityriasis rubra pilaris (PRP), 375
  compared to psoriasis, 370
  compared to secondary syphilis, 361
  compared to tinea corporis, 284, 361
  compared to tinea versicolor, 299
  compared to unilateral laterothoracic exanthem (ULE), 164
  with darker skin tones, 12
  diagnosis, 361
  introduction/etiology/epidemiology, 359
  prognosis, 362
  resources, 362
  signs and symptoms, 359–361, *360–361*
  treatment, 362
  when to worry or refer, 362
Pityriasis rubra pilaris (PRP)
  compared to atopic dermatitis, 375
  compared to juvenile plantar dermatosis, 61
  compared to pityriasis rosea, 375
  compared to psoriasis, 375
  diagnosis, 375
  introduction/etiology/epidemiology, 373
  prognosis, 376
  resources, 376
  signs and symptoms, 373–375, *374–375*
  treatment, 376
  when to worry or refer, 376
Plantar warts, 111
  compared to calluses, 115
Plant contact dermatitis, 56
Plaques, 1
  allergic contact dermatitis (ACD), *54*
  cutaneous larva migrans, 305
  hand, foot, and mouth disease (HFMD), *135*
  Henoch-Schönlein purpura (HSP), *814*
  lichen planus (LP), *347*
  meningococcemia, *212*
  morphea, 762, *763–764*
  nevus sebaceus, 685–688
  pityriasis rosea, 359–361, *360–361*
  polymorphous light eruption (PMLE), 843–845, *844*
  psoriasis, 363–370, *364–369*

scaling, 4
thrush, 263, *263*
tinea corporis, 281
tinea pedis, *292*
PLEVA. *See* Pityriasis lichenoides
Plexiform neurofibroma
  compared to congenital melanocytic nevi (CMN), 484
  compared to pigmentary mosaicism, hyperpigmented, 505
PMLE. *See* Polymorphous light eruption (PMLE)
Podofilox, 117
Podophyllin, 117
Polycystic ovary syndrome, acne vulgaris and, 68
Polymorphous light eruption (PMLE)
  compared to actinic prurigo, 845
  compared to hydroa vacciniforme, 845
  compared to juvenile dermatomyositis, 845
  compared to solar urticaria, 845
  compared to systemic lupus erythematosus (SLE), 784, 845
  diagnosis, 846
  introduction/etiology/epidemiology, 843
  prognosis, 846
  resources, 847
  signs and symptoms, 843–845, *844*
  treatment, 846
  when to worry or refer, 846
Port-wine stains, *2*
  compared to cutis marmorata, 386
  compared to infantile hemangioma, 400
  compared to morphea, 770
  with darker skin tones, 10
  signs and symptoms, 428, *429*
Postinfectious myopathy/myositis, compared to juvenile dermatomyositis (JDM), 757
Postinflammatory hypopigmentation
  compared to acanthosis nigricans, 469
  compared to café au lait macules, 479
  compared to piebaldism, 456
  compared to pityriasis alba, 456
  compared to tinea versicolor, 456
  compared to vitiligo, 456
  diagnosis, 456
  introduction/etiology/epidemiology, 455
  prognosis, 457
  resources, 457
  signs and symptoms, *455*, 455–456
  treating associated conditions, 457

treatment, 456
when to worry or refer, 457
Potassium hydroxide. *See* KOH preparation
PPGSS. *See* Papular-purpuric gloves-and-socks syndrome (PPGSS)
Prednicarbate, *22*
Prednisone, 277
Primary HSV gingivostomatitis, 92
Primary lesions, types of, 1, *2–6*, 4
Progeria, compared to morphea, 772
Propranolol, 402
Proteus syndrome, compared to vascular malformations, 434
PRP. *See* Pityriasis rubra pilaris (PRP)
Prurigo pigmentosa, compared to confluent and reticulated papillomatosis (CARP), 851
Pruritus
  childhood dermatitis herpetiformis, 545
  cutaneous larva migrans, 305
  infantile acropustulosis, 675
  lichen planus (LP), 345
  prevention, in atopic dermatitis, 40–41
  scabies, 325
  tinea corporis, 281
  tinea cruris, 287
  treatment, Gianotti-Crosti syndrome, 130
  unilateral laterothoracic exanthem (ULE), 161
  varicella, 166
Pseudomonas
  acute paronychia and, 173
  compared to cercarial dermatitis, 335, *336*
  folliculitis and, 185
Psoriasis, *4*
  compared to acrodermatitis enteropathica (AE), 798
  compared to acute paronychia, 175
  compared to atopic dermatitis, 39
  compared to candidal diaper dermatitis, 252
  compared to dermatomyositis, 370
  compared to head lice, 310
  compared to juvenile dermatomyositis (JDM), 757
  compared to juvenile plantar dermatosis, 61
  compared to kwashiorkor, 804
  compared to lichen planus (LP), 347, 370
  compared to lichen sclerosus et atrophicus (LSA), 840

Psoriasis, *continued*
    compared to lichen striatus, 351
    compared to neonatal lupus
        erythematosus (NLE), 785
    compared to onychomycosis, 268
    compared to perianal bacterial
        dermatitis, 199
    compared to pityriasis rosea, 370
    compared to pityriasis rubra pilaris
        (PRP), 375
    compared to scabies, 328
    compared to seborrheic dermatitis, 370,
        380
    compared to subacute cutaneous lupus
        erythematosus (SCLE), 785
    compared to tinea corporis, 284
    with darker skin tones, 10
    diagnosis, 370
    diaper dermatitis, 665–666
    distribution of lesions, 6
    introduction/etiology/epidemiology, 363
    prognosis, 371
    resources, 372
    scaling of, 9
    signs and symptoms, 363–370, *364–369*
    treating associated conditions, 371
    treatment, 370–371
    when to worry or refer, 371
Pulsed dye laser, 117
    for infantile hemangioma, 403
Purple urticaria, 723, *724*
Pustules, 4, *5*
    eosinophilic pustular folliculitis, *669,*
        669–670
    infantile acne, *80*
    infantile acropustulosis, *675*
    neonatal acne, *80*
    psoriasis, *366*
    scabies, *326*
    transient neonatal pustular melanosis,
        689–691
Pyloric atresia, JEB with, 553, *554*
Pyoderma gangrenosum, 6
Pyogenic granuloma
    compared to eruptive
        pseudoangiomatosis, 138
    compared to infantile hemangioma, 400,
        419
    compared to juvenile xanthogranuloma,
        419
    compared to spider angioma, 419
    compared to Spitz nevus, 419, 541
    compared to telangiectasias, 424

compared to vascular malformations, 433
diagnosis, 419
introduction/etiology/epidemiology, 417
prognosis, 420
resources, 420
signs and symptoms, 417–419, *418*
treatment, 419
when to worry or refer, 420

R
Rash. *See* Lesions
Raynaud phenomenon, compared to pernio/
    chilblains, 414
Reactive infectious mucocutaneous
        eruptions (RIME)
    compared to Kawasaki disease, 733, 826
    compared to linear immunoglobulin A
        dermatosis, 563
    compared to serum sickness–like
        eruption, 733
    compared to staphylococcal scalded skin
        syndrome (SSSS), 733
    compared to toxic epidermal necrolysis
        (TEN), 733, 739
    compared to urticaria, 733
    diagnosis, 733
    introduction/etiology/epidemiology,
        729–730
    prognosis, 734
    resources, 735
    signs and symptoms, *730–732*, 730–733
    treatment, 734
    when to worry or refer, 734
Recessive X-linked ichthyosis, signs and
        symptoms, 569, *570*
Recombinant interferon-alfa, 403
*Red Book: Report of the Committee on
        Infectious Diseases,* 168, 190,
        208, 214, 229
Retained food or formula compared to
        thrush, 264
Retapamulin, 176
Retinoids
    for acne vulgaris, *74,* 74–76
    for molluscum contagiosum, 110
    for neonatal and infantile acne, 81–82
Rheumatic fever, 228
Rheumatoid nodules, compared to
        granuloma annulare, 527
Rhipicephalus sanguineus, 217
Ribavirin, 145
Rickettsialpox, compared to varicella, 167
Rickettsia rickettsii, 217

RMSF. *See* Rocky Mountain spotted fever (RMSF)
Rocky Mountain spotted fever (RMSF)
  compared to atypical measles, 219
  compared to gonococcemia, 219
  compared to Henoch-Schönlein purpura, 219
  compared to measles, 144
  compared to meningococcemia, 213, 219
  compared to other bacteremias, 219
  compared to papular-purpuric gloves-and-socks syndrome (PPGSS), 149
  diagnosis, 220
  introduction/etiology/epidemiology, 217
  prognosis, 221
  resources, 221
  signs and symptoms, 217–219, *218*
  treatment, 220
  when to worry or refer, 221
Rosacea, compared to systemic lupus erythematosus (SLE), 784
Roseola infantum (exanthem subitum)
  diagnosis, 153
  introduction/etiology/epidemiology, 151
  prognosis, 153
  resources, 153
  signs and symptoms, 151–152, *152*
  treatment, 153
  when to worry or refer, 153
Rubella
  compared to congenital syphilis, 158
  compared to congenital thrombocytopenia, 158
  compared to cytomegalovirus infection, 158
  compared to enteroviral infection, 158
  compared to exanthematous drug eruption, 158
  compared to herpes simplex virus infection, 158
  compared to infectious mononucleosis, 158
  compared to measles, 144, 158
  compared to toxoplasmosis, 158
  diagnosis, 159
  introduction/etiology/epidemiology, 155
  prognosis, 159
  resources, 160
  signs and symptoms, 155–158, *156–157*
  treatment, 159
  when to worry or refer, 160
Ruxolitinib, 463

S

Salicylic acid therapy for warts, 116
Salmon patch, 427, *428*, 432
Sarcoidosis
  compared to granuloma annulare, 527
  compared to periorificial dermatitis, 85
Sarcoptes scabiei. *See* Scabies
Sawah itch. *See* Cercarial dermatitis
Scabies
  compared to acropustulosis of infancy, 328
  compared to arthropod bites, 328
  compared to atopic dermatitis, 39, 328
  compared to childhood dermatitis herpetiformis, 547
  compared to contact dermatitis, 328
  compared to cutaneous larva migrans, 307
  compared to cutaneous mastocytosis, 513
  compared to erythema toxicum, 673
  compared to impetigo, 328
  compared to incontinentia pigmenti, 580
  compared to Langerhans cell histiocytosis (LCH), 328, 833
  compared to neonatal/congenital candidiasis, 261
  compared to papular urticaria, 328
  compared to psoriasis, 328
  compared to seborrheic dermatitis, 328, 380
  compared to viral exanthem, 328
  diagnosis, 329, *329*
  introduction/etiology/epidemiology, 325
  mineral oil preparation for, 18, *19*
  prognosis, 330
  resources, 331
  signs and symptoms, 325–328, *326–327*
  treating associated conditions, 330
  treatment, 329–330
  when to worry or refer, 330
Scaling, 9
  acrodermatitis enteropathica (AE), *796, 796–797*
  asteatotic eczema, 49
  atopic dermatitis, *36, 38, 39*
  juvenile plantar dermatosis, *62*
  kwashiorkor, *803*
  pityriasis rubra pilaris (PRP), *374–375*
  seborrheic dermatitis, *378–379*
  tinea capitis, *272*
  tinea corporis, *282*
  tinea pedis, *292–293*
  tinea versicolor, *298*

Scalp electrode trauma, 652
Scarlet fever
  compared to *Arcanobacterium haemolyticum* infection, 227
  compared to erythema infectiosum/human parvovirus B19 infection (fifth disease), 124
  compared to exanthematous drug reaction, 716
  compared to infectious mononucleosis, 227
  compared to Kawasaki disease, 227, 826
  compared to parvovirus B19 infection, 227
  compared to staphylococcal scalded skin syndrome, 227
  compared to staphylococcal scarlet fever, 227
  compared to toxic shock syndrome, 227
  diagnosis, 228
  introduction/etiology/epidemiology, 223
  prognosis, 229
  resources, 229
  signs and symptoms, 223–227, *224–226*
  treating associated conditions, 228–229
  treatment, 228
  when to worry or refer, 229
Scarring, aplasia cutis congenita (ACC), 649, *650*
Scarring alopecia, compared to androgenetic alopecia, 617
SCLE. *See* Subacute cutaneous lupus erythematosus (SCLE)
Sclerema, compared to subcutaneous fat necrosis (SFN), 695
Scleroderma
  compared to juvenile dermatomyositis (JDM), 757
  compared to morphea, 771
Seabathers eruption, 335, *336*
Sebaceous hyperplasia, compared to neonatal acne, 81
Seborrheic dermatitis, 271
  compared to acrodermatitis enteropathica (AE), 798
  compared to allergic contact dermatitis (ACD), 57
  compared to atopic dermatitis, 39, 380
  compared to candidal diaper dermatitis, 252
  compared to head lice, 310
  compared to intertrigo, 678
  compared to irritant contact dermatitis, 50
  compared to kwashiorkor, 804
  compared to Langerhans cell histiocytosis (LCH), 380, 833
  compared to neonatal acne, 81
  compared to neonatal lupus erythematosus (NLE), 380, 785
  compared to perianal bacterial dermatitis, 199
  compared to periorificial dermatitis, 380
  compared to psoriasis, 370, 380
  compared to scabies, 328, 380
  compared to tinea capitis, 274
  diagnosis, 381
  diaper dermatitis, *659*, *662*
  distribution of lesions, 6
  introduction/etiology/epidemiology, 377
  prognosis, 381
  resources, 382
  signs and symptoms, 377–380, *378–379*
  treatment, 381
  when to worry or refer, 382
Secondary syphilis
  angular cheilitis/perlèche, 248
  compared to pityriasis lichenoides, 356
  compared to pityriasis rosea, 361
Segmental pigmentation disorder, 502
Selenium sulfide, 277, 300
Self-healing collodion baby, 655
Septic vasculitis, compared to Henoch-Schönlein purpura (HSP), 818
Serologic studies, 96, 783, 786, 827
Serpiginous erythematous tracts, cutaneous larva migrans, 305, *306*
Serum sickness–like reaction
  compared to erythema multiforme (EM), 710, 726
  compared to Kawasaki disease, 726, 826
  compared to *Mycoplasma pneumoniae*-induced rash and mucositis (MIRM), 733
  compared to reactive infectious mucocutaneous eruption (RIME), 733
  compared to Stevens-Johnson syndrome (SJS), 733
  compared to urticaria, 726, 745
  compared to urticarial drug eruption, 716
  compared to urticaria multiforme, 726
  diagnosis, 727
  introduction/etiology/epidemiology, 723
  prognosis, 727
  signs and symptoms, 723–726, *724–725*

treatment, 727
when to worry or refer, 727
Sexual abuse
  compared to lichen sclerosus et atrophicus (LSA), 840
  compared to perianal bacterial dermatitis, 199
Sexually transmitted diseases, molluscum contagiosum, 105
SFN. *See* Subcutaneous fat necrosis (SFN)
Shingles. *See* Herpes zoster
Signs and symptoms
  acanthosis nigricans, 467–469, *468*
  acne vulgaris, 68–70
  acquired melanocytic nevi, 471–474, *472–473*
  acrodermatitis enteropathica (AE), 795–798, *796–797*
  acute paronychia, 173–175, *174*
  albinism, 441–443, *442*
  allergic contact dermatitis (ACD), 53–57, *54–56*
  alopecia areata, 605–610, *606, 608–609*
  androgenetic alopecia, 615–617, *616*
  angular cheilitis/perlèche, 247, 247–248
  aplasia cutis congenita (ACC), 649–652, *650–651*
  atopic dermatitis, 33–38, *34–39*
  blistering distal dactylitis, *177,* 177–178
  café au lait macules, *477–478,* 477–479
  candidal diaper dermatitis, *251,* 251–252
  cercarial dermatitis, 333–335, *334*
  childhood dermatitis herpetiformis, *545–546,* 545–548
  chronic paronychia, 255–256, *255–256*
  collodion baby, 655–657, *656–657*
  congenital dermal melanocytosis, 493–494, *493–494*
  congenital melanocytic nevi (CMN), 481–484, *482–483*
  cutaneous larva migrans, 305–307, *306*
  cutaneous mastocytosis, 509–513, *510–512*
  cutis marmorata, *385,* 385–386
  cutis marmorata telangiectatica congenita (CMTC), 387–390, *388–389*
  dermoid cysts, 517–519, *518*
  diaper dermatitis, *659–667*
  drug hypersensitivity syndrome, 701–703, *702*
  ecthyma, 181–183, *182*
  ectodermal dysplasia, 599–601, *600–601*

eosinophilic pustular folliculitis, *669,* 669–670
ephelides, *487,* 487–488
epidermal nevi, 521–523, *522*
epidermolysis bullosa (EB), *552–556,* 552–557
eruptive pseudoangiomatosis, 136
erythema infectiosum/human parvovirus B19 infection (fifth disease), 121–124, *122–123*
erythema multiforme (EM), 707–710, *708–709*
erythema nodosum (EN), 809–811, *810*
erythema toxicum, *671–672,* 671–674
exanthematous and urticarial drug reactions, *714–715,* 714–716
fixed drug eruption, 720–721
folliculitis/furunculosis/carbunculosis, *186–187,* 186–188
Gianotti-Crosti syndrome, 127–129, *128–129*
granuloma annulare, *525–526,* 525–527
hand, foot, and mouth disease (HFMD), 132–133, *133–136*
Henoch-Schönlein purpura (HSP), 813–818, *814–817*
herpangina, 136
herpes simplex virus, 91–95, *92–94*
herpes zoster, 99–101, *100*
hyperhidrosis, 853–855, *854*
hypertrichosis and hirsutism, *620,* 620–621
ichthyosis, 569–574, *570–574*
impetigo, 191–194, *193–194*
incontinentia pigmenti, 577–580, *578–579*
infantile acne, 80, *80*
infantile acropustulosis, *675,* 675–676
infantile hemangioma, 393–400, *394–397, 399*
insect bites, 315–321, *316–320*
intertrigo, 677–678, *677–678*
irritant contact dermatitis, 48, *48–50*
juvenile dermatomyositis (JDM), 751–757, *752–755*
juvenile plantar dermatosis, 61, *62*
juvenile xanthogranuloma (JXG), 529–531, *530–531*
Kasabach-Merritt phenomenon (KMP), 407–409, *408*
Kawasaki disease, 821–826, *822–825*
kwashiorkor, 801–804, *802–803*
Langerhans cell histiocytosis (LCH), 829–834, *830–832*

Signs and symptoms, *continued*
lentigines, 489–491, *490*
lichen nitidus, 341–342, *341–342*
lichen planus (LP), 345–347, *346–347*
lichen sclerosus et atrophicus (LSA), 837–840, *838–839*
lichen striatus, 349–351, *350–351*
linear immunoglobulin A dermatosis, 561–564, *562*
loose anagen syndrome, 623–625, *624*
Lyme disease, 205–207, *206*
measles, 142–144, *143*
melanonychia striata, 497–499, *498*
meningococcemia, 211–213, *212*
miliaria, *681–682*, 681–683
molluscum contagiosum, 105–108, *106–108*
morphea, 762–772, *763–768*
neonatal acne, 80, *80*
neonatal/congenital candidiasis, 259–261, *260–261*
neurofibromatosis (NF), 583–587, *584–585*
nevus sebaceus, 685–687, *686–687*
onychomycosis, 267–268, *267–268*
papular-purpuric gloves-and-socks syndrome (PPGSS), 147–149, *148*
papular urticaria, 320, *320*
perianal bacterial dermatitis, 197–199, *198*
periorificial dermatitis, 83–85
pernio/chilblains, 410–414, *412–413*
pigmentary mosaicism
    hyperpigmented, 501–505, *502–504*
    hypopigmented, 445–448, *446–447*
pilomatricoma, 533–536, *534–535*
pityriasis alba, 451–452, *451–452*
pityriasis lichenoides, 353–356, *354–355*
pityriasis rosea, 359–361, *360–361*
pityriasis rubra pilaris (PRP), 373–375, *374–375*
polymorphous light eruption (PMLE), 843–845, *844*
postinflammatory hypopigmentation, *455*, 455–456
psoriasis, 363–370, *364–369*
pyogenic granuloma, 417–419, *418*
Rocky Mountain spotted fever (RMSF), *144, 149, 213*, 217–219, *218*
roseola infantum (exanthem subitum), 151–152, *152*
rubella, 155–158, *156–157*

scabies, 325–328, *326–327*
scarlet fever, 223–227, *224–226*
seborrheic dermatitis, 377–380, *378–379*
serum sickness–like reaction, 723–726, *724–725*
Spitz nevus, 539–541, *540–541*
staphylococcal scalded skin syndrome (SSSS), 231–233, *232*
Stevens-Johnson syndrome (SJS), *730–732*, 730–733
subcutaneous fat necrosis (SFN), 693–695, *694*
systemic lupus erythematosus (SLE), 777–785, *779–781, 783*
telangiectasias, *421*, 421–424, *423*
telogen effluvium, *630–631*, 630–632
thrush, *263*, 263–264
tinea capitis, 271–274, *272–273*
tinea corporis, 281–284, *282–283*
tinea cruris, 287–289, *288*
tinea pedis, 291–293, *292–293*
tinea versicolor, 297–299, *298*
toxic epidermal necrolysis (TEN), 737–739, *738*
toxic shock syndrome (TSS), 237–240, *238–239*
traction alopecia, 635–637, *636*
transient neonatal pustular melanosis, *689–690*, 689–691
trichotillomania, 639–644, *640–643*
tuberous sclerosis complex (TSC), 591–595, *592–593*
unilateral laterothoracic exanthem (ULE), 161–164, *162–163*
varicella, 165–167, *166*
vascular malformations, 427–431, *428–431*
vitiligo, 459–462, *460–461*
warts, 111–115
Silver-Russell syndrome, compared to neurofibromatosis (NF), 587
Silver syndrome, 480
Simple exanthematous drug eruption, compared to drug hypersensitivity syndrome, 703
Sinecatechins, 117
Sjögren-Larsson syndrome, 655
SJS. *See* Stevens-Johnson syndrome (SJS)
Skin of color
    appearance of lesions in, 10, *11–13*
    atopic dermatitis in, *35*, 37
    candidal diaper dermatitis in, 253

ecthyma in, *182*
erythema infectiosum/human parvovirus B19 infection (fifth disease) in, *122*
herpes zoster in, *100*
impetigo in, *193*
neonatal/congenital candidiasis in, *260*
pernio/chilblains in, *413*
warts in, *112*
SLE. *See* Systemic lupus erythematosus (SLE)
Smallpox, compared to varicella, 167
Soft-tissue malignancy
   compared to granuloma annulare, 527
   compared to hyperhidrosis, 855
   compared to infantile hemangioma, 400
   compared to Kasabach-Merritt phenomenon (KMP), 409
   compared to subcutaneous fat necrosis (SFN), 695
Solar urticaria, compared to polymorphous light eruption (PMLE), 845
Solid lesions, 1
Solitary mastocytoma, 509–515
   compared to juvenile xanthogranuloma (JXG), 531
Southern tick-associated rash illness (STARI), 207
Spider angioma
   compared to pyogenic granuloma, 419
   diagnosis, 424
   prognosis, 425
   signs and symptoms, 421, *421*
   treatment, 425
Spindle cell nevus, 539
Spinosad, 312
Spironolactone, 617
Spitz nevus
   compared to intradermal melanocytic nevus, 541
   compared to juvenile xanthogranuloma (JXG), 531, 541
   compared to pyogenic granuloma, 419, 541
   compared to telangiectasias, 424
   compared to verruca vulgaris, 541
   diagnosis, 542
   introduction/etiology/epidemiology, 539
   prognosis, 542
   resources, 542
   signs and symptoms, 539–541, *540–541*
   treatment, 542
   when to worry or refer, 542

SSSS. *See* Staphylococcal scalded skin syndrome (SSSS)
Staphylococcal folliculitis
   compared to erythema toxicum, 673
   compared to neonatal/congenital candidiasis, 261
Staphylococcal scalded skin syndrome (SSSS), 227
   compared to bullous impetigo, 233
   compared to cellulitis, 233
   compared to immersion burn, 233
   compared to Kawasaki disease, 233
   compared to *Mycoplasma pneumoniae*-induced rash and mucositis (MIRM), 733
   compared to reactive infectious mucocutaneous eruption (RIME), 733
   compared to Stevens-Johnson syndrome (SJS), 233, 733
   compared to streptococcal scarlet fever, 233
   compared to toxic epidermal necrolysis (TEN), 739
   compared to toxic shock syndrome (TSS), 233, 240
   diagnosis, 234
   introduction/etiology/epidemiology, 231
   prognosis, 234
   resources, 235
   signs and symptoms, 231–233, *232*
   treating associated conditions, 234
   treatment, 234
   when to worry or refer, 235
Staphylococcal scarlet fever
   compared to streptococcal scarlet fever, 227
   compared to toxic shock syndrome (TSS), 240
Staphylococcus aureus
   acute paronychia and, 173, 175
   atopic dermatitis, 33, 42, 44
   bedbugs and, 318
   blistering distal dactylitis and, 179
   ecthyma and, 181
   folliculitis and, 185
   impetigo and, 191
   perianal bacterial dermatitis and, 197
   pustulosis, compared to neonatal acne, 81
   scabies and, 325
   toxic shock syndrome (TSS) and, 237–240, *238–239*
   varicella and, 168

Stepwise management for atopic dermatitis, 41
Stevens-Johnson syndrome (SJS)
    compared to erythema multiforme (EM), 710
    compared to Kawasaki disease, 733, 826
    compared to linear immunoglobulin A dermatosis, 563
    compared to serum sickness–like eruption, 733
    compared to staphylococcal scalded skin syndrome (SSSS), 233, 733
    compared to toxic epidermal necrolysis (TEN), 733, 739
    compared to toxic shock syndrome (TSS), 240
    compared to urticaria, 733
    diagnosis, 733
    introduction/etiology/epidemiology, 729–730
    prognosis, 734
    resources, 735
    signs and symptoms, 730–732, 730–733
    treatment, 734
    when to worry or refer, 734
Streptococcal scarlet fever
    compared to staphylococcal scalded skin syndrome (SSSS), 233
    compared to toxic shock syndrome (TSS), 240
Streptococcus
    impetigo and, 191
    scarlet fever and, 223
Streptococcus pyogenes
    erythema nodosum (EN), 809
    impetigo and, 195
    psoriasis, 363
    scabies and, 325
    scarlet fever and, 223, 228
    toxic shock syndrome (TSS) and, 237–240, *238–239*
    varicella and, 168
Strongyloides stercoralis, 307
Sturge-Weber syndrome, compared to vascular malformations, 433
Subacute cutaneous lupus erythematosus (SCLE), *781*, 781–782
Subcutaneous fat necrosis (SFN)
    compared to cold panniculitis, 695
    compared to erysipelas, 695
    compared to malignancy, 695
    compared to myofibromatosis, 695
    compared to sclerema, 695
    diagnosis, 695, *696*
    introduction/etiology/epidemiology, 693
    prognosis, 697
    resources, 697
    signs and symptoms, 693–695, *694*
    treatment, 697
    when to worry or refer, 697
Sulfapyridine, 548
Sun allergy, 843
Sun poisoning, 843
Sun protection, 28–29
Sunscreen, 28–29
Surgery
    dermoid cysts, 519
    infantile hemangioma, 403
    pyogenic granuloma, 419
    warts, 117
Surgical scarlet fever, 223
Sweaty sock syndrome. *See* Juvenile plantar dermatosis
Swimmer's itch. *See* Cercarial dermatitis
Synergized pyrethrins, 312
Syphilis, angular cheilitis/perlèche, 248
Systemic corticosteroids
    for allergic contact dermatitis (ACD), 58
    for linear immunoglobulin A dermatosis, 564
    for urticaria, 746
Systemic lupus erythematosus (SLE)
    compared to atopic dermatitis, 785
    compared to drug reaction with eosinophilia and systemic symptoms (DRESS), 784
    compared to granuloma annulare, 785
    compared to juvenile dermatomyositis (JDM), 757, 784
    compared to juvenile idiopathic arthritis, systemic subtype, 784
    compared to polymorphous light eruption (PMLE), 784, 845
    compared to psoriasis, 785
    compared to rosacea, 784
    compared to seborrheic dermatitis, 785
    compared to tinea corporis, 785
    compared to drug hypersensitivity syndrome, 784
    diagnosis, 786–789
    discoid lupus erythematosus (DLE), 779, *779*–781
    introduction/etiology/epidemiology, 777
    lupus variants, 779–783
    other clinical findings, 778
    prognosis, 791

resources, 791
signs and symptoms, 777–785, *779–781,*
    783
subacute cutaneous lupus erythematosus
    (SCLE), *781,* 781–782
treating associated conditions, 790
treatment, 789–790
when to worry or refer, 791
Systemic-onset juvenile idiopathic arthritis,
    compared to Kawasaki disease,
    826
Systemic sclerosis, compared to morphea,
    771

T

Tap water iontophoresis, 856
Teeter-totter sign, *535*
Telangiectasias
    compared to cherry angioma, 424
    compared to pigmented purpura, 424
    compared to pyogenic granuloma, Spitz
        nevus, 424
    diagnosis, 424
    introduction/etiology/epidemiology, 421
    prognosis, 425
    resources, 426
    signs and symptoms, *421,* 421–424, *423*
    treatment, 425
    when to worry or refer, 426
Telogen effluvium
    compared to alopecia areata, 610, 632
    compared to androgenetic alopecia, 617
    compared to loose anagen syndrome,
        625, 632
    compared to tinea capitis, 632
    compared to traction alopecia, 632
    compared to trichotillomania, 632
    diagnosis, 632–633
    introduction/etiology/epidemiology,
        629–630
    prognosis, 633
    resources, 634
    signs and symptoms, *630–631,* 630–632
    treatment, 633
    when to worry or refer, 633
TEN. *See* Toxic epidermal necrolysis (TEN)
Tent sign, pilomatricoma, *535*
Terbinafine, 269, 277, *278,* 300
Therapeutics
    cryotherapy, 27
    moisturizers, 25–26
    sun protection, 28–29
    topical corticosteroids, *21–22,* 21–24, *24*
Thoracic sympathectomy, 855

Thrush
    compared to geographic tongue, 264
    compared to herpangina, 264
    compared to herpetic gingivostomatitis,
        264
    compared to Koplik spots of measles, 264
    compared to retained food or formula,
        264
    diagnosis, 264
    introduction/etiology/epidemiology, 263
    prognosis, 265
    resources, 265
    signs and symptoms, *263,* 263–264
    treatment, 264
    when to worry or refer, 265
Thyroglossal duct cyst, compared to
    pilomatricoma, 536
Ticks, 319
Timolol, 403
Tinea capitis, 16
    compared to alopecia areata, 274, 610
    compared to bacterial abscess, 274
    compared to bacterial folliculitis, 274
    compared to seborrheic dermatitis, 274
    compared to telogen effluvium, 632
    compared to traction alopecia, 274, 637
    compared to trichotillomania, 274, 644
    diagnosis, 275, *275–276*
    introduction/etiology/epidemiology, 271
    prognosis, 279
    resources, 279
    signs and symptoms, 271–274, *272–273*
    treating associated conditions, 279
    treatment, 276–277, *278*
    when to worry or refer, 279
    Wood lamp examination for, 20
Tinea corporis
    arrangement of lesions, 7, *8*
    compared to atopic dermatitis, 39
    compared to cutaneous larva migrans, 307
    compared to ecthyma, 284
    compared to granuloma annulare, 284,
        527
    compared to Lyme disease, 207
    compared to neonatal lupus
        erythematosus (NLE), 785
    compared to nummular eczema, 284
    compared to pityriasis rosea, 284, 361
    compared to psoriasis, 284
    compared to subacute cutaneous lupus
        erythematosus (SCLE), 785
    compared to unilateral laterothoracic
        exanthem (ULE), 164
    diagnosis, 284, *285*

Tinea corporis, *continued*
   introduction/etiology/epidemiology, 281
   prognosis, 285
   resources, 286
   scaling of, 9
   signs and symptoms, 281–284, *282–283*
   treatment, 285
   when to worry or refer, 286
Tinea cruris
   compared to candidiasis, 289
   compared to erythrasma, 289
   compared to intertrigo, 289, 678
   diagnosis, 289
   introduction/etiology/epidemiology, 287
   prognosis, 290
   resources, 290
   signs and symptoms, 287–289, *288*
   treatment, 289
   when to worry or refer, 290
Tinea pedis
   compared to contact dermatitis, 293
   compared to erythrasma, 293
   compared to juvenile plantar dermatosis, 61, 293
   compared to pitted keratolysis, 293
   diagnosis, 293
   introduction/etiology/epidemiology, 291
   prognosis, 294
   resources, 295
   signs and symptoms, 291–293, *292–293*
   treating associated conditions, 294
   treatment, 294
   when to worry or refer, 294
Tinea unguium, compared to chronic paronychia, 256
Tinea versicolor, 16, *17*
   compared to confluent and reticulated papillomatosis (CARP), 299, 851
   compared to pityriasis alba, 299, 452
   compared to pityriasis rosea, 299
   compared to postinflammatory hypopigmentation, 456
   compared to tuberous sclerosis complex (TSC), 594
   compared to vitiligo, 299, 462
   diagnosis, 299, *300*
   introduction/etiology/epidemiology, 297
   prognosis, 301
   resources, 301
   signs and symptoms, 297–299, *298*
   treatment, 300
   when to worry or refer, 301
   Wood lamp examination for, 20

Titanium dioxide, 28
Toilet seat dermatitis, *56*
Tolnaftate, 285, 294
Topical calcineurin
   for lichen sclerosus et atrophicus (LSA), 841
   for morphea, 773
Topical corticosteroids
   adverse effects, 24
   for allergic contact dermatitis (ACD), 58
   for alopecia areata, 611
   for atopic dermatitis, 42
   for cutaneous mastocytosis, 514
   frequency of application, 24
   for insect bites, 322
   for lichen planus (LP), 348
   for morphea, 773
   for periorificial dermatitis, 86
   by potency, 21, *21–22*
   selecting and prescribing, 22–23, *24*
   for vitiligo, 462
Toxic epidermal necrolysis (TEN), 729
   compared to acute generalized exanthematous pustulosis, 739
   compared to *Mycoplasma pneumoniae*-induced rash and mucositis (MIRM), 733, 739
   compared to reactive infectious mucocutaneous eruptions (RIME), 733, 739
   compared to staphylococcal scalded skin syndrome, 739
   compared to Stevens-Johnson syndrome (SJS), 733, 739
   diagnosis, 740
   introduction/etiology/epidemiology, 737
   prognosis, 741
   resources, 741
   signs and symptoms, 737–739, *738*
   treating associated conditions, 740
   treatment, 740
   when to worry or refer, 741
Toxic shock syndrome (TSS)
   compared to Kawasaki disease, 240, 826
   compared to scarlet fever, 227
   compared to staphylococcal scalded skin syndrome (SSSS), 233, 240
   compared to Stevens-Johnson syndrome, 240
   compared to streptococcal scarlet fever, 240
   compared to toxic epidermal necrolysis (TEN), 739

diagnosis, 240
introduction/etiology/epidemiology, 237
prognosis, 241
resources, 242
signs and symptoms, 237–240, *238–239*
treating associated conditions, 241
treatment, 241
when to worry or refer, 241
Toxoplasmosis, compared to rubella, 158
Trachyonychia, compared to onychomycosis, 268
Traction alopecia
    compared to alopecia areata, 610, 637
    compared to telogen effluvium, 632
    compared to tinea capitis, 274, 637
    compared to trichotillomania, 637, 644
    diagnosis, 637
    introduction/etiology/epidemiology, 635
    prognosis, 638
    resources, 638
    signs and symptoms, 635–637, *636*
    treating associated conditions, 637
    treatment, 637
    when to worry or refer, 638
Transient neonatal pustular melanosis
    compared to erythema toxicum, 673
    compared to neonatal/congenital candidiasis, 261
    diagnosis, 691
    introduction/etiology/epidemiology, 689
    prognosis, 691
    resources, 691
    signs and symptoms, *689–690*, 689–691
    treatment, 691
    when to worry or refer, 691
Trauma
    compared to acute paronychia, 175
    compared to angular cheilitis/perlèche, 248
    compared to aplasia cutis congenita (ACC), 652
Treatment and associated conditions
    acanthosis nigricans, 469
    acne vulgaris, *71–73*, 71–76, *74, 77*
    acquired melanocytic nevi, 474
    acrodermatitis enteropathica (AE), 799, *799*
    acute paronychia, 176
    albinism, 443–444
    allergic contact dermatitis (ACD), 58
    alopecia areata, 611–612
    androgenetic alopecia, 617
    angular cheilitis/perlèche, 249

aplasia cutis congenita (ACC), 652
atopic dermatitis, 40–45
blistering distal dactylitis, 179
café au lait macules, 479
candidal diaper dermatitis, 253
cercarial dermatitis, 337
childhood dermatitis herpetiformis, 548–549
chronic paronychia, 257
collodion baby, 657–658
confluent and reticulated papillomatosis (CARP), 851–852
congenital dermal melanocytosis, 495
congenital melanocytic nevi (CMN), 484–485
cutaneous mastocytosis, 514
cutis marmorata, 386
cutis marmorata telangiectatica congenita (CMTC), 390
dermoid cysts, 519
drug hypersensitivity syndrome, 704
ecthyma, 184
ectodermal dysplasia, 602
eosinophilic pustular folliculitis, 670
ephelides, 488
epidermal nevi, 524
epidermolysis bullosa (EB), 558
erythema infectiosum/human parvovirus B19 infection (fifth disease), 124
erythema multiforme (EM), 711
erythema nodosum (EN), 811
erythema toxicum, 674
exanthematous and urticarial drug reactions, 717
fixed drug eruption, 721
folliculitis/furunculosis/carbunculosis, 188–190
Gianotti-Crosti syndrome, 130
granuloma annulare, 527–528
hand, foot, and mouth disease (HFMD), 137
head lice, 312–313
Henoch-Schönlein purpura (HSP), 819
herpes simplex, 97
herpes zoster, 102
hyperhidrosis, 855–856
hypertrichosis and hirsutism, 621–622
ichthyosis, 574–575
impetigo, 195
incontinentia pigmenti, 581–582
infantile acne, 82
infantile acropustulosis, 676

Treatment and associated conditions, *continued*
  infantile hemangioma, 401–404
  insect bites, 322–323
  intertrigo, 679
  irritant contact dermatitis, 51–52
  juvenile dermatomyositis (JDM), 758–759
  juvenile plantar dermatosis, 63
  juvenile xanthogranuloma (JXG), 532
  Kasabach-Merritt phenomenon (KMP), 409–410
  Kawasaki disease, 827–828
  kwashiorkor, 805
  Langerhans cell histiocytosis (LCH), 834–835
  lentigines, 492
  lichen nitidus, 343
  lichen planus (LP), 348
  lichen sclerosus et atrophicus (LSA), 841
  lichen striatus, 351
  linear immunoglobulin A dermatosis, 564
  loose anagen syndrome, 626
  Lyme disease, 208
  measles, 145
  melanonychia striata, 499–500
  meningococcemia, 214
  miliaria, 683
  molluscum contagiosum, 109–110
  morphea, 773–774
  Mycoplasma pneumoniae-induced rash and mucositis (MIRM), 734
  neonatal acne, 81
  neonatal/congenital candidiasis, 262
  neurofibromatosis (NF), 588
  nevus sebaceus, 688
  papular-purpuric gloves-and-socks syndrome (PPGSS), 149
  perianal bacterial dermatitis, 200
  periorificial dermatitis, 86
  pernio/chilblains, 415
  pigmentary mosaicism
    hyperpigmented, 506
    hypopigmented, 449
  pilomatricoma, 536
  pityriasis alba, 453
  pityriasis lichenoides, 357
  pityriasis rosea, 362
  pityriasis rubra pilaris (PRP), 376
  polymorphous light eruption (PMLE), 846
  postinflammatory hypopigmentation, 456–457
  psoriasis, 370–371
  pyogenic granuloma, 419
  reactive infectious mucocutaneous eruptions (RIME), 734
  Rocky Mountain spotted fever (RMSF), 220
  roseola infantum (exanthem subitum), 153
  rubella, 159
  scabies, 329–330
  scarlet fever, 228
  seborrheic dermatitis, 381
  serum sickness–like reaction, 727
  Spitz nevus, 542
  staphylococcal scalded skin syndrome (SSSS), 234
  Stevens-Johnson syndrome (SJS), 734
  subcutaneous fat necrosis (SFN), 697
  systemic lupus erythematosus (SLE), 789–790
  telangiectasias, 425
  telogen effluvium, 633
  thrush, 264
  tinea capitis, 276–279, *278*
  tinea corporis, 285
  tinea cruris, 289
  tinea pedis, 294
  tinea versicolor, 300
  toxic epidermal necrolysis (TEN), 740
  toxic shock syndrome (TSS), 241
  traction alopecia, 637
  transient neonatal pustular melanosis, 691
  trichotillomania, 645
  tuberous sclerosis complex (TSC), 597
  unilateral laterothoracic exanthem (ULE), 164
  urticaria, 746–747
  varicella, 168
  vascular malformations, 432–435, *435–436*
  vitiligo, 462–463
  warts, 116–117
Triamcinolone, 249
Triamcinolone acetonide, *21*
Trichloroacetic acid, 117
Trichobezoar, 645
Trichobilharzia, 333
Trichophagia, 645
Trichophytic (Majocchi) granuloma, 281, 283

Trichophyton mentagrophytes, 291
Trichophyton rubrum, 267, 281, 291
Trichophyton tonsurans, 16, *16,* 271, 275, *275*
   Wood lamp examination for, 20
Trichorrhexis nodosa, 625
Trichothiodystrophy, 655
Trichotillomania
   compared to alopecia areata, 610, 644
   compared to loose anagen syndrome, 625
   compared to telogen effluvium, 632
   compared to tinea capitis, 274, 644
   compared to traction alopecia, 637, 644
   diagnosis, 644
   introduction/etiology/epidemiology, 639
   prognosis, 645
   resources, 646
   signs and symptoms, 639–644, *640–643*
   treating associated conditions, 645
   treatment, 645
   when to worry or refer, 645
Trimethoprim-sulfamethoxazole
   for acute paronychia, 176
   for head lice, 312
TSC. *See* Tuberous sclerosis complex (TSC)
TSS. *See* Toxic shock syndrome (TSS)
Tuberous sclerosis complex (TSC), 20
   compared to acne, 595
   compared to keratosis pilaris, 595
   compared to molluscum contagiosum, 595
   compared to nevus anemicus, 595
   compared to periorificial dermatitis, 595
   compared to piebaldism, 595
   compared to pigmentary mosaicism–hypomelanosis of Ito type, 595
   compared to pigmentary mosaicism–nevus depigmentosus type, 594
   compared to pityriasis alba, 594
   compared to tinea versicolor, 594
   compared to vitiligo, 594
   diagnosis, 596
   introduction/etiology/epidemiology, 591
   prognosis, 598
   resources, 598
   signs and symptoms, 591–595, *592–593*
   treating associated conditions, 597
   treatment, 597
   when to worry or refer, 598
Tufted angioma, 410
Tumors, 1
Tunga penetrans, 316
Tzanck test, 96, *96*

U

Ulcers, 4, 6
   aplasia cutis congenita (ACC), 649–653
   hand, foot, and mouth disease (HFMD), *133*
   infantile hemangioma, 404
Unilateral laterothoracic exanthem (ULE)
   compared to contact dermatitis, 164
   compared to Gianotti-Crosti syndrome, 164
   compared to papular eczema, 164
   compared to pityriasis rosea, 164
   compared to tinea corporis, 164
   diagnosis, 164
   introduction/etiology/epidemiology, 161
   prognosis, 164
   resources, 164
   signs and symptoms, 161–164, *162–163*
   treatment, 164
   when to worry or refer, 164
Unilateral nevoid telangiectasia, 421, *423*
   signs and symptoms, 422
Urticaria, 3. *See also* Papular urticaria
   compared to cutaneous mastocytosis, 513
   compared to erythema infectiosum/human parvovirus B19 infection (fifth disease), 124
   compared to erythema multiforme (EM), 710, 745
   compared to fixed drug eruption, 721
   compared to Henoch-Schönlein purpura (HSP), 745, 818
   compared to insect bites, 321
   compared to Lyme disease, 207
   compared to *Mycoplasma pneumoniae*-induced rash and mucositis (MIRM), 733
   compared to papular urticaria, 745
   compared to polymorphous light eruption (PMLE), 845
   compared to reactive infectious mucocutaneous eruption (RIME), 733
   compared to serum sickness–like reaction, 726, 745
   compared to Stevens-Johnson syndrome (SJS), 733
   compared to urticarial vasculitis, 745
   compared to urticaria multiforme, 745
   with darker skin tones, 10
   diagnosis, 746
   introduction/etiology/epidemiology, 743
   prognosis, 747

Urticaria, *continued*
   resources, 748
   signs and symptoms, 743–745, *744*
   solar, 845
   treating associated conditions, 747
   treatment, 746
   when to worry or refer, 747
Urticarial drug eruption. *See* Exanthematous and urticarial drug reactions
Urticarial vasculitis, compared to urticaria, 745
Urticaria multiforme
   compared to serum sickness–like reaction, 726
   compared to urticaria, 745
Urticaria pigmentosa, 509–515
UV therapy
   for morphea, 774
   for pityriasis lichenoides, 357
   for polymorphous light eruption (PMLE), 846
   for psoriasis, 371
   for vitiligo, 463

V

Valacyclovir, 102
Vancomycin, 241
Varicella, *4*
   compared to bullous insect bite reaction, 167
   compared to disseminated herpes zoster, 167
   compared to hand, foot, and mouth disease (HFMD), 138
   compared to herpes simplex virus infection, 167
   compared to other enteroviral exanthems, 167
   compared to pityriasis lichenoides, 356
   compared to rickettsialpox, 167
   compared to smallpox, 167
   diagnosis, 168
   introduction/etiology/epidemiology, 165
   prognosis, 169
   resources, 169
   signs and symptoms, 165–167, *166*
   treatment, 168
   when to worry or refer, 169
Varicella-zoster virus (VZV), 99. *See also* Varicella
   compared to impetigo, 194
Variola. *See* Smallpox, compared to varicella

Vascular malformations
   combined, 430, *431*
   compared to blue rubber bleb nevus syndrome, 435
   compared to bruising from birth trauma, 431
   compared to capillary malformation-arteriovenous malformation (CM-AVM) syndrome, 434, *435–436*
   compared to herpes simplex virus infection, 431
   compared to infantile hemangioma, 431
   compared to Klippel-Trénaunay syndrome, 433, *435*
   compared to macrocephaly-capillary malformation syndrome, 434
   compared to Maffucci syndrome, 435
   compared to phakomatosis pigmentovascularis (PPV), 433
   compared to proteus syndrome, 434
   compared to pyogenic granuloma, 433
   compared to Sturge-Weber syndrome, 433
   compared to warts, molluscum, 431
   diagnosis, 431–432
   introduction/etiology/epidemiology, 427
   prognosis, 436
   resources, 437
   signs and symptoms, 427–431, *428–431*
   treating associated conditions, 433–435, *435–436*
   treatment, 432–433
   when to worry or refer, 436
Vasculitis
   compared to ecthyma, 183
   compared to erythema nodosum (EN), 811
   compared to Henoch-Schönlein purpura (HSP), 818
Venous malformation
   compared to infantile hemangioma, 400
   compared to pilomatricoma, 536
   signs and symptoms, 428, *429*
   treatment, 432
Verruca vulgaris. *See* Warts
Vesicles, 4, *4*
   allergic contact dermatitis (ACD), 56
   crusting of, 9
   grouped, *7*
   hand, foot, and mouth disease (HFMD), *133*, 133–134, *135*

herpes simplex virus, 91–94, *91–94*
herpes zoster, *100*
incontinentia pigmenti, *578*
infantile acropustulosis, *675*
linear arrangement of, *7*
polymorphous light eruption (PMLE), 843–845, *844*
varicella, 165, *166*
Vincristine, 403
Viral exanthem. *See also* Nonspecific viral exanthem
  compared to drug hypersensitivity syndrome, 703
  compared to exanthematous drug reaction, 716
  compared to folliculitis/furunculosis/carbunculosis, 188
  compared to Kawasaki disease, 826
  compared to scabies, 328
  with darker skin tones, 10
Vitamin A treatment, 145
Vitamin D treatment, 575
Vitiligo, 8
  compared to albinism, 443
  compared to lichen sclerosus et atrophicus (LSA), 840
  compared to piebaldism, 462
  compared to pigmentary mosaicism, hypopigmented, 448
  compared to pityriasis alba, 452, 462
  compared to postinflammatory hypopigmentation, 456
  compared to tinea versicolor, 299, 462
  compared to tuberous sclerosis complex (TSC), 594
  compared to Waardenburg syndrome, 462
  diagnosis, 462
  introduction/etiology/epidemiology, 459
  prognosis, 463
  resources, 464
  signs and symptoms, 459–462, *460–461*
  treatment, 462–463
  when to worry or refer, 464
  Wood lamp examination for, 20

Vulvovaginitis, 197
  compared to lichen sclerosus et atrophicus (LSA), 840

W

Waardenburg syndrome
  compared to albinism, 443
  compared to vitiligo, 462
Warts
  arrangement of lesions, 7
  compared to acne vulgaris, 70
  compared to calluses, 115
  compared to epidermal nevi, 523
  compared to lichen nitidus, 342
  compared to molluscum contagiosum, 108
  compared to periorificial dermatitis, 85
  compared to Spitz nevus, 541
  compared to vascular malformations, 431
  introduction/etiology/epidemiology, 111
  resources, 118
  signs and symptoms, 111–115
  treatment, 116–117
  when to worry or refer, 117
Water-in-oil emulsions, 25
Watson syndrome, 480
Weber-Cokayne type of epidermolysis bullosa (EB), 552, *552*
Wet-wrap therapy, 44
Wheals, 1, *3*
Wood lamp examination, 20, *20*

X

Xerosis, atopic dermatitis, 38

Y

Yersinia enterocolitica, 809

Z

Zinc deficiency, 50
  acrodermatitis enteropathica (AE), 795
Zinc oxide, 28
Zosteriform herpes simplex, 94

2024 Red Book® 33rd edition!

The ultimate guide for effectively identifying, treating, and managing pediatric infectious diseases.

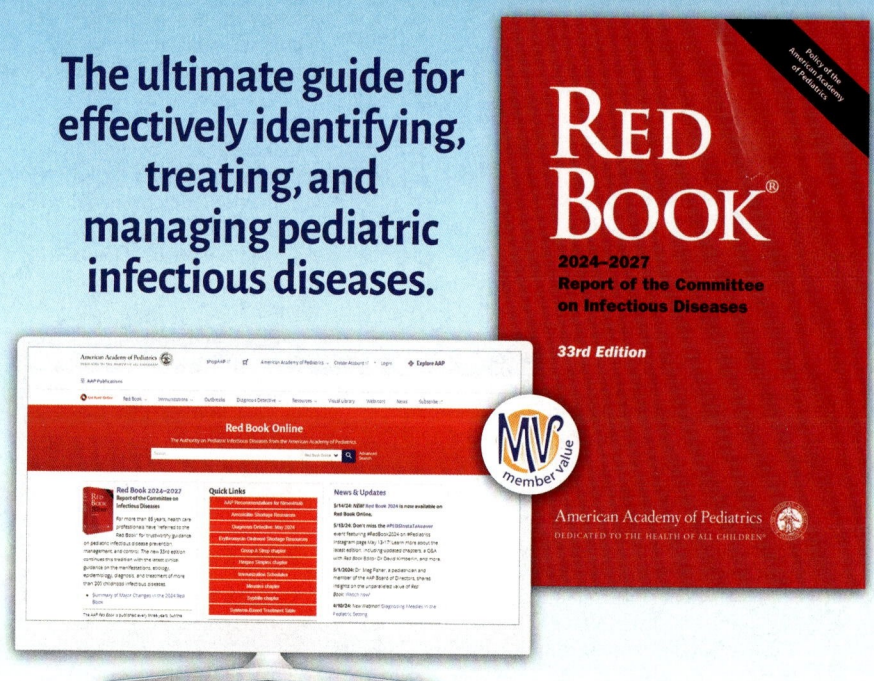

AAP Members
Request a print copy in addition to Red Book® Online as part of your member benefit!

Visit **aap.org/getredbook** and redeem your copy today!

A $20 service fee will be applied.

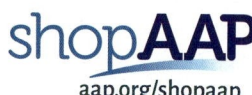
aap.org/shopaap

American Academy of Pediatrics
DEDICATED TO THE HEALTH OF ALL CHILDREN®

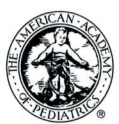